New Frontiers in Cancer Treatment

New Frontiers in Cancer Treatment

Editor: Adelina Brando

AMERICAN
MEDICAL PUBLISHERS
www.americanmedicalpublishers.com

AMERICAN
MEDICAL PUBLISHERS
www.americanmedicalpublishers.com

Cataloging-in-Publication Data

New frontiers in cancer treatment / edited by Adelina Brando.
p. cm.
Includes bibliographical references and index.
ISBN 979-8-88740-322-9
1. Cancer--Treatment. 2. Cancer. 3. Cancer--Treatment--Technological innovations.
4. Cancer--Diagnosis. I. Brando, Adelina.
RC270.8 .N49 2023
616.994 06--dc23

American Medical Publishers,
41 Flatbush Avenue,
1st Floor, New York,
NY 11217, USA

ISBN 979-8-88740-322-9 (Hardback)

Contents

Preface

I am honored to present to you this unique book which encompasses the most up-to-date data in the field. I was extremely pleased to get this opportunity of editing the work of experts from across the globe. I have also written papers in this field and researched the various aspects revolving around the progress of the discipline. I have tried to unify my knowledge along with that of stalwarts from every corner of the world, to produce a text which not only benefits the readers but also facilitates the growth of the field.

There are various types of therapies available for the treatment of cancer such as targeted therapy, chemotherapy, radiation therapy and immunotherapy. Chemotherapy makes use of drugs to eliminate cancer cells. Targeted therapy is a type of molecular medicine that stops cancer cells from growing by interfering with specific targeted molecules needed for carcinogenesis and tumor growth. It is available for lung cancer, colorectal cancer, multiple myeloma, lymphoma, head and neck cancer, breast cancer, prostate cancer, pancreatic cancer, and melanoma. Targeted cancer therapies are more successful and less damaging to normal cells than traditional treatments such as chemotherapy. Research related to cancer immunology has helped in creating several targeted therapies. They act as biological response modifiers or immunomodulators. The most successful targeted therapies target a protein or enzyme that possesses a mutation or any other genetic modification specific to cancer cells and not found in normal host tissues. The aim of this book is to present researches that have been instrumental in advancing cancer research and techniques of treating and managing cancer. It will provide innovative insights to all readers.

Finally, I would like to thank all the contributing authors for their valuable time and contributions. This book would not have been possible without their efforts. I would also like to thank my friends and family for their constant support.

Editor

1

Current Trends of Targeted Drug Delivery for Oral Cancer Therapy

Mingming Zhang[1†], *Jianqin Liang*[2†], *Yanyu Yang*[3*], *Huize Liang*[1], *Huaping Jia*[1*] and *Dawei Li*[4*]

[1] Strategic Support Force Characteristic Medical Center of Chinese People's Liberation Army, Beijing, China, [2] The 8th Medical Center, General Hospital of the Chinese People's Liberation Army, Beijing, China, [3] College of Materials Science and Engineering, Zhengzhou University, Zhengzhou, China, [4] The 4th Medical Center, General Hospital of the Chinese People's Liberation Army, Beijing, China

***Correspondence:**
Yanyu Yang
yyyang@zzu.edu.cn
Huaping Jia
jiahuaping12@126.com
Dawei Li
ldw309@126.com

† These authors have contributed equally to this work

Oral cancer is an aggressive tumor that invades the local tissue and can cause metastasis and high mortality. Conventional treatment strategies, e.g., surgery, chemotherapy, and radiation therapy alone or in combinations, possess innegligible issues, and significant side and adverse effects for the clinical applications. Currently, targeting drug delivery is emerging as an effective approach for oral delivery of different therapeutics. Herein we provide a state-of-the-art review on the current progress of targeting drug delivery for oral cancer therapy. Variously oral delivery systems including polymeric/inorganic nanoparticles, liposomes, cyclodextrins, nanolipids, and hydrogels-based forms are emphasized and discussed, and biomimetic systems with respect to oral delivery like therapeutic vitamin, exosomes, proteins, and virus-like particles are also described with emphasis on the cancer treatment. A future perspective is also provided to highlight the existing challenges and possible resolution toward clinical translation of current oral cancer therapies.

Keywords: oral cancer, drug delivery, nanoparticles, nanotechnology, OSCC (oral squamous cell carcinoma)

INTRODUCTION

Oral cancer refers to tumors that occur in the lips, hard palate, upper, and lower alveolar ridges, anterior two-thirds of the tongue, sublingual, buccal mucosa, posterior deltoid muscle of molars, and oral cavity (Vogel et al., 2010). More than 90% of oral cancers are carcinomas with squamous differentiation from the mucosal epithelium, thus called oral squamous cell carcinoma (OSCC), which is the sixth most common cancer worldwide with ~50% of the 5-year survival rate (Rivera, 2015; Manikandan et al., 2016). In 2018, 354,864 new cases of lip and oral cavity cancer were identified, and 177,384 people died from these types of cancer (Bray et al., 2018). Besides for the genetic and epigenetic mechanisms for the OSCC, environmental factors mainly including excessive alcohol intake and tobacco usage have significant roles in the multifactorial disease and carcinogenesis. In addition, human papillomavirus (HPV) associated with oropharyngeal squamous cell carcinoma and other factors (e.g., circadian clock disruption) also plays an important role in the initiation and progression of the OSCC therapy (Heck et al., 2009; Majchrzak et al., 2014; Nirvani et al., 2018; Adeola et al., 2019). Conventional therapy strategies for oral cancer mainly include surgery, chemotherapy and radiation therapy alone or in combinations, and have made important progress in oral cancer treatment, but these modalities possess innegligible issues and significant side and adverse effects. For instance, chemotherapy can cause nausea, vomiting, hair loss, infections and diarrhea in patients while radiation therapy can also bring about transient or permanent damage to healthy tissues, thus severely affecting the well-being and life quality.

Pathophysiology of oral cancer is important factor that should be intensively studied, wherein the genomic pathway plays a role in OSCC, that is, changes in the genome lead to changes in the expression of proteins, chemical mediators, and enzymes. Carcinogenesis is a process with multiple steps, which are characterized by the continuous stimulation of additional genetic defects and clonal expansion. Because oncogene was activated and tumor suppressor gene was inactivated, OSCC causes abnormal cell proliferation and death. Genetic changes mainly include gene amplification, oncogene overexpression, mutation, deletion and hypermethylation, leading to the inactivation of specific genes (e.g., p53 tumor suppressor genes).

In current therapies, anticancer drugs (e.g., 5-fluorouracil, paclitaxel, cisplatin, and docetaxel) are used alone or in combination, which have been employed in chrono-chemotherapy for oral cancer treatment (Catimel et al., 1994; Baselga et al., 2005; Bonner et al., 2006; Agüeros et al., 2009; Haddad et al., 2009). However, they are highly toxic to normal cells as intravenously administered with non-specific tissue distribution within the bodies, easily causing greater damages to healthy tissues with severely adverse reactions (Kruijtzer et al., 2002). In addition, low solubility, permeability, and poor bioavailability of these anticancer drugs in bodily fluids are also noted as limitations for oral chemotherapy. Therefore, development of new therapeutic regimen or modifications of current approaches are significantly urgent for improvement of human health and survival against the oral cancer and tissues.

To overcome the disadvantages of current treatment techniques, scientific community has turned toward nanotechnology to develop new and more effective nanotechnology-based drug carrier systems to optimize oral, buccal, and intravenous treatment routes. An innovative approach to improve the efficacy is the targeted drug delivery system that has great potentials to increase drug bioavailability and bio-distribution at the site of the primary tumor, showing promise in overcoming the complications of conventional anticancer agents and enhancing the therapeutic efficacy. Especially, naturally derived and synthetic polymers are exploited as two common candidates for delivering the chemotherapeutic agents into the tumor site, and the targeted drug delivery system is capable of releasing a bioactive molecule at a specific site to improve individual health outcomes for oral cancer. Thus, it is promising that targeted drug delivery system has the ability to reduce the severity/extent of side effects of some chemotherapeutic drugs, which can be exploited as a novel therapeutic strategy in oral, head, and neck cancer patients and beyond.

This review is aimed to summarize the current most relevant findings related to different drug delivery system for oral cancer therapy, and provide some potential of anticancer drug delivery approaches. Future perspectives and therapeutic strategies are also suggested. We believe this overview can be useful for promoting novel strategies that can be implemented in clinical management and applied pre-clinically for oral cancer therapy in the future.

NANOTECHNOLOGY-BASED CARRIERS FOR ORAL CANCER THERAPY

To address the issues of conventional chemotherapeutic agents, molecularly targeted therapies are urgently required for improving the drug efficiency and reducing the potential toxicity. Therefore, by means of the novel controlled nanodelivery systems, the drug-loaded nanoparticles with optimal size can express the smart manipulation of drug release behaviors once the microenvironment is slightly changed, which is utilized for the targeted therapy. Nanotechnology-based drug carriers have allowed for the selective methodologies for OSCC treatment (Huang et al., 2011; Calixto et al., 2014). Compared to the chemotherapeutic agents, targeted drug delivery systems are widely used for the controlled drug release with advanced advantages on improved therapeutic effect and reduced side effects, which can significantly amplify the main properties of the bioactive agent: absorption, metabolism, distribution and elimination. Various nanotechnology-based carriers based on nanoparticles, liposomes, cyclodextrins, nanolipids, and hydrogels are discussed here with their respective characteristics. In addition, biomimetic nanoparticles like vitamins, exosomes, peptides/proteins, and virus-like particles have also been utilized as potential carriers of chemotherapeutic agents for oral cancer therapy.

Nanoparticles for Oral Cancer Therapy

On account of the adjustable chemical and physical characteristics, nanoparticles show an increase in popularity on targeted drug delivery system with enhanced bioactivity and effective therapy, thus reducing its systemic toxicity for oral cancer therapy. These carriers mainly comprising of polymeric and inorganic nanoparticles can kill cancer cells by loading, stabilizing, and delivering the chemotherapeutic drugs with various loading contents and release profiles (Poonia et al., 2017).

Polymeric Nanoparticles for Oral Cancer Therapy

An ideal drug carrier should possess favorable biocompatibility, biodegradability and controlled drug release behaviors at specific sites. Naturally derived and synthetic polymers [e.g., polysaccharides, polycaprolactone (PCL), poly(lactic acid) (PLA), poly(glycolic acid) (PGA), and polyethylene glycol (PEG)] are series of suitable biomaterials for preparation of polymeric nanoparticles by many techniques like nanoprecipitation, emulsifications, and self-assembly (Panyam et al., 2002; Ravikumara et al., 2013; Du et al., 2014; Wang et al., 2015, 2016, 2018, 2019; Desai, 2018; Yang et al., 2018; Sun et al., 2019; Li et al., 2020; Zhou et al., 2020). They can be modified as chemo-preventive agents to be directly delivered into the affected sites within the oral cavity, so the malignant conversion is effectively prevented from oral epithelial dysplasia to frank carcinoma. For example, Endo et al. prepared a kind of polymeric nanoparticles to reduce the toxicity of cisplatin and improve OSCC therapy based on a PEG-poly(glutamic acid) block copolymer (Endo et al., 2013; Madhulaxmi et al., 2017). These cisplatin-loaded nanoparticles could activate the caspase-3 and caspase-7 pathways to induce apoptosis and killed the oral cancers. Compared to the oral cisplatin in solution, controlled release of cisplatin from nanoparticles could obviously decrease the nephrotoxicity and neurotoxicity both *in vitro* and *in vivo*. Zhu et al. developed an effective chemotherapeutic system for achieving co-delivery of anticancer drug sodium arsenite ($NaAsO_2$) and MTH1 inhibitor TH287 for the OSCC therapy (Li et al., 2017). By means of the self-assembly of an amphiphilic cationic hyperbranched poly(amine-ester) (HPAE), pH-sensitive HPAE nanoparticles were prepared in solutions that simultaneously encapsulated the $NaAsO_2$ and TH287. Under acidic microenvironments within the tumors, both of $NaAsO_2$ and TH287 were quickly released from nanoparticles, displaying effective inhibition of tumor proliferation by *in vitro* results (**Figure 1**).

Inorganic Nanoparticles for Oral Cancer Therapy

Inorganic nanoparticles are extensively employed due to their low toxicity, high tolerance of organic solvents and good bioavailability, and thus these inorganic nanoparticles (e.g., Au NPs, Ag NPs) have been applied in diagnostic and therapeutic fields for tumors with high efficacy, especially for their unique photo-thermal functions for oral cancer therapy (Subramani and Ahmed, 2012; Senapati et al., 2018). Sayed et al. described a design of an anti-epithelial growth factor receptor (EGFR) antibody-conjugated Au NPs for the therapeutic application of the OSCC therapy. *In vitro* experiments displayed that OSCC cells did not require high energy to produce photothermal destruction for anti-EGFR/Au conjugates, and clinical results showed that near-infrared (NIR) laser light could allow for effective delivery of anti-EGFR/Au conjugates into the malignant cells with the deep penetration, because Au NPs on the surface could be easily modified to absorb the NIR, thereby achieving the maximal therapeutic effects (El-Sayed et al., 2006). Lucky et al. prepared a kind of biocompatible up-conversion nanoparticles with encapsulation of PEGylated titanium dioxide (TiO_2), which enhanced tissue penetration using NIR and effectively targeted the EGFRs on the surface of OSCC cells to inhibit the tumor proliferation (Lucky et al., 2016; Marcazzan et al., 2018). For the inorganic nanoparticles systems, this photodynamic therapy (PDT) strategy was benefited for the oral cancer that required the deep penetration of antitumor drugs in the clinical practice.

Combinational (Polymeric-Inorganic) Nanoparticles for Oral Cancer Therapy

Combinational drug treatment is recognized as advanced therapeutic benefits for the targeted drug delivery system that allows for the reduced toxicity and improved therapeutic efficacy. Darwish et al. prepared a combinational chemo-photothermal therapy with vincristine (VCR) as phytochemical anticancer and plasmonic gold nanorods (GNRs) as photothermal reagents for the OSCC therapy (Darwish et al., 2020). Based on the self-assembly of amphiphilic poly (DL-lactide-co-glycolide) (PLGA)-PEG polymers, VCR was physically encapsulated into the polymeric corona through the chem-covalently assembly around silica coated gold nanorods (GNRs). The breakage of amide linkages impelled the sustainable VCR release under acidic intracellular environments, revealing the prepared combinational therapeutic nanoprobes were identified as promising candidates for potentially clinical translation (**Figure 2**).

Liposomes for Oral Cancer Therapy

Liposomes are a series of single- or multi-layer microscopic particles with the main component of a membrane-like lipid, phospholipids and cholesterol (Mezei and Gulasekharam, 1980; Ribeiro de Souza et al., 2012). Liposomes, as the non-toxic for the normal tissues or cells, are the most widely used drug delivery system to increase its accumulation at target sites, which have gained significant attention for the administration of drug release and utilization of drug delivery with highly efficient therapy (Lian and Ho, 2001). For example, Figueiró Longo et al. prepared a kind of liposomes that could tailor the release of aluminum phthalocyanine chloride using Swiss mice by the photodynamic therapy, exhibiting the effective treatment for the oral cancer (Figueiró Longo et al., 2012). Tedesco et al. proposed a kind of mixed lipid vesicles (LVs) based on the various ratios of 1,2-distearoyl-sn-glycero-3-phosphocholine and 1,2-dioleoyl-sn-glycero-3-phosphocholine for targeted drug delivery (Calori and Tedesco, 2016). These LVs could keep stability in solutions for more than 50 days. On account of the aluminum-phosphate specific interactions, LVs bonded with the AlClPc molecules that could distribute in the cellular organelles and suffer a disaggregation process after uptake by the OSCC, which could guide us for future deep study on the intracellular mechanism of PDT for oral cancer therapy (**Figure 3**).

Cyclodextrins for Oral Cancer Therapy

Cyclodextrins (CD), a family of cyclic oligosaccharides, are derived from the enzymatic degradation of starch, which can complex hydrophobic guest molecules (e.g., anticancer drugs of docetaxel, cisplatin, methotrexate, and paclitaxel) via the host-gust inclusion interactions (Rajewski and Stella, 1996). The interior lipophilic cavity prevents the hydrophobic molecules while the exterior polar surface contributes to the solubilising effects in aqueous solutions. Thus, these cyclodextrins and their derivatives are widely utilized as versatile multifunctional excipients with highly therapeutic efficiency and pharmacological activity for the targeted drug delivery system (Szente and Szejtli, 1999; Vyas and Saraf, 2008). Wang et al. reported a kind of soluble supramolecular complexes via the phospholipid compound technology and a hydroxypropyl-beta-cyclodextrin (HP-β-CD) inclusion technique, which obviously improved the solubility and oral bioavailability of two curcuminoids (**Figure 4**; Wang H. et al., 2020). The preparation of these supramolecular complexes was simple and the gastrointestinal absorption capacity was enhanced, expressing great potentials in the oral delivery for cargoes.

Nanolipids for Oral Cancer Therapy

Although nanoparticles are significantly applied for oral cancer, their potential cytotoxicity and low internalization into the tumor cells limit the therapeutic efficiency (Hoshyar et al.,

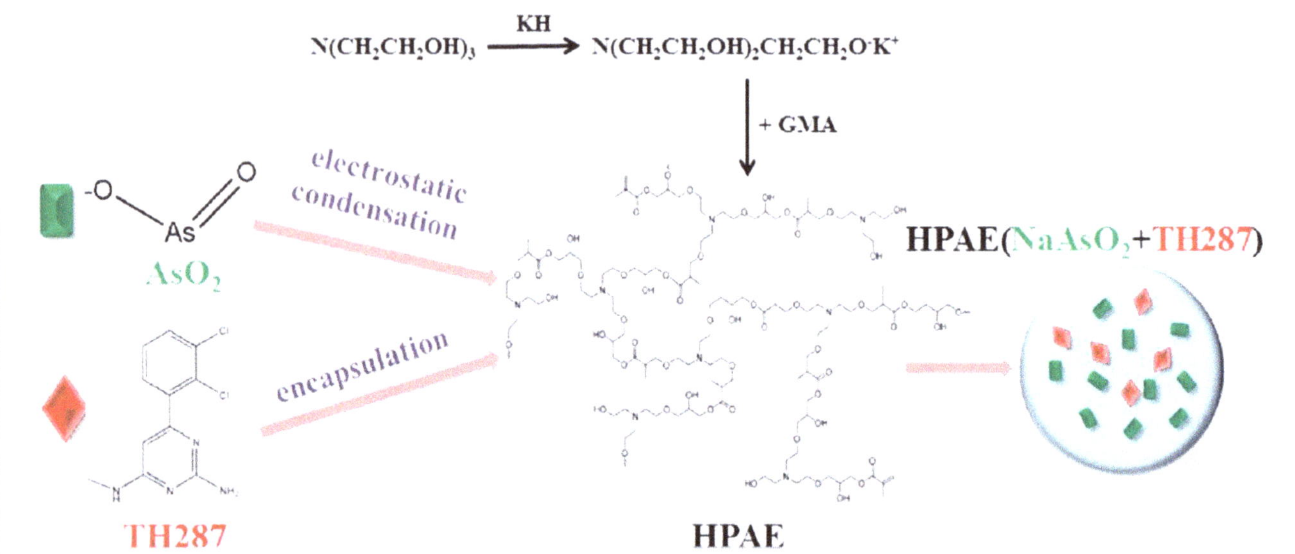

FIGURE 1 | Schematic fabrication of ($NaAsO_2$+TH287)-loaded HPAE nanoparticles. Reproduced from Li et al. (2017) with permission from Copyright 2017 Royal Society of Chemistry.

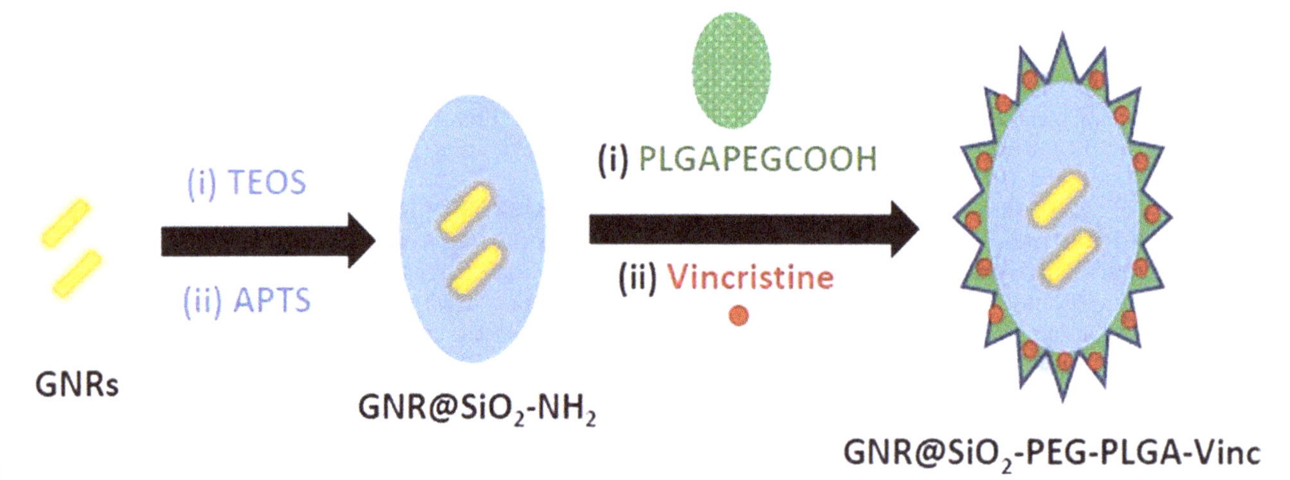

FIGURE 2 | Schematic combination (chemo-photothermal) therapeutic model for oral squamous carcinoma. Reproduced from Darwish et al. (2020) with permission from Copyright 2020 Elsevier.

2016). Nanolipid-based carriers are well-fabricated and widely applied to overcome this limitation for oral cancer therapy. These nanostructured lipid carriers consisting of solid and liquid lipids within a core matrix can distort their crystalline structures, provide the sufficient space and accommodate the local chemopreventive drugs in the amorphous clusters (Beloqui et al., 2016). Based on these advantages, nanolipids can improve the bioavailability, solubility and stability of drug carriers for therapeutic OSCC applications (Liu et al., 2011; Zhang et al., 2011; Iida et al., 2013; Zlotogorski et al., 2013).

Hydrogels for Oral Cancer Therapy

Hydrogels have a three-dimensional (3D) porous and interconnected structures that not only provide a biocompatible microenvironment for cell attachment and proliferation but also possess many unique advantages on the targeted drug delivery systems (Maitra and Kumar Shukla, 2014; Cao et al., 2018; Ketabat et al., 2018; Bao et al., 2019; Wang X. et al., 2020; Xu et al., 2020; Yan et al., 2020). Compared to the nanoparticle-based carriers, hydrogels provide sustained or triggered administration of both hydrophilic and hydrophobic agents and other biomolecules. In addition, hydrogel carriers allow for the

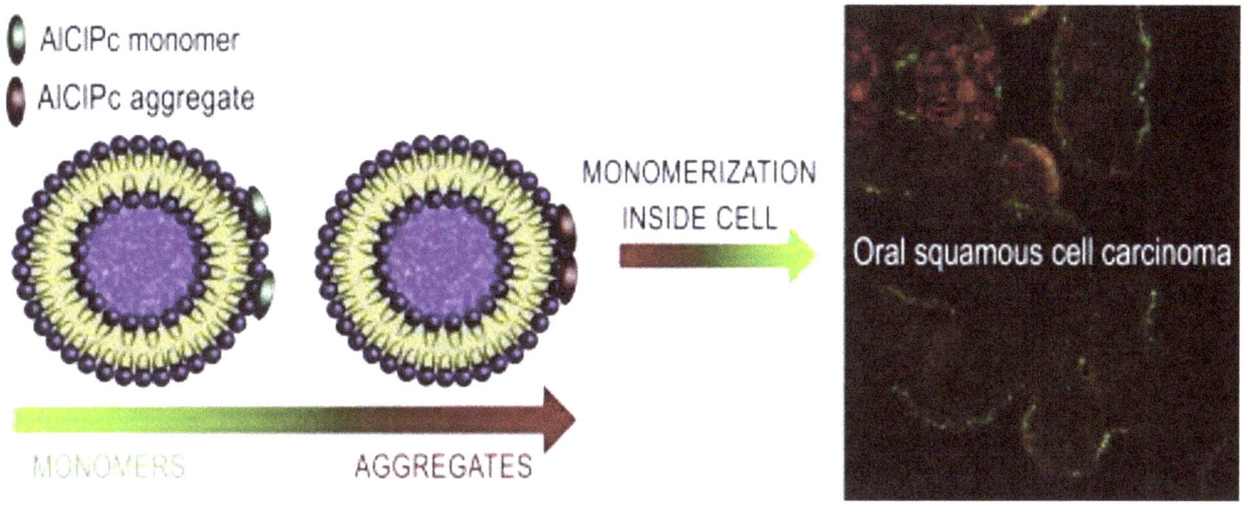

FIGURE 3 | Schematic image of lipid vesicles loading aluminum phthalocyanine chloride. Reproduced from Calori and Tedesco (2016) with permission from Copyright 2016 Elsevier.

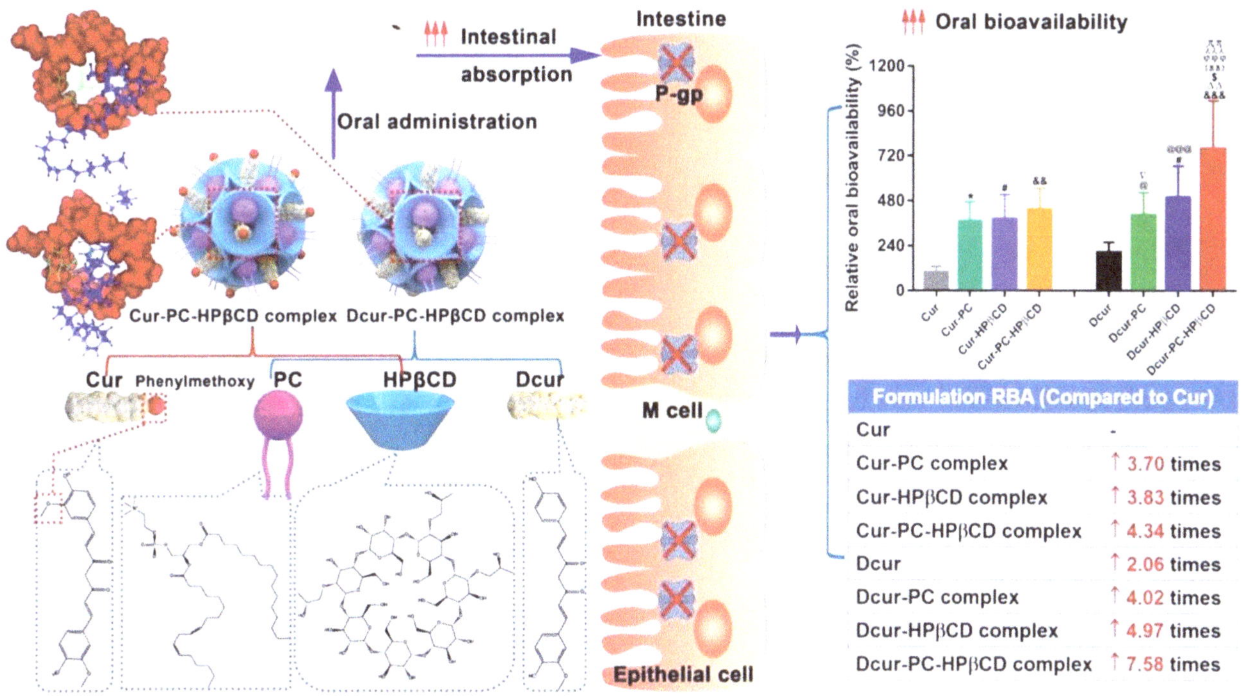

FIGURE 4 | Schematic image of HP-β-CD supramolecular complexes for oral delivery of curcuminoids. Reproduced from Wang H. et al. (2020) with permission from Copyright 2020 Elsevier.

co-administration of multiple drugs for achieving the synergistic anti-cancer effects with high drug loading content and low drug resistance (Li and Mooney, 2016; Ketabat et al., 2017; Sepantafar et al., 2017; Liu B. C. et al., 2020; Liu H. Y. et al., 2020; Tang et al., 2020; Yang et al., 2021). Another unique advantage is localized application for the targeted drug delivery systems, by which various hydrogel formulations can directly be implanted into the injury lesion location that can avoid the intravenous injection of small nanoparticles in the blood circulation. In this case, hydrogel carriers can tailor the drug release periods for a long time (several months) by controlling the hydrogel architectures, network pores, and gelation mechanisms (physical

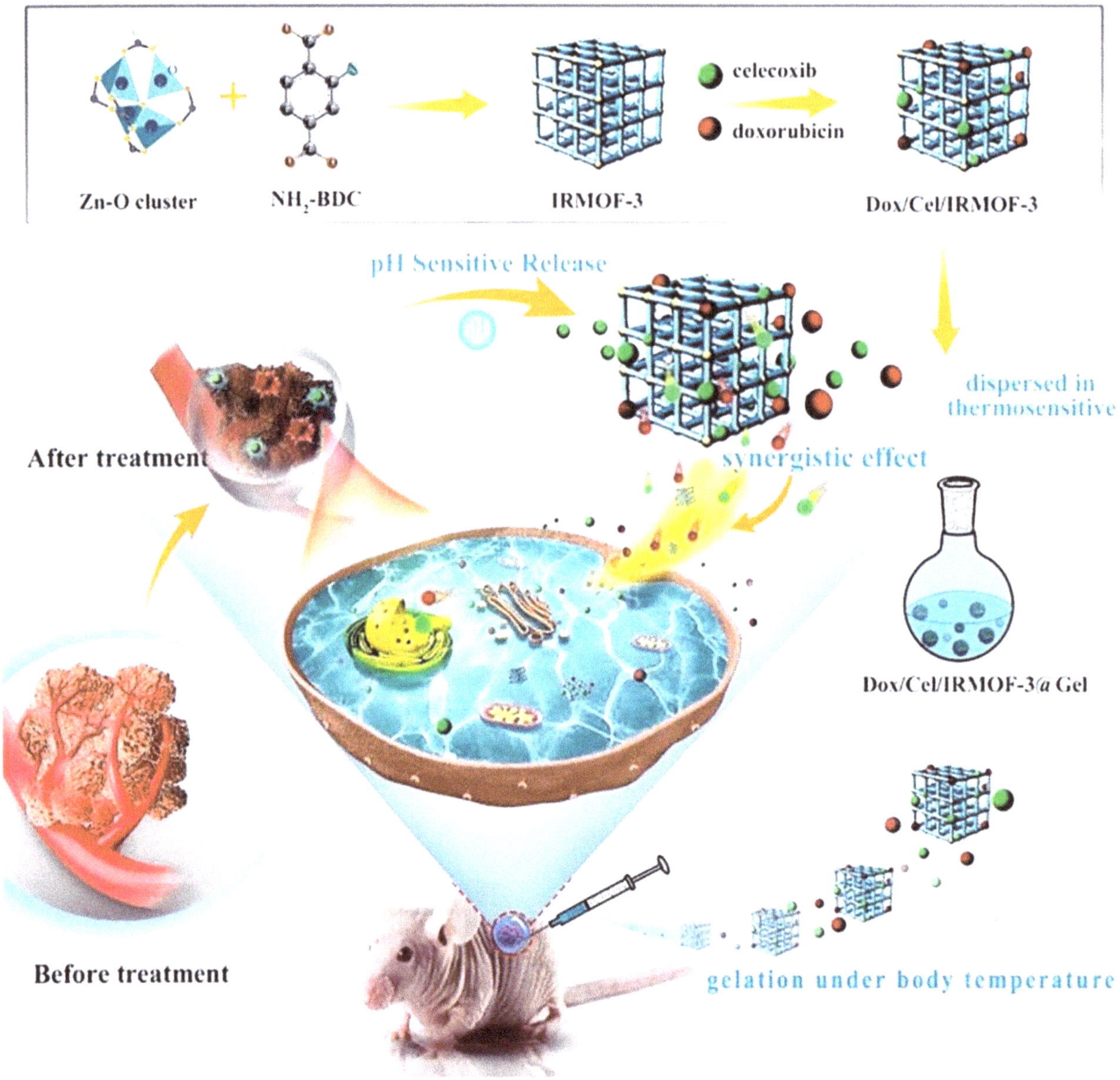

FIGURE 5 | Schematic illustration of DOX/Cel/MOFs@Gel as a novel injectable hydrogel for local dual drug delivery. Reproduced from Tan et al. (2020) with permission from Copyright 2020 Elsevier.

and chemical gelation) (Koutsopoulos and Zhang, 2012). For example, Tan et al. prepared an injectable thermosensitive hydrogel consisting of metal-organic frameworks (MOFs), doxorubicin (DOX) and celecoxib for oral cancer therapy (Tan et al., 2020). The loaded celecoxib possessed antiangiogenetic property that could improve the oral cancer therapy with the synergistic effect of DOX. In this system, DOX/Cel/MOFs@Gel exhibited high drug-loading capacity, pH-responsive release profile, and excellent tumor inhibition behavior by the *in vitro* and *in vivo* results (**Figure 5**). These injectable hydrogels had low toxicity and no apparent injury to the other tissues, possessing great potentials for fabrication of injectable implant platform for local oral cancer therapy.

BIOMIMETIC NANOPARTICLES FOR ORAL CANCER THERAPY

Although natural or synthetic materials have been applied as targeted drug carriers for the therapeutics, their low drug payloads, oral bioavailability, and delivery efficiency are still highly challenging that should be issued. Conclusively,

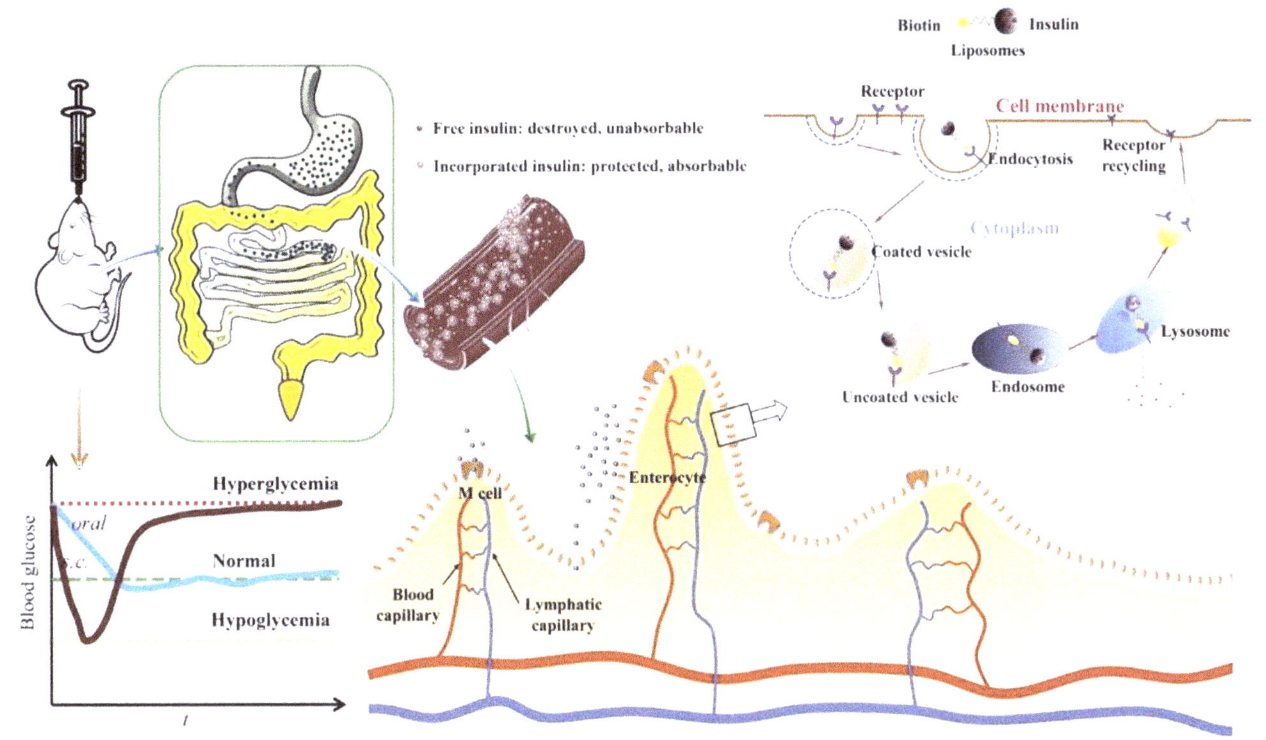

FIGURE 6 | Schematic images of the biotinylated liposomes with hypoglycemic effect and enhanced oral bioavailability of insulin for the oral delivery. Reproduced from Zhang et al. (2014) with permission from Copyright 2014 Elsevier.

biomimetic strategies are here investigated to illustrate the structure-property of biomimetic carriers to improve the bioavailability and targeting capability of therapeutic drugs.

Vitamin-Coated Nanoparticles for Oral Cancer Therapy

Vitamin B12 (VB12), due to the absorption pathway by receptor-mediated endocytosis, can form a complex with an intrinsic factor in the stomach, which are easily modified into the nanoparticles to improve the oral delivery efficiency. For example, Chalasani et al. found that compared with the pure nanoparticles, covalent conjugation of VB12 to insulin-loaded dextran caused a higher pharmacological availability using streptozotocin-induced diabetic animals. Similarly, VB12-modified nanoparticles based on trimethyl-chitosan or calcium phosphate improved the oral absorption of insulin (Chalasani et al., 2007a,b; Verma et al., 2016). In addition, Vitamin B7 is a non-endogenous vitamin and absorbed by Na^+-dependent and carrier-mediated endocytic mechanisms.

Wu et al. prepared a targeting biotinylated liposome for the oral insulin delivery, which effectively improved the drug bioavailability through the favorable cellular uptake and rapid gastrointestinal transport (Zhang et al., 2014). Vitamin B9, i.e., folic acid (FA), possessed unique abilities of high affinity and specificity to the folate receptor to increase the cellular uptake contents (**Figure 6**). By means of caveolinmediated endocytosis and modification with amphiphilic copolymers, an oral targeted delivery nanovehicle was fabricated and applied for the cancer therapy (Zheng et al., 2009; Liu et al., 2013).

Exosomes for Oral Cancer Therapy

Exosomes secreted by various cells (e.g., dendritic cells, macrophages, mesenchymal stem cells, endothelial, and epithelial cells) possess variously nanosized dimensions and natural formation, and therefore they have attracted great attentions by many researchers for the biological applications in recent years. Importantly, exosomes can deliver various biomolecules or chemotherapeutic agents for the intercellular exchange because of their effective adhesion abilities onto the cell membrane, suggestive of their potential roles as a novel vehicle for targeted drug delivery applications (Batrakova and Kim, 2015; Jiang and Gao, 2017; Zhao et al., 2020). For example, Tomita et al. demonstrated the a THP-1 and primary human macrophages (PHM)-derived exosomes to investigate the effects and sensitivity of macrophage secreted exosomes using 5 fluorouracil (5 FU) and cis diamminedichloroplatinum (CDDP) on the OSCC therapy (Tomita et al., 2020). The results found that these macrophage-derived exosomes decreased the proliferative inhibitory effects of 5 FU and CDDP and apoptosis in OSCC cells through activation of AKT/GSK-3β signaling pathway, playing important roles in reducing the sensitivity to chemotherapeutic agents in OSCC cells and improving the chemosensitivity of the tumor microenvironment in oral cancer. However, the exosomes also possess several limitations for the truly clinical applications, such as the effective separation and rigorous process for the purity, low loading capacity for the drug delivery and potential adverse immune for the biosafety (Ha et al., 2016), which should be addressed for the oral cancer therapy.

Peptides/Proteins for Oral Cancer Therapy

Synthetic peptides are also issued for the oral targeted delivery. Typically, CSKSSDYQC (CSK) peptide was employed to improve the hypoglycemic effect because of its goblet cell-targeting capacity (Sang et al., 2008). The studies found that CSK peptide-decorated chitosan NPs could effectively increase the oral bioavailability of other peptides and small agents by targeting intestinal goblet cells and promoting intestinal cellular uptake for oral delivery (Chen et al., 2018). Du et al. reported transferrin receptor specific nanocarriers conjugated with functional peptide, which increased intracellular uptake, alter intracellular trafficking, and enhance transcytosis in polarized cells for targeted oral drug delivery (Du et al., 2013).

Virus-Like Particles (VLPs) for Oral Cancer Therapy

VLPs are generally obtained by the self-assembly of viral capsids or viral-derived envelope proteins. On account of the surface biophysical and chemical properties, VLPs are easily regulated by altering VLP proteins through genetic and chemical engineering to provide their multifunction (Yang et al., 2019). Although VLPs are fully addressed to be effective as oral antigen carriers in immunization, they remain to be confirmed whether they have superior delivery characteristics in other oral cancer treatments (Chien et al., 2018; Ren et al., 2018; Serradell et al., 2019).

FUTURE OUTLOOK AND CONCLUSION

Considerable issues and advances have been developed with various nanotechnological strategies for oral cancer therapy. Based on these targeted drug delivery systems with tailored structures and various physicochemical properties, these carriers can load anticancer cargoes to target the malignant cells with high efficiency and less damage to the healthy cells, presenting a site-specific delivery behavior. Various forms of drug delivery have been deeply studied in this review as treatment options for the oral cancer, including polymeric/inorganic nanoparticles, liposomes, cyclodextrins, nanolipids, hydrogels, and several biomimetic forms. Taking advantages of their delicate regulations of structure-property relationship, most of these carriers expressed great potential alternative to overcome the limitations associated with oral drugs and conventional formulations. Nevertheless, for the currently targeted drug delivery systems, few clinic investigations were intensively performed thus far, which disclosed that improvement of clinical efficiency, well-control of drug release and reduction of side effects are highly challenging.

One of the main hindrances is the relatively complicated structures for most of drug carrier for the commercializations, causing severe problems like time-consuming and costly production. Even though, high-loading drug doses and ideal drug release profiles from these systems for the oral cancer therapy are still a major goal due to varied cellular mechanisms in OSCC scenario. In addition, other nanotechnologies on treatment of oral cancer should be introduced, such as ultrasounds, PTD, or PTT. For example, ultrasound-guided drug delivery has been a promising system to treat tumors since the ultrasound technology is simple, non-invasive, readily available, and spatial tailor of cargoes to the targeted sites with the high precision, which can be fabricated to respond to the thermal, mechanical effects of ultrasound or a combination of both.

Another important issue that needs to be solved in all cancer types, including oral cancer, is related to the clinic trials. Currently, most investigations are still focused on *in vitro* or *in vivo* studies. It is urgent to remind both clinicians and scientists to develop a full awareness of all the relative factors involved in the innovative strategy and guide appropriate clinical trials design, and further studies are needed to turn the concepts of nanotechnology toward practical applications in a multidisciplinary environment for oral cancer therapy. For instance, an advent of personalized medicine will lead to the advanced therapeutic outcomes, lower costs and high survival rates that benefit for both oncologists and patients in the near future.

AUTHOR CONTRIBUTIONS

YY and HJ initiated the project. MZ, JL, HL, and DL searched the data base, wrote, and finalized the manuscript. YY and DL made important suggestions and helped revising the paper. All authors reviewed and commented on the entire manuscript.

REFERENCES

Adeola, H. A., Papagerakis, P., and Papagerakis, S. (2019). System biology approaches and precision oral health: a circadian clock perspective. *Front. Physiol.* 10:399. doi: 10.3389/fphys.2019.00399

Agüeros, M., Ruiz-Gatón, L., Vauthier, C., Bouchemal, K., Espuelas, S., Irache, J. M., et al. (2009). Combined hydroxypropylbeta-cyclodextrin and poly(anhydride) nanoparticles improve the oral permeability of paclitaxel. *Eur. J. Pharm. Sci.* 38, 405–413. doi: 10.1016/j.ejps.2009.09.010

Bao, W. R., Lyu, J. R., Li, C. L., Zhang, J. F., Sun, T. N., Wang, X., et al. (2019). Fabrication of customized nanogel carriers from a UV-triggered dynamic self-assembly strategy. *Front. Chem.* 7:769. doi: 10.3389/fchem.2019.00769

Baselga, J., Trigo, J. M., Bourhis, J., Tortochaux, J., Cortés-Funes, H., Hitt, R., et al. (2005). Phase II multicenter study of the antiepidermal growth factor receptor monoclonal antibody cetuximab in combination with platinum-based chemotherapy in patients with platinum-refractory metastatic and/or recurrent squamous cell carcinoma of the head and neck. *J. Clin. Oncol.* 23, 568–5577. doi: 10.1200/JCO.2005.07.119

Batrakova, E. V., and Kim, M. S. (2015). Using exosomes, naturally-equipped nanocarriers, for drug delivery. *J. Control. Release* 219, 396–405. doi: 10.1016/j.jconrel.2015.07.030

Beloqui, A., Solinís, M. Á., Rodríguez-Gascón, A., Almeida, A. J., and Préat, V. (2016). Nanostructured lipid carriers: promising drug delivery systems for future clinics. *Nanomed. Nanotechnol. Biol. Med.* 12, 143–161. doi: 10.1016/j.nano.2015.09.004

Bonner, J. A., Harari, P. M., Giralt, J., Azarnia, N., Shin, D. M., Cohen, R. B., et al.

(2006). Radiotherapy plus cetuximab for squamous-cell carcinoma of the head and neck. *N. Engl. J. Med.* 354, 567–578. doi: 10.1056/NEJMoa053422

Bray, F., Ferlay, J., Soerjomataram, I., Siegel, R. L., Torre, L. A., and Jemal, A. (2018). Global cancer statistics 2018: GLOBOCAN estimates of incidence and mortality worldwide for 36 cancers in 185 countries. *CA Cancer J. Clin.* 68, 394–424. doi: 10.3322/caac.21492

Calixto, G., Bernegossi, J., Fonseca-Santos, B., and Chorilli, M. (2014). Nanotechnology-based drug delivery systems for treatment of oral cancer: a review. *Int. J. Nanomed.* 9, 3719–3735. doi: 10.2147/IJN.S61670

Calori, I. R., and Tedesco, A. C. (2016). Lipid vesicles loading aluminum phthalocyanine chloride: formulation properties and disaggregation upon intracellular delivery. *J. Photochem. Photobiol. B-Biol.* 160, 240–247. doi: 10.1016/j.jphotobiol.2016.03.050

Cao, C. Q., Wang, X., and Wu, D. C. (2018). Controlled cross-linking strategy for formation of hydrogels, microgels and nanogels. *Chinese J. Polym. Sci.* 36, 8–17. doi: 10.1007/s10118-018-2061-7

Catimel, G., Verweij, J., Mattijssen, V., Hanauske, A., Piccart, M., Wanders, J., et al. (1994). Docetaxel (Taxotere): an active drug for the treatment of patients with advanced squamous cell carcinoma of the head and neck. *EORTC early clinical trials group. Ann Oncol.* 5, 533–537. doi: 10.1093/oxfordjournals.annonc.a058908

Chalasani, K. B., Russell-Jones, G. J., Jain, A. K., Diwan, P. V., and Jain, S. K. (2007b). Effective oral delivery of insulin in animal models using vitamin B12-coated dextran nanoparticles. *J. Control. Release* 122, 141–150 doi: 10.1016/j.jconrel.2007.05.019

Chalasani, K. B., Russell-Jones, G. J., Yandrapu, S. K., Diwan, P. V., and Jain, S. K. (2007a). A novel vitamin B12-nanosphere conjugate carrier system for peroral delivery of insulin. *J. Controlled Release* 117, 421–429. doi: 10.1016/j.jconrel.2006.12.003

Chen, G., Svirskis, D., Lu, W., Ying, M., Huang, Y., and Wen, J. (2018). N-trimethyl chitosan nanoparticles and CSKSSDYQC peptide: N-trimethyl chitosan conjugates enhance the oral bioavailability of gemcitabine to treat breast cancer. *J. Control. Release* 277, 142–153. doi: 10.1016/j.jconrel.2018.03.013

Chien, M. H., Wu, S. Y., and Lin, C. H. (2018). Oral immunization with cell-free self-assembly virus-like particles against orange-spotted grouper nervous necrosis virus in grouper larvae, Epinephelus coioides. *Vet. Immunol. Immunopathol.* 197, 69–75. doi: 10.1016/j.vetimm.2018.01.012

Darwish, W. M., Abdoon, A. S., Shata, M. S., and Elmansy, M. (2020). Vincristine-loaded polymeric corona around gold nanorods for combination (chemo-photothermal) therapy of oral squamous carcinoma. *Reactive Funct. Polymers.* 151:104575. doi: 10.1016/j.reactfunctpolym.2020.10 4575

Desai, K. G. H. (2018). Polymeric drug delivery systems for intraoral site-specific chemoprevention of oral cancer. *J. Biomed. Mater. Res. Part B Appl. Biomater.* 106, 1383–1413. doi: 10.1002/jbm.b.33943

Du, F., Meng, H., Xu, K., et al. (2014). CPT loaded nanoparticles based on betacyclodextrin-grafted poly(ethylene glycol)/poly(L-glutamic acid) diblock copolymer and their inclusion complexes with CPT. *Colloids Surf. B Biointerfaces* 113, 230–236. doi: 10.1016/j.colsurfb.2013.0 9.015

Du, W., Fan, Y., Zheng, N., He, B., Yuan, L., Zhang, H., et al. (2013). Transferrin receptor specific nanocarriers conjugated with functional 7peptide for oral drug delivery. *Biomaterials* 34, 794–806. doi: 10.1016/j.biomaterials.2012.10.003

El-Sayed, I. H., Huang, X., and El-Sayed, M. A. (2006). Selective laser photo-thermal therapy of epithelial carcinoma using anti-EGFR antibody conjugated gold nanoparticles. *Cancer Lett.* 239, 129–135. doi: 10.1016/j.canlet.2005.07.035

Endo, K., Ueno, T., Kondo, S., Wakisaka, N., Murono, S., Ito, M., et al. (2013). Tumor-targeted chemotherapy with the nanopolymer-based drug NC-6004 for oral squamous cell carcinoma. *Cancer Sci.* 104, 369–374. doi: 10.1111/cas.12079

Figueiró Longo, J. P., Muehlmann, L. A., Velloso, N. V., Simioni, A. R., Lozzi, S. P., de Oliveira Cavalcanti, C. E., et al. (2012). Effects of photodynamic therapy mediated by liposomal aluminum-phthalocyanine chloride on chemically induced tongue tumors. *Chemotherapy* 1:103. doi: 10.4172/2167-7700.1000103

Ha, D., Yang, N., and Nadithe, V. (2016). Exosomes as therapeutic drug carriers and delivery vehicles across biological membranes: current perspectives and future challenges. *Acta Pharm. Sin. B.* 6, 287–296. doi: 10.1016/j.apsb.2016.02.001

Haddad, R., Sonis, S., Posner, M., Wirth, L., Costello, R., Braschayko, P., et al. (2009). Randomized phase 2 study of concomitant chemoradiotherapy using weekly carboplatin/paclitaxel with or without daily subcutaneous amifostine in patients with locally advanced head and neck cancer. *Cancer* 115, 4514–4523. doi: 10.1002/cncr.24525

Heck, J. E., Berthiller, J., Vaccarella, S., Winn, D. M., Smith, E. M., Shan'gina, O., et al. (2009). Sexual behaviours and the risk of head and neck cancers: a pooled analysis in the International Head and Neck Cancer Epidemiology (INHANCE) consortium. *Int. J. Epidemiol.* 39, 166–181. doi: 10.1093/ije/dyp350

Hoshyar, N., Gray, S., Han, H., and Bao, G. (2016). The effect of nanoparticle size on in vivo pharmacokinetics and cellular interaction. *Nanomedicine* 11, 673–692. doi: 10.2217/nnm.16.5

Huang, H., Barua, S., Sharma, G., Dey, S. K., and Rege, K. (2011). Inorganic nanoparticles for cancer imaging and therapy. *J. Control. Release.* 155, 344–357. doi: 10.1016/j.jconrel.2011.06.004

Iida, S., Shimada, J., and Sakagami, H. (2013). Cytotoxicity induced by docetaxel in human oral squamous cell carcinoma cell lines. *In Vivo* 27, 321–332.

Jiang, X. C., and Gao, J. Q. (2017). Exosomes as novel bio-carriers for gene and drug delivery. *Int. J. Pharm.* 521, 167–175. doi: 10.1016/j.ijpharm.2017.02.038

Ketabat, F., Karkhaneh, A., Mehdinavaz Aghdam, R., and Hossein Ahmadi Tafti, S. (2017). Injectable conductive collagen/alginate/polypyrrole hydrogels as a biocompatible system for biomedical applications. *J. Biomater. Sci. Polym. Ed.* 28, 794–805. doi: 10.1080/09205063.2017.1302314

Ketabat, F., Khorshidi, S., and Karkhaneh, A. (2018). Application of minimally invasive injectable conductive hydrogels as stimulating scaffolds for myocardial tissue engineering. *Polym. Int.* 67, 975–982. doi: 10.1002/pi.5599

Koutsopoulos, S., and Zhang, S. (2012). Two-layered injectable self-assembling peptide scaffold hydrogels for long-term sustained release of human antibodies. *J. Control. Release* 160, 451–458. doi: 10.1016/j.jconrel.2012.03.014

Kruijtzer, C. M., Beijnen, J. H., and Schellens, J. H. (2002). Improvement of oral drug treatment by temporary inhibition of drug transporters and/or cytochrome P450 in the gastrointestinal tract and liver: an overview. *Oncologist* 7, 516–530. doi: 10.1634/theoncologist.7-6-516

Li, D. W., Zhou, J., Zhang, M. M., Ma, Y. Z., Yang, Y. Y., Han, X., et al. (2020). Long-term delivery of alendronate through injectable tetra-peg hydrogel to promote osteoporosis therapy. *Biomater. Sci.* 8, 3138–3146. doi: 10.1039/D0BM00376J

Li, J., and Mooney, D. J. (2016). Designing hydrogels for controlled drug delivery. *Nat. Rev. Mater.* 1:16071. doi: 10.1038/natrevmats.2016.71

Li, X., Li, L., Huang, Y., Liu, B., Chi, H. R., Shi, L. L., et al. (2017). Synergistic therapy of chemotherapeutic drugs and MTH1 inhibitors using a pH-sensitive polymeric delivery system for oral squamous cell carcinoma. *Biomater. Sci.* 5, 2068–2078. doi: 10.1039/C7BM00395A

Lian, T., and Ho, R. J. (2001). Trends and developments in liposome drug delivery systems. *J. Pharm. Sci.* 90, 667–680. doi: 10.1002/jps.1023

Liu, B. C., Zhao, Y. R., Zhu, T. J., Gao, S., Ye, K. F., Zhou, F., et al. (2020). Biphasic double-network hydrogel with compartmentalized loading of bioactive glass for osteochondral defect repair. *Front. Bioeng. Biotechnol.* 8:752. doi: 10.3389/fbioe.2020.00752

Liu, D., Liu, Z., Wang, L., Zhang, C., and Zhang, N. (2011). Nanostructured lipid carriers as novel carrier for parenteral delivery of docetaxel. *Colloids Surf. B Biointerfaces* 85, 262–269. doi: 10.1016/j.colsurfb.2011.02.038

Liu, H. Y., Wang, X., Cao, Y. X., Yang, Y. Y., Yang, Y. T., Gao, Y. F., et al. (2020). Freezing-tolerant, highly sensitive strain and pressure sensors assembled from ionic conductive hydrogels with dynamic cross-links. *ACS Appl. Mater. Interfaces* 12, 25334–25344. doi: 10.1021/acsami.0c06067

Liu, X., Zhang, Y., Ma, D., Tang, H., and Yao, S. (2013). Biocompatible multi-walled carbon nanotube-chitosan–folic acid nanoparticle hybrids as GFP gene delivery materials. *Colloids Surf. B.* 111, 224–231. doi: 10.1016/j.colsurfb.2013.06.010

Lucky, S. S., Idris, N. M., Huang, K., Kim, J., Li, Z., Thong, P. S. P., et al. (2016). *In vivo* biocompatibility, biodistribution and therapeutic efficiency of titania coated upconversion nanoparticles for photodynamic therapy of solid oral cancers. *Theranostics.* 6, 1844–1865. doi: 10.7150/thno.15088

Madhulaxmi, M., Iyer, K., Periasamy, R., Gajendran, P., and Lakshmi, T. (2017). Role of cisplatin in oral squamous cell carcinoma-a review. *J Adv Pharm Educ Res.* 7, 39–42.

Maitra, J., and Kumar Shukla, V. (2014). Cross-linking in hydrogels-a review. *Am. J. Polym. Sci.* 4, 25–31. doi: 10.5923/j.ajps.20140402.01

Majchrzak, E., Szybiak, B., Wegner, A., Pienkowski, P., Pazdrowski, J., Luczewski, L., et al. (2014). Oral cavity and oropharyngeal squamous cell carcinoma in young adults: a review of the literature. *Radiol. Oncol.* 48, 1–10. doi: 10.2478/raon-2013-0057

Manikandan, M., Rao, A. K. D. M., Arunkumar, G., Manickavasagam, M., Rajkumar, K. S., Rajaraman, R., et al. (2016). Oral squamous cell carcinoma: microRNA expression profiling and integrative analyses for elucidation of tumourigenesis mechanism. *Mol. Cancer.* 15:28. doi: 10.1186/s12943-016-0512-8

Marcazzan, S., Varoni, E. M., Blanco, E., Lodi, G., and Ferrari, M. (2018). Nanomedicine, an emerging therapeutic strategy for oral cancer therapy. *Oral Oncol.* 76, 1–7. doi: 10.1016/j.oraloncology.2017.11.014

Mezei, M., and Gulasekharam, V. (1980). Liposomes-a selective drug delivery system for the topical route of administration. *Lotion dosage form. Life Sci.* 26, 1473–1477 doi: 10.1016/0024-3205(80)90268-4

Nirvani, M., Khuu, C., Utheim, T. P., Sand, L. P., and Sehic, A. (2018). Circadian clock and oral cancer. *Mol. Clin. Oncol.* 8, 219–226. doi: 10.3892/mco.2017.1518

Panyam, J., Zhou, W. Z., Prabha, S., Sahoo, S. K., and Labhasetwar, V. (2002). Rapid endo-lysosomal escape of poly(DL-lactide-co-glycolide) nanoparticles: implications for drug and gene delivery. *FASEB J.* 16, 1217–1226 doi: 10.1096/fj.02-0088com

Poonia, M., Ramalingam, K., Goyal, S., and Sidhu, K. S. (2017). Nanotechnology in oral cancer: a comprehensive review. *J. Oral Maxillofac. Pathol.* 3, 407–414. doi: 10.4103/jomfp.JOMFP_29_17

Rajewski, R. A., and Stella, V. J. (1996). Pharmaceutical applications of cyclodextrins. 2. *In vivo* drug delivery. *J. Pharm. Sci.* 85, 1142–1168. doi: 10.1021/js960075u

Ravikumara, N. R., Tiyaboonchai, W., and Madhusudhan, B. (2013). Fabrication and characterization of genistein encapsulated poly (D, L) lactic acid nanoparticles for pharmaceutical application. *Curr. Nanosci.* 9, 293–302. doi: 10.2174/1573413711309020021

Ren, Z., Zhao, Y., Liu, J., Ji, X., Meng, L., Wang, T., et al. (2018). Inclusion of membrane-anchored LTB or flagellin protein in H5N1 virus-like particles enhances protective responses following intramuscular and oral immunization of mice. *Vaccine* 36, 5990–5998. doi: 10.1016/j.vaccine.2018.08.053

Ribeiro de Souza, A. L., Kiill, C. P., dos Santos, F. K., et al. (2012). Nanotechnologybased drug delivery systems for dermatomycosis treatment. *Curr. Nanosci.* 8:512–519. doi: 10.2174/157341312801784311

Rivera, C. (2015). Essentials of oral cancer. *Int J Clin Exp Pathol.* 8, 11884–11894. doi: 10.5281/zenodo.192487

Sang, K. K., Woo, J. H., Kim, M. K., Woo, S. S., Choi, J. H., Lee, H. G., et al. (2008). Identification of a peptide sequence that improves transport of macromolecules across the intestinal mucosal barrier targeting goblet cells. *J. Biotechnol.* 135, 210–216. doi: 10.1016/j.jbiotec.2008.01.021

Senapati, S., Mahanta, A. K., Kumar, S., and Maiti, P. (2018). Controlled drug delivery vehicles for cancer treatment and their performance. *Signal Transduct. Target. Ther.* 3:7. doi: 10.1038/s41392-017-0004-3

Sepantafar, M., Maheronnaghsh, R., Mohammadi, H., Radmanesh, F., Hasani-sadrabadi, M. M., Ebrahimi, M., et al. (2017). Engineered hydrogels in cancer therapy and diagnosis. *Trends Biotechnol.* 35, 1074–1087. doi: 10.1016/j.tibtech.2017.06.015

Serradell, M. C., Rupil, L. L., Martino, R. A., Prucca, C. G., Carranza, P. G., Saura, A., et al. (2019). Efficient oral vaccination by bioengineering virus-like particles with protozoan surface proteins. *Nat. Commun.* 10:361. doi: 10.1038/s41467-018-08265-9

Subramani, K., and Ahmed, W. (2012). *Nanoparticulate Drug Delivery Systems for Oral Cancer Treatment, 1st Edn.* Amsterdam: Elsevier Inc.

Sun, G. F., Liu, J. H., Wang, X., Li, M., Cui, X., Zhang, L. C., et al. (2019). Fabrication of dual-sensitive poly(β-hydroxyl amine) micelles for controlled drug delivery. *Eur. Polym. J.* 114:338–345. doi: 10.1016/j.eurpolymj.2019.02.048

Szente, L., and Szejtli, J. (1999). Highly soluble cyclodextrin derivatives: chemistry, properties, and trends in development. *Adv. Drug Deliv. Rev.* 36, 17–28 doi: 10.1016/S0169-409X(98)00092-1

Tan, G. Z., Zhong, Y. T., Yang, L. L., Jiang, Y. D., Liu, J. Q., and Ren, F. (2020). A multifunctional MOF-based nanohybrid as injectable implant platform for drug synergistic oral cancer therapy. *Chem. Eng. J.* 390:124446. doi: 10.1016/j.cej.2020.124446

Tang, G. K., Zhou, B. Y., Li, F., Wang, W. H., Liu, Y., Wang, X., et al. (2020). Advances of naturally-derived and synthetic hydrogels for intervertebral disc regeneration. *Front. Bioeng. Biotechnol.* 8:745. doi: 10.3389/fbioe.2020.00745

Tomita, R., Sasabe, E., Tomomura, A., and Yamamoto, T. (2020). Macrophage-derived exosomes attenuate the susceptibility of oral squamous cell carcinoma cells to chemotherapeutic drugs through the AKT/GSK-3beta pathway. *Oncol. Rep.* 44, 1905–1916 doi: 10.3892/or.2020.7748

Verma, A., Sharma, S., Gupta, P. K., Singh, A., Teja, B. V., Dwivedi, P., et al. (2016). Vitamin B12 functionalized layer by layer calcium phosphate nanoparticles: a mucoadhesive and pH responsive carrier for improved oral delivery of insulin. *Acta Biomater.* 31, 288–300. doi: 10.1016/j.actbio.2015.12.017

Vogel, D. W. T., Zbaeren, P., and Thoeny, H. C. (2010). Cancer of the oral cavity and oropharynx. *Cancer Imaging.* 10, 62–72. doi: 10.1102/1470-7330.2010.0008

Vyas, A., and Saraf, S. (2008). Cyclodextrin based novel drug delivery systems. *J. Incl. Phenom. Macrocycl. Chem.* 62, 23–42. doi: 10.1007/s10847-008-9456-y

Wang, H., Luo, J. C., Zhang, Y. H., He, D., Jiang, R., Xie, X. M., et al. (2020). Phospholipid/hydroxypropyl-beta-cyclodextrin supramolecular complexes are promising candidates for efficient oral delivery of curcuminoids. *Int. J. Pharm.* 582:119301. doi: 10.1016/j.ijpharm.2020.119301

Wang, S. J., Jiang, D., Zhang, Z. Z., Chen, Y. R., Yang, Z. D., Zhang, J. Y., et al. (2019). Biomimetic nanosilica-collagen scaffolds for in situ bone regeneration: toward a cell-free, one-step surgery. *Adv. Mater.* 31:1904341. doi: 10.1002/adma.201904341

Wang, X., Gao, P. Y., Yang, Y. Y., Guo, G. X., and Wu, D. C. (2018). Dynamic and programmable morphology and size evolution via a living hierarchical self-assembly strategy. *Nat. Commun.* 9:2772. doi: 10.1038/s41467-018-05142-3

Wang, X., Yang, Y. Y., Gao, P. Y., Yang, F., Shen, H., Guo, H. X., et al. (2015). Synthesis, self-assembly and photoresponsive behavior of tadpole-shaped azobenzene polymers. *ACS Macro Lett.* 4, 1321–1326. doi: 10.1021/acsmacrolett.5b00698

Wang, X., Yang, Y. Y., Shi, Y., and Jia, F. (2020). Editorial: smart hydrogels in tissue engineering and regenerative medicine. *Front. Chem.* 8:245. doi: 10.3389/fchem.2020.00245

Wang, X., Yang, Y. Y., Zuo, Y. F., Yang, F., Shen, H., and Wu, D. C. (2016). Facile creation of fret systems from a ph-responsive AIE fluorescent vesicle. *Chem. Commun.* 52, 5320–5323. doi: 10.1039/C6CC01706A

Xu, B. B., Ye, J., Yuan, F. Z., Zhang, J. Y., Chen, Y. R., Fan, B. S., et al. (2020). Advances of stem cell-laden hydrogels with biomimetic microenvironment for osteochondral repair. *Front. Bioeng. Biotechnol.* 8:247. doi: 10.3389/fbioe.2020.00247

Yan, X., Chen, Y. R., Song, Y. F., Ye, J., Yang, M., Xu, B. B., et al. (2020). Advances in the application of supramolecular hydrogels for stem cell delivery and cartilage tissue engineering. *Front. Bioeng. Biotechnol.* 8:847. doi: 10.3389/fbioe.2020.00847

Yang, G., Chen, S., and Zhang, J. (2019). Bioinspired and biomimetic nanotherapies for the treatment of infectious diseases. *Front. Pharmacol.* 10:751. doi: 10.3389/fphar.2019.00751

Yang, Y. Y., Wang, X., Yang, F., Wang, L. N., and Wu, D. C. (2018). Highly elastic and ultratough hybrid ionic-covalent hydrogels with tunable structures and mechanics. *Adv. Mater.* 30:1707071. doi: 10.1002/adma.201707071

Yang, Y. Y., Yang, Y. T., Cao, Y. X., Wang, X., Chen, Y. R., Liu, H. Y., et al. (2021). Anti-freezing, resilient and tough hydrogels for sensitive and large-range strain and pressure sensors. *Chem. Eng. J.* 403:126431. doi: 10.1016/j.cej.2020.126431

Zhang, T., Chen, J., Zhang, Y., Shen, Q., and Pan, W. (2011). Characterization and evaluation of nanostructured lipid carrier as a vehicle for oral delivery of etoposide. *Eur. J. Pharm. Sci.* 43, 174–179. doi: 10.1016/j.ejps.2011.04.005

Zhang, X., Qi, J., Lu, Y., He, W., Li, X., and Wu, W. (2014). Biotinylated liposomes as potential carriers for the oral delivery of insulin. *Nanomedicine* 10, 167–176. doi: 10.1016/j.nano.2013.07.011

Zhao, X. G., Zhao, Y. H., Sun, X., Xing, Y., Wang, X., and Yang, Q. (2020). The immunomodulatory property of MSCs and MSC-derived exosomes in osteoarthritis. *Front. Bioeng. Biotechnol.* 11:1912. doi: 10.3389/fbioe.2020.575057

Zheng, Y., Cai, Z., Song, X., Chen, Q., Bi, Y., Li, Y., et al. (2009). Preparation and characterization of folate conjugated N-trimethyl chitosan nanoparticles as protein carrier targeting folate receptor: *in vitro* studies. *J. Drug Target.* 17, 294–303. doi: 10.1080/10611860902737920

Zhou, Z. X., Chen, Y. R., Zhang, J. Y., Jiang, D., Yuan, F. Z., Mao, Z. M., et al. (2020). Facile strategy on hydrophilic modification of poly (ε-caprolactone) scaffolds for assisting tissue-engineered meniscus constructs *in vitro*. *Front. Pharmacol.* 11:471. doi: 10.3389/fphar.2020.00471

2

MUS81 Inhibition Enhances the Anticancer Efficacy of Talazoparib by Impairing ATR/CHK1 Signaling Pathway in Gastric Cancer

Tao Wang†, Peng Zhang†, Chengguo Li, Weizhen Liu, Qian Shen, Lei Yang, Gengchen Xie, Jie Bai, Ruidong Li, Kaixiong Tao and Yuping Yin**

Department of Gastrointestinal Surgery, Union Hospital, Tongji Medical College, Huazhong University of Science and Technology, Wuhan, China

***Correspondence:**
Yuping Yin
yinyuping2017@hust.edu.cn
Kaixiong Tao
kaixiongtao@hust.edu.cn

†These authors have contributed equally to this work

MUS81 is a critical endonuclease involved in heterodimer formation with Eme1/Mms4 and an important DNA damage repair regulatory molecule. Our previous study suggested that MUS81 was overexpressed and its high expression was positively correlated with gastric cancer metastasis. However, the therapeutic potential of targeting MUS81 in gastric cancer requires further exploration. Therefore, in this study, the Cancer Genome Atlas (TCGA) data were analyzed and showed that MUS81 is a key regulator of cell cycle distribution and DNA damage repair in gastric cancer. *In vitro* and *in vivo*, MUS81 knockdown significantly enhanced the anticancer effect of the PARP inhibitor talazoparib. Mechanistically, MUS81 inhibition impaired the activation of the ATR/CHK1 cell cycle signaling pathway and promoted gastric cancer cells with talazoparib-induced DNA damage to continue mitosis. Moreover, addition of the bromodomain-containing protein 4 inhibitor AZD5153 increased the anticancer effect of talazoparib *via* MUS81 inhibition in gastric cancer cells, and this combination effect was largely impaired when MUS81 was knocked down. In conclusion, these data suggested that MUS81 regulated ATR/CHK1 activation, a key signaling pathway in the G2M checkpoint, and targeting MUS81 enhanced the antitumor efficacy of talazoparib. Therefore, AZD5153 combined with talazoparib may represent a promising therapeutic strategy for patients with MUS81 proficient gastric cancer.

Keywords: gastric cancer, MUS81, PARP inhibitor, BRD4 inhibitor, DNA damage

INTRODUCTION

Gastric cancer is one of the most prevalent forms of cancers and the third leading cause of cancer-related deaths worldwide (1). For early gastric cancer, radical surgical resection is currently the main treatment. However, among patients newly diagnosed with gastric cancer, 70% of them have advanced gastric cancer, and surgery combined with chemoradiotherapy is the standard treatment

---

Abbreviations: ATR, ataxia telangiectasia and Rad3-related; BRCA, breast cancer susceptibility gene; CHK1, checkpoint kinase 1; DSB, double-strand break; HR, homologous recombination repair; PARP, poly (ADP-ribose) polymerase; SSB, single-strand break; TCGA, the Cancer Genome Atlas; Xpf, Xeroderma pigmentosum type F/Cockayne syndrome.

(2). Limited by the high heterogeneity of gastric cancer biology and genetics, the effect of traditional chemotherapy regimens for gastric cancer has less than optimal results (3). Therefore, more effective treatment strategies need to be explored.

PARP inhibitors block the single-strand break (SSB) repair pathway by targeting PARP, causing homologous recombination deficiency malignant tumors to be synthetically lethal (4, 5). MUS81 belongs to the Xpf family of structure-specific endonucleases (6). It acts as a DNA replication pressure sensor, regulating the DNA replication forks reactivation, further affecting important DNA damage repair pathways, such as cell non-homologous end joining and homologous recombination repair (HR) (6, 7). Inhibition of MUS81 expression in ovarian cancer, significantly impairs cell HR activity (8, 9). Our previous research showed that MUS81 was overexpressed in gastric cancer cells and might promote gastric cancer cell invasion and metastasis (10). However, the therapeutic value of targeting MUS81 requires further investigation.

In this study, whether MUS81 silencing enhances talazoparib sensitivity, was evaluated in gastric cancer, and the mechanism of MUS81 knockdown sensitizing the anticancer effect of talazoparib was characterized. Furthermore, it was observed that AZD5153 sensitized the anticancer effect of talazoparib in gastric cancer *via* down-regulating the expression of MUS81. This is the first report to show that AZD5153 sensitizes the efficacy of talazoparib in gastric cancer by increasing DNA damage and apoptosis.

MATERIALS AND METHODS

Cell Lines, Cell Culture, and Antibodies

SGC7901 and BGC823 cells were purchased from the National Collection of Authenticated Cell Cultures of China. RPMI-1640 medium (Gibco, USA) containing 10% FBS (Gibco BRL, USA) was used to cultivate cells at 37°C in a 5% CO_2 atmosphere.

The primary antibodies against histone H2AX (γ-H2AX)^{S139} (9718S), ATR (13934S), p-ATR^{T1989} (30632S), CHK1 (2360), p-CHK1^{S317} (12302S), p-Histone H3^{Ser10} (53348S), Ki67 (9449S), and GAPDH (5174S) were obtained from Cell Signaling Technology (MA, USA). Antibodies against cleaved PARP (ab32064) were obtained from Abcam (MA, USA). HRP-conjugated secondary antibodies (SA00001-1 and SA00001-2) and anti-MUS81 antibodies were purchased from Proteintech (Wuhan, China).

Cell Survival Assay

SGC7901 and BGC823 cells (1×10^3 cells/well) were seeded in 96-well plates, and then treated with 0 to 1 μmol/L of talazoparib for 5 d. After drug treatment, the cell proliferation rate was determined using the CellTiter™ AQueous assay (MTS, Promega). Ten microliters of CellTiter 96® AQueous One Solution Reagent was added to each well. After incubating for 1 h at 37°C , the absorbance was read at 490 nm using a microplate reader. The cell proliferation rate was calculated using the following formula: (mean optical density (OD) treated well [–blank])/(mean OD control well [–blank]) × 100. Five technical replicates were prepared for each sample in three separate experiments.

Clonogenic Assay

Cells (1×10^3 cells/well) were seeded into 6-well plates and exposed to different concentrations of talazoparib (0 or 100 nmol/L) for 10 d. Cells fixation and staining were performed as previously described (11). Finally, cell clones in 6-well plates were evaluated by ImageJ. The experiments were carried out three times.

Western Blot Analysis

Western blotting was performed as described previously (12). RIPA buffer (V900854, Sigma, MO, USA) containing phosphatase inhibitors (G2007, Servicebio, Wuhan, China) and protease (B14001, Bimake, TX, USA) was used to lyse cells. Equivalent proteins were separated by 7.5%–12.5% SDS-PAGE. Finally, protein bands were detected using the ECL detection reagent (Thermo Fisher Scientific, USA). The results were analyzed using ImageJ. Experiments were performed three times.

Apoptosis and Cell Cycle Analysis

Cells (2×10^5 cells/well) were seeded into 6-well plates and exposed to DMSO or talazoparib (1 μmol/L) for 3 d. To examine apoptosis, the cells were harvested by trypsinization and washed twice with PBS at 4°C . The cells were resuspended in 100 μL Annexin V binding buffer, and 5 μL 7-AAD and 5 μL allophycocyanin-Annexin V were added. After the cells were incubated for 15 min in the dark at room temperature, 100 μL Annexin V binding buffer was added, and the proportion of apoptotic cells was analyzed by flow cytometry.

Cell cycle detection was performed as described previously (13). These experiments were performed using three biological replicates.

Immunofluorescence Assay

Coverslips were coated with 0.01% poly-L-lysine and exposed to DMSO, talazoparib (0.5 μmol/L), AZD5153 (1 μmol/L), or their combination after the cells were plated. After two days of treatment, immunofluorescence was performed by staining with primary antibodies against γ-H2AX (1:100), p-Histone H3 (1:1600), or p-CHK1 (1:800) as previously described (14). Then, the coverslips were incubated with DAPI and CY3-conjugated secondary antibodies. Finally, coverslips were scanned using a fluorescence microscope (Nikon, Tokyo, Japan). The reproducibility of the results was confirmed by at least three separate experiments.

Cell Transfection and RNA Interference

Two different shRNA sequences were used for MUS81 knockdown. Lentivirus (GeneChem Co. Ltd., China) targeting the sequence of human MUS81 (shRNA #1: 5′-TACCAACAAA CAGCAAGTGGG-3′, shRNA #2: 5′-CACGCGCTTCGTATTT CAGAA-3′) was purchased from GeneChem Co. Ltd. (Shanghai, China). The corresponding control shRNA sequence was 5′-TTCTCCGAACGTGTCACGT-3′. Lentiviral infection was conducted as described previously (15). Stable GC cell lines transfected with scramble shRNA, shRNA #1, or shRNA #2 were selected for 7 d with 4 μg/mL puromycin.

Two specific MUS81 siRNAs were purchased from RiboBio (Guangzhou, China). The negative control siRNA sequence is 5'-GGGUAUCGACGAUUACAAA-3', and the sequences of siRNA #1 and siRNA #2 targeting MUS81 are 5'-TACCAACAAACAGCAAGTGGG-3' and 5'-CACGCGCTTCGTATTTCAGAA-3', respectively. Transient transfection was performed using Lipofectamine 2000 (Thermo Fisher Scientific, USA) and siRNAs for 24 h. Western blotting was used to verify the knockdown effect of MUS81.

In Vivo Experiments

The Institutional Animal Care and Use Committee of Tongji Medical College, Huazhong University of Science and Technology approved all animal experiments in this study. A total of 20 five-week-old BALB/c-null mice were purchased from HFK Biotechnology (Beijing, China). SGC7901^{shCtrl} and SGC7901^{shMUS81} cells were resuspended in PBS to obtain a concentration of 1×10^7 cells/mL, and then each mouse was subcutaneously injected 150 μL of the solution in the right flank. When the tumor volume reached 100 mm^3, the mice were randomly divided into four groups: control, MUS81-knockdown, talazoparib-treated, and MUS81-knockdown plus talazoparib-treated groups (five mice per group). Mice in the talazoparib group was administered talazoparib (0.33 mg/kg) by gavage for 21 consecutive days. The control group was administered the same dose of DMSO and PBS by gavage. After treatment, the mice were sacrificed, tumors were collected and embedded in paraffin, and immunohistochemically stained.

Immunohistochemistry

Immunohistochemistry was performed using an antibody against Ki67 or γ-H2AX at a dilution of 1:200 as previously described (16). A brown signal was defined as a positive reaction in the cells. The results of immunohistochemical staining using a mean score were compared, considering both the intensity of staining and the proportion of tumor cells; the staining intensity score was 3, strong; 2, moderate; 1, weak; and 0, negative. The positive cell frequency was defined as 4 (76%–100%), 3 (51%–75%), 2 (26%–50%), 1 (1%–25%), and 0 (none). Immunohistochemical staining was performed for each component and the final score was obtained *via* multiplying the score of staining intensity and the score of positive cell frequency. Scores 0–7 were defined as negative staining, and 8–12 were defined as positive staining.

Statistical Analyses

Statistical analysis was performed using GraphPad Prism version 9. A *t*-test was performed for intergroup comparisons and data are presented as the mean ± standard deviation (SD). *P* values less than 0.05 were considered significantly different and all tests were two-tailed.

RESULTS

MUS81 Was Highly Expressed and Enriched in DNA Damage Repair Pathways in Gastric Cancer

Using TCGA database, the differential expression of DNA damage repair network-related molecules was analyzed in 18 common malignant tumors; MUS81 was significantly highly expressed in gastric cancer (**Figures 1A, B**). Based on the gene set enrichment analysis in malignant tumors, MUS81 may play a critical role in many signaling pathways, such as the cell cycle regulation and DNA damage response pathways (**Figures 1C, D**). These results suggested that targeting MUS81 is a potential treatment strategy in the clinical treatment of gastric cancer.

MUS81 Knockdown Promoted Apoptosis and Anticancer Efficacy of Talazoparib *In Vitro*

Next, SGC7901 and BGC823 cells were infected with the lentivirus vector (LV)-shMUS81. Western blotting was used to examine MUS81 protein levels in SGC7901 and BGC823 cells infected with LV-shMUS81 and LV-Ctrl. MUS81 protein levels were significantly decreased in MUS81 knockdown cells (**Figure 2A**).

MUS81 is an important DNA damage repair regulatory molecule and MUS81 deficiency impairs cell HR (8, 17). To explore whether down-regulation of MUS81 expression in gastric cancer cells affected the antitumoral efficacy of PARP inhibitors, MTS assay was performed and the data were analyzed to construct the dose-inhibition efficiency curves of the PARP inhibitor talazoparib in different groups. As shown in **Figure 2B**, cell proliferation of the LV-shMUS81 group was significantly decreased compared to that of the LV-Ctrl group in both SGC7901 and BGC823 cells, and the clone formation rate in the LV-shMUS81 group was significantly lower than that in the LV-Ctrl group after talazoparib treatment (71.69% ± 3.61% versus 12.38% ± 2.21% and 65.34% ± 3.22% versus 7.67% ± 1.53%, respectively, $P < 0.01$ for all) (**Figure 2C**).

To further confirm whether the antitumor effect of PARP inhibitors increased by MUS81 knockdown was due to increased apoptosis, flow cytometry was performed to measure the apoptosis rate of gastric cancer cells. Seventy-two hours after talazoparib treatment, a marked increase in apoptotic SGC7901 and BGC823 cells was revealed in the LV-shMUS81 group compared to that in the LV-Ctrl group (39.67% ± 2.08% versus 20.67% ± 1.50% and 48.69% ± 5.51% versus 17.34% ± 2.00%, respectively, $P < 0.01$ for all) (**Figure 2D**). In addition, western blotting also showed that the expression of cleaved PARP, a marker of apoptosis, increased significantly after exposure to talazoparib in the LV-shMUS81 group (**Figure 2E**).

MUS81 Inhibition Pushed Cells Into Mitosis From G2M Checkpoint Arrest Induced by Talazoparib and Increased DNA Damage Caused by Talazoparib in Gastric Cancer Cells

To further investigate the mechanism by which MUS81 knockdown enhanced the sensitivity of SGC7901 and BGC823 cells to talazoparib, flow cytometry was performed for cell cycle analysis. Cell cycle analysis showed that talazoparib treatment induced significant G2M phase arrest in SGC7901 and BGC823 cells (**Figure 3A**). However, after stably transfecting with shMUS81, SGC7901 and BGC823 cells that were arrested by talazoparib in the G2M phase continued to mitosis, and the

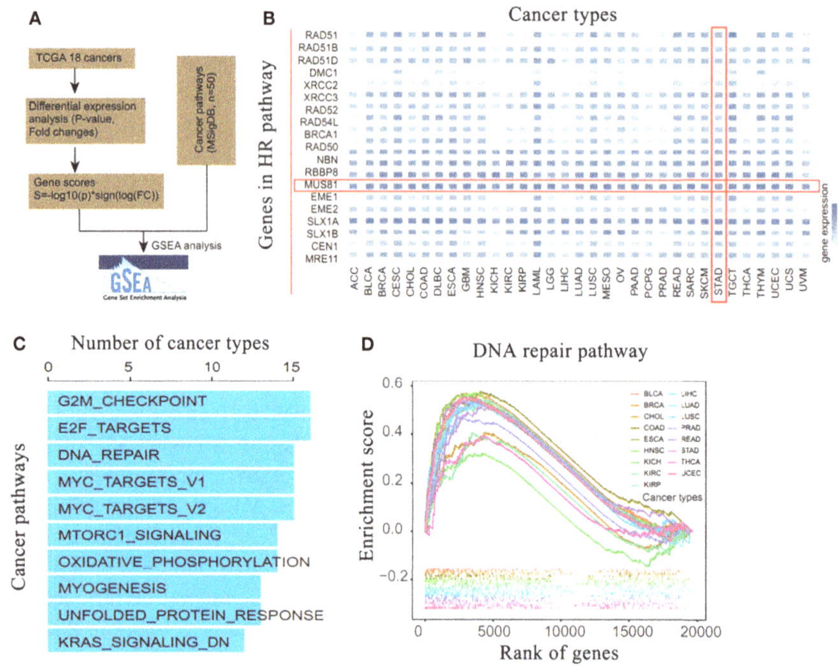

FIGURE 1 | MUS81 is overexpressed in gastric cancer and is enriched in DNA damage repair pathways in malignant tumors. **(A)** Bioinformatics analysis process. **(B)** Analysis of the differential expression of DNA damage and repair-related molecules in 18 common malignant tumors in TCGA database suggests that MUS81 is overexpressed in gastric cancer. **(C)** Gene set enrichment analysis of MUS81-related enrichment signaling pathways in malignant tumors. **(D)** Enrichment of MUS81 in DNA damage repair pathways in malignant tumors.

proportion of G0/G1 phase cells increased significantly (**Figure 3A**). To verify the effect of MUS81 knockdown on cell mitosis, the LV-shMUS81 and LV-Ctrl groups were stained for p-Histone H3 (Ser10), a mitosis marker, following treatment with talazoparib. MUS81 knockdown pushed gastric cancer cells with talazoparib-induced DNA damage into mitosis (**Figure 3B**).

Next, whether MUS81 deficiency impaired cellular DNA repair ability was tested. In this study, a DNA damage model was established using talazoparib. γ-H2AX expression was significantly increased after talazoparib treatment in LV-shMUS81 cells (**Figures 3C, D**). These data indicated that MUS81 knockdown increased talazoparib-induced DNA damage in gastric cancer cells.

MUS81 Deficiency Impaired ATR/CHK1 Activation Induced by Talazoparib in Gastric Cancer

Having observed a defective G2M phase checkpoint in MUS81-deficient cells, whether MUS81 deficiency impaired the DNA damage checkpoint signaling pathway was further examined. Because CHK1 is a key G2/M checkpoint regulator, cells were exposed to talazoparib and CHK1 phosphorylation (Ser317) was examined by immunofluorescence and western blotting. In SGC7901 and BGC823 LV-Ctrl cells, CHK1 phosphorylation (Ser317) significantly increased after treatment with talazoparib. However, relatively reduced CHK1 phosphorylation (Ser317) was observed in response to talazoparib in LV-shMUS81 cells (**Figure 4A**).

CHK1 (Ser317) can be phosphorylated by ATR phosphorylation, and CHK1 phosphorylation prompts cells to enter G2M phase arrest for DNA repair (18–21). Therefore, whether MUS81 deficiency affected ATR activation was examined. Western blotting showed that MUS81 knockdown significantly decreased ATR activation and reduced the CHK1 activation response to talazoparib (**Figures 4B, C**). These results indicated that MUS81 knockdown impaired the G2M phase checkpoint of cells by suppressing ATR/CHK1 signaling.

MUS81 Knockdown Enhanced Anticancer Efficacy of Talazoparib in Gastric Cancer *In Vivo*

To demonstrate that MUS81 knockdown increases the antitumor effect of talazoparib *in vivo*, nude mice bearing MUS81-deficient and parental xenograft gastric cancer were treated daily with and without oral 0.33 mg/kg talazoparib. Talazoparib showed outstanding anticancer effect in the MUS81-deficient gastric cancer model (**Figure 5A**); the antitumor effect was most significant after 21 d of treatment (**Figure 5B**). There was no significant difference in the body weight among the four groups of nude mice (**Figure 5C**).

IHC studies indicated that after treatment with talazoparib, tumor tissues from the MUS81-deficient group showed lower Ki67 expression, suggesting lower proliferation ability compared to that of the parental xenograft group (**Figure 5D**). Furthermore, the expression of γ-H2AX was analyzed. As

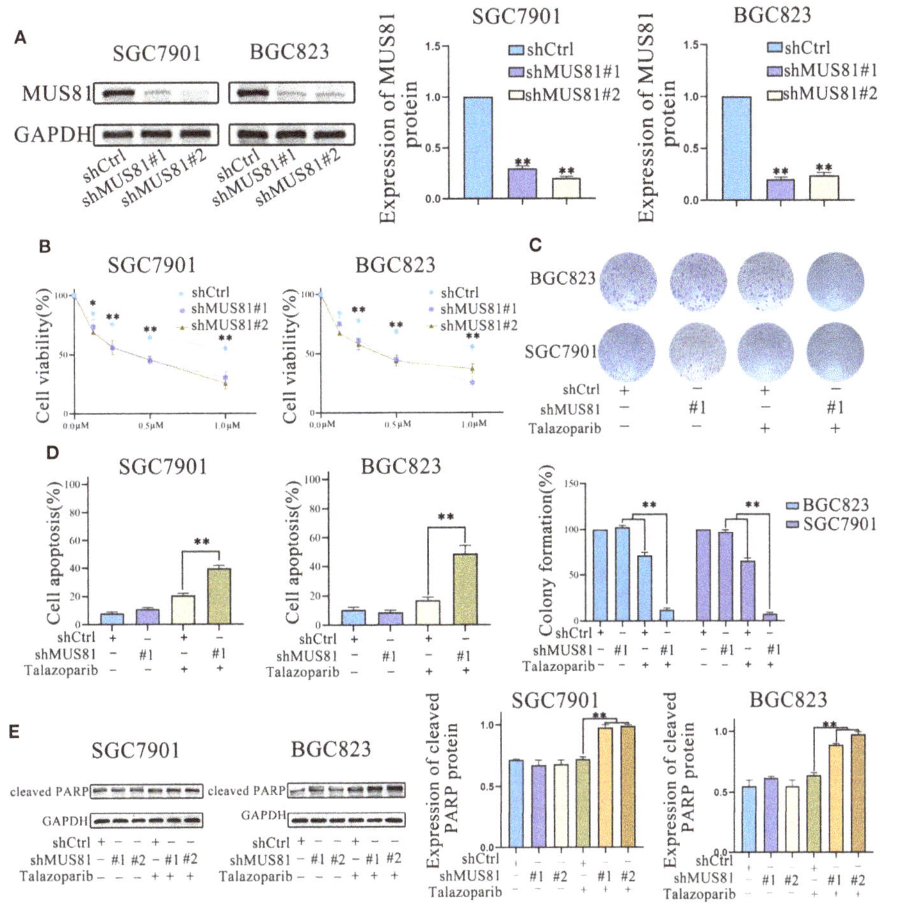

FIGURE 2 | MUS81 knockdown promotes apoptosis and talazoparib anticancer efficacy *in vitro*. **(A)** Western blotting of MUS81 protein expression after transfection with the lentivirus expressing short hairpin RNA (shRNA) targeting the sequence of human MUS81 for 24 h. **$P < 0.01$. **(B, C)** Viability of SGC7901 and BGC823 cells transfected with lentivirus expressing shMUS81 #1, shMUS81 #2 or shCtrl, as determined using MTS and colony formation assays (t-test). *$P < 0.05$. **$P < 0.01$. **(D)** Cells treated with DMSO or talazoparib (1 μmol/L) for 3 d to evaluate apoptosis by flow cytometry (*t*-test). **$P < 0.01$. **(E)** Expression of apoptosis-related proteins in SGC7901 and BGC823 cells treated with DMSO or talazoparib (0.5 μmol/L) for 24 h, as evaluated by western blotting (*t*-test). **$P < 0.01$.

expected, MUS81 knockdown tumor cells showed higher expression of γ-H2AX than control cells in response to talazoparib (**Figure 5D**). Overall, these data represented excellent antitumor efficacy of talazoparib in the MUS81-deficient gastric cancer xenograft model.

AZD5153 Sensitized the Anticancer Effect of Talazoparib in a MUS81-Dependent Manner in Gastric Cancer Cells

Our previous study has shown that the BRD4 inhibitor AZD5153 downregulates MUS81 expression (10). Thus, it was hypothesized that AZD5153 might sensitize the talazoparib antitumor effect in gastric cancer cells by regulating MUS81 expression. To verify the potential synergy between AZD5153 and talazoparib, the effects of monotherapy and combination therapy were assessed in SGC7901 and BGC823 cell lines. MTS data showed that the AZD5153/talazoparib combination was synergistic with a combination index of less than 0.5 in LV-Ctrl cell lines. Interestingly, in the MUS81 knockdown cell line, the AZD5153/talazoparib combination effect was significantly impaired (**Figures 6A, B**).

Next, western blotting showed that AZD5153 significantly reduced MUS81 expression. Furthermore, similar to talazoparib therapy in MUS81 knockdown cells, the AZD5153/talazoparib combination therapy significantly improved the expression of γ-H2AX and cleaved PARP in LV-Ctrl cells (**Figures 6C, D**). These data suggested that the efficacy of AZD5153 sensitized talazoparib in gastric cancer cells may be attributed to its ability to downregulate MUS81. AZD5153/talazoparib combination therapy promoted DNA damage and apoptosis in SGC7901 and BGC823 cells (**Figure 7**).

DISCUSSION

Among DNA damage repair pathways, PARP plays an indispensable role in the repair of DNA SSBs (22, 23). PARP

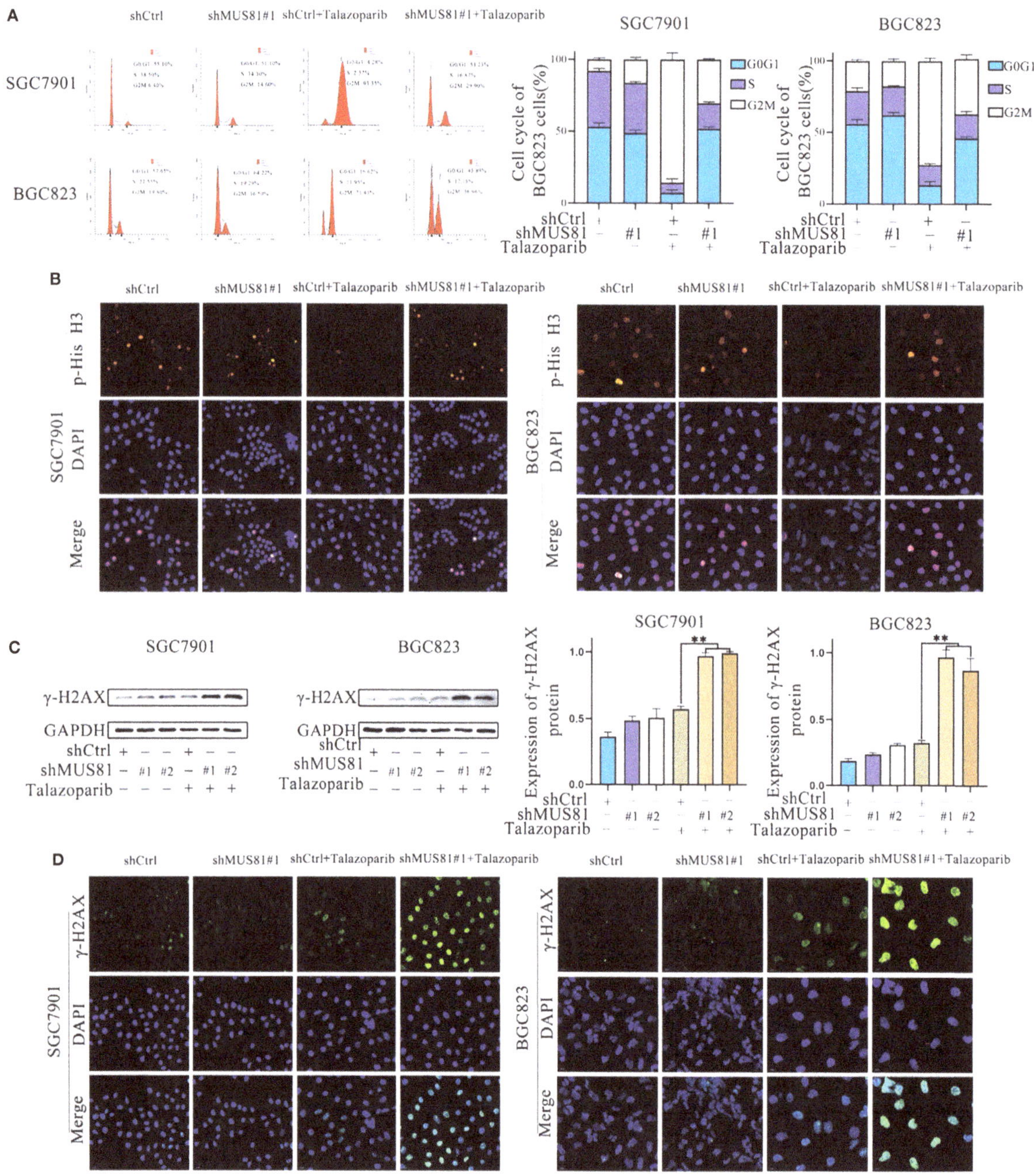

FIGURE 3 | MUS81 inhibition may increase talazoparib-induced DNA damage in gastric cancer cells. **(A)** Cells treated with DMSO or talazoparib (1 μmol/L) for 3 d to evaluate cell cycle distribution by flow cytometry (*t*-test). $^{**}P < 0.01$. **(B)** Immunofluorescence to detect the expression of p-Histone H3 (Ser10) in DMSO or talazoparib-treated (0.5 μmol/L) cells for 2 d. Magnification, 400×. **(C)** Western blot analysis of γ-H2AX expression after treatment with 0.5 μmol/L talazoparib for 24 h (t-test). $^{**}P < 0.01$. **(D)** Immunofluorescence to detect the expression of γ-H2AX in DMSO or talazoparib-treated (0.5 μmol/L) cells for 2 d. Magnification, 400×. $^{**}P < 0.01$.

inhibitors impair SSB repair to cause tumor cells to transform into DNA DSBs in the S phase, which leads to cell death due to mitotic catastrophe or apoptosis in tumors with BRCA1 and BRCA2 mutations as well as an HR deficiency (24). However, in gastric cancer, mutation rates in HRD genes (BRCA1 and BRCA2) are low, and individual PARP inhibitors have limited efficacy (25). Therefore, it is urgent to explore other targets to enhance the antitumor effect of PARP inhibitors and to expand the beneficiary population in gastric cancer. The DNA endonuclease MUS81 is a member of the endonuclear

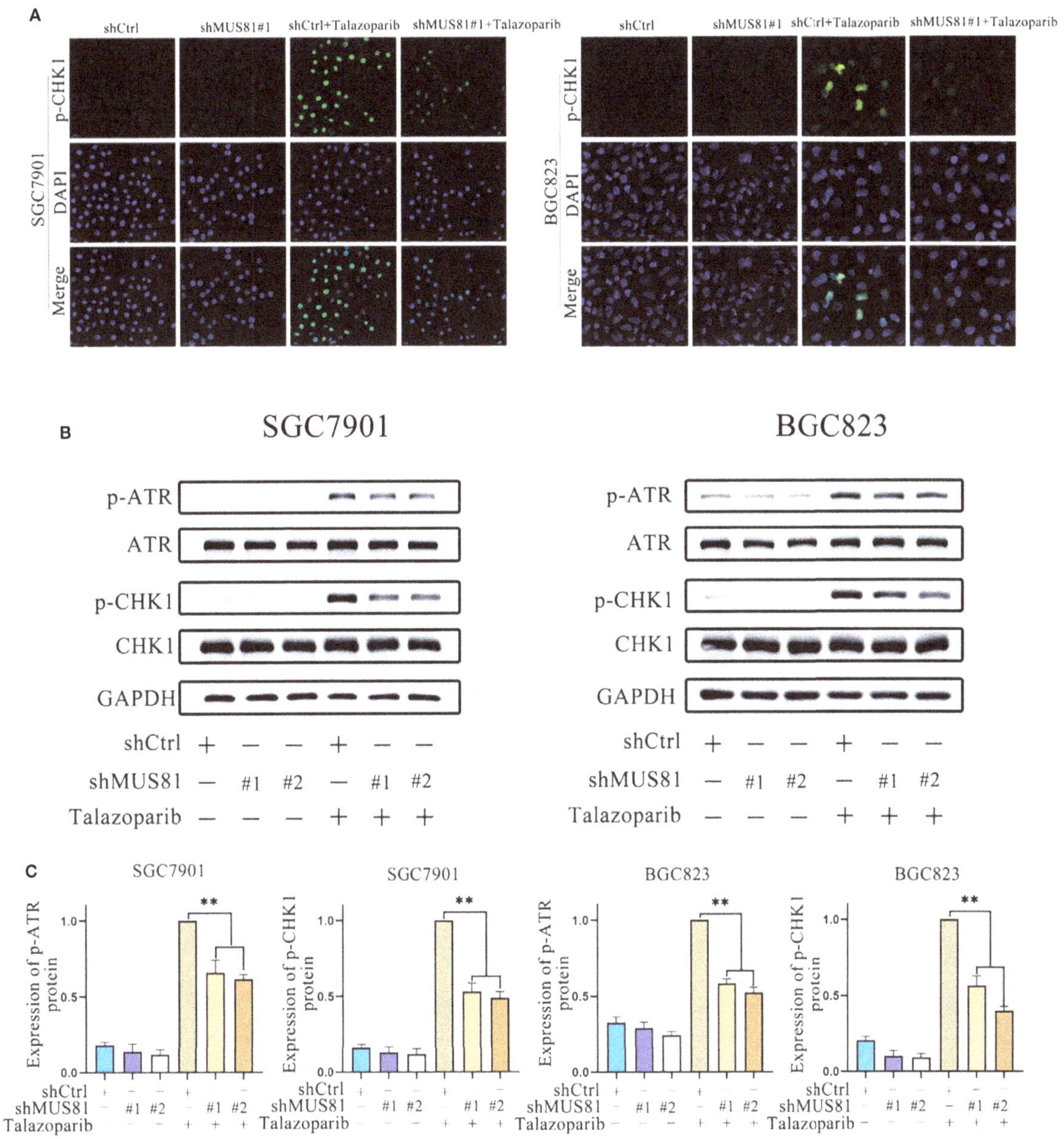

FIGURE 4 | MUS81 deficiency impairs ATR/CHK1 activation induced by talazoparib in gastric cancer. **(A)** Immunofluorescence to detect p-CHK1 expression in talazoparib-treated (0.5 μmol/L) cells for 2 d. Magnification, 400×. **(B, C)** Western blot analysis examining the expression of p-ATR and p-CHK1 after treatment with 0.5 μmol/L talazoparib for 24 h (*t*-test). $^{**}P < 0.01$.

XPF family, which has been implicated in DNA repair *via* HR (7, 26–28). In the present study, MUS81 was involved in DNA damage repair and cell cycle regulation pathways in gastric cancer. MUS81 knockdown enhanced the cytotoxic effects of talazoparib-induced apoptosis in gastric cancer cells.

DNA damage checkpoints mainly include G1-S and G2-M, which regulate whether the cell continues mitosis or performs DNA repair or apoptosis (29, 30). Our research showed that talazoparib causes DNA damage in tumor cells, activates G2-M checkpoints, and leads to G2-M phase arrest. A previous study showed that MUS81 knockdown reverses the G2-M block caused by epirubicin in liver cancer cells (31). The current study also confirmed that MUS81 knockdown reversed G2-M block caused by talazoparib in gastric cancer, which might cause tumor cells to continue mitosis with unrepaired DNA and eventually lead to cell death. This research showed that talazoparib had significant antitumor effects in a MUS81-deficient SGC7901 xenograft model, and there was no significant difference in the body weight among the four groups of nude mice during the treatment.

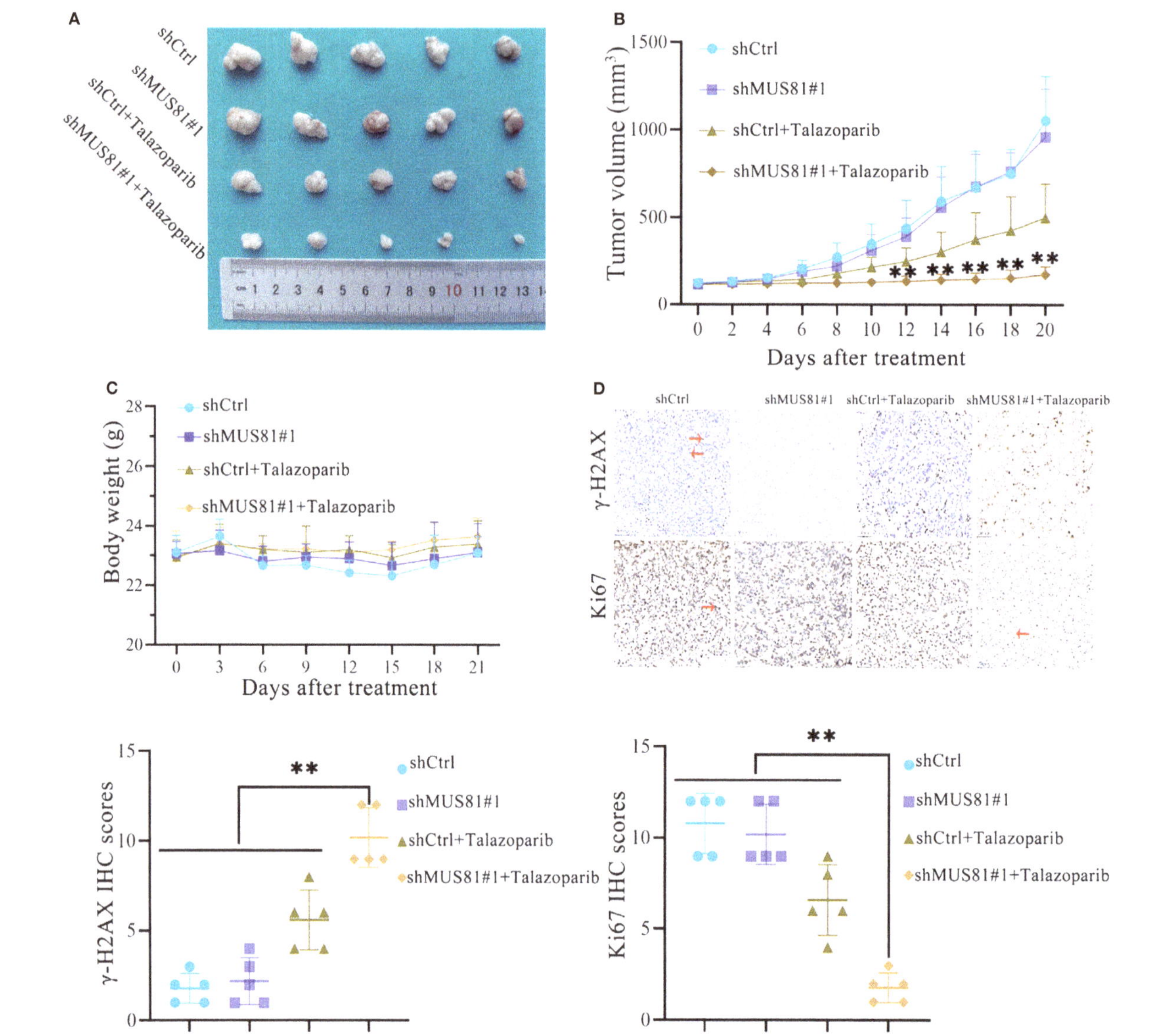

FIGURE 5 | MUS81 knockdown enhances the anticancer efficacy of talazoparib in gastric cancer *in vivo*. **(A, B)** Tumor volume of each group on the indicated days of treatment (*t*-test). $^{**}P < 0.01$. **(C)** Weight of nude mice on indicated days of treatment (*t*-test). **(D)** Representative images of γ-H2AX and Ki-67 immunohistochemistry (*t*-test). Positive expression (→). Negative expression (←). Magnification, 200×. $^{**}P < 0.01$.

In addition, it was observed that MUS81 knockdown reduced the activation of ATR and CHK1 in gastric cancer cells induced by talazoparib. ATR is one of the central regulators that control cellular responses to DNA damage (32, 33). In the G2 phase, activation of the ATR/CHK1 pathway blocks cells from continuing mitosis with damaged DNA (34, 35). Our previous study has shown that the CHK1 inhibitor LY2606368 impairs HR-mediated DNA damage repair, thereby sensitizing the antitumor efficacy of PARP inhibitors (36). Therefore, MUS81 knockdown promoted talazoparib-induced DNA damage by regulating the ATR/CHK1 pathway.

Overall, these findings indicated that sensitivity of gastric cancer to talazoparib relied on MUS81 inactivation. Our previous research has shown that AZD5153, a novel BRD4 inhibitor, downregulates MUS81 expression, and reduces the migration of gastric cancer cells *in vitro* and *in vivo* (10). Therefore, talazoparib combined with AZD5153 was applied to treat gastric cancer. In LV-Ctrl gastric cancer cells, combined MUS81 and AZD5153 treatment achieved the same antitumor effect as MUS81 knockdown combined with talazoparib treatment. Our previous work confirmed that AZD5153 inhibits the expression of sirt5 and impairs the MUS81 transcription function in gastric cancer cells (10); however,

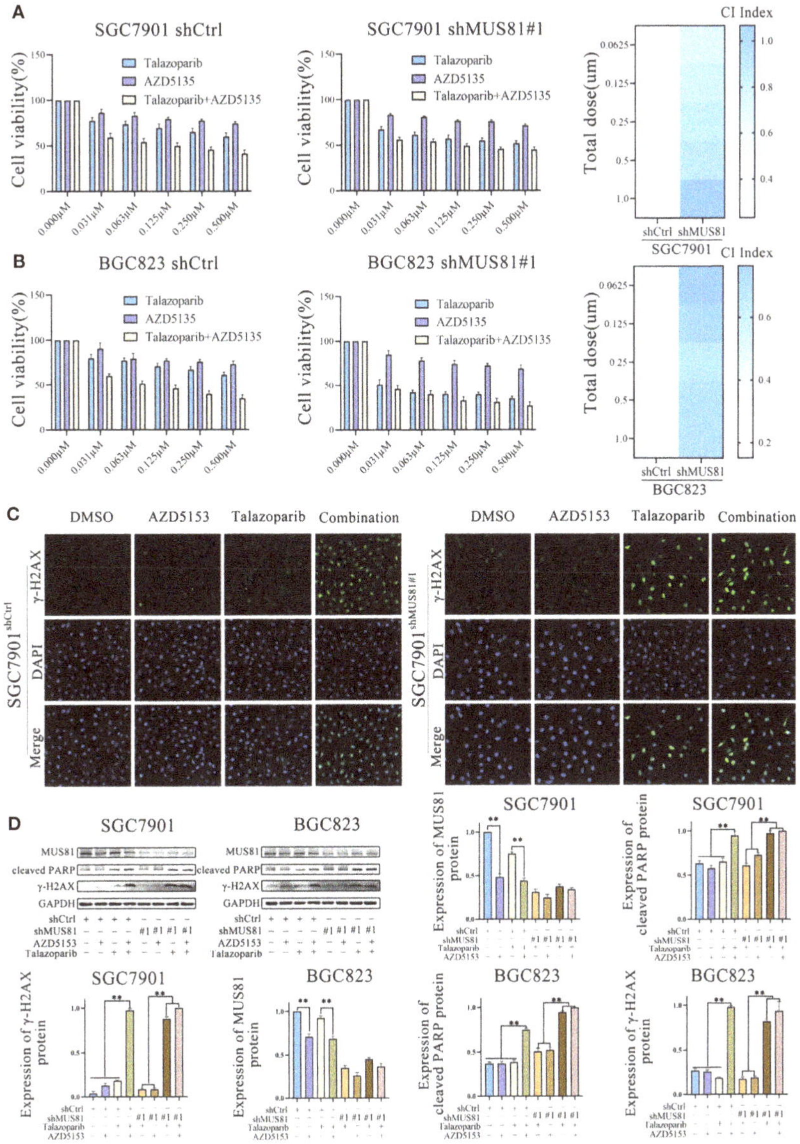

FIGURE 6 | AZD5153 sensitizes the talazoparib anticancer effect in a MUS81-dependent manner in gastric cancer cells. **(A, B)** Viability of cells treated with monotherapy and combination therapy for 5 d, as determined using MTS (*t*-test). At five gradually increasing concentrations (0.0625 μmol/L to 1.000 μmol/L), the mean CI of SGC7901^{shCtrl} cells were 0.26, 0.23, 0.25, 0.26, and 0.36, respectively; the mean CI of SGC7901^{shMU81} cells were 0.69, 0.75, 0.81, 0.87, and 1.07, respectively; the mean CI of BGC823^{shCtrl} cells were 0.23, 0.15, 0.18, 0.21, and 0.29, respectively; the mean CI of BGC823^{shMU81} cells were 0.76, 0.69, 0.62, 0.67, and 0.67, respectively. The difference between shMU81 and shCtrl groups was statistically significant (all $P < 0.01$). **(C)** Immunofluorescence to detect the expression of phosphorylated checkpoint kinase 1 (p-CHK1) in cells treated with DMSO, AZD5153 (1 μmol/L), talazoparib (0.5 μmol/L), or combination therapy for 2 d. Magnification, 400×. **(D)** Western blot analysis examining the expression of MUS81, cleaved PARP, and γ-H2AX in gastric cancer cells after treatment with DMSO, AZD5153 (1 μmol/L), talazoparib (0.5 μmol/L), or combination therapy for 2 d (*t*-test). $^{**}P < 0.01$.

the underlying mechanism by which AZD5153 regulates MUS81 remains to be explored. In future, the combined use of AZD5153 and talazoparib in clinical trials may further verify their efficacy in the treatment of gastric cancer and may improve the prognosis of patients with advanced gastric cancer. However, *in vivo* experiments need to be conducted to examine whether AZD5153 can enhance the lethality of talazoparib to normal cells. Additionally, the combination therapy's therapeutic window remains to be confirmed by further studies.

In conclusion, MUS81 was overexpressed in gastric cancer cells and was closely related to cell cycle regulation and DNA damage repair pathways. Moreover, MUS81 was a key molecule that

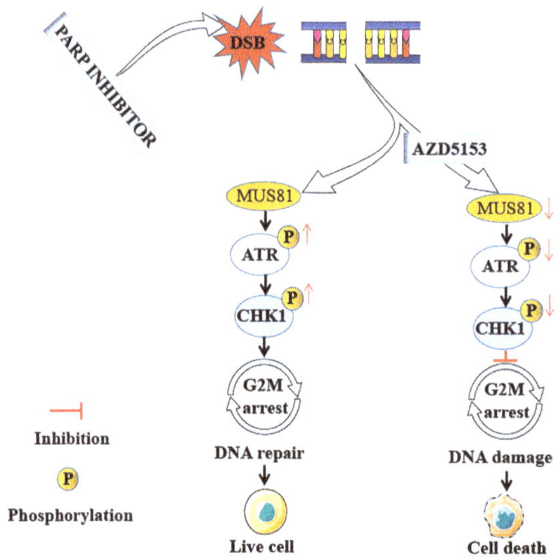

FIGURE 7 | Schema of the antitumor effect of AZD5153 sensitizing gastric cancer cells to talazoparib. AZD5153 inhibits the ATR/CHK1 pathway activated by DNA damage by downregulating MUS81 expression, causing gastric cancer cells to continue mitosis with damaged DNA, ultimately leading to cell death.

enhanced the talazoparib antitumor effect in gastric cancer cells. MUS81 targeting markedly induced DNA damage and promoted cell apoptosis after talazoparib treatment by inhibiting ATR/CHK1 pathway activation. Importantly, AZD5153 enhanced the talazoparib antitumor effect in gastric cancer cells by reducing MUS81 expression. Taken together, talazoparib in combination with AZD5153 may be a promising treatment strategy for MUS81 overexpressed gastric cancer.

AUTHOR CONTRIBUTIONS

TW and PZ conducted the experiments, performed the data analysis and wrote the paper. CL, WL, QS, and LY performed the experiments. GX, JB, and RL analyzed data. YY and KT revised the manuscript and designed the experiment. All authors contributed to the article and approved the submitted version.

REFERENCES

Bray F, Ferlay J, Soerjomataram I, Siegel RL, Torre LA, Jemal A. Global Cancer Statistics 2018: GLOBOCAN Estimates of Incidence and Mortality Worldwide for 36 Cancers in 185 Countries. *CA Cancer J Clin* (2018) 68 (6):394–424. doi: 10.3322/caac.21492

Wagner AD, Syn NL, Moehler M, Grothe W, Yong WP, Tai BC, et al. Chemotherapy for Advanced Gastric Cancer. *Cochrane Database Syst Rev* (2017) 8(8):CD004064. doi: 10.1002/14651858.CD004064.pub4

Padmanabhan N, Ushijima T, Tan P. How to Stomach an Epigenetic Insult: The Gastric Cancer Epigenome. *Nat Rev Gastroenterol Hepatol* (2017) 14 (8):467–78. doi: 10.1038/nrgastro.2017.53

Negrini S, Gorgoulis VG, Halazonetis TD. Genomic Instability–An Evolving Hallmark of Cancer. *Nat Rev Mol Cell Biol* (2010) 11(3):220–8. doi: 10.1038/nrm2858

Pearl LH, Schierz AC, Ward SE, Al-Lazikani B, Pearl FM. Therapeutic Opportunities Within the DNA Damage Response. *Nat Rev Cancer* (2015) 15(3):166–80. doi: 10.1038/nrc3891

Ho CK, Mazo⊠n G, Lam AF, Symington LS. Mus81 and Yen1 Promote Reciprocal Exchange During Mitotic Recombination to Maintain Genome Integrity in Budding Yeast. *Mol Cell* (2010) 40(6):988–1000. doi: 10.1016/j.molcel.2010.11.016

Di Marco S, Hasanova Z, Kanagaraj R, Chappidi N, Altmannova V, Menon S, et al. RECQ5 Helicase Cooperates With MUS81 Endonuclease in Processing Stalled Replication Forks at Common Fragile Sites During Mitosis. *Mol Cell* (2017) 66(5):658–71. doi: 10.1016/j.molcel.2017.05.006

Lu R, Xie S, Wang Y, Zheng H, Zhang H, Deng M, et al. MUS81 Participates in the Progression of Serous Ovarian Cancer Associated With Dysfunctional DNA Repair System. *Front Oncol* (2019) 9:1189. doi: 10.3389/ fonc.2019.01189

Zhong A, Zhang H, Xie S, Deng M, Zheng H, Wang Y, et al. Inhibition of MUS81 Improves the Chemical Sensitivity of Olaparib by Regulating MCM2 in Epithelial Ovarian Cancer. *Oncol Rep* (2018) 39(4):1747–56. doi: 10.3892/ or.2018.6229

Yin Y, Liu W, Shen Q, Zhang P, Wang L, Tao R, et al. The DNA Endonuclease Mus81 Regulates ZEB1 Expression and Serves as a Target of BET4 Inhibitors in Gastric Cancer. *Mol Cancer Ther* (2019) 18(8):1439–50. doi: 10.1158/1535- 7163.MCT-18-0833

Huang Y, Zhang J, Hou L, Wang G, Liu H, Zhang R, et al. LncRNA AK023391 Promotes Tumorigenesis and Invasion of Gastric Cancer Through Activation of the PI3K/Akt Signaling Pathway. *J Exp Clin Cancer Res* (2019) 36(1):194. doi: 10.1186/s13046-017-0666-2

Nam HJ, Kim HP, Yoon YK, Song SH, Min AR, Han SW, et al. The Irreversible Pan-HER Inhibitor PF00299804 Alone or Combined With Gemcitabine Has an Antitumor Effect in Biliary Tract Cancer Cell Lines. *Invest New Drugs* (2012) 30(6):2148–60. doi: 10.1007/s10637-011-9782-6

Zhang J, Wang G, Chu SJ, Zhu JS, Zhang R, Lu WW, et al. Loss of Large Tumor Suppressor 1 Promotes Growth and Metastasis of Gastric Cancer Cells Through Upregulation of the YAP Signaling. *Oncotarget* (2016) 7(13):16180– 93. doi: 10.18632/oncotarget.7568

Chen X, Li L, Liu F, Hoh J, Kapron CM, Liu J. Cadmium Induces Glomerular Endothelial Cell-Specific Expression of Complement Factor H *via* the -1635 AP-1 Binding Site. *J Immunol* (2019) 202(4):1210–8. doi: 10.4049/ jimmunol.1800081

Fang Z, Cao B, Liao JM, Deng J, Plummer KD, Liao P, et al. SPIN1 Promotes Tumorigenesis by Blocking the Ul18 (Universal Large Ribosomal Subunit Protein 18)-MDM2-P53 Pathway in Human Cancer. *Elife* (2018) 7:e31275. doi: 10.7554/eLife.31275

Jia X, Guo T, Li Z, Zhang M, Feng Y, Dong B, et al. Clinicopathological and Immunomicroenvironment Characteristics of Epstein-Barr Virus-Associated Gastric Cancer in a Chinese Population. *Front Oncol* (2021) 10:586752. doi: 10.3389/fonc.2020.586752

Ghamrasni SE, Cardoso R, Li L, Guturi KK, Bjerregaard VA, Liu Y, et al. Rad54 and Mus81 Cooperation Promotes DNA Damage Repair and Restrains Chromosome Missegregation. *Oncogene* (2016) 35(37):4836–45. doi: 10.1038/onc.2016.16

Jazayeri A, Falck J, Lukas C, Bartek J, Smith GC, Lukas J, et al. ATM- and Cell Cycle-Dependent Regulation of ATR in Response to DNA Double-Strand Breaks. *Nat Cell Biol* (2006) 8(1):37–45. doi: 10.1038/ncb1337

Kozlov SV, Graham ME, Peng C, Chen P, Robinson PJ, Lavin MF. Involvement of Novel Autophosphorylation Sites in ATM Activation. *EMBO J* (2006) 25(15):3504–14. doi: 10.1038/sj.emboj.7601231

Nam EA, Zhao R, Glick GG, Bansbach CE, Friedman DB, Cortez D. Thr-1989 Phosphorylation Is a Marker of Active Ataxia Telangiectasia-Mutated and Rad3-Related (ATR) Kinase. *J Biol Chem* (2011) 286(33):28707–14. doi: 10.1074/ jbc. M111.248914

Liu S, Shiotani B, Lahiri M, Maréchal A, Tse A, Leung CC, et al. ATR Autophosphorylation as a Molecular Switch for Checkpoint Activation. *Mol Cell* (2011) 43(2):192–202. doi: 10.1016/j.molcel.2011.06.019

Powell SN, Bindra RS. Targeting the DNA Damage Response for Cancer Therapy. *DNA Repair (Amst)* (2009) 8(9):1153–65. doi: 10.1016/j.dnarep.2009.04.011

Pascal JM, Ellenberger T. The Rise and Fall of Poly(ADP-Ribose): An Enzymatic Perspective. *DNA Repair (Amst)* (2015) 32:10–6. doi: 10.1016/ j.dnarep.2015.04.008

Hoevenaar WHM, Janssen A, Quirindongo AI, Ma H, Klaasen SJ, Teixeira A, et al. Degree and Site of Chromosomal Instability Define Its Oncogenicpotential. *Nat Commun* (2020) 11(1):1501. doi: 10.1038/s41467-020-15279-9

Alexandrov LB, Nik-Zainal S, Siu HC, Leung SY, Stratton MR. A Mutational Signature in Gastric Cancer Suggests Therapeutic Strategies. *Nat Commun* (2015) 6:8683. doi: 10.1038/ncomms9683 McCabe N, Turner NC, Lord CJ, Kluzek K, Bialkowska A, Swift S, et al. Defificiency in the Repair of DNA Damage by Homologous Recombination and Sensitivity to Poly(ADP-Ribose) Polymerase Inhibition. *Cancer Res* (2006) 66(16):8109–15. doi: 10.1158/0008-5472.CAN-06-0140

Kikuchi K, Narita T, Pham VT, Iijima J, Hirota K, Keka IS, et al. Structure- Specific Endonucleases Xpf and Mus81 Play Overlapping But Essential Roles in DNA Repair by Homologous Recombination. *Cancer Res* (2013) 73 (14):4362–71. doi: 10.1158/0008-5472.CAN-12-3154

Lai X, Broderick R, Bergoglio V, Zimmer J, Badie S, Niedzwiedz W, et al. MUS81 Nuclease Activity Is Essential for Replication Stress Tolerance and Chromosome Segregation in BRCA2-Deficient Cells. *Nat Commun* (2017) 8:15983. doi: 10.1038/ncomms15983

Abroudi A, Samarasinghe S, Kulasiri D. A Comprehensive Complex Systems Approach to the Study and Analysis of Mammalian Cell Cycle Control System in the Presence of DNA Damage Stress. *J Theor Biol* (2017) 429:204–28. doi: 10.1016/j.jtbi.2017.06.018

Sancar A, Lindsey-Boltz LA, Unsal-Kaçmaz K, Linn S. Molecular Mechanisms of Mammalian DNA Repair and the DNA Damage Checkpoints. *Annu Rev Biochem* (2004) 73:39–85. doi: 10.1146/annurev.biochem.73.011303.073723

Wu F, Chen WJ, Yan L, Tan GQ, Li WT, Zhu XJ, et al. Mus81 Knockdown Improves Chemosensitivity of Hepatocellular Carcinoma Cells by Inducing S- Phase Arrest and Promoting Apoptosis Through CHK1 Pathway. *Cancer Med* (2016) 5(2):370–85. doi: 10.1002/cam4.588

Ciccia A, Elledge SJ. The DNA Damage Response: Making It Safe to Play With Knives. *Mol Cell* (2010) 40(2):179–204. doi: 10.1016/j.molcel.2010.09.019

Jackson SP, Bartek J. The DNA-Damage Response in Human Biology and Disease. *Nature* (2009) 461(7267):1071–8. doi: 10.1038/nature08467

Cortez D, Guntuku S, Qin J, Elledge SJ. ATR and ATRIP: Partners in Checkpoint Signaling. *Science* (2001) 294(5547):1713–6. doi: 10.1126/ science.1065521

Brown EJ. The ATR-Independent DNA Replication Checkpoint. *Cell Cycle* (2003) 2(3):188–9. doi: 10.4161/cc.2.3.395

Yin Y, Shen Q, Zhang P, Tao R, Chang W, Li R, et al. Chk1 Inhibition Potentiates the Therapeutic Efficacy of PARP Inhibitor BMN673 in Gastric Cancer. *Am J Cancer Res* (2017) 7(3):473–83.

3

Toxicological Properties of 7-Methylguanine and Preliminary Data on its Anticancer Activity

*Kirill Kirsanov[1,2], Timur Fetisov[1], Elena Antoshina[1], Lubov Trukhanova[1], Tatiana Gor'kova[1], Olga Vlasova[1], Irina Khitrovo[1], Ekaterina Lesovaya[1,3], Nataliya Kulbachevskaya[1], Tatiana Shcherbakova[4], Gennady Belitsky[1], Marianna Yakubovskaya[1], Vytas Švedas[4,5] and Dmitry Nilov[4]**

[1]Blokhin Cancer Research Center, Moscow, Russia, [2]Peoples' Friendship University of Russia, Moscow, Russia, [3]Pavlov Ryazan State Medical University, Ryazan, Russia, [4]Belozersky Institute of Physicochemical Biology, Lomonosov Moscow State University, Moscow, Russia, [5]Faculty of Bioengineering and Bioinformatics, Lomonosov Moscow State University, Moscow, Russia

***Correspondence:**
Dmitry Nilov
nilovdm@gmail.com

7-Methylguanine (7-MG) competitively inhibits the DNA repair enzyme poly(ADP-ribose) polymerase (PARP) and RNA-modifying enzyme tRNA-guanine transglycosylase (TGT) and represents a potential anticancer drug candidate. Furthermore, as a natural compound, it could escape the serious side effects characteristic for approved synthetic PARP inhibitors. Here we present a comprehensive study of toxicological and carcinogenic properties of 7-MG. It was demonstrated that 7-MG does not induce mutations or structural chromosomal abnormalities, and has no blastomogenic activity. A treatment regimen with 7-MG has been established in mice (50 mg/kg per os, 3 times per week), exerting no adverse effects or changes in morphology. Preliminary data on the 7-MG anticancer activity obtained on transplantable tumor models support our conclusions that 7-MG can become a promising new component of chemotherapy.

Keywords: 7-Methylguanine, inhibitor, cancer, carcinogenicity, toxicity

INTRODUCTION

7-Methylguanine (7-MG) (Shapiro et al., 1968) is a degradation product of nucleic acids which is present in small amounts in human urine (Bromberg et al., 1957a; Bromberg et al., 1957b; Lothrop and Uziel, 1983; Svoboda and Kasai, 2004; Rodríguez-Gonzalo et al., 2013; Raćkowska et al., 2019) and may be considered an indicator of whole-body RNA turnover (Sander et al., 1986a; Sander et al., 1986b; Sander et al., 1986c; Topp et al., 1987). In mRNA the guanosine cap is methylated due to methyltransferase activity, that is required for maturation and translation (Shuman, 2002; Shafer et al., 2005; Topisirovic et al., 2011; Varshney et al., 2016). Furthermore, 7-MG adducts are normally present in DNA, exposed to various exogenous and endogenous methylating agents, and their number is increasing on aging (Park and Ames, 1988; Tan et al., 1990; Mustonen and Hemminki, 1992; O'Connor, 1993; Tamae et al., 2009). There is no evidence, however, for synthesis of nucleotides from free 7-MG base or for its direct incorporation into nucleic acids (Craddock et al., 1968; Kaina et al., 1983; Kerr, 1985; Kerr, 1990). A certain proportion of 7-MG is converted to

Abbreviations: 7-MG, 7-methylguanine; PARP, poly(ADP-ribose) polymerase; TGT, tRNA-guanine transglycosylase.

8-hydroxy-7-methylguanine by xanthine oxidase or demethylated (Weissmann and Gutman, 1957; Borowitz et al., 1965; Litwack and Weissmann, 1966; Skupp and Ayvazian, 1969).

Recently we have shown that 7-MG inhibits DNA repair enzymes poly(ADP-ribose) polymerases, PARP1 and PARP2, in a competitive manner and accelerates apoptotic death of cancer cells induced by cisplatin and doxorubicin (Nilov et al., 2016; Nilov et al., 2018a; Nilov et al., 2020a). These PARP enzymes bind to DNA breaks and synthesize a signal polymer poly (ADP-ribose) from NAD^+ molecules to activate the excision repair proteins (Hassler and Ladurner, 2012; Drenichev and Mikhailov, 2015; Ray Chaudhuri and Nussenzweig, 2017; Alemasova and Lavrik, 2019; Nilov et al., 2020b). Inhibitors of PARP1/2, therefore, can exert anti-proliferative effect and be combined with DNA damaging agents (Cepeda et al., 2006; Martin et al., 2008; Ferraris, 2010; Lord et al., 2015; Nilov et al., 2018b). We have demonstrated that 7-MG forms substrate-specific interactions with the Gly863 and Tyr907 residues in the PARP1/2 active site and suppresses DNA-dependent PARP activity in three different assays (biochemical assay with radiolabeled NAD^+, fluorescence anisotropy assay, and Förster resonance energy transfer microscopy assay with nucleosome particles) (Nilov et al., 2016; Nilov et al., 2020a). This results in the formation of nonproductive PARP–nucleosome complexes and likely prevents further steps in DNA repair, replication and transcription, leading to cancer cell death (Maluchenko et al., 2019; Nilov et al., 2020a). 7-MG is also known as a competitive inhibitor of RNA-modifying enzyme tRNA-guanine transglycosylase (TGT) which substitutes the guanine base with 7-deazaguanine derivative queuine (Farkas et al., 1984; Johannsson et al., 2018). In a recent paper, it was shown that TGT deficiency could significantly suppress the proliferation and migration of cancer cells (Zhang et al., 2020). From the point of view of polypharmacology, such a multitarget (PARP1/2, TGT) mechanism of a drug candidate may be promising, if adverse effects are negligible (Bolognesi, 2013; Medina-Franco et al., 2013).

FDA-approved synthetic PARP1/2 inhibitors olaparib, rucaparib, niraparib (Frampton, 2015; Mittica et al., 2018; Zimmer et al., 2018) can cause side effects likely related to the nonselective interaction with numerous NAD^+-binding proteins and nonspecific effects on the organism. Myelodysplastic syndrome/acute myeloid leukemia occurred in some patients after treatment with above-mentioned synthetic inhibitors, and some cases were fatal (Malyuchenko et al., 2015; Sonnenblick et al., 2015; Wang et al., 2016; Ohmoto and Yachida, 2017; Jain and Patel, 2019). 7-MG, being a natural compound, may have a more favorable toxicity profile, which is also supported by QSAR modeling (Nilov et al., 2016; Nilov et al., 2018a). In this article, we present the results of a comprehensive experimental study of toxicological and carcinogenic properties of 7-MG that establish the basis for further testing of its anticancer activity.

MATERIALS AND METHODS

Toxicology Studies

Six-week-old female CBA, BALB/c, and C57BL/6 mice were obtained from the Stolbovaya farm of the Federal Medical Biological Agency (http://www.scbmt.ru). These mouse strains are widely used in toxicology studies and in studies involving transplantable tumor models. 7-MG (Sigma-Aldrich, product No. 67073) was administered orally by gavage in experiments A and B (**Figure 1**). In experiment A, CBA mice were divided randomly to four treatment groups of 10 animals: control group I, drinking water (3 times per week for 4 weeks); group II, 50 mg/kg 7-MG (3 times per week for 4 weeks); group III, 200 mg/kg 7-MG (3 times per week for 1 week); group IV, 600 mg/kg 7-MG (single dose). Animals were euthanized by cervical dislocation 1 week after the last treatment. In experiment B, mice of each strain (CBA, BALB/c, C57BL/6) were divided into two groups, group I (drinking water) and group II (600 mg/kg 7-MG), and euthanized 4 weeks after single-dose administration. Lungs, heart, liver, spleen, thymus, kidneys, adrenal glands, pancreas, stomach, small and large intestines were collected from euthanized mice and inspected. The tissues were processed for light microscopy by fixing in 10% buffered formalin, dehydrating, and embedding in paraffin. Histological analysis was performed on sections stained by hematoxylin-eosin. Organ lesions were detected on the examined sections (representative microphotographs of the found abnormalities are shown in **Supplementary Figure S1**), and the number of lesions per animal was counted.

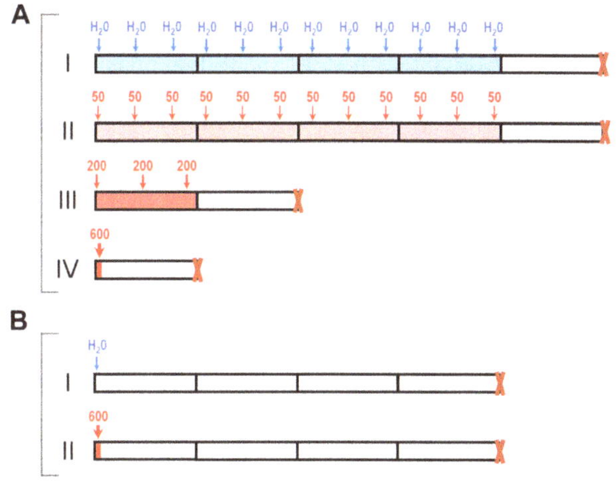

FIGURE 1 | Toxicology study of 7-MG: schematic representation of experiments. **(A)** CBA mice were treated either with water (group I) or with single and multiple doses of 7-MG (groups II–IV, total dose for each group was 600 mg/kg); **(B)** CBA, BALB/c, or C57BL/6 mice were treated with water (groups I) or a single 600 mg/kg dose of 7-MG (group II), and euthanized 4 weeks later.

Carcinogenicity Studies

The Ames test was performed in *S. typhimurium* strains TA98 and TA100 as described previously (Maron and Ames, 1983). Three 7-MG doses (1.4, 7.0, and 35.0 µg/plate) were tested with and without rat liver S9 fraction. Distilled water was used as a negative control; 3,4-benzopyrene (4.4 µg/plate), 2-acetylaminofluorene (22.0 µg/plate), 4,9-diazapyrene derivative (8.8 µg/plate), and sodium azide (8.8 µg/plate) served as positive controls. Plates were incubated for 72 h and then revertant colonies were counted. The comet assay was performed as described previously (Singh et al., 1988). Immortalized human kidney epithelial cells (NKE-hTERT) were treated with different concentrations of 7-MG (0.02 and 0.2 mg/ml) for 24 h and then embedded in agarose on microscope slides. After cell lysis and electrophoresis, slides were stained with DNA dye (Vista Green) and the number of comets was counted. Distilled water was used as a negative control and cisplatin (25 μg/ml) served as a positive control. The somatic mutation and recombination test in *D. melanogaster* was based on previous work (Kirsanov et al., 2011). Five wild type males and 10 $wts^{P4}/TM3$ females were placed into vials for breeding. Heterozygous larvae were treated with 7-MG (1 and 2 mg/vial); distilled water and oxoplatin (0.2 mg/vial) were used as controls. Adult F1 males and females were examined for the presence of tumors using a binocular microscope.

The chromosomal aberration assay was performed using standard procedure (Albertini et al., 2000). C57BL/6 mice were divided to groups of 5 animals and treated with 7-MG (50–250 mg/kg per os). Distilled water was used as a negative control and cyclophosphamide (50 mg/kg i.p.) served as a positive control. Bone marrow cells were collected 24 h after the treatment; to arrest proliferating cells at metaphase, animals received colchicine (0.004% i.p.) 3 h prior to euthanasia. Cells were obtained from the femurs, stained on slides with Giemsa, and analyzed by microscopy.

Anticancer Activity

Six-week-old female CBA mice were obtained from the Stolbovaya farm. Uterine sarcoma US-322 and cervical squamous cell carcinoma RShM-5 (originally derived from CBA mice exposed to 1,2-dimethylhydrazine and 3-methylcholanthrene, respectively) (Treshalina et al., 2000; Turusov et al., 2005; Bunyatyan et al., 2019) were inoculated subcutaneously by injecting 0.5 ml of tumor cell suspension (0.1 g/ml in PBS) into the right axillary cavity. Mice with US-322 were divided into three treatment groups of 10 animals: control group I, PBS (s.c., 3 times per week); group II, 7-MG (50 mg/kg per os, 3 times per week); group III, cisplatin (2.5 mg/kg s.c., 2 times within a week after inoculation). Mice with RShM-5 were divided into five groups of 10 animals: group I, PBS (s.c., 3 times per week); group II, 7-MG (50 mg/kg per os, 3 times per week); group III, 7-MG for 1 week (50 mg/kg per os, 3 times within a week after inoculation); group IV, cisplatin (1.5 mg/kg s.c., 3 times within a week after inoculation); group V, cisplatin + 7-MG (1.5 mg/kg s.c. + 50 mg/kg per os, 3 times within a week after inoculation). For the combined treatment, 7-MG was administered 3 h prior to cisplatin. The length and width of a subcutaneous tumor were measured with a digital çaliper, and the tumor volume was calculated as 1/2 (length×width^2).

The animal protocols were approved by the Local Committee for Ethics of Animal Experimentation (Blokhin Cancer Research Center, decision 2019-5 dated 11 February 2019), experiments were conducted in accordance with resolution 81 of the Eurasian Economic Commission and directive 2010/63/EU (on the protection of animals used for scientific purposes).

TABLE 1 | Histological abnormalities of internal organs (+) in CBA mice treated with 7-MG.

Group	Lungs	Liver	Spleen	Intestine
I control	–	–	–	–
II 50 mg/kg[a]	–	–	–	–
III 200 mg/kg[a]	–	–	–	+
IV 600 mg/kg	+	+	+	+

[a]*Multiple-dose administration.*

Statistical Analysis

Statistical significance of the difference between animal groups was assessed with the Pearson's chi-squared test (study of anticancer activity, study of chromosomal abnormalities in mice), Student's *t*-test (analysis of organ weights), and Fisher's exact test (study of blastomogenic activity in flies). Significant differences between cells in the comet assay were assessed with the Fisher's exact test. Data processing was carried out using the Statistica software (StatSoft Inc.).

RESULTS

Toxicology Studies

The adverse effects of 7-MG that can result either from a single or multiple exposures were assessed using four groups of female CBA mice, as presented in **Figure 1A**. A maximum dose of 600 mg/kg was chosen based on mouse/rat oral LD_{50} values (40–500 mg/kg) predicted for 7-MG with QSAR software ACD/Percepta (www.acdlabs.com). Oral administration of 7-MG to group II (50 mg/kg, 3 times per week for 4 weeks), group III (200 mg/kg, 3 times per week for 1 week), and group IV (600 mg/kg, single dose) was not lethal to any of the animals. Visual observation revealed no apparent lesions or abnormalities of internal organs in treated mice. However, a significant elevation in spleen weight was produced in group IV (**Supplementary Table S1**). Histological analysis of the heart, thymus, kidney, adrenal gland, pancreas and stomach showed no abnormalities in all treatment groups. Lung, liver, and spleen tissues were affected only in group IV (**Table 1**). In this group, small lymphoid infiltrates developed in the lungs and liver (**Supplementary Figures S1A,B**). The splenic white pulp had poorly defined follicles and lacked germinal centers, and the red pulp was infiltrated with lymphoid cells (**Supplementary Figure S1C**). In addition, focal lymphoid hyperplasia of the small and large intestines was found in groups III and IV (**Supplementary Figure S1D**).

The stimulating effect on lymphoid tissue caused by a single 600 mg/kg dose of 7-MG was then investigated in more detail using different mouse strains: CBA, BALB/c and C57BL/6. Animals were administered with either water or 7-MG (600 mg/kg), and samples of lung, liver, spleen, and intestine were collected after 4 weeks (**Figure 1B**). Microscopic examination revealed the persistence of lymphoid lesions produced by a high dose of 7-MG in all strains. Lung, liver and intestine abnormalities were found in

TABLE 2 | Study of the mutagenicity of 7-MG in *S. typhimurium* strains TA98 (detects frameshift mutagens) and TA100 (detects mutagens that cause base-pair substitutions).

Tested compound	Dose, μg/plate	TA98				TA100			
		−S9		+S9		−S9		+S9	
		M	MA	M	MA	M	MA	M	MA
Control	—	9 ± 1	—	16 ± 5	—	43 ± 9	—	53 ± 2	—
BP	4.4			139 ± 15	+			623 ± 23	+
AAF	22.0			448 ± 53	+			433 ± 33	+
DP	8.8	248 ± 42	+						
AZ	8.8					397 ± 31	+		
7-MG	1.4	11 ± 3	—	16 ± 0.4	—	45 ± 1	—	56 ± 3	—
	7.0	10 ± 1	—	14 ± 3	—	35 ± 8	—	44 ± 8	—
	35.0	11 ± 1	—	14 ± 2	—	41 ± 3	—	56 ± 2	—

7-MG, 3,4-benzopyrene (BP), 2-acetylaminofluorene (AAF), 4,9-diazapyrene derivative (DP), and sodium azide (AZ) were tested with and without rat liver S9 fraction. The number of revertant colonies (M) was counted to assess the mutagenic activity (MA). MA was considered positive if M in the treated plates exceeded that in the control more than twice.

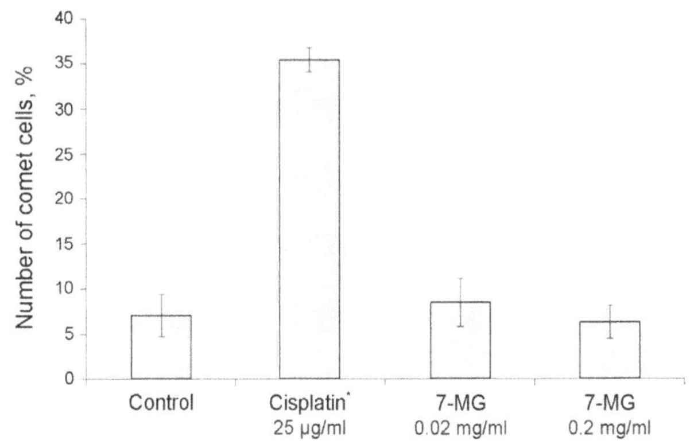

FIGURE 2 | Study of the ability of 7-MG to produce DNA strand breaks in immortalized human kidney epithelial cells using the comet assay (500 cells were analyzed per slide). *Significant difference from the control cells (Fisher's exact test, $p < 0.05$).

nearly all animals (**Supplementary Table S2**), and the splenic microarchitecture was affected in 33% of CBA mice, 30% of BALB/c, and 60% of C57BL/6. However, 7-MG treatment was not lethal to any of the animals and had no significant effect on body weight (**Supplementary Figure S2**). The median lethal dose (LD_{50}) is therefore expected to be substantially greater than 600 mg/kg, which allows us to classify 7-MG as only slightly toxic inhibitor.

These results lead to a conclusion that 50 mg/kg administration 3 times per week may be an optimal regimen, which is devoid of adverse effects and can be readily applied in further testing for anticancer activity of 7-MG in mice (see the **Section 3.3**).

Carcinogenicity Studies

The mutagenic and carcinogenic properties of 7-MG have been studied using various short term tests: the Ames test (uses bacterial strains to assess the mutagenic potential) (Maron and Ames, 1983), comet assay (detects DNA strand breaks at the level of the individual cell) (Collins, 2004), chromosomal aberration assay (detects structural chromosomal abnormalities in mice) (Albertini et al., 2000), and somatic mutation and recombination test (uses *Drosophila melanogaster* to assess the mutagenic, recombinogenic and blastomogenic potential) (Sidorov et al., 2001). The mutagenicity of 7-MG was tested in *Salmonella typhimurium* strains, TA98 and TA100, both with and without metabolic activation by rat liver S9 fraction. It was demonstrated that 7-MG does not induce frameshift mutations or base-pair substitutions (**Table 2**). The comet assay showed that 7-MG does not produce DNA damage in immortalized human kidney epithelial cells (**Figure 2; Supplementary Figure S3**), and the chromosomal aberration assay showed that it does not induce chromatid or chromosome breaks in bone marrow cells of C57BL/6 mice (**Table 3; Supplementary Figure S4**). The somatic mutation and recombination test detected no blastomogenic activity of 7-MG in *wts*/+ heterozygotes of *D. melanogaster* (**Table 4**).

Anticancer Activity

In previous sections, the following findings were made: 1) 7-MG is not carcinogenic and 2) it can be safely administered in an appropriate dosage. As molecular mechanisms of 7-MG are known (PARP1/2 and TGT inhibition), a thorough investigation of its anticancer properties could be initiated *in vivo*, involving various transplantable tumor models and a set of existing drugs as active controls. Below are two illustrative examples demonstrating the utility of 7-MG as a component of chemotherapy.

Preliminary studies of 7-MG anticancer activity at a safe dose were carried out using mouse transplantable tumor models of uterine sarcoma US-322 (**Figure 3, Supplementary Table S3**) and cervical cancer RShM-5 (**Figure 4, Supplementary Table S4**). Tumor nodes appeared in all control group animals within 3 and 7 days after inoculation, respectively. The US-322 model demonstrated a statistically significant inhibition of tumor growth by the treatment with 7-MG, 50 mg/kg 3 times per week (**Figure 3**, group II), and the effect of 7-MG was comparable to cisplatin (group III). In the case of RShM-5 model, an ineffective dose of cisplatin was used to test the ability of 7-MG to sensitize the tumor to DNA-damaging agents. It was revealed that the combined treatment with cisplatin and 7-MG within a week after inoculation inhibits tumor growth, whilst 7-MG or cisplatin administration alone

TABLE 3 | Study of the ability of 7-MG to induce chromosomal aberrations in C57BL/6 mice.

Group		Dose, mg/kg	Number of damaged cells per 500 cells			
			Chromatid breaks	Chromosome breaks	Multiple aberrations	Total number
1 day	I control, males	–	8	0	0	8
	II cyclophosphamide, males	50	30	1	11	42[a]
	III 7-MG, males	50	7	0	0	7
	IV 7-MG, males	250	7	0	0	7
5 days	V control, males	–	9	0	0	9
	VI control, females	–	10	0	0	10
	VII 7-MG, males	5 × 50[b]	7	0	0	7
	VIII 7-MG, females	5 × 50	9	0	0	9

Bone marrow cells were collected 24 h after the last treatment.
[a]Significant difference from the control group (Pearson's chi-squared test, $p < 0.01$).
[b]50 mg/kg per day.

TABLE 4 | Study of the blastomogenic activity of 7-MG in *D. melanogaster*.

Tested compound	Dose, mg/vial	Number of flies	Number of tumors	Tumor frequency, %
Control	–	452	14	3.1
Oxoplatin	0.2	564	128	22.7[a]
7-MG	1.0	488	14	2.9
	2.0	405	9	2.2

[a]Significant difference from the control (Fisher's exact test, $p < 0.01$).

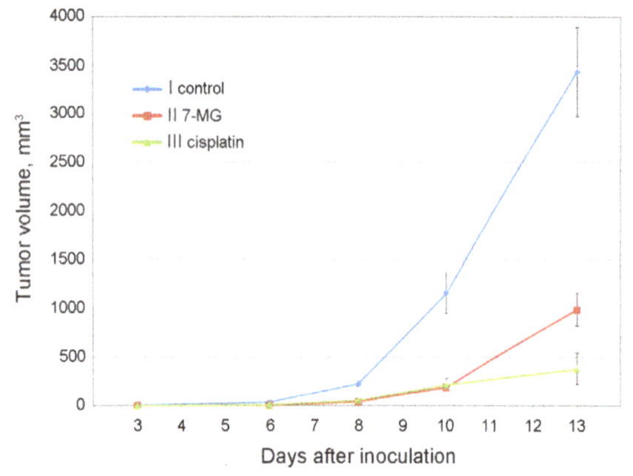

FIGURE 3 | Dynamics of US-322 tumor growth in female CBA mice at different treatment regimens.

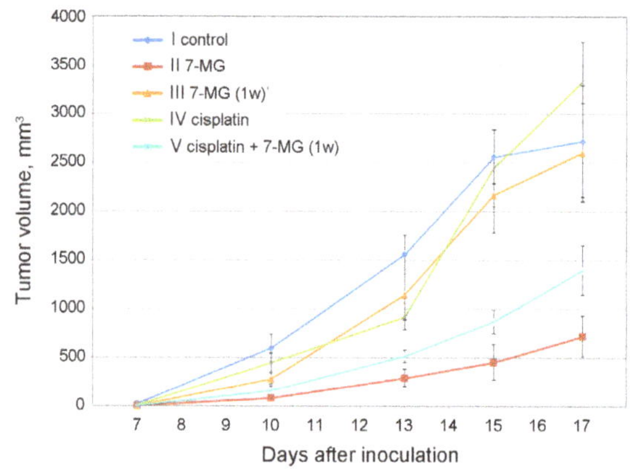

FIGURE 4 | Dynamics of RShM-5 tumor growth in female CBA mice at different treatment regimens. *7-MG was given for 1 week only.

exerted no significant effect (**Figure 4**, groups III–V). It is noteworthy that single-agent 7-MG treatment extended to more than 1 week (group II) had an even more pronounced antitumor effect compared to 1 week of combined treatment. Furthermore, group III (7-MG given for 1 week) clearly demonstrates that interruption of the 7-MG treatment results in accelerated tumor growth starting from the 10th day.

DISCUSSION

PARP1/2 inhibitors represent a novel class of anticancer agents. Although initially proposed for treatment of BRCA-deficient tumors in women (breast or ovarian cancer), these inhibitors have also demonstrated efficacy in other models such as prostate and gastric cancers (Underhill et al., 2011; Sachdev et al., 2019). Soft tissue sarcomas were also shown to be sensitive to PARP inhibition combined with genotoxic chemotherapy (Ordóñez et al., 2015). The strong PARP1/2 suppression seems to be inherently toxic due to an important role played by these proteins in the organism, but attempts are continuing to find the proper balance between efficacy and toxicity of inhibitors. Fatigue, anemia, nausea and neutropenia together with a risk of myelodysplastic syndrome/acute myeloid leukemia accompany the use of synthetic PARP1/2 inhibitors (Walsh, 2018). The recently described inhibitor 7-MG is a natural nitrogenous base that could escape the serious side effects and become a promising new component of chemotherapy. Additionally, 7-MG inhibits the RNA-modifying enzyme TGT, which may enhance its anticancer activity.

The primary aim of this research was to outline the safety profile of 7-MG *in vivo*. We have established an oral regimen for 7-MG treatment in CBA mice (50 mg/kg, 3 times per week for up to 4 weeks) that exerts no adverse effects or changes in morphology. Adverse events were detected only at a maximum single dose of 600 mg/kg, in the form of small lymphoid infiltrates of non-inflammatory origin in the lungs and liver. These lesions may be resulted from the excessive inhibition of PARP (Beneke and Möröy, 2001; Ricks et al., 2015; Dasa et al., 2018) at concentrations much higher than therapeutic levels. The safety of 7-MG was also confirmed by the examination in four short-term carcinogenicity assays where it showed no mutagenic or blastomogenic effects.

Preliminary data obtained on mouse transplantable tumor models (uterine sarcoma, cervical carcinoma) demonstrated that 7-MG significantly reduces tumor growth at a safe dose and can also potentiate the activity of cisplatin. The interruption of the 7-MG treatment results in accelerated tumor growth, which highlights the advantages of a multiple-dose regimen. The molecular mechanism of 7-MG is fundamentally different from that of drugs like cisplatin. It acts by modulating the enzyme activity instead of causing DNA damage, and the multiple exposure to 7-MG is needed for the effective modulation. The present study of the natural 7-MG compound has confirmed its safety and potential tumor suppressing activity in mice. For further development, it would be important to identify the most sensitive tumors for the 7-MG treatment as well as to select DNA-damaging agents for the combination treatment.

AUTHOR CONTRIBUTIONS

Conceptualization and funding acquisition, DN; investigation, KK, TF, EA, LT, TG, OV, IK, EL, NK, and TS; writing—original draft, KK, EL, and DN; supervision and writing—review and editing, GB, MY, and VŠ.

REFERENCES

Albertini, R. J., Anderson, D., Douglas, G. R., Hagmar, L., Hemminki, K., Merlo, F., et al. (2000). IPCS Guidelines for the Monitoring of Genotoxic Effects of Carcinogens in Humans. International Programme on Chemical Safety. *Mutat. Res.* 463, 111–172. doi:10.1016/s1383-5742(00)00049-1

Alemasova, E. E., and Lavrik, O. I. (2019). Poly(ADP-ribosyl)ation by PARP1: Reaction Mechanism and Regulatory Proteins. *Nucleic Acids Res.* 47, 3811–3827. doi:10.1093/nar/gkz120

Beneke, R., and Möröy, T. (2001). Inhibition of poly(ADP-Ribose) Polymerase Activity Accelerates T-Cell Lymphomagenesis in P53 Deficient Mice. *Oncogene* 20, 8136–8141. doi:10.1038/sj.onc.1205056

Bolognesi, M. L. (2013). Polypharmacology in a Single Drug: Multitarget Drugs. *Curr. Med. Chem.* 20, 1639–1645. doi:10.2174/0929867311320130004

Borowitz, I. J., Bloom, S. M., Rothschild, J., and Sprinson, D. B. (1965). Methylated Purines and Pyrimidines. I. Syntheses of 8-Hydroxy-7-Methylguanine and Methylation of a 5-(benzylideneamino) Pyrimidine. *Biochemistry* 4, 650–655. doi:10.1021/bi00880a006

Bromberg, P. A., Gutman, A. B., and Weissmann, B. (1957). The Purine Bases of Human Urine. II. Semiquantitative Estimation and Isotope Incorporation. *J. Biol. Chem.* 224, 423–434. doi:10.1016/s0021-9258(18)65041-0

Bromberg, P. A., Gutman, A. B., and Weissmann, B. (1957). The Purine Bases of Human Urine. I. Separation and Identification. *J. Biol. Chem.* 224, 407–422. doi:10.1016/s0021-9258(18)65040-9

Bunyatyan, N. D., Oborotova, N. A., Nikolaeva, L. L., Saprykina, N. S., Borisova, L. M., Kiseleva, M. P., et al. (2019). Comparative Analysis of Bioactivity of the Russian-made Antitumor Substances of the Nitrosourea Group. *Bull. Exp. Biol. Med.* 166, 456–460. doi:10.1007/s10517-019-04371-w

Cepeda, V., Fuertes, M. A., Castilla, J., Alonso, C., Quevedo, C., Soto, M., et al. (2006). Poly(ADP-ribose) Polymerase-1 (PARP-1) Inhibitors in Cancer Chemotherapy. *Recent Pat. Anticancer Drug Discov.* 1, 39–53. doi:10.2174/157489206775246430

Collins, A. R. (2004). The Comet Assay for DNA Damage and Repair: Principles, Applications, and Limitations. *Mol. Biotechnol.* 26, 249–261. doi:10.1385/MB:26:3:249

Craddock, V. M., Mattocks, A. R., and Magee, P. N. (1968). The Fate of 7[14C]-Methylguanine after Administration to the Rat. *Biochem. J.* 109, 75–78. doi:10.1042/bj1090075

Dasa, S. S. K., Diakova, G., Suzuki, R., Mills, A. M., Gutknecht, M. F., Klibanov, A. L., et al. (2018). Plectin-targeted Liposomes Enhance the Therapeutic Efficacy of a PARP Inhibitor in the Treatment of Ovarian Cancer. *Theranostics* 8, 2782–2798. doi:10.7150/thno.23050

Drenichev, M. S., and Mikhailov, S. N. (2015). Poly(ADP-ribose)--a Unique Natural Polymer Structural Features, Biological Role and Approaches to the Chemical Synthesis. *Nucleosides Nucleotides Nucleic Acids* 34, 258–276. doi:10.1080/15257770.2014.984073

Farkas, W. R., Jacobson, K. B., and Katze, J. R. (1984). Substrate and Inhibitor Specificity of tRNA-Guanine Ribosyltransferase. *Biochim. Biophys. Acta* 781, 64–75. doi:10.1016/0167-4781(84)90124-6

Ferraris, D. V. (2010). Evolution of poly(ADP-Ribose) Polymerase-1 (PARP-1) Inhibitors. From Concept to Clinic. *J. Med. Chem.* 53, 4561–4584. doi:10.1021/jm100012m

Frampton, J. E. (2015). Olaparib: A Review of its Use as Maintenance Therapy in Patients with Ovarian Cancer. *BioDrugs* 29, 143–150. doi:10.1007/s40259-015-0125-6

Hassler, M., and Ladurner, A. G. (2012). Towards a Structural Understanding of PARP1 Activation and Related Signalling ADP-Ribosyl-Transferases. *Curr. Opin. Struct. Biol.* 22, 721–729. doi:10.1016/j.sbi.2012.08.005

Jain, P. G., and Patel, B. D. (2019). Medicinal Chemistry Approaches of Poly ADP-Ribose Polymerase 1 (PARP1) Inhibitors as Anticancer Agents - A Recent Update. *Eur. J. Med. Chem.* 165, 198–215. doi:10.1016/j.ejmech.2019.01.024

Johannsson, S., Neumann, P., and Ficner, R. (2018). Crystal Structure of the Human tRNA Guanine Transglycosylase Catalytic Subunit QTRT1. *Biomolecules* 8, 81. doi:10.3390/biom8030081

Kaina, B., Heindorff, K., and Aurich, O. (1983). O6-methylguanine, but Not N7-Methylguanine or N3-Methyladenine, Induces Gene Mutations, Sister-Chromatid Exchanges and Chromosomal Aberrations in Chinese Hamster Cells. *Mutat. Res.* 108, 279–292. doi:10.1016/0027-5107(83)90126-4

Kerr, S. J. (1985). Induction of Adipocyte Formation in 10T1/2 Cells by 1-methylguanine and 7-methylguanine. *Tumour Biol.* 6, 115–121.

Kerr, S. J. (1990). Methylated Oxypurines and Induction of Differentiation of Murine Erythroleukemia Cells. *Mol. Cell. Biochem.* 92, 37–44. doi:10.1007/BF00220717

Kirsanov, K. I., Lesovaya, E. A., Sidorov, R. A., Belitsky, G. A., and Yakubovskaya, M. G. (2011). Analysis of Blastomogenic Activity of Mammal Carcinogens in Drosophila Using the Wts P4 Allele and RNA Interference-Induced P53 Silencing. *Russ. J. Genet.* 47, 409–416. doi:10.1134/s1022795411040065

Litwack, M. D., and Weissmann, B. (1966). Source of Urinary 8-Hydroxy-7-Methylguanine in Man. *Biochemistry* 5, 3007–3012. doi:10.1021/bi00873a033

Lord, C. J., Tutt, A. N., and Ashworth, A. (2015). Synthetic Lethality and Cancer Therapy: Lessons Learned from the Development of PARP Inhibitors. *Annu. Rev. Med.* 66, 455–470. doi:10.1146/annurev-med-050913-022545

Lothrop, C. D., Jr., and Uziel, M. (1983). RNA Turnover in Cultured Hamster Embryo Cells: Identification of Modified Nucleoside End Products. *J. Cell. Physiol.* 114, 111–116. doi:10.1002/jcp.1041140118

Maluchenko, N., Nilov, D., Feofanov, A., Lys, A., Kutuzov, M., Gerasimova, N., et al. (2019). 7-Methylguanine Traps PARP-1 on Nucleosomes: spFRET Microscopy Study. *Microsc. Microanal.* 25, 1282–1283. doi:10.1017/S1431927619007141

Malyuchenko, N. V., Kotova, E. Y., Kulaeva, O. I., Kirpichnikov, M. P., and Studitskiy, V. M. (2015). PARP1 Inhibitors: Antitumor Drug Design. *Acta Naturae* 7, 27–37. doi:10.32607/20758251-2015-7-3-27-37

Maron, D. M., and Ames, B. N. (1983). Revised Methods for the Salmonella Mutagenicity Test. *Mutat. Res.* 113, 173–215. doi:10.1016/0165-1161(83)90010-9

Martin, S. A., Lord, C. J., and Ashworth, A. (2008). DNA Repair Deficiency as a Therapeutic Target in Cancer. *Curr. Opin. Genet. Dev.* 18, 80–86. doi:10.1016/j.gde.2008.01.016

Medina-Franco, J. L., Giulianotti, M. A., Welmaker, G. S., and Houghten, R. A. (2013). Shifting from the Single to the Multitarget Paradigm in Drug Discovery. *Drug Discov. TodayToday* 18, 495–501. doi:10.1016/j.drudis.2013.01.008

Mittica, G., Ghisoni, E., Giannone, G., Genta, S., Aglietta, M., Sapino, A., et al. (2018). PARP Inhibitors in Ovarian Cancer. *Recent Pat. Anticancer Drug Discov.* 13, 392–410. doi:10.2174/1574892813666180305165256

Mustonen, R., and Hemminki, K. (1992). 7-Methylguanine Levels in DNA of Smokers' and Non-smokers' Total White Blood Cells, Granulocytes and Lymphocytes. *Carcinogenesis* 13, 1951–1955. doi:10.1093/carcin/13.11.1951

Nilov, D., Maluchenko, N., Kurgina, T., Pushkarev, S., Lys, A., Kutuzov, M., et al. (2020a). Molecular Mechanisms of PARP-1 Inhibitor 7-methylguanine. *Int. J. Mol. Sci.* 21, 2159. doi:10.3390/ijms21062159

Nilov, D. K., Pushkarev, S. V., Gushchina, I. V., Manasaryan, G. A., Kirsanov, K. I., and Švedas, V. K. (2020b). Modeling of the Enzyme-Substrate Complexes of Human poly(ADP-Ribose) Polymerase 1. *Biochem. (Mosc)* 85, 99–107. doi:10.1134/S0006297920010095

Nilov, D. K., Tararov, V. I., Kulikov, A. V., Zakharenko, A. L., Gushchina, I. V., Mikhailov, S. N., et al. (2016). Inhibition of poly(ADP-Ribose) Polymerase by Nucleic Acid Metabolite 7-methylguanine. *Acta Naturae* 8, 108–115. doi:10.32607/20758251-2016-8-2-108-115

Nilov, D., Kirsanov, K., Antoshina, E., Maluchenko, N., Feofanov, A., Kurgina, T., et al. (2018a). 7-Methylguanine: A Natural DNA Repair Inhibitor and a Promising Anticancer Compound. *FEBS Open Bio* 8. doi:10.1002/2211-5463.12453

Nilov, D. K., Yashina, K. I., Gushchina, I. V., Zakharenko, A. L., Sukhanova, M. V., Lavrik, O. I., et al. (2018b). 2,5-Diketopiperazines: A New Class of poly(ADP-Ribose)polymerase Inhibitors. *Biochem. (Mosc)* 83, 152–158. doi:10.1134/S0006297918020074

O'Connor, T. R. (1993). Purification and Characterization of Human 3-Methyladenine-DNA Glycosylase. *Nucleic Acids Res.* 21, 5561–5569. doi:10.1093/nar/21.24.5561

Ohmoto, A., and Yachida, S. (2017). Current Status of poly(ADP-Ribose) Polymerase Inhibitors and Future Directions. *Onco Targets Ther.* 10, 5195–5208. doi:10.2147/OTT.S139336

Ordóñez, J. L., Amaral, A. T., Carcaboso, A. M., Herrero-Martín, D., del Carmen García-Macías, M., Sevillano, V., et al. (2015). The PARP Inhibitor Olaparib Enhances the Sensitivity of Ewing Sarcoma to Trabectedin. *Oncotarget* 6, 18875–18890. doi:10.18632/oncotarget.4303

Park, J. W., and Ames, B. N. (1988). 7-Methylguanine Adducts in DNA Are Normally Present at High Levels and Increase on Aging: Analysis by HPLC with Electrochemical Detection. *Proc. Natl. Acad. Sci. U. S. A.* 85, 7467–7470. doi:10.1073/pnas.85.20.7467

Raćkowska, E., Bobrowska-Korczak, B., and Giebułtowicz, J. (2019). Development and Validation of a Rapid LC-MS/MS Method for Determination of Methylated Nucleosides and Nucleobases in Urine. *J. Chromatogr. B Anal. Technol. Biomed. Life Sci.* 1128, 121775. doi:10.1016/j.jchromb.2019.121775

Ray Chaudhuri, A., and Nussenzweig, A. (2017). The Multifaceted Roles of PARP1 in DNA Repair and Chromatin Remodelling. *Nat. Rev. Mol. Cell Biol.* 18, 610–621. doi:10.1038/nrm.2017.53

Ricks, T. K., Chiu, H. J., Ison, G., Kim, G., McKee, A. E., Kluetz, P., et al. (2015). Successes and Challenges of PARP Inhibitors in Cancer Therapy. *Front. Oncol.* 5, 222. doi:10.3389/fonc.2015.00222

Rodríguez-Gonzalo, E., Hernández-Prieto, R., García-Gómez, D., and Carabias-Martínez, R. (2013). Capillary Electrophoresis-Mass Spectrometry for Direct Determination of Urinary Modified Nucleosides. Evaluation of Synthetic Urine as a Surrogate Matrix for Quantitative Analysis. *J. Chromatogr. B Anal. Technol. Biomed. Life Sci.* 942–943, 21–30. doi:10.1016/j.jchromb.2013.10.022

Sachdev, E., Tabatabai, R., Roy, V., Rimel, B. J., and Mita, M. M. (2019). PARP Inhibition in Cancer: An Update on Clinical Development. *Target. Oncol.* 14, 657–679. doi:10.1007/s11523-019-00680-2

Sander, G., Hülsemann, J., Topp, H., Heller-Schöch, G., and Schöch, G. (1986). Protein and RNA Turnover in Preterm Infants and Adults: A Comparison Based on Urinary Excretion of 3-methylhistidine and of Modified One-Way RNA Catabolites. *Ann. Nutr. Metab.* 30, 137–142. doi:10.1159/000177186

Sander, G., Topp, H., Heller-Schöch, G., Wieland, J., and Schöch, G. (1986). Ribonucleic Acid Turnover in Man:RNA Catabolites in Urine as Measure for the Metabolism of Each of the Three Major Species of RNA. *Clin. Sci.* 71, 367–374. doi:10.1042/cs0710367

Sander, G., Topp, H., Wieland, J., Heller-Schöch, G., and Schöch, G. (1986). Possible Use of Urinary Modified RNA Metabolites in the Measurement of RNA Turnover in the Human Body. *Hum. Nutr. Clin. Nutr.* 40, 103–118.

Shafer, B., Chu, C., and Shatkin, A. J. (2005). Human mRNA Cap Methyltransferase: Alternative Nuclear Localization Signal Motifs Ensure Nuclear Localization Required for Viability. *Mol. Cell. Biol.* 25, 2644–2649. doi:10.1128/MCB.25.7.2644-2649.2005

Shapiro, R. (1968). "Chemistry of Guanine and its Biologically Significant Derivatives,". Editors J. N. Davidson and W. E. Cohn (New York, USA: Academic Press).*Prog. Nucleic Acid Res. Mol. Biol.*, Vol. 8, 73–112. doi:10.1016/s0079-6603(08)60544-9

Shuman, S. (2002). What Messenger RNA Capping Tells Us about Eukaryotic Evolution. *Nat. Rev. Mol. Cell Biol.* 3, 619–625. doi:10.1038/nrm880

Sidorov, R. A., Ugnivenko, E. G., Khovanova, E. M., and Belitsky, G. A. (2001). Induction of Tumor Clones in *D. melanogaster Wts*/+ Heterozygotes with Chemical Carcinogens. *Mutat. Res.* 498, 181–191. doi:10.1016/s1383-5718(01)00277-7

Singh, N. P., McCoy, M. T., Tice, R. R., and Schneider, E. L. (1988). A Simple Technique for Quantitation of Low Levels of DNA Damage in Individual Cells. *Exp. Cell Res.* 175, 184–191. doi:10.1016/0014-4827(88)90265-0

Skupp, S., and Ayvazian, J. H. (1969). Oxidation of 7-methylguanine by Human Xanthine Oxidase. *J. Lab. Clin. Med.* 73, 909–916.

Sonnenblick, A., de Azambuja, E., Azim, H. A., Jr., and Piccart, M. (2015). An Update on PARP Inhibitors-Mmoving to the Adjuvant Setting. *Nat. Rev. Clin. Oncol.* 12, 27–41. doi:10.1038/nrclinonc.2014.163

Svoboda, P., and Kasai, H. (2004). Simultaneous HPLC Analysis of 8-hydroxydeoxyguanosine and 7-methylguanine in Urine from Humans and Rodents. *Anal. Biochem.* 334, 239–250. doi:10.1016/j.ab.2004.08.021

Tamae, K., Kawai, K., Yamasaki, S., Kawanami, K., Ikeda, M., Takahashi, K., et al. (2009). Effect of Age, Smoking and Other Lifestyle Factors on Urinary 7-methylguanine and 8-hydroxydeoxyguanosine. *Cancer Sci.* 100, 715–721. doi:10.1111/j.1349-7006.2009.01088.x

Tan, B. H., Bencsath, F. A., and Gaubatz, J. W. (1990). Steady-state Levels of 7-methylguanine Increase in Nuclear DNA of Postmitotic Mouse Tissues during Aging. *Mutat. Res.* 237, 229–238. doi:10.1016/0921-8734(90)90004-b

Topisirovic, I., Svitkin, Y. V., Sonenberg, N., and Shatkin, A. J. (2011). Cap and Cap-Binding Proteins in the Control of Gene Expression. *Wiley Interdiscip. Rev. RNA.* 2, 277–298. doi:10.1002/wrna.52

Topp, H., Sander, G., Heller-Schöch, G., and Schöch, G. (1987). Determination of 7-methylguanine, N2,N2-Dimethylguanosine, and Pseudouridine in Ultrafiltrated Serum of Healthy Adults by High-Performance Liquid Chromatography. *Anal. Biochem.* 161, 49–56. doi:10.1016/0003-2697(87)90650-6

Treshalina, H. M., Lukasheva, E. V., Sedakova, L. A., Firsova, G. A., Guerassimova, G. K., Gogichaeva, N. V., et al. (2000). Anticancer Enzyme L-Lysine α-Oxidase: Properties and Application Perspectives. *Abab* 88, 267–274. doi:10.1385/abab:88:1-3:267

Turusov, V. S., Siniak, IuE., Grigor'ev, A. I., Zaridze, D. G., Antoshina, E. E., Trukhanova, L. S., et al. (2005). Low-deuterium Water Effect on Transplantable Tumors. *Vopr. Onkol.* 51, 99–102.

Underhill, C., Toulmonde, M., and Bonnefoi, H. (2011). A Review of PARP Inhibitors: from Bench to Bedside. *Ann. Oncol.* 22, 268–279. doi:10.1093/annonc/mdq322

Varshney, D., Petit, A. P., Bueren-Calabuig, J. A., Jansen, C., Fletcher, D. A., Peggie, M., et al. (2016). Molecular Basis of RNA Guanine-7 Methyltransferase (RNMT) Activation by RAM. *Nucleic Acids Res.* 44, 10423–10436. doi:10.1093/nar/gkw637

Walsh, C. (2018). Targeted Therapy for Ovarian Cancer: the Rapidly Evolving Landscape of PARP Inhibitor Use. *Minerva Ginecol.* 70, 150–170. doi:10.23736/S0026-4784.17.04152-1

Wang, Y. Q., Wang, P. Y., Wang, Y. T., Yang, G. F., Zhang, A., and Miao, Z. H. (2016). An Update on poly(ADP-Ribose)polymerase-1 (PARP-1) Inhibitors: Opportunities and Challenges in Cancer Therapy. *J. Med. Chem.* 59, 9575–9598. doi:10.1021/acs.jmedchem.6b00055

Weissmann, B., and Gutman, A. B. (1957). The Identification of 6-succinoaminopurine and of 8-Hydroxy-7-Methylguanine as Normal Human Urinary Constituents. *J. Biol. Chem.* 229, 239–250. doi:10.1016/s0021-9258(18)70612-1

Zhang, J., Lu, R., Zhang, Y., Matuszek, Ż., Zhang, W., Xia, Y., et al. (2020). tRNA Queuosine Modification Enzyme Modulates the Growth and Microbiome Recruitment to Breast Tumors. *Cancers (Basel)* 12, 628. doi:10.3390/cancers12030628

Zimmer, A. S., Gillard, M., Lipkowitz, S., and Lee, J. M. (2018). Update on PARP Inhibitors in Breast Cancer. *Curr. Treat. Options Oncol.* 19, 21. doi:10.1007/s11864-018-0540-2

4

Dual-Targeted Therapy Circumvents Non-Genetic Drug Resistance to Targeted Therapy

Wei Wang[1], Yue Sun[1], Xiaobo Liu[1], Shaji K. Kumar[2], Fengyan Jin[3†] and Yun Dai[1*†]*

[1] Laboratory of Cancer Precision Medicine, The First Hospital of Jilin University, Changchun, China, [2] Division of Hematology, Mayo Clinic College of Medicine, Rochester, MN, United States, [3] Department of Hematology, The First Hospital of Jilin University, Changchun, China

***Correspondence:**
Yun Dai
daiyun@jlu.edu.cn;
daiyun62@hotmail.com
Fengyan Jin
fengyanjin@jlu.edu.cn

The introduction of various targeted agents into the armamentarium of cancer treatment has revolutionized the standard care of patients with cancer. However, like conventional chemotherapy, drug resistance, either preexisting (primary or intrinsic resistance) or developed following treatment (secondary or acquired resistance), remains the Achilles heel of all targeted agents with no exception, *via* either genetic or non-genetic mechanisms. In the latter, emerging evidence supports the notion that intracellular signaling pathways for tumor cell survival act as a mutually interdependent network *via* extensive cross-talks and feedback loops. Thus, dysregulations of multiple signaling pathways usually join forces to drive oncogenesis, tumor progression, invasion, metastasis, and drug resistance, thereby providing a basis for so-called "bypass" mechanisms underlying non-genetic resistance in response to targeted agents. In this context, simultaneous interruption of two or more related targets or pathways (an approach called dual-targeted therapy, DTT), *via* either linear or parallel inhibition, is required to deal with such a form of drug resistance to targeted agents that specifically inhibit a single oncoprotein or oncogenic pathway. Together, while most types of tumor cells are often addicted to two or more targets or pathways or can switch their dependency between them, DTT targeting either intrinsically activated or drug-induced compensatory targets/pathways would efficiently overcome drug resistance caused by non-genetic events, with a great opportunity that those resistant cells might be particularly more vulnerable. In this review article, we discuss, with our experience, diverse mechanisms for non-genetic resistance to targeted agents and the rationales to circumvent them in the treatment of cancer, emphasizing hematologic malignancies.

Keywords: targeted agent, non-genetic mechanism, dual-targeted therapy, parallel inhibition, drug resistance, cancer, linear inhibition, hematologic malignancy

INTRODUCTION

Targeted therapy refers to the treatment specifically targeting a protein (oncoprotein in most cases) or dysregulated pathway that drives oncogenesis. Imatinib mesylate (Gleevec), a tyrosine kinase inhibitor (TKI) targeting BCR-ABL fusion oncoprotein for treating Ph+ chronic myelogenous leukemia (CML) (1), is considered as the first targeted agent for this approach. Another prototypic targeted agent is all-trans retinoic acid (ATRA), which acts to override the differentiation block mediated by PML-RARα fusion protein due to t(15;17) translocation in promyelocytic leukemia (PML) cells, resulting in the high efficacy of ATRA in treatment of PML (2). These successes have ignited enthusiasm to identify numerous novel molecular targets and develop a tremendous number of the first-in-class or best-in-class agents selectively against these targets. In consequence, we have witnessed an explosive increase in the number of targeted agents approved for the treatment of various cancer types, including both hematologic malignancies and solid tumors. The introduction of targeted therapy into the armamentarium for cancer treatment has initiated an era of precision medicine, which has been advanced with astonishing speed afterwards (3).

The notion of resistance to targeted agents is intimately associated with the concept of oncogene addiction (4), one of cancer hallmarks initially described in 2000 and subsequently updated and expanded (5–7). Although the mechanism by which oncogene addiction occurs remains to be elucidated with certainty, one concept holds that the genes responsible for malignant transformation may have certain lethal effects that must be overridden in order for transformed cells to survive (4). For example, c-Myc, a well-described oncogene that promotes cell proliferation, may exert a pro-apoptotic action in some circumstances. Under these conditions, over-expression of the anti-apoptotic gene Bcl-2 is required for survival of c-Myc-driven transformed cells (8). Then, such cells become dependent on Bcl-2 and thus susceptible to strategies targeting Bcl-2. In addition, transformed cells are equipped with powerful anti-stress properties to adapt not only intracellular stresses (e.g., oxidative, replicative, metabolic, etc.) during oncogenesis but also various extracellular insults (e.g., hypoxic, inflammatory, etc.) in tumor microenvironment, both of which must be overcome in order to preserve their survival and proliferative advantages over their normal counterparts (6). Moreover, oncogene addiction is dynamic due to clonal selection or evolution under therapeutic pressure, an event stemmed from tumor heterogeneity (9–11). It is common that new genetic alterations (e.g., point mutations) of either primary targeted oncogene or other related oncogenes occur during treatment with targeted agents, thus conferring resistance to those agents *via* such a genetic mechanism involving the change of addicting oncogene (named *de novo* mutation). Even more problematically, only a few types of cancer are addicted to only one oncogene for transformation and tumor cell survival, while the vast majority of malignancies rely on multiple alterations involving oncogenic and non-oncogenic proteins or pathways (12). Thus, the mechanisms of drug resistance are often multifaceted and highly heterogeneous at intratumoral or intercellular levels, as well as from genetic and non-genetic point of view (11, 13, 14). Of note, in addition to the well-recognized genetic mechanism, non-genetic mechanisms of drug resistance have been emerging as a much broader (not only for TKIs but also for non-TKI targeted agents) and more complicated challenge in cancer treatment.

In this review, we do not intend to provide a comprehensive overview of current understanding of overall mechanisms for resistance to targeted agents or strategies to circumvent them; a number of reviews dealing with these subjects have been published (9, 10, 12–15). Instead, we aim to focus on the non-genetic mechanisms by which tumor cells escape the lethal effects of targeted agents, and how rational strategies can be designed to solve this problem, with our experience.

THE ORIGIN OF DRUG RESISTANCE - INTRINSIC VERSUS ACQUIRED

As in the case of more conventional chemotherapeutic agents, resistance to targeted agents may be either intrinsic or acquired (**Figure 1**) (16). During targeted therapy, most patients carrying the driver genetic alterations (e.g., EGFR mutations in non-small cell lung cancer (NSCLC) and fusion protein BCR/ABL in CML) would respond to corresponding targeted agents thus be benefited, while some patients do not respond well and thus are considered to experience primary or intrinsic resistance. However, only a few diseases like CML are addicted to single

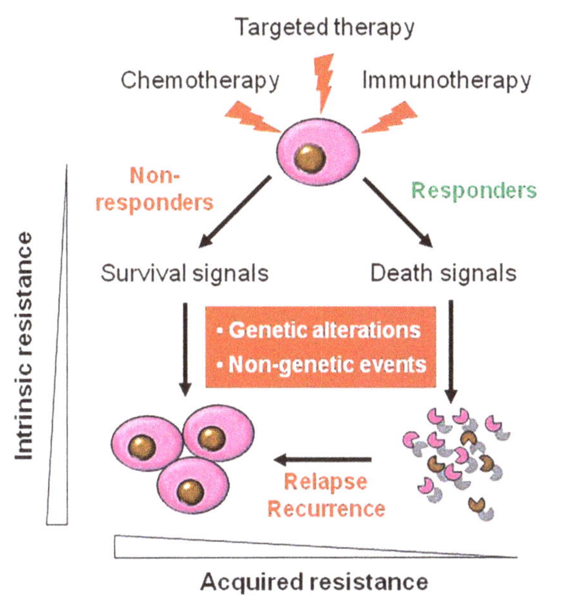

FIGURE 1 | Diverse types of drug resistance to targeted therapy. During targeted therapy as well as conventional chemotherapy and novel immunotherapy, most patients carrying the driver genetic alterations respond to corresponding targeted agents, who are known as responders, while some patients who do not respond well, who are known as non-responder, due to intrinsic (primary) resistance. However, virtually all responders will eventually relapse and become resistant to agents targeting the original oncoproteins (as well as other targeted agents in most cases) due to acquired (secondary) resistance. Mechanistically, both intrinsic and acquired resistance stem from either genetic (e.g., *de novo* mutations) or non-genetic mechanisms, or both.

oncogene (e.g., BCR-ABL), most cancer types rely on multiple oncogenic alterations, with only partial dependency upon an individual target or pathway. Patients with NSCLC expressing certain activating EGFR mutations are much more likely to respond to EGFR inhibitors (17), and thus such tumors appear to be particularly addicted to EGFR signaling for survival. Unfortunately, some patients with NSCLC carrying EGFR mutations do not respond to EGFR inhibitors, suggesting EGFR mutation-independent mechanisms such as co-occurrence of KRAS mutations (18). Similarly, patients with colon cancer carrying KRAS mutations are unlikely to respond to TKIs directed against EGFR (19). A likely explanation for this phenomenon is that activation of the Ras/Raf/MEK/ERK pathway, which lies downstream of EGFR may bypass the addiction to EGFR activation. This may also apply to the case of the PTEN/PI3K/AKT/mTOR pathway, which is activated downstream of EGFR (20, 21). The development or pre-existence of PTEN mutations may, as in the case of mutant RAS, relieve transformed cells from their dependency on EGFR signaling. In this context, interventions capable of interrupting the PTEN/PI3K/AKT pathway (e.g., by PI3K inhibitors) have been shown to be effective in this setting (22). While the mechanisms underlying this phenomenon remain to be fully elucidated, one speculative possibility is that for reasons not yet understood, the activating mutations do not require or induce activation of "orthogonal" protective pathways (4). Alternatively, in the case of KRAS mutation that is commonly considered "undruggable" (11, 23), the activation of wild-type RAS by multiple receptor tyrosine kinases (RTKs) can confer resistance to mutated-KRAS (e.g., KRAS-G12C) inhibitors (in addition to *de novo* KRAS mutations) (24), suggesting a role of "horizontal" protective pathways (4). Consequently, inhibition of such activated compensatory signaling pathways in a linear or parallel manner may render interruption of the mutant RTK particularly lethal. More importantly, it should be kept in mind that although TKIs display significant activity in patients carrying oncogenic mutations, these targeted agents are not curative, and patients ultimately die of their disease. This raises a possibility that even in the case of susceptible disease with oncogenic mutations, interrupting complementary survival signaling pathways in combination with TKIs may improve patient outcome further.

Virtually all of patients who initially respond to targeted agents eventually develop acquired resistance to these agents, with no exception thus far. Such resistance may stem from *de novo* mutations in oncoprotein that prevent drug binding to their active sites (e.g., ATP-binding site in most cases) (25). The classic example is the development of point mutations (e.g., T315I or T790M) in the ATP binding pocket of BCR/ABL or EGFR, thereby conferring resistance to TKIs by preventing their binding to targets (26). Thus, *de novo* mutation represents a primary genetic mechanism for acquired TKI resistance (1). Furthermore, such new genetic alterations are not necessary to occur only in original targets, but also involve other oncoproteins (27). For example, acquired RET fusion proteins (e.g., CCDC6-RET fusion) in NSCLC cells bearing both primary and acquired EGFR mutations (e.g., del19 and L858R/T790M) confer resistance to both first- and second-generation TKIs (e.g., AZD9291/osimertinib) (18, 28). Similar phenomenon has also been observed in the case of acquired resistance to FGFR inhibitors in different cancer types bearing FGFR mutations or fusions (29). Both *de novo* FGFR gatekeeper mutations and activation of alternate RTKs account for acquired resistance to FGFR inhibitors. However, the distinction between acquired versus intrinsic resistance may be blurred in view of evidence that resistant cells carrying "*de novo*" mutations may pre-exist, while they remain dormant (like leukemic stem cells, LSCs) but expand after leukemic blasts carrying primary targets (e.g., BCR-ABL) are selectively eliminated by targeted therapy and eventually become dominant, a process known as clonal selection or evolution (11). A main strategy to overcome such mechanisms of drug resistance, either intrinsic or acquired, is to develop new-generation of TKIs active against mutant oncoproteins (26). However, although second- and third-generation TKIs are active to bind to and target these mutants, other *de novo* mutations (e.g., gatekeeper mutations such as T315I in BCR-ABL, which cannot be effectively targeted thus far) confer resistance to these next-generation TKIs again (26). Almost identical phenomena have been observed in the case of solid tumors, such as TKIs targeting activating EGFR mutations and EML4-ALK fusion protein in NSCLC (12). Another potentially promising strategy directed against either intrinsic or acquired mechanisms of resistance involves inhibition of critical pathways downstream of the original target (termed linear inhibition; see below). For example, because many kinases, including Aurora kinase A and Polo-like kinase 1 (PLK-1), operate downstream of BCR/ABL, inhibitors of Aurora kinases or PLK-1 may bypass the resistant barrier (e.g., T315I gatekeeper mutation of BCR/ABL) to induce apoptosis in imatinib mesylate-resistant cells (30–32). The advantage of such a strategy is that inhibiting such a downstream target or pathway eliminates the need to circumvent the primary resistance mechanism (e.g., *de novo* mutation), whatever its origin (intrinsic or acquired).

Similar mechanisms may also apply to immunotherapy such as monoclonal antibodies (MoAbs) targeting cell surface receptors like HER2 in breast cancer and CD20 in lymphoma. For example, in the case of MoAbs (e.g., the HER2 MoAb trastuzumab), resistance can be acquired *via* genetic alterations in the receptor (e.g., the presence of its mutant forms that do not bind to the MoAb), competition with endogenous ligands, activation of parallel or downstream pathways, or other immunological mechanisms (10, 33).

THE NATURE OF RESISTANCE - GENETIC VS NON-GENETIC

Mechanistically, drug resistance to targeted agents, either intrinsic or acquired, can be divided into genetic (target-dependent) versus non-genetic (target-independent) (**Figure 1**) (34). In this classification, the former is primarily related to oncogene addiction, while the latter often reflects the ability of transformed cells to escape or adapt to the lethal actions of targeted agents due to acquisition of the perturbations that protect tumor cells from lethality of targeted agents, a "bypass" mechanism (12, 27). For the genetic mechanism, the development of *de novo* mutations that prevent binding of a targeted agent to its target of interest represents a primary resistance mechanism as discussed above (35). Other mechanisms also involve addiction to multiple targets/pathways and pharmacokinetic reasons preventing achievement of effective plasma concentrations (36). For the non-genetic mechanism, replacement or substitution of tumor cell dependency often involves the activation of a complementary pathway, an event capable of transmitting alternative signals sufficient to survive from the lethal consequences of interrupting the primary pathway by a targeted agent (10).

A typical example is that the lethal consequences of blocking the Ras/Raf/MEK/ERK pathway (e.g., by BRAF inhibitors) can be compromised by the activation of the PI3K/AKT pathway in tumor cells (20, 21). Alternatively, up-regulation of anti-apoptotic proteins or down-regulation of their pro-apoptotic counterparts can abrogate the lethality of various targeted agents (especially including most TKIs) (37, 38). In general, such a non-genetic form of resistance involves a fundamental change that makes neoplastic cells no longer dependent upon primary oncogenic signals, which originally drive transformation, for their survival. Thus, the strategies to overcome drug resistance *via* increasing the degree or duration of target inhibition by pharmacokinetic means (36) or developing more potent next-generation agents are most likely to fail in this circumstance. Since tumor cells has developed, in response to a targeted agent, such a non-genetic mechanism that makes them independent of their oncogenic drivers for survival, the identification of alternative targets responsible for or involved in this form of resistance and the development of fundamentally different approaches are required to prime resistant tumor cells for death.

In this context, dysregulation of the apoptosis-regulatory machinery mediated by the Bcl-2 family represents a universal non-genetic mechanism for drug resistance to targeted agents. It has been well documented that the Bcl-2 family of pro- and anti-apoptotic proteins is ultimately responsible for determining the fate of tumor cells. Anti-apoptotic proteins (e.g., Bcl-2, Bcl-xL, Mcl-1, and A1) are often multi-domain proteins that promote cell survival either directly by preserving mitochondrial integrity, or indirectly by binding to and blocking the activity of pro-apoptotic proteins (an event known as neutralization) (37, 38). The pro-apoptotic proteins include multi-domain (e.g., Bak and Bax) and BH3-only proteins (e.g., Bim, Bid, Bik, Bad, Puma, Noxa, and Hrk) (37). Based on their mechanisms of action, these pro-apoptotic proteins can be further subdivided into activator (e.g., Bim, Bid, and Puma), which directly triggers mitochondrial injury, and sensitizer (e.g., Bad), which antagonize the functions of anti-apoptotic proteins (39). The lethal actions of various targeted agents that disrupt oncogenic signaling pathways are considered to be integrated at the level of pro- and anti-apoptotic proteins (40). For example, the intracellular levels and disposition of Bim and Bad is regulated *via* their phosphorylation by multiple upstream kinases involving major signaling pathways, particularly Ras/Raf/MEK/ERK and PI3K/AKT/mTOR (20, 41). Thus, simultaneous interruption of these pathways results in accumulation of Bad and Bim in tumor cells and thus enhances lethality (42). On the other hand, co-administration of Bcl-2 inhibitors can circumvent resistance to targeted agents due to increased expression of anti-apoptotic proteins (43). An alternative strategy is to bypass the barrier of the intrinsic, mitochondrial apoptotic pathway (due to up-regulation of anti-apoptotic proteins or down-regulation of pro-apoptotic proteins) by triggering the extrinsic apoptotic cascade *via* up-regulating and activating death receptors (44–46). Moreover, in addition to apoptosis, multiple other forms of programmed cell death (PCD e.g., necroptosis, ferroptosis, pyroptosis, etc.) with almost entirely distinctive mechanisms have been identified (47, 48), which may provide much more choices to develop therapeutic approaches, particularly for enhancing apoptosis and overcoming the resistance to apoptosis based on these unique mechanisms.

Another common non-genetic mechanism is related to autophagy, a term literally meaning "self-eating". Autophagy is a process in which cellular constituents are catabolized in the lysosome, which provides a source of energy to maintain critical cellular functions (49, 50). Autophagy thus functions as a cytoprotective mechanism to protect cells from environmental insults as well as anti-cancer treatment (particularly targeted therapy) (50). Under conditions in which autophagy protects cells from the lethal effects of targeted agents, co-administration of autophagy antagonists may dramatically increase the lethality of targeted agents (51). However, autophagy can also contribute to cell death under other circumstances. Instead of simply inhibiting autophagy, targeting the key step (e.g., cargo-loading mediated by SQSTM1/p62) leads to "inefficient" autophagy, which may more selectively kill malignant cells (52). While it could be a challenge to develop small molecule inhibitors for this kind of autophagy adaptor proteins, nanocarriers may represent an alternative and promising approach to deliver siRNA and shRNA specifically targeting molecular components that regulate autophagy (e.g., Beclin-1, LC3-II, ATGs, or even SQSTM1/p62) (53).

THE DTT STRATEGY TO OVERCOME RESISTANCE - LINEAR VS PARALLEL INHIBITION

Despite the diversity for the nature of resistance, it is certain that strategies will have to be tailored specifically to the mechanism(s) responsible for resistance. For example, improving drug pharmacokinetics through optimizing drug doses or schedules as well as ameliorating drug design (36, 54), or developing next-generation agents capable of inhibiting mutants resistant to first-generation inhibitors (55), is capable of overcoming target-dependent (genetic) resistance, but most likely not going to work for target-independent (non-genetic) resistance. For the latter, emerging evidence supports that dual-targeted therapy

(DTT), which is here defined as inhibition of two or more survival-related targets or signaling pathways, represents a promising strategy, for target-dependent and particularly target-independent forms of resistance (55). In general, inhibition of multiple targets *via* DTT includes at least two ways - parallel versus linear inhibition.

Parallel Inhibition

DTT that simultaneously inhibits two or more complementary oncogenic pathways, which cooperate to maintain transformed cell survival or confer resistance (intrinsic or acquired), may be effective when targeting either single pathway is no longer capable of triggering cell death. This kind of DTT is considered a parallel inhibition approach to overcome resistance to primary targeted agents (56). A classic example of such an approach involves the Ras/Raf/MEK/ERK and PI3K/AKT/mTOR pathways (21), both of which prevent cell death by promoting phosphorylation, at different amino acid residues, and subsequent degradation of pro-death proteins (e.g., Bim and Bad). In this context, several studies have demonstrated that regimens combining PI3K or AKT inhibitors and MEK1/2 inhibitors potently induce cell death in both solid tumor and hematologic malignancies (20, 22, 40, 57). Another example is to combine the second-generation EGFR TKI osimertinib, which is active against the most important *de novo* mutation T790M that confers resistance to first-generation EGFR TKIs, with RET inhibition to overcome resistance to osimertinib due to acquired RET fusion in NSCLC (28). Similarly, simultaneous inhibition of canonical and non-canonical NF-κB pathways can also potentiate lethality in drug-sensitive and -resistant cells (58). Moreover, a DTT approach, known as dual targeting of epigenetic therapy that combines a DNMT inhibitor with a HDAC inhibitor to simultaneously target two epigenetic mechanisms (e.g., DNA methylation and histone acetylation, respectively), has already been used to treat several myeloid malignancies (59). This approach may be extended to include agents targeting other epigenetic mechanisms (e.g., histone methylation) as well (60). Notably, as these therapeutics primarily target epigenetic modifications of DNA or histones involving the transcription-regulatory machinery, they would theoretically influence numerous downstream targets with various functions and signaling pathways. Thus, they could be good candidates suitable for the development of the DTT regimens. However, the caution needs to be taken that they may also increase the incidence of adverse effects due to the diversity of their targets.

Numerous links have been found between the cell cycle- and survival-regulatory machineries. For example, the Ras/Raf/MEK/ERK pathway has been implicated in the regulation of G2/M progression and in the disposition of cyclin D1, which is involved in the progression from G0/G1 into cell cycle (61). A DTT strategy targeting the cell cycle and survival signaling pathways involves inhibition of cell cycle checkpoints, most notably Chk1 or Wee1. Chk1 and Wee1 are key components of the DNA damage response (DDR), which trigger cell cycle arrest in cells subjected to genotoxic insults, allowing repair to occur if the damage is fixable, or apoptosis if it is not (62–64). This "self-checking" mechanism may be particularly important in maintaining survival of tumor cells harboring driver oncogenic mutations (64–66). Thus, Chk1 has been an attractive target for therapeutic intervention because it is involved in virtually all DNA damage checkpoints, and may also contribute to cell survival in a more direct manner (67). Most strategies involving the inhibitors of Chk1 or Wee1, as well as many other key components of various DDR pathways, have been combining them with various DNA-damaging agents (68). In this area, an elegant review article recently published has provided an overview of the advances and current status for the development of agents targeting DDR in various types of cancer (69). However, we observed that Chk1 inhibition triggers a compensatory activation of the Ras/Raf/MEK/ERK pathway in both hematologic malignancies and solid tumors, which may limit the lethal effect of Chk1 inhibitors (70, 71). Notably, abrogation of this signaling pathway at downstream sites (e.g., by MEK1/2 inhibitors) or more upstream sites (e.g., by farnesyltransferase or Src inhibitors) dramatically increases Chk1 inhibitor lethality (70–76). This phenomenon has been specifically attributed to potentiation of Chk1 inhibitor-mediated DNA damage (77), as well as up-regulation of the pro-apoptotic protein Bim, due to prevention of its phosphorylation and degradation *via* the ubiquitin-proteasome system (UPS) (78, 79). Such observations raise a possibility that in transformed cells, disruption of cell cycle checkpoints, which are often dysregulated in neoplasia, triggers a compensatory activation of the Ras/Raf/MEK/ERK pathway allowing them to survive, though the link between them remains unknown. Consequently, a DTT approach *via* parallel inhibition of these two critical survival pathways can lower the threshold for DNA damage-induced cell death (**Figure 2**), thus improving the anti-tumor activity of Chk1 inhibitors alone or in combination with conventional DNA-damaging agents (80, 81).

As a key family of anti-apoptotic proteins, Bcl-2 or its relatives (e.g., Bcl-xL and Mcl-1) are highly expressed in various types of cancer, particularly hematologic malignancies (e.g., lymphoma, leukemia, and multiple myeloma/MM), therefore representing one of the most attractive therapeutic targets (37, 38). However, it has taken a long time to develop the Bcl-2 inhibitor venetoclax (formerly ABT-199), which has been approved for the treatment of CLL and AML (82). One potential hurdle stems from a phenomenon that pro-apoptotic BH3-only proteins (e.g., Bim) released from one anti-apoptotic protein (e.g., Bcl-2) would bind to another anti-apoptotic protein (e.g., Mcl-1), thus disabling the lethal action of agents (e.g., Bcl-2 inhibitors) targeting only one arm of the apoptosis-regulatory machinery (83). Consequently, the activity of Bcl-2 inhibitors is inversely related to expression of Mcl-1 in tumor cells (83, 84). A corollary of this notion is that agents or interventions capable of down-regulating or inhibiting Mcl-1 could increase the activity of Bcl-2 inhibitors (85–87). Indeed, multiple such agents have been demonstrated to synergistically interact with Bcl-2 inhibitors in various hematologic malignancies. For example, CDK inhibitors that target transcription-regulatory CDKs (e.g.,

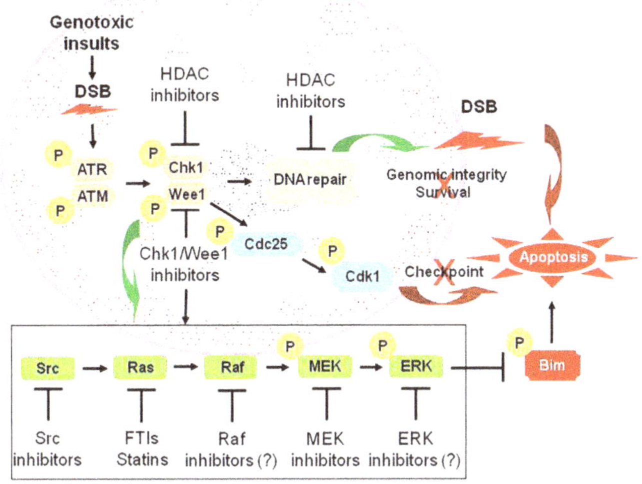

FIGURE 2 | An example for the DTT approach *via* parallel inhibition. As DNA damage checkpoint and the Ras/Raf/MEK/ERK pathway represent two separate mechanisms for maintaining genomic integrity and survival of tumor cells under intracellular and extracellular stresses (e.g., genotoxic insults caused by conventional DNA-damaging chemotherapeutics). Treatment with Chk1 (or Wee1) inhibitors promotes DNA damage by abrogating checkpoints *via* Cdc25-mediated dephosphorylation of Cdk1 at inhibitory sites, an effect that could be potentiated by HDAC inhibitors *via* down-regulation of multiple genes involving DNA damage checkpoint and repair (linear inhibition). However, they also triggers activation of the Ras/Raf/MEK/ERK pathway *via* a not-yet-defined crosstalk between these two pathways, which most likely accounts for non-genetic resistance to Chk1 (or Wee1) inhibitors. Thus, a DTT approach *via* parallel inhibition of both DNA damage checkpoint (pathway #1) and its complementary Ras/Raf/MEK/ERK signaling cascade (pathway #2; e.g., by inhibitors of Src, Ras, Raf, MEK, and ERK, which act to prevent phosphorylation and degradation of pro-apoptotic proteins such as Bim, thus priming tumor cells for death induced by targeted agents like Chk1/Wee1 inhibitors), leads to unfixable DNA damage and thus triggers robust apoptosis. DSB, double-stranded break; P, phosphorylation.

CDK9 and CDK7) and thus down-regulate Mcl-1 by disrupting the transcriptional regulatory apparatus (e.g., P-TEFb) *via* inhibiting the phosphorylation of the carboxy-terminal domain (CTD) of RNA Pol II (88–90). Analogous phenomenon has also found in the case of Mcl-1 down-regulation by B-Raf or MEK1/2 inhibitors (86, 91), or Bcl-xL down-regulation by PI3K/AKT inhibitors (92). An alternative approach is to up-regulate pro-apoptotic proteins (e.g., Bim) that prime tumor cells (e.g., by pre-occupying or saturating anti-apoptotic proteins) for death induced by Bcl-2 inhibitors (93). For example, HDAC inhibitors can up-regulate Bim in transformed cells (94), thus potentiating the activity of Bcl-2 inhibitors (95). Similarly, MEK1/2 and proteasome inhibitors prevent phosphorylation and following UPS-mediated degradation of Bim, thereby synergistically interacting with Bcl-2 inhibitors in hematologic malignancies (e.g., MM and lymphoma) (43, 96, 97).

Because the majority of targeted agents have multiple targets, attempts to understand the basis for interactions between them have been hindered by their complexity. Nevertheless, due to a variety of factors (e.g., the development of resistance or the presence or emergence of compensatory survival pathways), the need to interrupt two or more such pathways to achieve meaningful clinical benefits is now generally acknowledged. In addition, up-regulated expression of targeted oncogenic proteins also contributes to acquired resistance as observed in the case of mutant RTK-driven malignancies (1). Conventional strategies to circumvent this mechanism of acquired resistance include increasing drug doses, optimizing dosing schedules, or developing more potent next-generation kinase inhibitors active against mutant oncoproteins (55). However, these approaches may not be efficient enough, at least in certain circumstances, to overcome such a target-dependent mechanism of resistance. In this scenario, DTT combining targeted agents with inhibitors of other relevant targets/pathways *via* parallel inhibition provide an alternative, probably more effective, strategy to circumvent this resistance mechanism.

Linear Inhibition

An alternative approach for overcoming resistance is to inhibit multiple targets involving two or more "orthogonal" pathways. In the other words, it attacks critical targets downstream of the primary target or its *de novo* mutant form, therefore circumventing target-independent (non-genetic) resistance (56). Such a DTT approach can be considered a "linear inhibition" strategy, which either improves the anti-tumor efficacy of targeted therapy (e.g., TKIs) or more importantly, overcomes its acquired resistance *via* a bypass mechanism. Linear inhibition often refers to blockade of a single pathway at two or more separate sites. For example, DTT can lower the threshold for cell death triggered by the primary targeted agent by inhibiting additional survival- or proliferation-regulatory pathways. In this case, dual inhibition of the driver oncogene and its downstream target (e.g., anti-apoptotic proteins of the Bcl-2 family), which is required for survival of tumor cells under oncogene-related stress (e.g., oxidative, replicative, metabolic, etc.) or in response to inhibition of the primary target, could yield a synergistic effect in both sensitive and resistant cells (98).

Clinical observations have shed light on the reciprocal nature of resistance versus sensitivity to targeted agents in a linear manner. For example, CML with overexpression and activation of other kinases (e.g., the Src family kinases such as Lyn, Hck, and Fyn) at downstream signaling cascade of BCR-ABL signaling are likely resistant to TKIs directed against BCR-ABL (99). Furthermore, these Src family kinases can phosphorylate BCR-ABL to alter its oncogenicity, a positive feedback to amplify this oncogenic signal. Thus, increased expression and activity of the downstream kinases of targeted oncoproteins may play an important role in determining the clinical response to TKIs and patient outcome. This may provide an explanation for the fact that multi-kinase inhibitors often display better activity against TKI-sensitive and -resistant tumor cells than those targeting only one kinase. For example, dasatinib, a dual-specific TKI targeting both BCR-ABL and the Src family kinases (e.g., Lyn) (26) is active against both imatinib-sensitive and -resistant CML *via* target-dependent or -independent mechanisms (99). In the latter, Lyn up-regulation and activation are associated with expression of Bcl-2, which is often silenced in BCR-ABL-positive CML cells, which in turn confers imatinib resistance (100). Thus, Bcl-2 inhibitors are able to overcome this form of imatinib resistance, suggesting a shift of oncogene addiction from BCR-ABL to Bcl-2 in these imatinib-resistant CML cells. Because Bcl-2 is a crucial survival factor for CML stem cells that are not addicted to BCR-ABL (26, 101), the most important factor for disease recurrence and TKI resistance (102), DTT targeting both RTK (e.g., BCR-ABL) and Bcl-2 thus represents a rational approach to circumvent acquired TKI resistance (100, 101). Other examples include simultaneous inhibition of PI3K and AKT or mTOR (103), inhibition of BCR/ABL and its downstream targets (e.g., Aurora kinase A and PLK-1) (30, 31), EGFR and MEK1/2 inhibitors (20), etc.

HDAC inhibitors, a class of epigenetic therapeutics, are truly pleiotropic agents that exert their anti-tumor activity through diverse mechanisms, including up-regulation of death receptors, generation of reactive oxygen species (ROS), disruption of multiple cell cycle checkpoints and DNA repair processes, down-regulation of survival-related proteins, and induction of pro-apoptotic proteins, among many others (104–106). Based on their multifaceted functions, it is not surprising that HDAC inhibitors have been shown to interact synergistically with multiple targeted agents as well as more conventional therapeutics, therefore representing an ideal candidate for the development of DTT (parallel or linear inhibition) (106, 107). A prototypical example for linear inhibition is activation of the NF-κB pathway as a compensatory response to HDAC inhibition. HDACs are responsible for deacetylation of multiple histones (primarily involving transcriptional regulation of gene expression) as well as numerous non-histone proteins involving cell cycle, DDR, DNA repair, cellular signaling, apoptosis, autophagy, RNA processing and stability, protein folding and aggregation, etc. (108). In this case, HDAC has also been named as lysine (K) deacetylase (KDAC). Among multiple proteins involved in cell survival decisions (105, 109), one such protein is RelA/p65, the most abundant component of the canonical NF-κB pathway, which plays an important role in drug resistance (acquired in particular) involving both solid tumor and hematologic malignancies (110, 111). Under basal conditions, RelA is bound by IκBα and sequestered in the cytoplasm, thus keeping the NF-κB pathway inactivated. Upon stimulation (e.g., by TNF-α), the activation of the IKK complex (consisting of IKKα/IKK1, IKKβ/IKK2, and IKKγ/NEMO) results in IKKβ phosphorylation (activation), which in turn phosphorylates IκBα and leads to its degradation *via* the UPS (112). This unleashes RelA, which then translocates into the nucleus where it is acetylated by histone (or lysine) acetyltransferases (HATs or KATs) and exerts its role as a transcription factor. RelA is then deacetylated by nuclear HDACs (e.g., HDAC1-3), an event required for binding of *de novo* synthesized IκBα and thus its nuclear export (113), as RelA itself lacks a nuclear export sequence. This process accounts for terminating NF-κB signal, thus making NF-κB activation as a short-term and reversible response in the case of TNF-α. However, hyperacetylation of RelA due to failure of its deacetylation (e.g., by HDAC inhibitors) leads to sustained NF-κB activation as observed in leukemic cells exposed to HDAC inhibitors (114), which in turn limits anti-tumor activity of HDAC inhibitors (115). Moreover, exposure to HDAC inhibitors also increases RelA phosphorylation (e.g., S365), an event mediated by IKKβ, which promotes its nuclear entry and susceptibility for acetylation by HATs (116). Notably, disruption of such compensatory NF-κB activation at either upstream (e.g., by IKK inhibitors that block phosphorylation of both IκBα and RelA) or downstream sites (e.g., by proteasome inhibitors that prevent IκBα degradation) interferes with RelA acetylation and nuclear import, resulting in down-regulation of NF-κB-dependent genes such as XIAP, cIAP1/2, Bcl-xL, and SOD2 (115–119). This intervention markedly increases the lethal action of HDAC inhibitors, suggesting another linear inhibition-based DTT approach (**Figure 3**). One of the examples for this approach is the combination of the HDAC inhibitor panobinostat and the proteasome inhibitor bortezomib, which has been approved to treat relapsed and refractory MM that are resistant to front-line therapy in virtually all cases. Similar phenomenon has also been observed in other hematologic malignancies (e.g., CLL and AML) when either pan-HDAC or class I HDAC inhibitors are utilized) (120, 121).

It is worth noting that DTT may be particularly appropriate when inhibition of a single component of the targeting pathway is incomplete and insufficient to trigger cell death. In this case, simultaneous interruption of this pathway at a second, downstream site may reduce survival signals below the threshold necessary to support survival. However, interruption of such a pathway at both upstream and downstream sites may be redundant, and could, at least theoretically, be counterproductive. For example, the lethal consequence of interruption of an upstream node may depend upon signaling imbalances stemming from activation of downstream targets. Thus, interruption of such conflicting signals could instead potentially attenuate the lethal consequences.

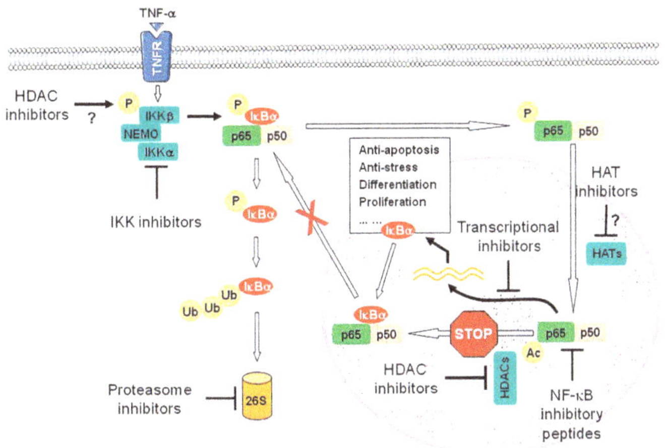

FIGURE 3 | An example for the DTT approach *via* linear inhibition. While HDAC inhibitors exhibit anti-tumor activity *via* multiple mechanisms of action, exposure to HDAC inhibitors however activates the NF-κB pathway *via* post-translational modifications of RelA/p65, a major component of this critical survival pathway, including phosphorylation mediated by IKKβ (the mechanism for IKK activation by HDAC inhibitors remains unclear) and then acetylation mediated by HATs, but failure of its deacetylation due to inhibition of nuclear HDACs (e.g., HDAC1-3). Hyperacetylation of RelA/p65 prevents its nuclear export *via* binding of *de novo* synthesized IκBα, a downstream gene of NF-κB, resulting in sustained activation of NF-κB signal and therefore counteracting the lethal action of HDAC inhibitors. Thus, a DTT approach *via* linear inhibition of this non-genetic survival pathway at multiple sites can eliminate such an "off-target" effect of HDAC inhibitors and improve their efficacy as anti-tumor epigenetic therapy, though HDAC inhibitors often display limited single-agent activity. Disruption of these sites could involve IKK inhibitors that block phosphorylation of both IκBα and RelA/p65 (preventing IκBα degradation *via* the UPS and subsequent RelA/p65 entering into the nucleus), proteasome inhibitors that block proteasomal degradation of IκBα, (thus sequestering RelA/p65 in the cytoplasm), transcriptional inhibitors (e.g., inhibitors of CDK7 and CDK9) that block the expression of NF-κB-dependent genes), inhibitory peptides directly targeting RelA/p65 or its partner p50, and probably HAT inhibitors that block acetylation of RelA/p65. P, phosphorylation; Ub, ubiquitination; Ac, acetylation; 26S, 26S proteasome.

CONCLUSION AND FUTURE DIRECTIONS

To date, the bulk of evidence suggests that targeting a single oncogenic target or pathway would most likely be insufficient to achieve meaningful clinical responses and long-term survival of patients with most cancer types, despite a few exceptions (e.g., BCR/ABL inhibitors in CML and EGFR or ALK inhibitors in NSCLC). Diverse DTT approaches combining a targeted agent with another targeted agent, chemotherapy, or immunotherapy have been required for effective treatment and even cures of cancer (56), including hematologic malignancies such as diffuse large B-cell lymphoma (DLBCL), Hodgkin's lymphoma, acute myeloid and lymphoid leukemia, and MM. Although it seems logic that targeted agents may have the capacity to enhance the activity of conventional cytotoxic agents, results with this strategy have not yet realized their potential. On the other hand, the rational combination of targeted agents, particularly those targeting complementary survival signaling or cell cycle regulatory pathways, in a parallel or linear inhibition manner, represents another promising DTT approach (**Table 1**). The notion of targeting two or more survival pathways specifically implicated in transformation offers the prospect of personalized therapy and the potential for therapeutic selectivity.

According to our and others' experience, optimization of a DTT approach requires addressing a number of unanswered questions. Among them, a key question is whether a targeted agent should have single agent activity in a particular disease in order to be of benefit in a DTT regimen. It is conceivable, although not formally proven yet, that a targeted agent inactive alone may also be able to potentiate the activity of another targeted agent if it disables a critical compensatory pathway. For example, while the HDAC inhibitor panobinostat does not show single agent activity in MM, it however enhances the efficacy of the proteasome inhibitor bortezomib in this setting, a DTT regimen approved to treat relapsed MM. Another key question is what a role of targeted agents that disrupts so-called "orthogonal" pathways downstream of driver oncogenes should play in the DTT strategies. They may ameliorate the otherwise lethal effects of oxidative, proteotoxic, DNA damage-related and other forms of stress due to the activation of oncogenes such as RAS and c-Myc. Although such inhibitors may not be as specific as those directly targeting oncoproteins that drive transformation (e.g., BCR/ABL in CML, FLT3 mutations in AML, and EGFR mutation or EML4-ALK fusion protein in NSCLC), they may disrupt the mechanisms required for maintaining survival of transformed cells and thus play an important adjunctive role in various DTT approaches. Notably, unlike in the case of TKIs, the mechanisms for drug resistance (either intrinsic or acquired) to non-TKI agents (e.g., proteasome inhibitors and IMiDs, the frontline therapy in MM treatment) remain largely unclear, most likely involving diverse and even more complicated non-genetic mechanisms (162, 163), although multiple DTT regimens (with undefined mechanisms for synergism) have already be successfully used in clinical practice.

TABLE 1 | Dual-targeted therapy (DDT) in hematologic malignancies and other cancers.

DDT strategy	Targeting pathway	MOA	Cancer type	Refs
Chk1/Wee1 inhibitor-based combinations				
Chk1 inhibitors + MEK inhibitors, FTIs, or Src inhibitors	DNA damage checkpoint & Ras/Raf/MEK/ERK pathway	Prevention of Bim phosphorylation and degradation; promotion of DNA damage; targeting myeloma stem cells; anti-angiogenesis; disrupting Ras farnesylation; activation of SEK1/JNK pathway	AML, MM, glioblastoma, breast, prostate	(70–78, 122–127)
Chk1 or Wee1 inhibitors + HDAC inhibitors	Epigenetic regulation & DNA damage checkpoints	DDR inhibition; disruption of DNA replication	AML	(63, 64)
Chk1 inhibitors + PARP1 inhibitors	DNA damage checkpoints & DNA repair	Potentiation of DNA damage	Breast, ovarian	(69, 128, 129)
HDAC inhibitor-based combinations				
HDAC inhibitors + DNMT inhibitors	DNA methylation & histone acetylation	Dual inhibition of HDACs and DNMTs; targeting CSCs	AML (approved), breast	(130, 131)
HDAC inhibitors + NAE inhibitors	DNA damage checkpoint & NEDD8	NF-κB inhibition; Bim up-regulation; inhibition of DNA repair	AML	(79)
HDAC inhibitors + TRAIL	Epigenetic regulation & extrinsic apoptotic cascade	Upregulation of DR4 and DR5	AML	(44, 132)
HDAC inhibitors + TKIs	Epigenetic regulation & oncogenic signaling	Disruption of chaperone function; overcoming TKI resistance	AML, CML, lung	(133–138)
HDAC inhibitors + Aurora kinase inhibitors	Epigenetic regulation & cell cycle	Potentiation of aurora kinase inhibition; overcoming TKI resistance	CML, kidney	(30, 139)
HDAC inhibitors + CDK inhibitors	Epigenetic regulation & cell cycle	Downregulation of Mcl-1 and p21^{CIP1} *via* inhibition of RNA Pol II	AML	(140, 141)
HDAC inhibitors + IKK inhibitors	Epigenetic regulation & NF-κB pathway	Prevention of NF-κB activation by blocking RelA acetylation	AML, MM	(115, 116)
HDAC inhibitors + Bcl-2 antagonists	Epigenetic regulation & apoptosis-regulatory pathway	Up-regulation and reactivation of Bim; autophagy inhibition	AML, MM	(51, 82, 95)
HDAC inhibitors + HSP90 antagonists	Epigenetic regulation & HSP90	p21^{CIP1} upregulation; Mcl-1 downregulation; inhibition of Bcr/Abl and its downstream STAT5	AML, CML	(142, 143)
HDAC inhibitors + IAP antagonists	Non-canonical NF-κB pathway & extrinsic apoptotic cascade	NF-κB inhibition; caspase 8 activation	MM	(46)
HDAC inhibitors + MLL-menin antagonists	DNA damage checkpoint & MLL-menin interaction	Disruption of DNA damage checkpoint and DNA repair	AML	(144)
Proteasome inhibitor-based combinations				
Proteasome inhibitors + HDAC inhibitors	UPS & epigenetic regulation	NF-κB inhibition; aggresome disruption; ER stress; Bim upregulation; ROS	MM (approved), CLL, ALL pancreatic cancer	(119–121, 145–148)
Proteasome inhibitors + CDK inhibitors	UPS & cell cycle	Bim upregulation; SAPK/JNK activation; NF-κB inhibition; Induction of ER stress	CML, AML, MM	(117, 149–151)
Proteasome inhibitors + Bcl-2 antagonists	UPS & apoptosis-regulatory pathway	Mcl-1 downregulation; SAPK/JNK activation; BAK activation; ROS	MM, MCL, DLBCL,CLL	(43, 96, 152, 153)
Proteasome inhibitors + IAP antagonist	UPS & cIAPs	Inhibition of canonical and non-canonical NF-κB pathways; Bcl-xL downregulation	MM	(58)
Proteasome inhibitors + XPO-1 inhibitor	UPS & NF-κB pathway	Nuclear localization of IκBα; overcome drug resistance	MM (approved)	(154, 155)
Bcl-2 antagonist-based combinations				
Bcl-2 antagonists + MEK inhibitors	Apoptosis-regulatory pathway & Ras/Raf/MEK/ERK pathway	Downregulation of Mcl-1	AML,	(86)

(Continued)

TABLE 1 | Continued

DDT strategy	Targeting pathway	MOA	Cancer type	Refs
Bcl-2 antagonists + CDK inhibitors	Apoptosis- or autophagy-regulatory pathways & transcription-regulatory machinery	Mcl-1 downregulation by RNA Pol II inhibition; down-regulation of SQSTM1/p62 (inefficient autophagy); up-regulation of pro-apoptotic BH3-only proteins; BAK/BAX activation; ROS; JNK activation	AML, MM	(51, 85, 87, 89, 90, 97, 156)
Bcl-2 inhibitors + sorafenib	Apoptosis-regulatory pathways & oncogenic signaling	Mcl-1 downregulation; Bim upregulation	AML	(157)
Bcl-2 inhibitors + TKIs	Apoptosis-regulatory pathways & oncogenic signaling	Overcoming TKI resistance; Lyn inhibition; targeting CSCs	CML, Ph+ ALL	(100, 101, 158)
MEK inhibitor-based combinations				
MEK inhibitors + TKI	Ras/Raf/MEK/ERK pathway & Bcr/Abl	Co-inhibition of Bcr/Abl downstream signals	CML	(159)
MEK inhibitors + AKT/mTOR inhibitors	Ras/Raf/MEK/ERK pathway & P13K/AKT/mTOR pathway	Prevention of feedback ERK activation; prevention of BAD degradation; Bim upregulation	AML, Prostate cancer, breast cancer, melanoma, colon cancer, glioblastoma	(20, 22, 41, 57)
MEK inhibitors + proteasome inhibitors	Ras/Raf/MEK/ERK pathway & UPS	ERK inhibition; RANKL inhibition	MM	(160)
MEK inhibitors + sorafenib	Ras/Raf/MEK/ERK pathway	Bim upregulation; Mcl-1 downregulation	DLBCL	(161)

MOA, mechanism of action; DDR, DNA damage response; HDAC, histone deacetylase; DNMT, DNA methyltransferase; CDK, cyclin-dependent kinase; NAE, NEDD8 activating enzyme; TKI, tyrosine kinase inhibitor; CSC, cancer stem cell; AML, acute myeloid leukemia, CML, chronic myeloid leukemia; MM, multiple myeloma, MCL, mantle cell lymphoma; DLBCL, diffuse large B-cell lymphoma; CLL, chronic lymphocytic leukemia; ALL, acute lymphoblastic leukemia.

The bulk of attention in this area of DTT has focused on the simultaneous interruption of two complementary survival pathways to achieve enhanced efficacy of targeted therapy thus far. However, some of the successful DTT approaches have involved more than two agents e.g., R-CHOP in DLBCL and several triplet regimens in MM. In this case, emerging evidence suggests that simultaneous interruption of more than two pathways may be required for maximal cell killing of transformed cells, or in the other words, to reduce the size of minimal residue disease (MRD), a main cause for disease recurrence (15). A future paradigm for such a DTT approach may combine targeted agents with more than two separate but somehow complementary mechanisms of action involving both linear and parallel inhibition, such as an inhibitor directly targeting oncoprotein (e.g., TKI) in conjunction with an inhibitor targeting potential compensatory survival pathway (parallel inhibition) and an inhibitor of an "orthogonal" pathway (linear inhibition).

Last, a curative approach may ultimately depend upon the eradication of both tumor cells (e.g., leukemic blasts) and cancer stem cells (CSCs e.g., leukemia-initiating cells) (164). Notably, CSCs seem not to addict to the oncogenic target or pathway for transformation (e.g., BCR/ABL for CML blasts but not CSCs) (165) but depend upon their unique survival pathways (166, 167). Indeed, a DTT approach combining inhibitors of such pathways for CSC survival and maintenance with agents targeting oncoproteins directly implicated in oncogenesis may yield results superior to those obtained with either agent alone or may overcome both genetic and non-genetic resistance (164, 167). A logical extension of this DTT approach would be to incorporate inhibitors of CSC-related pathways into the multi-agent regimens targeting two or more pathways described above. It is also worth mentioning that although resistance (either intrinsic or acquired) to immunotherapy (particularly immune checkpoint inhibitors such as PD-1 and PD-L1 MoAbs) has its unique mechanisms (e.g., those related to immune response and its regulatory machineries) (168), the principle of diverse resistance mechanisms and DTT approaches discussed above may also be implicated in this novel type of "targeted" therapy. Non-genetic mechanisms may also contribute to resistance to novel forms of targeted agents (e.g., PROTACs that act to degrade, rather than inhibit, targeted proteins) (169). In addition, with recent applications of single-cell sequencing techniques, dissection of intratumoral heterogeneity has helped identify distinctive targets and pathways in different clusters (clones) of tumor cells within the same tumor (170, 171). On the one hand, this could explain why many agents targeting a single oncoprotein (even though it drives malignant transformation or oncogenesis) presumably existed in dominant clones are not sufficient enough to kill the meaningful number of tumor cells. On the other hand, it provides a great opportunity for developing the DTT approaches that target multiple oncoproteins or survival pathways existed in different clones to achieve maximal killing of tumor cells. Given the large number of agents capable of inhibiting numerous targets currently available, DTT (linear or parallel inhibition, or both) may offer a chance of achieving the best response and long-lasting remissions or even cures of some cancer types, especially hematologic malignancies, otherwise considered fatal. Future progress in this effort is awaited with considerable anticipation.

AUTHOR CONTRIBUTIONS

YD and FJ conceptualized, wrote, edited, and revised the manuscript. YD and WW gathered and analyzed the literatures, and prepared the figures. YS and XL contributed to literature search and collection. SKK contributed to writing, editing, and revising the manuscript. All authors contributed to the article and approved the submitted version.

REFERENCES

Braun TP, Eide CA, Druker BJ. Response and Resistance to BCR-ABL1- Targeted Therapies. *Cancer Cell* (2020) 37:530–42. doi: 10.1016/ j.ccell.2020.03.006

de The H. Differentiation Therapy Revisited. *Nat Rev Cancer* (2018) 18:117– 27. doi: 10.1038/nrc.2017.103

Bedard PL, Hyman DM, Davids MS, Siu LL. Small Molecules, Big Impact: 20 Years of Targeted Therapy in Oncology. *Lancet* (2020) 395:1078–88. doi: 10.1016/ S0140-6736(20)30164-1

Orlando E, Aebersold DM, Medová M, Zimmer Y. Oncogene Addiction as a Foundation of Targeted Cancer Therapy: The Paradigm of the MET Receptor Tyrosine Kinase. *Cancer Lett* (2019) 443:189–202. doi: 10.1016/ j.canlet.2018.12.001

Hanahan D, Weinberg RA. The Hallmarks of Cancer. *Cell* (2000) 100:57–70. doi: 10.1016/s0092-8674(00)81683-9

Luo J, Solimini NL, Elledge SJ. Principles of Cancer Therapy: Oncogene and Non-Oncogene Addiction. *Cell* (2009) 136:823–37. doi: 10.1016/ j.cell.2009.02.024

Hanahan D. Hallmarks of Cancer: New Dimensions. *Cancer Discov* (2022) 12:31–46. doi: 10.1158/2159-8290.CD-21-1059

Vaux DL, Cory S, Adams JM. Bcl-2 Gene Promotes Haemopoietic Cell Survival and Cooperates With C-Myc to Immortalize Pre-B Cells. *Nature* (1988) 335:440–2. doi: 10.1038/335440a0

Lim Z-F, Ma PC. Emerging Insights of Tumor Heterogeneity and Drug Resistance Mechanisms in Lung Cancer Targeted Therapy. *J Hematol Oncol* (2019) 12:134. doi: 10.1186/s13045-019-0818-2

Aleksakhina SN, Kashyap A, Imyanitov EN. Mechanisms of Acquired Tumor Drug Resistance. *Biochim Biophys Acta Rev Cancer* (2019) 1872:188310. doi: 10.1016/j.bbcan.2019.188310

Michael JV, Goldfinger LE. Concepts and Advances in Cancer Therapeutic Vulnerabilities in RAS Membrane Targeting. *Semin Cancer Biol* (2019) 54:121–30. doi: 10.1016/j.semcancer.2017.11.021

Lovly CM, Shaw AT. Molecular Pathways: Resistance to Kinase Inhibitors and Implications for Therapeutic Strategies. *Clin Cancer Res* (2014) 20:2249–56. doi: 10.1158/1078-0432.CCR-13-1610

Holohan C, Van Schaeybroeck S, Longley DB, Johnston PG. Cancer Drug Resistance: An Evolving Paradigm. *Nat Rev Cancer* (2013) 13:714–26. doi: 10.1038/nrc3599

Chatterjee N, Bivona TG. Polytherapy and Targeted Cancer Drug Resistance. *Trends Cancer* (2019) 5: 170 – 82. doi: 10 .1016 / j.trecan.2019.02.003

Vasan N, Baselga J, David M, Hyman DM. A View on Drug Resistance in Cancer. *Nature* (2019) 575:299–309. doi: 10.1038/s41586-019-1730-1

Wang X, Zhang H, Chen X. Drug Resistance and Combating Drug Resistance in Cancer. *Cancer Drug Resist* (2019) 2:141–60. doi: 10.20517/ cdr.2019.10

Sharma SV, Bell DW, Settleman J, Haber DA. Epidermal Growth Factor Receptor Mutations in Lung Cancer. *Nat Rev Cancer* (2007) 7:169–81. doi: 10.1038/ nrc2088

Oxnard GR, Hu Y, Mileham KF, Husain H, Costa DB, Tracy P, et al. Assessment of Resistance Mechanisms and Clinical Implications in Patients With EGFR T790M-Positive Lung Cancer and Acquired Resistance to Osimertinib. *JAMA Oncol* (2018) 4:1527–34. doi: 10.1001/jamaoncol.2018.2969

Raponi M, Winkler H, Dracopoli NC. KRAS Mutations Predict Response to EGFR Inhibitors. *Curr Opin Pharmacol* (2008) 8:413–8. doi: 10.1016/ j.coph.2008.06.006

She QB, Solit DB, Ye Q, O'Reilly KE, Lobo J, Rosen N. The BAD Protein Integrates Survival Signaling by EGFR/MAPK and PI3K/Akt Kinase Pathways in PTEN-Deficient Tumor Cells. *Cancer Cell* (2005) 8:287–97. doi: 10.1016/j. ccr.2005.09.006

Fruman DA, Rommel C. PI3K and Cancer: Lessons, Challenges and Opportunities. *Nat Rev Drug Discov* (2014) 13:140–56. doi: 10.1038/nrd4204

Kinkade CW, Castillo-Martin M, Puzio-Kuter A, Yan J, Foster TH, Gao H, et al. Targeting AKT/mTOR and ERK MAPK Signaling Inhibits Hormone-Refractory Prostate Cancer in a Preclinical Mouse Model. *J Clin Invest* (2008) 118:3051–64. doi: 10.1172/JCI34764

Timar J, Kashofer K. Molecular Epidemiology and Diagnostics of KRAS Mutations in Human Cancer. *Cancer Metastasis Rev* (2020) 39:1029–38. doi: 10.1007/ s10555-020-09915-5

Awad MM, Liu S, Rybkin II, Arbour KC, Dilly J, Zhu VW, et al. Acquired Resistance to KRASG12C Inhibition in Cancer. *N Engl J Med* (2021) 384:2382–93. doi: 10.1056/NEJMoa2105281

Gottesman MM, Lavi O, Hall MD, Gillet J-P. Toward a Better Understanding of the Complexity of Cancer Drug Resistance. *Annu Rev Pharmacol Toxicol* (2016) 56:20.1–20.18. doi: 10.1146/annurev-pharmtox- 010715-103111

Jabbour E, Kantarjian H. Chronic Myeloid Leukemia: 2020 Update on Diagnosis, Therapy and Monitoring. *Am J Hematol* (2020) 95:691–709. doi: 10.1002/ ajh.25792

Shaikh M, Shinde Y, Pawara P, Noolvi M, Surana S, Ahmad I, et al. Emerging Approaches to Overcome Acquired Drug Resistance Obstacles to Osimertinib in Non-Small-Cell Lung Cancer. *J Med Chem* (2022) 65:1008- 46.. doi: 10.1021/ acs.jmedchem.1c00876

Piotrowska Z, Isozaki H, Lennerz JK, Gainor JF, Lennes IF, Zhu VW, et al. Landscape of Acquired Resistance to Osimertinib in EGFR-Mutant NSCLC and Clinical Validation of Combined EGFR and RET Inhibition With Osimertinib and BLU-667 for Acquired RET Fusion. *Cancer Discov* (2018) 8:1529–39. doi: 10.1158/2159-8290.CD-18-1022

Lau DK, Jenkins L, Weickhardt A. Mechanisms of Acquired Resistance to Fibroblast Growth Factor Receptor Targeted Therapy. *Cancer Drug Resist* (2019) 2:568–79. doi: 10.20517/cdr.2019.42

Dai Y, Chen S, Venditti CA, Pei X-Y, Nguyen TK, Dent P, et al. Vorinostat Synergistically Potentiates MK-0457 Lethality in Chronic Myelogenous Leukemia Cells Sensitive and Resistant to Imatinib Mesylate. *Blood* (2008) 112:793–804. doi: 10.1182/blood-2007-10-116376

Gleixner KV, Ferenc V, Peter B, Gruze A, Meyer RA, Hadzijusufovic E, et al. Polo-Like Kinase 1 (Plk1) as a Novel Drug Target in Chronic Myeloid Leukemia: Overriding Imatinib Resistance With the Plk1 Inhibitor BI 2536. *Cancer Res* (2010) 70:1513–23. doi: 10.1158/0008-5472.CAN-09-2181

Giles FJ, Swords RT, Nagler A, Hochhaus A, Ottmann OG, DA Rizzieri DA, et al. MK-0457, an Aurora Kinase and BCR–ABL Inhibitor, is Active in Patients With BCR–ABL T315I Leukemia. *Leukemia* (2013) 27:113–7. doi: 10.1038/ leu.2012.186

Choong GM, Cullen GD, O'Sullivan CC. Evolving Standards of Care and New Challenges in the Management of HER2-Positive Breast Cancer. *CA Cancer J Clin* (2020) 70:355–74. doi: 10.3322/caac.21634

Ma L, Shan Y, Bai R, Xue L, Eide CA, Ou J, et al. A Therapeutically Targetable Mechanism of BCR-ABL Independent Imatinib Resistance in Chronic Myeloid Leukemia. *Sci Transl Med* (2014) 6:252ra121. doi: 10.1126/ scitranslmed.3009073

Marusyk A, Janiszewska M, Polyak K. Intratumor Heterogeneity: The Rosetta Stone of Therapy Resistance. *Cancer Cell* (2020) 37:471–84. doi: 10.1016/j. ccell.2020.03.007

Laramy JK, Kim M, Parrish KE, Sarkaria JN, Elmquist WF. Pharmacokinetic Assessment of Cooperative Efflux of the Multitargeted Kinase Inhibitor Ponatinib Across the Blood-Brain Barrier. *J Pharmacol Exp Ther* (2018) 365:249–61. doi: 10.1124/jpet.117.246116

Basu A. The Interplay Between Apoptosis and Cellular Senescence: Bcl-2 Family Proteins as Targets for Cancer Therapy. *Pharmacol Ther* (2022) 230:107943.. doi: 10.1016/j.pharmthera.2021.107943

Wang H, Guo M, Wei H, Chen Y. Targeting MCL-1 in Cancer: Current Status and Perspectives. *J Hematol Oncol* (2021) 14:67. doi: 10.1186/s13045- 021-01079-1

Green DR. At the Gates of Death. *Cancer Cell* (2006) 9:328–30. doi: 10.1016/ j.ccr.2006.05.004

Watanabe D, Nogami A, Okada K, Akiyama H, Umezawa Y, Miura O. FLT3-ITD Activates RSK1 to Enhance Proliferation and Survival of AML Cells by Activating Mtorc1 and Eif4b Cooperatively With PIM or PI3K and by Inhibiting Bad and BIM. *Cancers (Basel)* (2019) 11:1827. doi: 10.3390/ cancers11121827

Carracedo A, Ma L, Teruya-Feldstein J, Rojo F, Salmena L, Alimonti A, et al. Inhibition of Mtorc1 Leads to MAPK Pathway Activation Through a PI3K-Dependent Feedback Loop in Human Cancer. *J Clin Invest* (2008) 118:3065– 74. doi: 10.1172/JCI34739

Han Z, Liang J, Li Y, He J. Drugs and Clinical Approaches Targeting the Antiapoptotic Protein: A Review. *BioMed Res Int* (2019) 2019:1212369. doi: 10.1155/2019/1212369

Pei XY, Dai Y, Grant S. The Proteasome Inhibitor Bortezomib Promotes

Mitochondrial Injury and Apoptosis Induced by the Small Molecule Bcl-2 Inhibitor HA14-1 in Multiple Myeloma Cells. *Leukemia* (2003) 17:2036–45. doi: 10.1038/sj.leu.2403109

Insinga A, Monestiroli S, Ronzoni S, Gelmetti V, Marchesi F, Viale A, et al. Inhibitors of Histone Deacetylases Induce Tumor-Selective Apoptosis Through Activation of the Death Receptor Pathway. *Nat Med* (2005) 11:71–6. doi: 10.1038/nm1160

Dai Y, Dent P, Grant S. Tumor Necrosis Factor-Related Apoptosis-Inducing Ligand (TRAIL) Promotes Mitochondrial Dysfunction and Apoptosis Induced by 7-Hydroxystaurosporine and Mitogen-Activated Protein Kinase Kinase Inhibitors in Human Leukemia Cells That Ectopically Express Bcl-2 and Bcl-xL. *Mol Pharmacol* (2003) 64:1402–9. doi: 10.1124/ mol.64.6.1402

Zhou L, Zhang Y, Meads MB, Dai Y, Ning Y, Hu X, et al. LCL161 Interacts Synergystically With Panobinostat in Multiple Myeloma Cells Through non-Canonical NF-*k*B- and Caspase-8-Dependent Mechanisms. *Blood Adv* (2021) 5:3776–88. doi: 10.1182/bloodadvances.2020003597

Chen X, Zeh HJ, Kang R, Kroemer G, Tang D. Cell Death in Pancreatic Cancer: From Pathogenesis to Therapy. *Nat Rev Gastroenterol Hepatol* (2021) 18:804–23. doi: 10.1038/s41575-021-00486-6

Ye L, Jin F, Kumar SK, Dai Y. The Mechanisms and Therapeutic Targets of Ferroptosis in Cancer. *Expert Opin Ther Targets* (2021) 25:965–86. doi: 10.1080/14728222.2021.2011206

Zhao YG, Codogno P, Zhang H. Machinery, Regulation and Pathophysiological Implications of Autophagosome Maturation. *Nat Rev Mol Cell Biol* (2021) 22:733–50. doi: 10.1038/s41580-021-00392-4

Dai Y, Grant S. BCL2L11/Bim as a Dual-Agent Regulating Autophagy and Apoptosis in Drug Resistance. *Autophagy* (2015) 11:416–8. doi: 10.1080/ 15548627.2014.998892

Chen S, Zhang Y, Zhou L, Leng Y, Lin H, Kmieciak M, et al. A Bim- Targeting Strategy Overcomes Adaptive Bortezomib-Resistance in Multiple Myeloma Through a Novel Link Between Autophagy and Apoptosis. *Blood* (2014) 124:2687–97. doi: 10.1182/blood-2014-03-564534

Chen S, Zhou L, Zhang Y, Leng Y, Pei X-Y, Lin H, et al. Targeting SQSTM1/ p62 Induces Cargo-Loading Failure and Converts Autophagy to Apoptosis *Via* NBK/Bik. *Mol Cell Biol* (2014) 34:3435–49. doi: 10.1128/MCB.01383-13

Paskeh MDA, Entezari M, Clark C, Zabolian A, Ranjbar E, Farahani MV, et al. Targeted Regulation of Autophagy Using Nanoparticles: New Insight Into Cancer Therapy. *Biochim Biophys Acta Mol Basis Dis* (2021) 1868:166326. doi: 10.1016/j.bbadis.2021.166326

Ward RA, Fawell S, Floc'h N, Flemington V, McKerrecher D, Smith PD. Challenges and Opportunities in Cancer Drug Resistance. *Chem Rev* (2021) 121:3297–351. doi: 10.1021/acs.chemrev.0c00383

Cree IA, Charlton P. Molecular Chess? Hallmarks of Anti-Cancer Drug Resistance. *BMC Cancer* (2017) 17:10. doi: 10.1186/s12885-016-2999-1

Sabnis AJ, Bivona TG. Principles of Resistance to Targeted Cancer Therapy: Lessons From Basic and Translational Cancer Biology. *Trends Mol Med* (2019) 25:185–97. doi: 10.1016/j.molmed.2018.12.009

Rahmani M, Anderson A, Habibi JR, Crabtree TR, Mayo M, Harada H, et al. The BH3-Only Protein Bim Plays a Critical Role in Leukemia Cell Death Triggered by Concomitant Inhibition of the PI3K/Akt and MEK/ERK1/2 Pathways. *Blood* (2009) 114:4507–16. doi: 10.1182/blood-2008-09-177881

Zhou L, Zhang Y, Leng Y, Dai Y, Kmieciak M, Kramer L, et al. The IAP Antagonist Birinapant Potentiates Bortezomib Anti-Myeloma Activity *In Vitro* and *In Vivo*. *J Hematol Oncol* (2019) 12:25. doi: 10.1186/s13045-019- 0713-x

Yang T, Liu X, Kumar SK, Jin F, Dai Y. Decoding DNA Methylation in Epigenetics of Multiple Myeloma. *Blood Rev* (2022) 51:100872. doi: 10.1016/ j.blre.2021.100872

Yang C, Zhang J, Ma Y, Wu C, Cui W, Wang L. Histone Methyltransferase and Drug Resistance in Cancers. *J Exp Clin Cancer Res* (2020) 39:173. doi: 10.1186/ s13046-020-01682-z

Wu PK, Becker A, Park JI. Growth Inhibitory Signaling of the Raf/ MEK/ERK Pathway. *Int J Mol Sci* (2020) 21:5436. doi: 10.3390/ ijms21155436

Dai Y, Pei XY, Rahmani M, Conrad DH, Dent P, Grant S. Interruption of the NF-kappaB Pathway by Bay 11-7082 Promotes UCN-01-Mediated Mitochondrial Dysfunction and Apoptosis in Human Multiple Myeloma Cells. *Blood* (2004) 103:2761–70. doi: 10.1182/blood-2003-09-3037

Dai Y, Chen S, Kmieciak M, Zhou L, Lin H, Pei XY, et al. The Novel Chk1 Inhibitor MK-8776 Sensitizes Human Leukemia Cells to HDAC Inhibitors by Targeting the Intra-S Checkpoint and DNA Replication and Repair. *Mol Cancer Ther* (2013) 12:878–89. doi: 10.1158/1535-7163.MCT-12-0902

Zhou L, Zhang Y, Chen S, Kmieciak M, Leng Y, Lin H, et al. A Regimen Combining the Wee1 Inhibitor AZD1775 With HDAC Inhibitors Targets Human Acute Myeloid Leukemia Cells Harboring Various Genetic Mutations. *Leukemia* (2015) 29:807–18. doi: 10.1038/leu.2014.296

Sirbu BM, Cortez D. DNA Damage Response: Three Levels of DNA Repair Regulation. *Cold Spring Harb Perspect Biol* (2013) 5:a012724. doi: 10.1101/ cshperspect.a012724

Jia R, Kutzner L, Koren A, Runggatscher K, Májek P, Müller AC, et al. High-Throughput Drug Screening Identifies the ATR-CHK1 Pathway as a Therapeutic Vulnerability of CALR Mutated Hematopoietic Cells. *Blood Cancer J* (2021) 11:137. doi: 10.1038/s41408-021-00531-2

Mull BB, Livingston JA, Patel N, Bui T, Hunt KK, Keyomarsi K. Specific, Reversible G1 Arrest by UCN-01 *In Vivo* Provides Cytostatic Protection of Normal Cells Against Cytotoxic Chemotherapy in Breast Cancer. *Br J Cancer* (2020) 122:812–22. doi: 10.1038/s41416-019-0707-z

Klomp JE, Lee YS, Goodwin CM, Papke B, Klomp JA, Waters AM, et al. CHK1 Protects Oncogenic KRAS-Expressing Cells From DNA Damage and Is a Target for Pancreatic Cancer Treatment. *Cell Rep* (2021) 37:110060. doi: 10.1016/j. celrep.2021.110060

Chang HR, Jung E, Cho S, Jeon Y-J, Kim Y. Targeting non-Oncogene Addiction for Cancer Therapy. *Biomolecules* (2021) 11:129. doi: 10.3390/ biom11020129

Dai Y, Yu C, Singh V, Tang L, Wang Z, McInistry R, et al. Pharmacological Inhibitors of the Mitogen-Activated Protein Kinase (MAPK) Kinase/MAPK Cascade Interact Synergistically With UCN-01 to Induce Mitochondrial Dysfunction and Apoptosis in Human Leukemia Cells. *Cancer Res* (2001) 61:5106–15.

Dai Y, Landowski TH, Rosen ST, Dent P, Grant S. Combined Treatment With the Checkpoint Abrogator UCN-01 and MEK1/2 Inhibitors Potently Induces Apoptosis in Drug-Sensitive and -Resistant Myeloma Cells Through an IL-6-Independent Mechanism. *Blood* (2002) 100:3333–43. doi: 10.1182/ blood-2002-03-0940

Dai Y, Rahmani M, Pei XY, Khanna P, Han SI, Mitchell C, et al. Farnesyltransferase Inhibitors Interact Synergistically With the Chk1 Inhibitor UCN-01 to Induce Apoptosis in Human Leukemia Cells Through Interruption of Both Akt and MEK/ERK Pathways and Activation of SEK1/JNK. *Blood* (2005) 105:1706–16. doi: 10.1182/blood- 2004-07-2767

Pei XY, Dai Y, Rahmani M, Li W, Dent P, Grant S. The Farnesyltransferase Inhibitor L744832 Potentiates UCN-01-Induced Apoptosis in Human Multiple Myeloma Cells. *Clin Cancer Res* (2005) 11:4589–600. doi: 10.1158/1078-0432.CCR-04-2346

Dai Y, Khanna P, Chen S, Pei XY, Dent P, Grant S. Statins Synergistically Potentiate 7-Hydroxystaurosporine (UCN-01) Lethality in Human Leukemia and Myeloma Cells by Disrupting Ras Farnesylation and Activation. *Blood* (2007) 109:4415–23. doi: 10.1182/blood-2006-09-047076

Dai Y, Chen S, Shah R, Pei X-Y, Wang L, Almenara JA, et al. Disruption of Src Function Potentiates Chk1 Inhibitor-Induced Apoptosis in Human Multiple Myeloma Cells *In Vitro* and *In Vivo*. *Blood* (2011) 117:1947–57. doi: 10.1182/ blood-2010-06-291146

Pei X-Y, Dai Y, Youssefian LE, Chen S, Bodie WW, Takabatake Y, et al. Cytokinetically Quiescent (G0/G1) Human Multiple Myeloma Cells are Susceptible to Simultaneous Inhibition of Chk1 and MEK1/2. *Blood* (2011) 118:5189–200. doi: 10.1182/blood-2011-02-339432

Dai Y, Chen S, Pei X-Y, Almenara JA, Kramer LB, Venditti CA, et al. Interruption of the Ras/MEK/ERK Signaling Cascade Enhances Chk1 Inhibitor-Induced DNA Damage *In Vitro* and *In Vivo* in Human Multiple Myeloma Cells. *Blood* (2008) 112:2439–49. doi: 10.1182/blood-2008-05- 159392

Pei XY, Dai Y, Tenorio S, Lu J, Harada H, Dent P, et al. MEK1/2 Inhibitors Potentiate UCN-01 Lethality in Human Multiple Myeloma Cells Through a Bim-Dependent Mechanism. *Blood* (2007) 110:2092–101. doi: 10.1182/ blood-2007-04-083204

Zhou L, Chen S, Zhang Y, Kmieciak M, Leng Y, Li L, et al. The NAE Inhibitor Pevonedistat Interacts With the HDAC Inhibitor Belinostat to Target AML Cells by Disrupting the DDR. *Blood* (2016) 127:2219–30. doi: 10.1182/ blood-2015-06-653717

Dai Y, Grant S. Molecular Pathways Feature: New Insights Into Checkpoint Kinase 1 in the DNA Damage Response Signaling Network. *Clin Cancer Res* (2010) 16:376–83. doi: 10.1158/1078-0432.CCR-09-1029

Dent P, Tang Y, Yacoub A, Dai Y, Fisher PB, Grant S. CHK1 Inhibitors in Combination Chemotherapy: Thinking Beyond the Cell Cycle. *Mol Interv* (2011) 11:133–40. doi: 10.1124/mi.11.2.11

Chen K, Yang Q, Zha J, Deng M, Zhou Y, Fu G, et al. Preclinical Evaluation of a Regimen Combining Chidamide and ABT-199 in Acute Myeloid Leukemia. *Cell Death Dis* (2020) 11:778. doi: 10.1038/s41419-020-02972-2

Dai Y, Grant S. Targeting Multiple Arms of the Apoptotic Regulatory Machinery. *Cancer Res* (2007) 67:2908–11. doi: 10.1158/0008-5472.CAN- 07-0082

Deng J, Carlson N, Takeyama K, Cin PD, Shipp M, Letai A. BH3 Profiling Identifies Three Distinct Classes of Apoptotic Blocks to Predict Response to ABT-737 and Conventional Chemotherapeutic Agents. *Cancer Cell* (2007) 12:171–85. doi: 10.1016/j.ccr.2007.07.001

Chen S, Dai Y, Harada H, Dent P, Grant S. Mcl-1 Down-Regulation Potentiates ABT-

737 Lethality by Cooperatively Inducing Bak Activation and Bax Translocation. *Cancer Res* (2007) 67(2):782–91. doi: 10.1158/0008- 5472.CAN-06-3964

Konopleva M, Contractor R, Tsao T, Samudio I, Ruvolo PP, Kitada S, et al. Mechanisms of Apoptosis Sensitivity and Resistance to the BH3 Mimetic ABT-737 in Acute Myeloid Leukemia. *Cancer Cell* (2006) 10:375–88. doi: 10.1016/j.ccr.2006.10.006

Lin X, Morgan-Lappe S, Huang X, Li L, Zakula DM, Vernetti LA, et al. 'Seed' Analysis of Off-Target siRNAs Reveals an Essential Role of Mcl-1 in Resistance to the Small-Molecule Bcl-2/Bcl-XL Inhibitor ABT-737. *Oncogene* (2007) 26:3972–9. doi: 10.1038/sj.onc.1210166

Dai Y, Jin F, Wu W, Kumar SK. Cell Cycle Regulation and Hematologic Malignancies. *Blood Sci* (2019) 1:34–43. doi: 10.1097/BS9.0000 000000000009

Zhou L, Zhang Y, Sampath D, Leverson J, Dai Y, Kmieciak M, et al. Flavopiridol Enhances ABT-199 Sensitivity in Unfavourable-Risk Multiple Myeloma Cells *In Vitro* and *In Vivo*. *Br J Cancer* (2018) 118:388–97. doi: 10.1038/bjc.2017.432

Zhang Y, Zhou L, Bandyopadhyay D, Sharma K, Allen AJ, Kmieciak M, et al. The Covalent CDK7 Inhibitor THZ1 Potently Induces Apoptosis in Multiple Myeloma Cells *In Vitro* and *In Vivo*. *Clin Cancer Res* (2019) 25:6195–205. doi: 10.1158/1078-0432.CCR-18-3788

Rahmani M, Davis EM, Bauer C, Dent P, Grant S. Apoptosis Induced by the Kinase Inhibitor BAY 43-9006 in Human Leukemia Cells Involves Down- Regulation of Mcl-1 Through Inhibition of Translation. *J Biol Chem* (2005) 280:35217–27. doi: 10.1074/jbc.M506551200

Qian J, Zou Y, Rahman JSM, Lu B, Massion PP. Synergy Between Phosphatidylinositol 3-Kinase/Akt Pathway and Bcl-xL in the Control of Apoptosis in Adenocarcinoma Cells of the Lung. *Mol Cancer Ther* (2009) 8:101–9. doi: 10.1158/1535-7163.MCT-08-0973

Potter DS, Letai A. To Prime, or Not to Prime: That is the Question. *Cold Spring Harb Symp Quant Biol* (2016) 81:131–40. doi: 10.1101/sqb.2016.81.030841

Zhao Y, Tan J, Zhuang L, Jiang X, Liu ET, Yu Q, et al. Inhibitors of Histone Deacetylases Target the Rb-E2F1 Pathway for Apoptosis Induction Through Activation of Proapoptotic Protein Bim. *Proc Natl Acad Sci USA* (2005) 102:16090–5. doi: 10.1073/pnas.0505585102

Chen S, Dai Y, Pei X-Y, Grant S. Bim Upregulation by Histone Deacetylase Inhibitors Mediates Interactions With the Bcl-2 Antagonist ABT-737: Evidence for Distinct Roles for Bcl-2, Bcl-Xl, and Mcl-1. *Mol Cell Biol* (2009) 29:6149–69. doi: 10.1128/MCB.01481-08

Paoluzzi L, Gonen M, Bhagat G, Furman RR, Gardner JR, Scotto L, et al. The BH3-Only Mimetic ABT-737 Synergizes the Antineoplastic Activity of Proteasome Inhibitors in Lymphoid Malignancies. *Blood* (2008) 112:2906– 16. doi: 10.1182/blood-2007-12-130781

Chen S, Dai Y, Pei XY, Myers J, Wang L, Kramer LB, et al. CDK Inhibitors Up-Regulate BH3-Only Proteins to Sensitize Human Myeloma Cells to BH3 Mimetic Therapies. *Cancer Res* (2012) 72:4225–37. doi: 10.1158/0008- 5472.CAN-12-1118

Dai Y, Grant S. Chapter 10: Rational Combination of Targeted Agents to Overcome Cancer Cell Resistance. In: Gioeli D, editor. *Targeted Therapies: Mechanisms of Resistance, Molecular and Translational Medicine*. New York, NY: Springer Science+Business Media, LLC. (2011). doi: 10.1007/978-1- 60761-478-4_10

Wu J, Meng F, Kong L-Y, Peng Z, Ying Y, Bornmann WG, et al. Association Between Imatinib-Resistant BCR-ABL Mutation-Negative Leukemia and Persistent Activation of LYN Kinase. *J Natl Cancer Inst* (2008) 100:926–39. doi: 10.1093/jnci/djn188

Dai Y, Rahmani M, Corey SJ, Dent P, Grant S. A Bcr/Abl-Independent, Lyn-Dependent Form of Imatinib Mesylate (STI-571) Resistance Is Associated With Altered Expression of Bcl-2. *J Biol Chem* (2004) 279:34227–39. doi: 10.1074/jbc.M402290200

Carter BZ, Mak PY, Mu H, Zhou H, Mak DH, Schober W, et al. Combined Targeting of BCL-2 and BCR-ABL Tyrosine Kinase Eradicates Chronic Myeloid Leukemia Stem Cells. *Sci Transl Med* (2016) 8:355ra117. doi: 10.1126/scitranslmed.aag1180

Shibue T, Weinberg RA. EMT, CSCs, and Drug Resistance: The Mechanistic Link and Clinical Implications. *Nat Rev Clin Oncol* (2017) 14:611–29. doi: 10.1038/nrclinonc.2017.44

Bhatt AP, Bhende PM, Sin S-H, Roy D, Dittmer DP, Damania B, et al. Dual Inhibition of PI3K and mTOR Inhibits Autocrine and Paracrine Proliferative Loops in PI3K/Akt/mTOR-Addicted Lymphomas. *Blood* (2010) 115:4455– 63. doi: 10.1182/blood-2009-10-251082

Bose P, Dai Y, Grant S. Histone Deacetylase Inhibitor (HDACI) Mechanisms of Action: Emerging Insights. *Pharmacol Ther* (2014) 143:323–36. doi: 10.1016/j.pharmthera.2014.04.004

Dai Y, Bose P, Grant S. Chapter 16 – Cell-Cycle Regulation and Hematologic Disorders. In: Kaushansky K, et al, editors. *Williams Hematology, 9th Edition*. New York, NY: McGraw-Hill Education. (2015).

Jenke R, Reßing N, Hansen FK, Aigner A, Büch T. Anticancer Therapy With HDAC Inhibitors: Mechanism-Based Combination Strategies and Future Perspectives. *Cancers (Basel)* (2021) 13:634. doi: 10.3390/ cancers13040634

Grant S, Dai Y. Histone Deacetylase Inhibitors and Rational Combination Therapies. *Adv Cancer Res* (2012) 116:199–37. doi: 10.1016/B978-0-12- 394387-3.00006-9

Narita T, Weinert BT, Choudhary C. Functions and Mechanisms of Non- Histone Protein Acetylation. *Nat Rev Mol Cell Biol* (2019) 20:156–74. doi: 10.1038/s41580-018-0081-3

Nebbioso A, Carafa V, Conte M, Tambaro FP, Abbondanza C, Martens J, et al. C-Myc Modulation and Acetylation Is a Key HDAC Inhibitor Target in Cancer. *Clin Cancer Res* (2017) 23:2542–55. doi: 10.1158/1078-0432.CCR- 15-2388

Xia Y, Shen S, Verma IM. NF-*k*B, an Active Player in Human Cancers. *Cancer Immunol Res* (2014) 2:823–30. doi: 10.1158/2326- 6066.CIR-14-0112

Lantermann AB, Chen D, McCutcheon K, Hoffman K, Frias E, Ruddy D, et al. Inhibition of Casein Kinase 1 Alpha Prevents Acquired Drug Resistance to Erlotinib in EGFR-Mutant Non-Small Cell Lung Cancer. *Cancer Res* (2015) 75:4937–48. doi: 10.1158/0008-5472.CAN-15-1113

Juvekar A, Manna S, Ramaswami S, Chang T-P, Vu H-Y, Ghosh CC, et al. Bortezomib Induces Nuclear Translocation of I*k*B*a* Resulting in Gene- Specific Suppression of NF-*k*B–Dependent Transcription and Induction of Apoptosis in CTCL. *Mol Cancer Res* (2011) 9:183–94. doi: 10.1158/1541- 7786.MCR-10-0368

Chen LF, Greene WC. Regulation of Distinct Biological Activities of the NF-kappaB Transcription Factor Complex by Acetylation. *J Mol Med (Berl)* (2003) 81:549–57. doi: 10.1007/s00109-003-0469-0

Dai Y, Rahmani M, Grant S. An Intact NF-kappaB Pathway is Required for Histone Deacetylase Inhibitor-Induced G1 Arrest and Maturation in U937 Human Myeloid Leukemia Cells. *Cell Cycle* (2003) 2:467–72. doi: 10.4161/ cc.2.5.465

Dai Y, Rahmani M, Dent P, Grant S. Blockade of Histone Deacetylase Inhibitor-Induced RelA/p65 Acetylation and NF-kappaB Activation Potentiates Apoptosis in Leukemia Cells Through a Process Mediated by Oxidative Damage, XIAP Downregulation, and C-Jun N-Terminal Kinase 1 Activation. *Mol Cell Biol* (2005) 25:5429–44. doi: 10.1128/mcb.25.13.5429- 5444.2005

Dai Y, Chen S, Wang L, Pei XY, Funk VL, Kramer LB, et al. Disruption of IKK-Mediated RelA Serine 536 Phosphorylation Sensitizes Human Multiple Myeloma Cells to HDAC Inhibitors. *J Biol Chem* (2011) 286:34036–50. doi: 10.1074/jbc.M111.284216

Dai Y, Rahmani M, Grant S. Proteasome Inhibitors Potentiate Leukemic Cell Apoptosis Induced by the Cyclin-Dependent Kinase Inhibitor Flavopiridol Through a SAPK/JNK- and NF-KappaB-Dependent Process. *Oncogene* (2003) 22:7108–22. doi: 10.1038/sj.onc.1206863

Dai Y, Guzman M, Chen S, Yeung S-K, Dent P, Jordan CT, et al. The NF (Nuclear Factor)-kB Inhibitor Parthenolide Interacts With Histone Deacetylase Inhibitors to Induce MKK7/JNK1-Dependent Apoptosis in Human Acute Myeloid Leukaemia Cells. *Br J Haematol* (2010) 151:70–83. doi: 10.1111/j.1365-2141.2010.08319.x

Pei XY, Dai Y, Grant S. Synergistic Induction of Oxidative Injury and Apoptosis in Human Multiple Myeloma Cells by the Proteasome Inhibitor Bortezomib and Histone Deacetylase Inhibitors. *Clin Cancer Res* (2004) 10:3839–52. doi: 10.1158/1078-0432.CCR-03-0561

Dai Y, Chen S, Kramer LB, Funk VL, Dent P, Grant S. Interactions Between Bortezomib and Romidepsin and Belinostat in Chronic Lymphocytic Leukemia Cells. *Clin Cancer Res* (2008) 14:549–58. doi: 10.1158/1078- 0432.CCR-07-1934

Dai Y, Chen S, Wang L, Pei X-Y, Kramer LB, Dent P, et al. Bortezomib Interacts Synergistically With Belinostat in Human AML and ALL Cells in Association With Perturbation in NF-*k*B and Bim. *Br J Haematol* (2011) 153:222–35. doi: 10.1111/j.1365-2141.2011.08591.x

Pei X-Y, Dai Y, Felthousen J, Chen S, Takabatake Y, Liang L, et al. Circumvention of Mcl-1-Dependent Drug Resistance by Simultaneous Chk1 and MEK1/2 Inhibition in Human Multiple Myeloma Cells. *PloS One* (2014) 9:e89064. doi: 10.1371/journal.pone.0089064

Tang Y, Dai Y, Grant S, Dent P. Enhancing CHK1 Inhibitor Lethality in Glioblastoma. *Cancer Biol Ther* (2012) 13:379–88. doi: 10.4161/cbt.19240

Mitchell C, Hamed HA, Cruickshanks N, Tang Y, Bareford MD, Hubbard N, et al. Simultaneous Exposure of Transformed Cells to SRC Family Inhibitors and CHK1 Inhibitors Causes Cell Death. *Cancer Biol Ther* (2011) 12:215–28. doi: 10.4161/cbt.12.3.16218

Hamed H, Hawkins W, Mitchell C, Gilfor D, Zhang G, Pei XY, et al. Transient Exposure of Carcinoma Cells to RAS/MEK Inhibitors and UCN- 01 Causes Cell Death *In Vitro* and *In Vivo*. *Mol Cancer Ther* (2008) 7:616–29. doi: 10.1158/1535-7163.MCT-07-2376

Pei X-Y, Li W, Dai Y, Dent P, Grant S. Dissecting the Roles of Chk1/cdc2 and MEK1/2/ERK1/2 in Relation to UCN-01-Induced Apoptosis in Human Multiple Myeloma Cells. *Mol Pharmacol* (2006) 70:1965–73. doi: 10.1124/mol.106.028373

Hawkins W, Mitchell C, McKinstry R, Gilfor D, Starkey J, Dai Y, et al. Transient Exposure of Mammary Tumors to PD184352 and UCN-01 Causes Tumor Cell Death *In Vivo* and Prolonged Suppression of Tumor Regrowth. *Cancer Biol Ther* (2005) 4:1275–84. doi: 10.4161/cbt.4.11.2286

Booth L, Cruickshanks N, Ridder T, Dai Y, Grant S, Dent P. PARP and CHK Inhibitors Interact to Cause DNA Damage and Cell Death in Mammary Carcinoma Cells. *Cancer Biol Ther* (2013) 14:458–65. doi: 10.4161/cbt.24424

Tang Y, Hamed HA, Poklepovic A, Dai Y, Grant S, Dent P. Poly(ADP-Ribose) Polymerase 1 Modulates the Lethality of CHK1 Inhibitors in Mammary Tumors. *Mol Pharmacol* (2012) 82:322–32. doi: 10.1124/mol.112.078907

Pathania R, Ramachandran S, Mariappan G, Thakur P, Shi H, Choi J-H, et al. Combined Inhibition of DNMT and HDAC Blocks the Tumorigenicity of Cancer Stem-Like Cells and Attenuates Mammary Tumor Growth. *Cancer Res* (2016) 76:3224–35. doi: 10.1158/0008-5472.CAN-15-2249

Blagitko-Dorfs N, Schlosser P, Greve G, Pfeifer D, Meier R, Baude A, et al. Combination Treatment of Acute Myeloid Leukemia Cells With DNMT and HDAC Inhibitors: Predominant Synergistic Gene Downregulation Associated With Gene Body Demethylation. *Leukemia* (2019) 33:945–56. doi: 10.1038/s41375-018-0293-8

Rosato RR, Almenara JA, Dai Y, Grant S. Simultaneous Activation of the Intrinsic and Extrinsic Pathways by Histone Deacetylase (HDAC) Inhibitors and Tumor Necrosis Factor-Related Apoptosis-Inducing Ligand (TRAIL) Synergistically Induces Mitochondrial Damage and Apoptosis in Human Leukemia Cells. *Mol Cancer Ther* (2003) 2:1273–84.

Workman P, Burrows F, Neckers L, Rosen N. Drugging the Cancer Chaperone HSP90: Combinatorial Therapeutic Exploitation of Oncogene Addiction and Tumor Stress. *Ann N Y Acad Sci* (2007) 1113:202–16. doi: 10.1196/annals.1391.012

Yu C, Rahmani M, Almenara J, Subler M, Krystal G, Conrad C, et al. Histone Deacetylase Inhibitors Promote STI571-Mediated Apoptosis in STI571-Sensitive and -Resistant Bcr/Abl+ Human Myeloid Leukemia Cells. *Cancer Res* (2003) 63:2118–26.

Fiskus W, Pranpat M, Balasis M, Bali P, Estrella V, Kumaraswamy S, et al. Cotreatment With Vorinostat (Suberoylanilide Hydroxamic Acid) Enhances Activity of Dasatinib (BMS-354825) Against Imatinib Mesylate-Sensitive or Imatinib Mesylate-Resistant Chronic Myelogenous Leukemia Cells. *Clin Cancer Res* (2006) 12:5869–78. doi: 10.1158/1078-0432.CCR-06-0980

Bali P, George P, Cohen P, Tao J, Guo F, Sigua C, et al. Superior Activity of the Combination of Histone Deacetylase Inhibitor LAQ824 and the FLT-3 Kinase Inhibitor PKC412 Against Human Acute Myelogenous Leukemia Cells With Mutant FLT-3. *Clin Cancer Res* (2004) 10:4991–7. doi: 10.1158/ 1078-0432.CCR-04-0210

Witta SE, Gemmill RM, Hirsch FR, Coldren CD, Hedman K, Ravdel L, et al. Restoring E-Cadherin Expression Increases Sensitivity to Epidermal Growth Factor Receptor Inhibitors in Lung Cancer Cell Lines. *Cancer Res* (2006) 66:944–50. doi: 10.1158/0008-5472.CAN-05-1988

Nguyen T, Dai Y, Attkisson E, Kramer L, Jordan N, Nguyen N, et al. HDAC Inhibitors Potentiate the Activity of the BCR/ABL Kinase Inhibitor KW- 2449 in Imatinib-Sensitive or -Resistant BCR/ABL+ Leukemia Cells *In Vitro* and *In Vivo*. *Clin Cancer Res* (2011) 17:3219–32. doi: 10.1158/1078- 0432.CCR-11-0234

Cha TL, Chuang MJ, Wu ST, Sun G-H, Chang S-Y, Yu D-S, et al. Dual Degradation of Aurora A and B Kinases by the Histone Deacetylase Inhibitor LBH589 Induces G2-M Arrest and Apoptosis of Renal Cancer Cells. *Clin Cancer Res* (2009) 15:840–50. doi: 10.1158/1078-0432.CCR-08-1918

Almenara J, Rosato R, Grant S. Synergistic Induction of Mitochondrial Damage and Apoptosis in Human Leukemia Cells by Flavopiridol and the Histone Deacetylase Inhibitor Suberoylanilide Hydroxamic Acid (SAHA). *Leukemia* (2002) 16:1331–43. doi: 10.1038/sj.leu.2402535

Grant S, Kolla S, Sirulnik A, Shapiro G, Supko J, Cooper B, et al. Phase I Trial of Vorinostat (SAHA) in Combinatin With Alvocidib (Flavopiridol) in Patients With Refractory, Relapsed, or (Selected) Poor-Prognosis AML or Refractory Anemia With Excess Blasts-2 (RAEB-2). *Blood* (2008) 112:2986. doi: 10.1182/blood.V112.11.2986.2986

Rahmani M, Yu C, Dai Y, Reese E, Ahmed W, Dent P, et al. Coadministration of the Heat Shock Protein 90 Antagonist 17- Allylamino- 17-Demethoxygeldanamycin With Suberoylanilide Hydroxamic Acid or Sodium Butyrate Synergistically Induces Apoptosis in Human Leukemia Cells. *Cancer Res* (2003) 63:8420–7.

Rahmani M, Reese E, Dai Y, Bauer C, Kramer LB, Huang M, et al. Cotreatment With Suberanoylanilide Hydroxamic Acid and 17-Allylamino 17-Demethoxygeldanamycin Synergistically Induces Apoptosis in Bcr-Abl+ Cells Sensitive and Resistant to STI571 (Imatinib Mesylate) in Association With Down-Regulation of Bcr-Abl, Abrogation of Signal Transducer and Activator of Transcription 5 Activity, and Bax Conformational Change. *Mol Pharmacol* (2005) 67:1166–76. doi: 10.1124/mol.104.007831

Ye J, Zha J, Shi Y, Li Y, Yuan D, Chen Q, et al. Co-Inhibition of HDAC and MLL-Menin Interaction Targets MLL-Rearranged Acute Myeloid Leukemia Cells *Via* Disruption of DNA Damage Checkpoint and DNA Repair. *Clin Epigenetics* (2019) 11:137. doi: 10.1186/s13148-019-0723-0

Mitsiades CS, Mitsiades NS, McMullan CJ, Poulaki V, Shringarpure R, Hideshima T, et al. Transcriptional Signature of Histone Deacetylase Inhibition in Multiple Myeloma: Biological and Clinical Implications. *Proc Natl Acad Sci USA* (2004) 101:540–5. doi: 10.1073/pnas.2536759100

Badros A, Burger AM, Philip S, Niesvizky R, Kolla SS, Goloubeva O, et al. Phase I Study of Vorinostat in Combination With Bortezomib for Relapsed and Refractory Multiple Myeloma. *Clin Cancer Res* (2009) 15:5250–7. doi: 10.1158/1078-0432.CCR-08-2850

Bali P, Pranpat M, Bradner J, Balasis M, Fiskus W, Guo F, et al. Inhibition of Histone Deacetylase 6 Acetylates and Disrupts the Chaperone Function of Heat Shock Protein 90: A Novel Basis of Antileukemia Activity of Histone Deacetylase Inhibitors. *J Biol Chem* (2005) 280:26729–34. doi: 10.1074/ jbc.C500186200

Nawrocki ST, Carew JS, Dunner KJr., Boise LH, Paul J, Chiao PJ, et al. Bortezomib Inhibits PKR-Like Endoplasmic Reticulum (ER) Kinase and Induces Apoptosis *Via* ER Stress in Human Pancreatic Cancer Cells. *Cancer Res* (2005) 65:11510–9. doi: 10.1158/0008-5472.CAN-05-2394

Dai Y, Rahmani M, Pei XY, Dent P, Grant S. Bortezomib and Flavopiridol Interact Synergistically to Induce Apoptosis in Chronic Myeloid Leukemia Cells Resistant to Imatinib Mesylate Through Both Bcr/Abl-Dependent and -Independent Mechanisms. *Blood* (2004) 104:509–18. doi: 10.1182/blood- 2003-12-4121

Holkova B, Perkins EB, Ramakrishnan V, Tombes MB, Shrader E, Talreja N, et al. Phase I Trial of Bortezomib (PS-341; NSC 681239) and Alvocidib (Flavopiridol; NSC 649890) in Patients With Recurrent or Refractory B-Cell Neoplasms. *Clin Cancer Res* (2011) 17:3388–97. doi: 10.1158/1078- 0432.CCR-10-2876

Holkova B, Kmieciak M, Perkins EB, Bose P, Baz RC, Roodman GD, et al. Phase I Trial of Bortezomib (PS-341; NSC 681239) and "Nonhybrid" (Bolus) Infusion Schedule of Alvocidib (Flavopiridol; NSC 649890) in Patients With Recurrent or Refractory Indolent B-Cell Neoplasms. *Clin Cancer Res* (2014) 20:5652–62. doi: 10.1158/1078-0432.CCR-14-0805

Perez-Galan P, Roue G, Villamor N, Campo E, Colomer D. The BH3- Mimetic GX15-070 Synergizes With Bortezomib in Mantle Cell Lymphoma by Enhancing Noxa-Mediated Activation of Bak. *Blood* (2007) 109:4441–9. doi: 10.1182/blood-2006-07-034173

Trudel S, Li ZH, Rauw J, Tiedemann RE, Wen XY, Stewart AK. Preclinical Studies of the Pan-Bcl Inhibitor Obatoclax (GX015-070) in Multiple Myeloma. *Blood* (2007) 109:5430–8. doi: 10.1182/blood-2006-10-047951

Turner JG, Kashyap T, Dawson JL, Gomez J, Bauer AA, Grant S, et al. XPO1 Inhibitor Combination Therapy With Bortezomib or Carfilzomib Induces Nuclear Localization of *IkBa* and Overcomes Acquired Proteasome Inhibitor Resistance in Human Multiple Myeloma. *Oncotarget* (2016) 7:78896–909. doi: 10.18632/oncotarget.12969

Turner JG, Dawson JL, Grant S, Shain KH, Dalton WS, Dai Y, et al. Treatment of Acquired Drug Resistance in Multiple Myeloma by Combination Therapy With XPO1 and Topoisomerase II Inhibitors. *J Hematol Oncol* (2016) 9:73. doi: 10.1186/s13045-016-0304-z

Zhang Y, Zhou L, Leng Y, Dai Y, Orlowski R, Grant S. Positive Transcription Elongation Factor B (P-TEFb) is a Therapeutic Target in Human Multiple Myeloma. *Oncotarget* (2017) 8:59476–9. doi: 10.18632/oncotarget.19761

Zhang W, Konopleva M, Ruvolo VR, McQueen T, Evans RL, Bornmann WG, et al. Sorafenib Induces Apoptosis of AML Cells *Via* Bim-Mediated Activation of the Intrinsic Apoptotic Pathway. *Leukemia* (2008) 22:808–18. doi: 10.1038/sj.leu.2405098

Massimino M, Tirrò E, Stella S, Pennisi MS, Vitale SR, Puma A, et al. Targeting BCL-2 as a Therapeutic Strategy for Primary P210 BCR- ABL1-Positive B-ALL Cells. *In Vivo* (2020) 34:511–6. doi: 10.21873/ invivo.11802

Yu C, Krystal G, Varticovksi L, McKinstry R, Rahmani M, Dent P, et al. Pharmacologic Mitogen-Activated Protein/Extracellular Signal-Regulated Kinase Kinase/Mitogen-Activated Protein Kinase Inhibitors Interact Synergistically With STI571 to Induce Apoptosis in Bcr/Abl-Expressing Human Leukemia Cells. *Cancer Res* (2002) 62:188–99.

Tai YT, Fulciniti M, Hideshima T, Song W, Leiba M, Li X-F, et al. Targeting MEK Induces Myeloma Cell Cytotoxicity and Inhibits Osteoclastogenesis. *Blood* (2007) 110:1656–63. doi: 10.1182/blood-2007-03-081240

Nguyen TK, Jordan N, Friedberg J, Fisher RI, Dent P, Grant S. Inhibition of MEK/ERK1/2 Sensitizes Lymphoma Cells to Sorafenib-Induced Apoptosis. *Leuk Res* (2010) 34:379–86. doi: 10.1016/j.leukres.2009.07.013

Jin F, Li W, Turner JG, Dai Y. Novel Mechanisms of Action for Immunomodulatory Drugs (IMiDs) Against Multiple Myeloma: From a Tragedy to a Therapy. *Int J Hematol Ther* (2015) 2:1–6. doi: 10.15436/2381- 1404.15.008

Davis LN, Sherbenou DW. Emerging Therapeutic Strategies to Overcome Drug Resistance in Multiple Myeloma. *Cancers (Basel)* (2021) 13:1686. doi: 10.3390/cancers13071686

Jones CL, Stevens BM, D'Alessandro A, Reisz JA, Culp-Hill R, Nemkov T, et al. Inhibition of Amino Acid Metabolism Selectively Targets Human Leukemia Stem Cells. *Cancer Cell* (2018) 34:724–40.e4. doi: 10.1016/ j.ccell.2018.10.005

Perl A, Carroll M. BCR-ABL Kinase is Dead; Long Live the CML Stem Cell. *J Clin Invest* (2011) 121:22–5. doi: 10.1172/JCI43605

Tanaka Y, Takeda R, Fukushima T, Mikami K, Tsuchiya S, Tamura M, et al. Eliminating Chronic Myeloid Leukemia Stem Cells by IRAK1/4 Inhibitors. *Nat Commun* (2022) 13:271. doi: 10.1038/s41467-021-27928-8

Zhou J, Wang S, Nie D, Lai P, Li Y, Li Y, et al. Super-Enhancer Landscape Reveals Leukemia Stem Cell Reliance on X-Box Binding Protein 1 as a Therapeutic Vulnerability. *Sci Trans Med* (2021) 13:eabh3462. doi: 10.1126/ scitranslmed.abh3462

Fujiwara Y, Mittra A, Naqash AR, Takebe N. A Review of Mechanisms of Resistance to Immune Checkpoint Inhibitors and Potential Strategies for Therapy. *Cancer Drug Resist* (2020) 3:252–75. doi: 10.20517/cdr.2020.11

Zhang L, Riley-Gillis B, Vijay P, Shen Y. Acquired Resistance to BET- PROTACs (Proteolysis-Targeting Chimeras) Caused by Genomic Alterations in Core Components of E3 Ligase Complexes. *Mol Cancer Ther* (2019) 18:1302–11. doi: 10.1158/1535-7163.MCT-18-1129

Contreras-Trujillo H, Eerdeng J, Akre S, Jiang D, Contreras J, Gala B, et al. Deciphering Intratumoral Heterogeneity Using Integrated Clonal Tracking and Single-Cell Transcriptome Analyses. *Nat Commun* (2021) 12:6522. doi: 10.1038/s41467-021-26771-1

Hinohara K, Polyak K. Intratumoral Heterogeneity: More Than Just Mutations. *Trends Cell Biol* (2019) 29:569–79. doi: 10.1016/j.tcb.2019.03.003

5

Olaparib Combined with Dacomitinib in Osimertinib-Resistant Brain and Leptomeningeal Metastases from Non-Small Cell Lung Cancer

Hui Zhang[1,2†], Yong Wang[3†], Huaguo Wu[4], Shizhen Zhou[3], Shuo Li[5], Xiangji Meng[3], Rongjie Tao[2] and Jinming Yu[1,6*]*

[1] Tianjin Cancer Institute, Key Laboratory of Cancer Prevention and Therapy, National Clinical Research Center for Cancer, Tianjin Medical University Cancer Institute and Hospital, Tianjin's Clinical Research Center for Cancer, Tianjin Medical University, Tianjin, China, [2] Department of Medical Oncology, Shandong Cancer Hospital and Institute, Shandong First Medical University and Shandong Academy of Medical Science, Jinan, China, [3] Department of Neurosurgery, Shandong Cancer Hospital and Institute, Shandong First Medical University and Shandong Academy of Medical Science, Jinan, China, [4] Department of Head and Neck Surgery, Shandong Cancer Hospital and Institute, Shandong First Medical University and Shandong Academy of Medical Science, Jinan, China, [5] School of Medicine and Life Science, University of Jinan-Shandong Academy of Medical Science, Jinan, China, [6] Department of Radiation Oncology, Shandong Cancer Hospital and Institute, Shandong First Medical University and Shandong Academy of Medical Science, Jinan, China

***Correspondence:**
Jinming Yu
sdyujinming@163.com
Rongjie Tao
Drtaorongjie@163.com

†These authors have contributed equally to this work

Lung cancer patients with brain and leptomeningeal metastases usually have poor prognosis. For those patients with EGFR mutations, osimertinib, a third-generation tyrosine kinase inhibitor (TKI), is the first choice of treatment. However, drug resistance to osimertinib frequently occurs; and to date, the available follow-up treatment strategies have limited efficacy. In this case study, we report that treatments with olaparib, a Poly (ADP-ribose) polymerase (PARP) inhibitor, combined with dacomitinib, a second-generation EGFR TKI, benefited a lung cancer patient with osimertinib-resistant brain and leptomeningeal metastases. This 55-year-old male patient was found to have a pL858R mutation on EGFR exon 21 combined with TP53 and ERBB2 mutations after developing drug resistance to osimertinib treatment. Based on the genetic testing results, he was treated with olaparib and dacomitinib, and obtained 6 months of progression-free survival (PFS) and 13 months of overall survival (OS) after the diagnosis of leptomeningeal metastasis. This case report represents the first study applying PARP inhibitor in combination with dacomitinib in the treatment of leptomeningeal metastases after osimertinib resistance.

Keywords: olaparib, dacomitinib, osimertinib-resistant, brain and leptomeningeal metastases, non-small cell lung cancer

INTRODUCTION

Patients with central nervous system (CNS) metastases from non-small cell lung cancer (NSCLC) usually have very poor prognosis (1, 2). The median survival of patients in this population is usually less than 1 year despite the emerging advancement in treatment options (3–5). It has been reported that in patients with NSCLC, up to 50% would develop brain metastases (BM) during the course of their illness (5) and 3-5% would develop leptomeningeal metastases (LM) (6). The incidence could be higher in those with anaplastic lymphoma kinase (ALK)-rearrangement or epidermal growth factor receptor (EGFR) mutations (7). Currently, a combinational strategy of multidisciplinary therapies involving systemic and intrathecal chemotherapy, radiotherapy, and targeted therapies (such as osimertinib and bevacizumab) is preferred for NSCLC patients with brain and leptomeningeal metastases (2, 8). However, the reported survival time remains unsatisfied and more investigation on treatment strategies is needed.

Osimertinib (AZD9291), a third-generation oral irreversible EGFR tyrosine kinase inhibitor (TKI) (9), has been approved by the United States Food and Drug Administration (FDA) and the European Medicines Agency (EMA) for patients with acquired EGFR T790M mutation (10). In preclinical studies, osimertinib exhibited greater penetration of the mouse blood-brain barrier than gefitinib, rociletinib, or afatinib at clinically relevant doses and showed some effectiveness for treating the first or second-generation EGFR-TKI resistant leptomeningeal metastases from EGFR-mutant lung cancer (11, 12). In clinical studies, osimertinib also showed significant intracranial activity (13, 14). In the most recent prospective phase II study which evaluated the efficacy of osimertinib 160 mg in T790M-positive BM or LM of NSCLC patients who progressed on prior EGFR TKI treatment, the median overall survival was 16.9 months in the BM cohort and 13.3 months in the LM cohort (14).

In spite of the success of osimertinib as a therapy for patients with NSCLC and its potential efficacy for CNS metastases, acquired resistance involving EGFR-dependent or EGFR-independent mechanisms inevitably occurs and hampers its clinical benefits (15). It is estimated that when osimertinib is used as a first-line treatment, resistance develops approximately after 19 months of treatment; and when it is used as a second-line treatment, resistance could occur after 11 months (16). The mechanisms of resistance to osimertinib are complicated, but most of them involved in EGFR exon 20 mutations (C797S, M766Q, S768I, L718 V, and others) leading to disruption of osimertinib binding sites, alternative pathway activation, aberrant downstream signaling and lineage plasticity leading to small cell transformation, such as *MET* and *ERBB2* amplifications, inactivation of *TP53* and/or *RB1*, and so on (15, 16). The good treatment option for patients who develop resistance to osimertinib remains a critical unresolved issue in the field. Current clinical trials are focusing on targeting alternative pathways (resistance mediated by *MET*, *ERBB2*, and C979S mutation) and combination of VEGF inhibitions with EGFR-TKIs (clinical trials: NCT03392246, NCT03784599, NCT04181060, NCT03909334, and so on.) (16, 17).

Poly (ADP-ribose) polymerase 1 (PARP1) is an important DNA repair enzyme of the base excision repair (BER) pathway and represents a critical target in cancer treatments (18). FDA has approved four PARP inhibitors (Olaparib, Rucaparib, Niraparib, and Talazoparib) for treatments of ovarian and breast cancers (19). To date, very few studies have reported their efficacies in lung adenocarcinoma. A pre-clinical study by Lynnette Marcar et al. showed that compared to TKI sensitive cells, TKI (gefitinib and osimertinib) resistant EGFR mutant NSCLC cells were more sensitive to PARP inhibitors, indicating the potential efficacy of PARP inhibitors in treating osimertinib-resistant NSCLC (20). A phase I clinical trial investigating the efficacy of the PARP inhibitor, niraparib, together with osimertinib in treating patients with stage IV EGFR-mutated NSCLC is ongoing (NCT03891615).

In this case study, we report that the treatment using PARP inhibitor olaparib in combination with dacomitinib, a second generation EGFR-TKI, benefited a NSCLC patient with osimertinib-resistant brain and leptomeningeal metastases who had EGFR mutations combined with TP53 and ERBB2 mutations.

CASE PRESENTATION

A 55-year-old male underwent thoracoscopic-assisted small-incision radical resection of lung cancer in October 11, 2017 after diagnosis of lung adenocarcinoma (stage pT1bN0M0, IA) (**Figure 1**). His postoperative regular magnetic resonance imaging (MRI) and computerized tomography (CT) examinations showed no obvious abnormalities. Two years later (on October 12, 2019), the patient started to experience headache, blurred vision, and hearing loss. On October 31, 2019, his brain MRI exam showed multiple brain masses including multiple metastases in the lateral ventricle, right frontal lobe, and cerebellar hemisphere (**Figure 2A**). His genetic testing revealed the L858R mutation in exon 21 of EGFR. His positron emission tomography (PET) CT scan suggested bone metastasis (**Figure S1**). The patient was then treated with osimertinib (80 mg oral administration daily), bevacizumab (7.5mg/kg q3w), and bisphosphonate (4mg q3w). After treatment for 1 month, his symptom of headache almost disappeared, but he developed blurred vision and unstable walking on both feet. On 2020-1-4, the patient complained increased blurred vision and occasional headache. On 2020-4-21, his brain MRI (**Figure 2B**) showed multiple dot-line enhancements (masses) in the cerebellar sulci, suggesting meningeal metastasis. On 2020-4-30, the patient underwent cerebrospinal fluid (CSF) cytology examination and cancer cells were found in the cerebrospinal fluid, which was in line with the characteristics of adenocarcinoma cells (**Figure 2C**). His CSF genetic testing results in May 2020 showed that mutations were EGFR p.L858R, TP53 p.R273C and ERBB2 p.S442L (**Figure 3A**). The patient was then treated with whole brain radiotherapy (40Gy/20 fractions). Between July 2020 and December 2020, the patient was treated with osimertinib (80 mg oral administration daily), anlotinib (12mg d1-14, q3w), pemetrexed (500mg/kg q4w), and temozolomide (300mg d1-5, q4w). Then, the patient experienced less headache. The re-test of the CSF samples showed that the mutations included EGFR

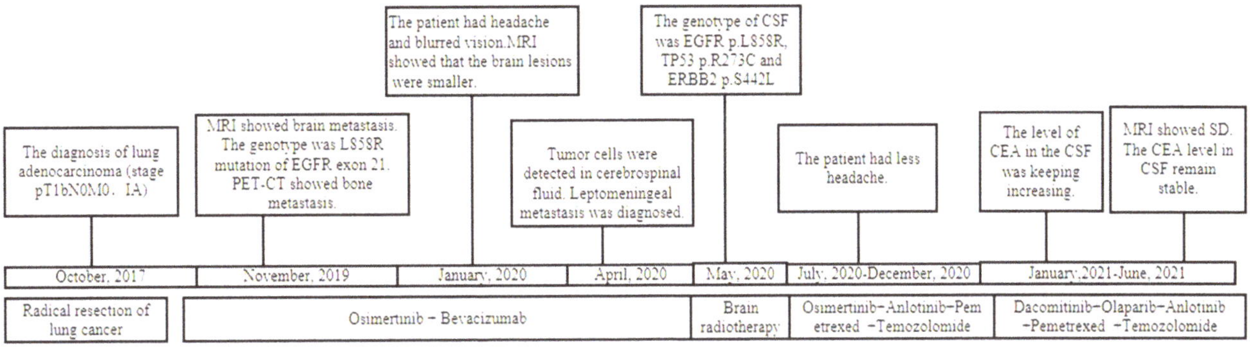

FIGURE 1 | Summary of the diagnosis and treatment process.

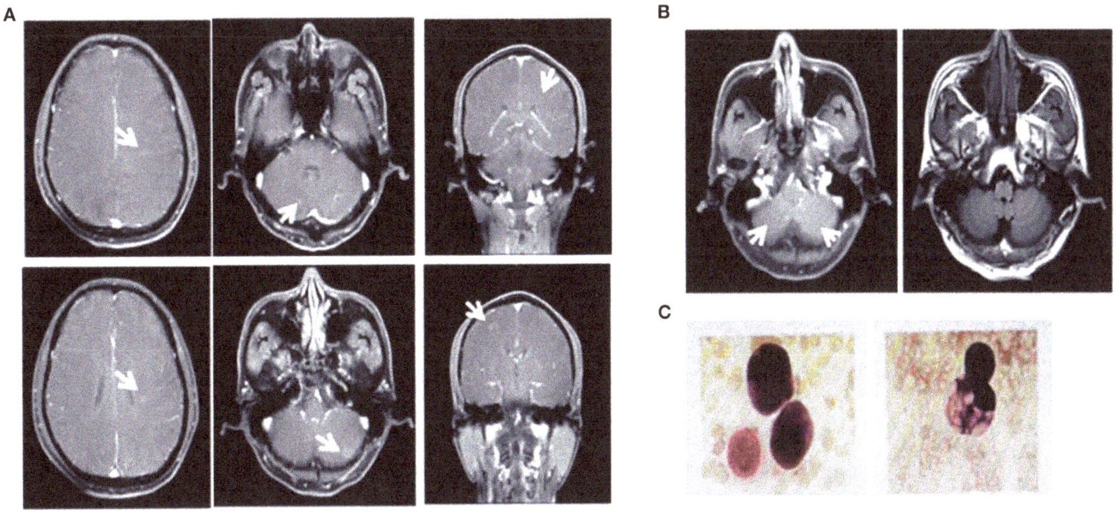

FIGURE 2 | Diagnosis of brain metastases. **(A)** On October 31, 2019, the magnetic resonance imaging (MRI) examination of the patient showed multiple brain masses including multiple metastases in the lateral ventricle, right frontal lobe, and cerebellar hemisphere. Diagnosis of leptomeningeal metastases. **(B)** On April 21, 2020, MRI T1 enhancement and FLARE examination showed that the cerebellar sulci had multiple line-like and spot-like enhancements, suggesting meningeal metastasis. **(C)** On April 30, 2020, retest of the cerebrospinal fluid (CSF) showed the presence of cancer cells with the characteristics of adenocarcinoma cells.

p.L858R, TP53, ERBB2, and others (October 28, 2021). (**Figure 3A**). In January 2021, due to the continued elevated levels of tumor marker carcinoembryonic antigen (CEA) in his CSF (**Figure 3B**) and based on his CSF genetic test results, his treatment was switched to dacomitinib (30mg po qd), olaparib (100mg po bid), anlotinib (8mg po d1-14,q3w), pemetrexed (500mg/m^2, q3w), and temozolomide (200mg/m^2 d1-5, q4w). The patient's condition was stable after adjusting the treatment plan. His level of CEA was stable (**Figure 3B**), and his brain MRI showed no progression of the brain metastasis. The efficacy evaluation during the treatment period is shown in **Figure 4**. In addition, after switching to targeted therapy, the patient no longer experienced obvious headache and dizziness, and his quality of life was significantly improved. Although he had the 2nd degree bone marrow suppression, there was no obvious functional damage of the liver and kidney during the process of treatment. The patient died of cachexia caused by the tumor in June 2021. Based upon, targeted drug therapy helped this patient obtain 6 months of progression-free survival (PFS). After the diagnosis of CNS metastases, although he was no longer sensitive to osimertinib, his overall survival reached 13 months which might be benefited from the treatment of olaparib in combination with dacomitinib.

DISCUSSION

This case represents the first study applying PARP inhibitor combined with dacomitinib for treating CNS metastases from NSCLC after osimertinib resistance. Using this new treatment strategy in combination with other chemotherapeutic drugs and

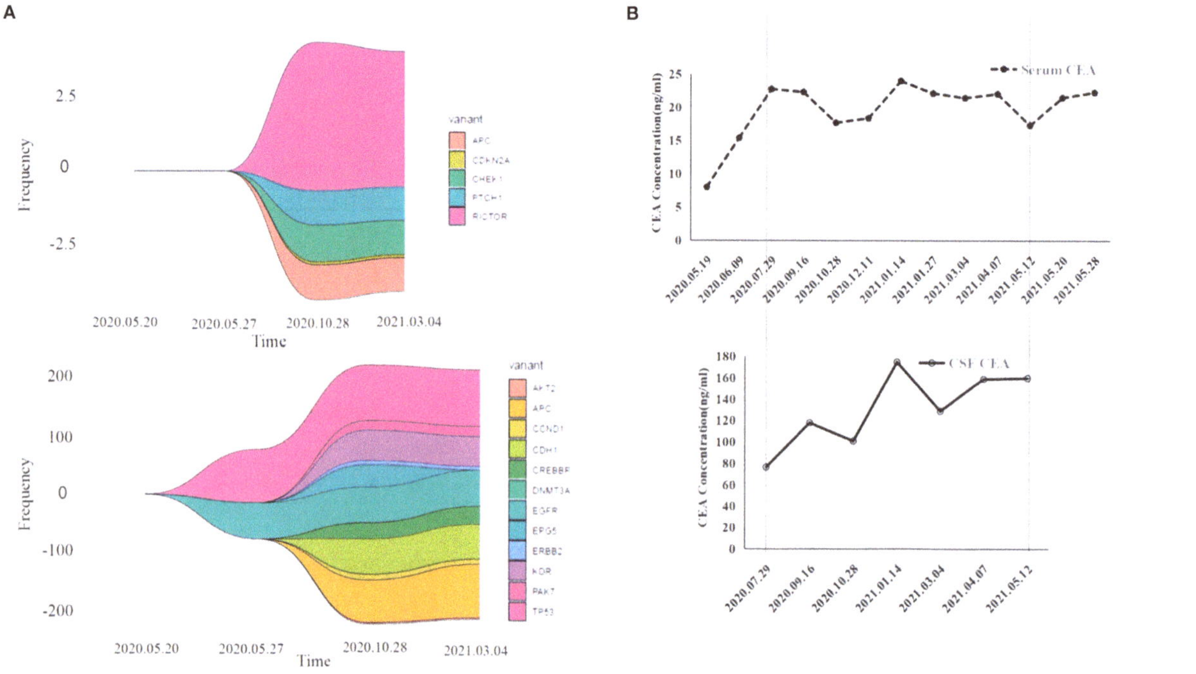

FIGURE 3 | Gene detection diagram and levels of carcinoembryonic antigen (CEA) during treatment. **(A)** Gene detection diagram during the treatment was shown. Different colors represent different genes and different wave widths. The number on the vertical axis represents the mutation frequency (wave width). **(B)** The levels of CEA, including serum CEA and cerebrospinal fluid CEA, were shown.

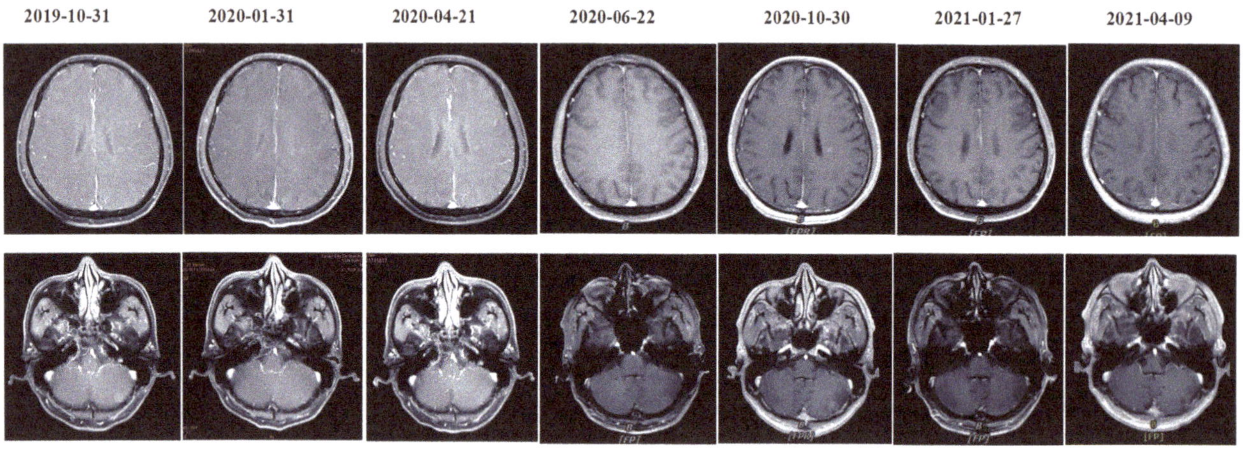

FIGURE 4 | MRI imaging changes at different time points during the treatment process.

radiotherapy, the patient eventually obtained 6 months of progression-free survival and 13 months of overall survival after the diagnosis of leptomeningeal metastasis, which is markedly longer than the median survival reported in previous studies (3, 4, 21).

Unlike a previous case report which showed that dacomitinib, the second-generation TKI, did not benefit a patient who developed mutations after later-line osimertinib treatment (22), the present case with ERBB2 mutations showed a different outcome. This patient also had mutations in TP53, a gene that is essential for DNA repair. Given the effects of PARP inhibitors in DNA repair pathway, this patient was treated with olaparib and seemed to be benefited from this combined targeted therapy.

This case report also highlighted the importance of CSF genetic testing in the diagnoses of CNS metastases. For this patient, his plasma genetic testing in May 2020 was negative for EGFR mutations; however, his CSF samples were positive and showed mutations in EGFR p.L858R, TP53, and ERBB2, which helped determining his subsequent treatment strategies (dacomitinib and olaparib). This case suggests that CSF genetic testing is necessary for patients who may have CNS metastases. Indeed, CSF-derived cell free DNA holds promise for diagnosis and characterization of CNS tumors or metastases (23). In a study involving 26 lung cancer patients with leptomeningeal metastasis and known EGFR mutations in the primary tumor, mutations in driver genes were detected in 100% (26/26), 84.6% (22/26), and 73.1% (19/26) of samples from CSF cell-free DNA (cfDNA), CSF precipitates, and plasma, respectively (24). Therefore, genetic profiling of CSF samples could help the diagnoses of patients with CNS metastases and improve their treatment outcomes.

For cancer patients, a significant increase in CEA level is often related to meningeal metastases (25). Therefore, CEA levels in CSF samples could be an indicator for the prognosis. In this case, the CEA levels in the CSF samples were notably higher than that in the blood. After targeted therapy, his CEA levels were stable, which was consistent with his MRI test results.

CNS metastases frequently occur in patients with lung cancer; and these patients often have an extremely poor prognosis. Due to the poor penetration of the blood-brain barrier, the first- and second- generation of EGFR-TKIs have low efficacy in the treatment of BM and LM in NSCLC. Although the third generation of EGFR-TKI, osimertinib, has shown increased penetration into the blood-brain barrier and enhanced clinical activity in patients with CNS metastasis, unfortunately, similar to the first- and second- generation of EGFR-TKIs, drug resistance to osimertinib commonly occurs after over 1 year of treatment. As reviewed by Alessandro Leonetti et al., the known mechanisms of resistance to osimertinib include EGFR modifications, activation of bypass signaling pathways mediated by MET, ERBB2, ALK, IGFR1, FGFR, and others, downstream pathway activation, epithelial-to-mesenchymal transition, histologic transformation, oncogenic gene fusions and cell-cycle gene aberrations (15).

Currently, platinum-based chemotherapy remains the standard of care after osimertinib resistance develops. Several early phase clinical trials for overcoming osimertinib resistance in NSCLC patients are ongoing. The strategies in these trials are mainly targeting specific known resistance mechanisms, including MET-inhibitors, MEK inhibitors, or combination of VEGF-inhibition with EGFR-TKIs (16). According to the phase Ib TATTON study involving patients with advanced EGFR-mutant NSCLC, osimertinib with either the MEK1/2 inhibitors (selumetinib or durvalumab), MET-inhibitor (savolitinib), or the PDL1-inhibitor (durvalumab) seemed to be safe and tolerable by patients (26). Currently the phase II clinical trial testing osimertinib plus savolitinib in EGFRm+/MET+ NSCLC patients following prior osimertinib (SAVANNAH) is still ongoing (NCT03778229). In another phase II study recruiting patients with advanced NSCLC who progressed on first-line osimertinib therapy (ORCHARD; NCT03944772), up to 9 experimental modules are tested: including Osimertinib + Savolitinib, Osimertinib + Gefitinib, Osimertinib + Necitumumab, Carboplatin + Pemetrexed + Durvalumab, Osimertinib + Alectinib, Osimertinib + Selpercatinib, Etoposide + Durvalumab + Carboplatin or Cisplatin, Osimertinib + Pemetrexed + Carboplatin or Cisplatin, Osimertinib + Selumetinib. However, the estimated primary completion date is set to be in the year of 2025. Therefore, whether these strategies could be beneficial to NSCLC patients with CNS metastasis and osimertinib resistance remains unclear. Immunotherapy using immune checkpoint inhibitors has been utilized in EGFR-mutated NSCLC patients, though its efficacy seemed to be not as good as in other cancers (27). Currently it is not clear whether immunotherapy has beneficial effects in NSCLC patients with Osimertinib resistance. However, it should be noted that interstitial lung disease-like events could occur when combining checkpoint inhibitors with osimertinib according to the phase Ib TATTON trial which assessed treatment of osimertinib in combination with durvalumab (26).

This case report in the patient with mutations in EGFR pL858R, TP53, and ERBB2 supported that dacomitinib, a second-generation EGFR-TKI, together with olaparib, a PARP inhibitor, may benefit NSCLC patient with CNS metastases after developing osimertinib resistance. The possible mechanisms could be as followed. First, dacomitinib is a selective inhibitor for ERBB2. It has been reported that dacomitinib could suppress the proliferation of Ba/F3 cells expressing T790M in *cis* to different deletions in exon 19 (IC50: 140-330 nmol/L) (28). Since this patient was tested positive for ERBB2 mutation in his CSF samples, dacomitinib might be the most relevant drug and he obtained the beneficial treatment result. Second, as suggested in the *in vitro* and *in vivo* experiments by Lynnette Marcar et al., the PARP inhibitor could increase reactive oxygen species (ROS) production and induce oxidative damage in osimertinib-resistant EGFR mutant NSCLC cells (20). Third, in triple-negative breast cancer, it has been shown that TP53 mutations combined with BRCA1 mutations are very frequent and may be sensitive to PARP inhibitors (29). Therefore, PARP inhibitors may also benefit NSCLC patients with TP53 mutations, which requires further evaluation. Moreover, it is known that P-glycoprotein (P-gp) is one of the proteins expressed naturally on the plasma membrane of endothelial cells in the blood-brain barrier (BBB), that could restrict substrate compounds from entering the brain (30). PARP inhibitors including olaparib, veliparib, and CEP-8983 are P-glycoprotein substrates (31). Therefore, olaparib may help enhance the antagonizing effect of dacomitinib on multidrug resistance, by inhibiting the efflux activity of ABCB1 and ABCG2 transporters (32).

In summary, exploring treatment strategies for patients with acquired osimertinib drug resistance is critical, particularly for patients with CNS metastases. The cerebrospinal fluid genetic testing plays an important role in guiding individualized treatment of patients with CNS metastases, as appropriate targeted treatments could be selected based on testing results. PARP inhibitors, olaparib, combined with EGFR-TKIs, may benefit patients with CNS metastases of NSCLC, and this combination strategy of multiple-target therapy is safe and holds promise for clinical application.

AUTHOR CONTRIBUTIONS

HZ, YW, XM, and SZ collected the clinical and pathological data. HW and HZ wrote the manuscript. JY and RT assisted in revising the manuscript. All authors contributed to the article and approved the submitted version.

REFERENCES

Dawe DE, Greenspoon JN, Ellis PM. Brain Metastases in Non-Small-Cell Lung Cancer. *Clin Lung Cancer* (2014) 15(4):249–57. doi: 10.1016/j.cllc. 2014.04.008

Cheng H, Perez-Soler R. Leptomeningeal Metastases in Non-Small-Cell Lung Cancer. *Lancet Oncol* (2018) 19(1):e43–55. doi: 10.1016/S1470-2045(17) 30689-7

Morris PG, Reiner AS, Szenberg OR, Clarke JL, Panageas KS, Perez HR, et al. Leptomeningeal Metastasis From Non-Small Cell Lung Cancer: Survival and the Impact of Whole Brain Radiotherapy. *J Thorac Oncol* (2012) 7(2):382–5. doi: 10.1097/JTO.0b013e3182398e4f

Wu YL, Zhou L, Lu Y. Intrathecal Chemotherapy as a Treatment for Leptomeningeal Metastasis of Non-Small Cell Lung Cancer: A Pooled Analysis. *Oncol Lett* (2016) 12(2):1301–14. doi: 10.3892/ol.2016.4783

Page S, Milner-Watts C, Perna M, Janzic U, Vidal N, Kaudeer N, et al. Systemic Treatment of Brain Metastases in Non-Small Cell Lung Cancer. *Eur J Cancer* (2020) 132:187–98. doi: 10.1016/j.ejca.2020.03.006

Remon J, Le Rhun E, Besse B. Leptomeningeal Carcinomatosis in Non-Small Cell Lung Cancer Patients: A Continuing Challenge in the Personalized Treatment Era. *Cancer Treat Rev* (2017) 53:128–37. doi: 10.1016/j.ctrv. 2016.12.006

Li YS, Jiang BY, Yang JJ, Tu HY, Zhou Q, Guo WB, et al. Leptomeningeal Metastases in Patients With Nsclc With Egfr Mutations. *J Thorac Oncol* (2016) 11(11):1962–9. doi: 10.1016/j.jtho.2016.06.029

Mantovani C, Gastino A, Cerrato M, Badellino S, Ricardi U, Levis M. Modern Radiation Therapy for the Management of Brain Metastases From Non-Small Cell Lung Cancer: Current Approaches and Future Directions. *Front Oncol* (2021) 11:772789. doi: 10.3389/fonc.2021.772789

Cross DA, Ashton SE, Ghiorghiu S, Eberlein C, Nebhan CA, Spitzler PJ, et al. Azd9291, an Irreversible Egfr Tki, Overcomes T790m-Mediated Resistance to Egfr Inhibitors in Lung Cancer. *Cancer Discov* (2014) 4(9):1046–61. doi: 10.1158/2159-8290.CD-14-0337

Odogwu L, Mathieu L, Goldberg KB, Blumenthal GM, Larkins E, Fiero MH, et al. Fda Benefit-Risk Assessment of Osimertinib for the Treatment of Metastatic Non-Small Cell Lung Cancer Harboring Epidermal Growth Factor Receptor T790m Mutation. *Oncologist* (2018) 23(3):353–9. doi: 10.1634/theoncologist.2017-0425

Ballard P, Yates JW, Yang Z, Kim DW, Yang JC, Cantarini M, et al. Preclinical Comparison of Osimertinib With Other Egfr-Tkis in Egfr-Mutant Nsclc Brain Metastases Models, and Early Evidence of Clinical Brain Metastases Activity. *Clin Cancer Res* (2016) 22(20):5130–40. doi: 10.1158/1078-0432.CCR-16- 0399

Nanjo S, Ebi H, Arai S, Takeuchi S, Yamada T, Mochizuki S, et al. High Efficacy of Third Generation Egfr Inhibitor Azd9291 in a Leptomeningeal Carcinomatosis Model With Egfr-Mutant Lung Cancer Cells. *Oncotarget* (2016) 7(4):3847–56. doi: 10.18632/oncotarget.6758

Yang JCH, Kim SW, Kim DW, Lee JS, Cho BC, Ahn JS, et al. Osimertinib in Patients With Epidermal Growth Factor Receptor Mutation-Positive Non- Small-Cell Lung Cancer and Leptomeningeal Metastases: The Bloom Study. *J Clin Oncol* (2020) 38(6):538–47. doi: 10.1200/JCO.19.00457

Park S, Lee MH, Seong M, Kim ST, Kang JH, Cho BC, et al. A Phase Ii, Multicenter, Two Cohort Study of 160 Mg Osimertinib in Egfr T790m- Positive Non-Small-Cell Lung Cancer Patients With Brain Metastases or Leptomeningeal Disease Who Progressed on Prior Egfr Tki Therapy. *Ann Oncol* (2020) 31(10):1397–404. doi: 10.1016/j.annonc.2020.06.017

Leonetti A, Sharma S, Minari R, Perego P, Giovannetti E, Tiseo M. Resistance Mechanisms to Osimertinib in Egfr-Mutated Non-Small Cell Lung Cancer. *Br J Cancer* (2019) 121(9):725–37. doi: 10.1038/s41416-019-0573-8

Schmid S, Li JJN, Leighl NB. Mechanisms of Osimertinib Resistance and Emerging Treatment Options. *Lung Cancer* (2020) 147:123–9. doi: 10.1016/j.lungcan.2020.07.014

Sequist LV, Han JY, Ahn MJ, Cho BC, Yu H, Kim SW, et al. Osimertinib Plus Savolitinib in Patients With Egfr Mutation-Positive, Met-Amplified, Non-Small-Cell Lung Cancer After Progression on Egfr Tyrosine Kinase Inhibitors: Interim Results From a Multicentre, Open-Label, Phase 1b Study. *Lancet Oncol* (2020) 21(3):373–86. doi: 10.1016/S1470-2045(19)30785-5

Chen A. Parp Inhibitors: Its Role in Treatment of Cancer. *Chin J Cancer* (2011) 30(7):463–71. doi: 10.5732/cjc.011.10111

Rose M, Burgess JT, O'Byrne K, Richard DJ, Bolderson E. Parp Inhibitors: Clinical Relevance, Mechanisms of Action and Tumor Resistance. *Front Cell Dev Biol* (2020) 8:564601. doi: 10.3389/fcell.2020.564601

Marcar L, Bardhan K, Gheorghiu L, Dinkelborg P, Pfaffle H, Liu Q, et al. Acquired Resistance of Egfr-Mutated Lung Cancer to Tyrosine Kinase Inhibitor Treatment Promotes Parp Inhibitor Sensitivity. *Cell Rep* (2019) 27 (12):3422–32 e4. doi: 10.1016/j.celrep.2019.05.058

Marcinowska-Suchowierska E, Lorenc R, Brzozowski R. [Effect of Long-Term Irradiation of the Skin on Calcium-Phosphate Metabolism and the 25-Oh-D Level in Patients With Chronic Diseases of the Digestive System]. *Przegl Lek* (1988) 45(8):614–9.

Li HS, Yang GJ, Wang Y. Case Report: Dacomitinib May Not Benefit Patients Who Develop Rare Compound Mutations After Later-Line Osimertinib Treatment. *Front Oncol* (2021) 11:649843. doi: 10.3389/fonc.2021.649843

McEwen AE, Leary SES, Lockwood CM. Beyond the Blood: Csf-Derived Cfdna for Diagnosis and Characterization of Cns Tumors. *Front Cell Dev Biol* (2020) 8:45. doi: 10.3389/fcell.2020.00045

Li YS, Jiang BY, Yang JJ, Zhang XC, Zhang Z, Ye JY, et al. Unique Genetic Profiles From Cerebrospinal Fluid Cell-Free DNA in Leptomeningeal Metastases of Egfr-Mutant Non-Small-Cell Lung Cancer: A New Medium of Liquid Biopsy. *Ann Oncol* (2018) 29(4):945–52. doi: 10.1093/annonc/ mdy009

Kang SJ, Kim KS, Ha YS, Huh SY, Lee JH, Kim JK, et al. Diagnostic Value of Cerebrospinal Fluid Level of Carcinoembryonic Antigen in Patients With Leptomeningeal Carcinomatous Metastasis. *J Clin Neurol* (2010) 6(1):33–7. doi: 10.3988/jcn.2010.6.1.33

Oxnard GR, Yang JC, Yu H, Kim SW, Saka H, Horn L, et al. Tatton: A Multi- Arm, Phase Ib Trial of Osimertinib Combined With Selumetinib, Savolitinib, or Durvalumab in Egfr-Mutant Lung Cancer. *Ann Oncol* (2020) 31(4):507–16. doi: 10.1016/j.annonc.2020.01.013

Jin R, Zhao J, Xia L, Li Q, Li W, Peng L, et al. Application of Immune Checkpoint Inhibitors in Egfr-Mutant Non-Small-Cell Lung Cancer: From Bed to Bench. *Ther Adv Med Oncol* (2020) 12:1758835920930333. doi: 10.1177/1758835920930333

Lavacchi D, Mazzoni F, Giaccone G. Clinical Evaluation of Dacomitinib for the Treatment of Metastatic Non-Small Cell Lung Cancer (Nsclc): Current Perspectives. *Drug Des Devel Ther* (2019) 13:3187–98. doi: 10.2147/ DDDT. S194231

Na B, Yu X, Withers T, Gilleran J, Yao M, Foo TK, et al. Therapeutic Targeting of Brca1 and Tp53 Mutant Breast Cancer Through Mutant P53 Reactivation. *NPJ Breast Cancer* (2019) 5:14. doi: 10.1038/s41523-019-0110-1

Aryal M, Fischer K, Gentile C, Gitto S, Zhang YZ, McDannold N. Effects on P-Glycoprotein Expression After Blood-Brain Barrier Disruption Using Focused Ultrasound and Microbubbles. *PloS One* (2017) 12(1):e0166061. doi: 10.1371/journal.pone.0166061

Lawlor D, Martin P, Busschots S, Thery J, O'Leary JJ, Hennessy BT, et al. Parp Inhibitors as P-Glyoprotein Substrates. *J Pharm Sci* (2014) 103(6):1913–20. doi: 10.1002/jps.23952

Fan YF, Zhang W, Zeng L, Lei ZN, Cai CY, Gupta P, et al. Dacomitinib Antagonizes Multidrug Resistance (Mdr) in Cancer Cells by Inhibiting the Efflux Activity of Abcb1 and Abcg2 Transporters. *Cancer Lett* (2018) 421:186– 98. doi: 10.1016/j.canlet.2018.01.021

6

Anti-Tumor Effect of Simvastatin in Combination with DNA Methyltransferase Inhibitor on Gastric Cancer via GSDME-Mediated Pyroptosis

Ying Xia[1,2,3,4†], Yong Jin[1,4†], Daxiang Cui[5], Xia Wu[6], Cunfeng Song[5], Weilin Jin[5,7*] and Hai Huang[1,4*]*

[1]Center for Clinical Laboratories, The Affiliated Hospital of Guizhou Medical University, Guiyang, China, [2]Department of Pathophysiology, School of Basic Medical Science, Guizhou Medical University, Guiyang, China, [3]Department of Clinical Laboratory, The First Affiliated Hospital of Guizhou University of Traditional Chinese Medicine, Guiyang, China, [4]School of Clinical Laboratory Science, Guizhou Medical University, Guiyang, China, [5]Shanghai Engineering Research Center for Intelligent Diagnosis and Treatment Instrument, Department of Instrument Science and Engineering, School of Electronic Information and Electrical Engineering, Institute of Nano Biomedicine and Engineering, Shanghai Jiao Tong University, Shanghai, China, [6]Guizhou Provincial People's Hospital, Guiyang, China, [7]Institute of Cancer Neuroscience, Medical Frontier Innovation Research Center, The First Hospital of Lanzhou University, The First Clinical Medical College of Lanzhou University, Lanzhou, China

***Correspondence:**
Cunfeng Song
songcf@sjtu.edu.cn
Weilin Jin
ldyy_jinwl@lzu.edu.cn
Hai Huang
huanghai828@gmc.edu.cn

[†]These authors have contributed equally to this work

Gasdermin E (GSDME) is one of the executors of pyroptosis, a type of programmed lytic cell death, which can be triggered by caspase-3 activation upon stimulation. Silenced GSDME expression due to promoter hypermethylation is associated with gastric cancer (GC), which is confirmed in the present study by bioinformatics analysis and methylation-specific PCR (MSP) test of GC cell lines and clinical samples. GC cell lines and mouse xenograft models were used to investigate the pyroptosis-inducing effect of the common cholesterol-depleting, drug simvastatin (SIM), allied with upregulating GSDME expression by doxycycline (DOX)- inducible Tet-on system or DNA methyltransferase inhibitor 5-Aza-2′-deoxycytidine (5-Aza-CdR). Cell viability assessment and xenograft tumour growth demonstrated that the tumour inhibition effects of SIM can be enhanced by elevated GSDME expression. Morphological examinations and assays measuring lactate dehydrogenase (LDH) release and caspase-3/GSDME protein cleavage underlined the stimulation of pyroptosis as an important mechanism. Using short hairpin RNA (shRNA) knockdown of caspase-3 or GSDME, and caspase-3-specific inhibitors, we provided evidence of the requirement of caspase-3/GSDME in the pyroptosis process triggered by SIM. We conclude that reactivating GSDME expression and thereby inducing cancer cell-specific pyroptosis could be a potential therapeutic strategy against GC.

Keywords: GSDME, pyroptosis, DNA methyltransferase inhibitor, gastric cancer, simvastatin

INTRODUCTION

Gastric cancer (GC) is ranked third in cancer mortality and poses a serious threat to human health (Mattiuzzi and Lippi, 2020). To date, surgery and chemoradiotherapy remain the first-line treatment towards GC, but many patients still suffer from poor prognosis and low 5-year survival rate due to severe adverse effects and acquired drug resistance (Yang et al., 2022). Induction of pyroptosis has been emerging as a novel therapeutic strategy against a variety of malignant tumours including GC (Zhou and Fang, 2019; Tan et al., 2021a; Li et al., 2021; Shao et al., 2021), because of its dual function of cytotoxicity and immunogenicity.

Pyroptosis is a gasdermin (GSDM)-dependent programmed cell death featuring membrane rupture formed by translocated GSDM fragments originated from caspase cleavage (Xia et al., 2020). One important characteristic of pyroptosis is the release of cellular contents such as pro-inflammatory cytokines interleukin-1β (IL-1β) and interleukin-18 (IL-18), which actively regulate the immune profile of the tumour microenvironment (Tan et al., 2021b). Gasdermin D (GSDMD) and gasdermin E (GSDME) are the best-studied pyroptotic effectors in the GSDM family. Their sheared N-terminals perforate cell membrane in a similar manner but differ in the activation cascades (Jorgensen and Miao, 2015; Hou et al., 2021). The anti-tumour action of Cucurbitacin B was found to involve the activation of GSDMD-dependent pyroptosis of non-small cell lung cancer (NSCLC) cells *in vitro* and *in vivo* (Yuan et al., 2021). GSDME, located on chromosome 7p15 and also named deafness autosomal dominant 5 (DFNA5) due to its association with hereditary hearing loss (Van Laer et al., 1998), has been implicated as a putative tumour suppressor (Rogers et al., 2017; Wang et al., 2017). Cleaved by the activated caspase-3, the N-terminal of GSDME (GSDME-N) inserts into the membrane lipids and forms pores to trigger pyroptosis (Wang et al., 2017).

In contrast to the substantial investment of time and resources into developing a new drug from scratch repurposing approved drugs can significantly accelerate the clinical translation of basic research (Pushpakom et al., 2019), as exemplified in the quest for drugs to induce pyroptosis. The histamine 2 antagonist famotidine is found to induce GSDME-, not GSDMD-, mediated cell pyroptosis by activation of NLRP3 inflammasome form, leading to increase Caspase-1 activation and IL-18 release in GC cells (Huang et al., 2021). In recent years, studies and clinical trials exploiting the preventive and therapeutic potential of statin in cancer treatment are flourishing. Statin is a class of HMG-CoA reductase inhibitors and the most commonly prescribed cholesterol-reducing drugs thanks to their safety, efficacy, and low cost (Jiang et al., 2021a). In particular, it was shown that simvastatin (SIM), one of the six statin medicines, elicits its anti-cancer effects through not only lowering of cholesterol content, but also activation of caspase-3 (Deng et al., 2019; Alhakamy et al., 2020; Sun et al., 2020) and consequently apoptosis or pyroptosis (Peng et al., 2020; Xu et al., 2021). Moreover, the SIM-induced pyroptosis is confirmed to be cancer cell-specific in lung cancer, without causing toxicity to normal cells (Wang et al., 2018).

However, the death of tumour cells *via* pyroptosis is often dampened by epigenetic silencing of GSDME, as hypermethylation of GSDME promoter is found in about 52%–65% of primary cancers (Op de Beeck et al., 2011) including colorectal cancer (Kim et al., 2008a; Yokomizo et al., 2012) and GC (Akino et al., 2007). Studies have used hypomethylating agents such as decitabine (DAC) (Fan et al., 2019) or 5-aza-2′-deoxycytidine (5-Aza-CdR) (Kim et al., 2008b) to restore the transcription of the GSDME gene and reinstate the sensitivity of various cancer cells, including GC cells, to chemotherapy (Akino et al., 2007). In this study, using GC cell lines MGC-803 and HGC-27 and mouse xenograft GC models, we aim to seek the optimal antitumor effects of SIM-induced pyroptosis, in tandem with upregulating GSDME gene expression.

MATERIALS AND METHODS

Patient Samples

The surgical specimens of 20 paired GC tissues and adjacent non-cancerous tissues were collected from the Departments of Gastrointestinal Surgery, Affiliated Hospital of Guizhou Medical University. Use of the clinical samples were approved by the Affiliated Hospital of Guizhou Medical University Ethics Committee, approval number: 2020 (106). Written informed consent was acquired from all patients. The clinicopathological characteristics of the patients are shown in **Supplementary Table S1**.

Cell Culture and Reagents

The GC cell lines AGS, MKN45, and HGC-27 were obtained from the Chinese Academy of Sciences (Shanghai, China). The GC cell line MGC-803 was from the Institute of Nano Biomedicine and Engineering, Shanghai Engineering Research Centre (Shanghai, China). The cells were cultured in Dulbecco's modified Eagle's medium (HyClone, Logan, UT, United States) containing 10% foetal bovine serum (FBS, Gibco BRL, Gaithersburg, MD, United States), 100 U/ml penicillin, and 100 mg/ml streptomycin (Invitrogen, Carlsbad, CA, United States). All cells were incubated at 37°C in 5% CO_2. SIM (Cat. HY-17502) and 5-Aza-CdR (Cat. HY-0004) were purchased from MedChemExpress (Shanghai, China). Doxorubicin hydrochloride (DOX, Cat. ST039A) was from Beyotime Biotechnology (Shanghai, China). 3, 3′-Dioctadecyloxacarbocyanine perchlorate (DIO, Cat. 40725ES10) was from YEASEN (Shanghai, China). Caspase-3 inhibitors (Ac-DMPD-CMK [DMPD] and Ac-DMLD-CMK [DMLD]) were courtesy of Professor Li-Juan Cao (China Pharmaceutical University, Nanjing, China). DOX and 5-Aza-CdR were dissolved in phosphate-buffered saline (PBS, Servicebio, Cat. G0002-2L) and stored at −20°C. SIM, DIO, and the caspase-3 inhibitors were dissolved in dimethyl sulfoxide (DMSO, Sigma, Cat. D2650) and stored at −20°C.

Cell Treatment

Cells were seeded in 10 cm-diameter culture plates. Once the cells were 80% confluent, they were treated with certain concentration of SIM or with equal volumes of DMSO as control, for 48 h. For the inhibitor experiments, DMPD (5 μM) or DMLD (5 μM) was added to the cells 6 h before SIM treatment. For the SIM and 5-Aza-CdR combination experiments, MGC-803 and HGC-27 cells were incubated in medium containing 1 μM 5-Aza-CdR, refreshed daily for 72 h (Akino et al., 2007; Yanokura et al., 2020) before treatmen with 5 μM SIM (MGC-803 cells) or 20 μM SIM (HGC-27 cells) in the new medium for another 48 h.

Cell Viability Assay

Cell proliferation was measured by a Cell Counting Kit-8 (CCK8) Assay Kit following manufacturer's instructions (YEASEN, Cat. 40203ES60). The data is presented as the percent (%) of viable cells relative to the control.

Lactate Dehydrogenase Release Assay

Cellular toxicity was detected using an LDH Cytotoxicity Assay kit, following the manufacturer's instructions (Beyotime Biotechnology, Cat. C0017). Cellular membrane integrity was evaluated by the amount of LDH leaking from the damaged cell membrane and presented as fold changes to the control.

Transmission Electron Microscopy (TEM)

MGC-803 cells were treated with SIM (5 μM) and after 48 h incubation, they were harvested and fixed in 2.5% glutaraldehyde in PBS (pH 7.4) at 4°C, and post-fixed with 1.3% osmic tetroxide. Subsequently, the cells were dehydrated in graded alcohols, transferred to propylene oxide, and embedded in epoxy resin. Thereafter, ultrathin sections were stained with uranyl acetate followed by lead citrate. Finally, sections were transferred to copper grids and observed with an 80-kV transmission electron microscope (Wang et al., 2021).

Plasmids Lentivirus Transfection

All plasmids (Tet-on overexpression GSDME plasmid, the plasmids of GSDME-shRNA and caspase 3-shRNA knockdown and their control plasmids) were constructed by Public Protein/Plasmid Library. The procedure for lentivirus transfection has already been described previously (Zhou et al., 2019). For GSDME gene expression induction, 1 μg/ml of DOX was used in the medium for 4 days incubation (Croft et al., 2011). Stable low-expression or over-expression of GSDME in MGC-803 cells and HGC-27 cells were detected by real-time quantitative PCR (RT-qPCR) and Western blotting.

RNA Extraction and Real-Time quantitative PCR

Total RNA was extracted from the frozen tissue or cultured cells with TRIzol (Invitrogen, Cat. 15596018), following the manufacturer's instructions. Expression of the target genes was quantified with reverse transcription and RT-qPCR kits (Takara, Cat. DRR820A), normalized to the housekeeping gene β-actin. The relative gene expression levels were determined by the comparative threshold cycle ($2^{-\Delta\Delta CT}$) method. **Supplementary Table S1** shows the primers used in the RT-qPCR.

Western Blotting

Protein lysates were processed in RIPA-buffer (Beyotime, Cat. P0013C) supplemented with phosphatase inhibitor cocktail (Beyotime, Cat. P1050) and protease inhibitors (Beyotime, Cat. P1010). The protein was quantified by bicinchoninic acid (BCA) analysis (Beyotime, Cat. P0012). The protein extracts (30 μg/lane) were separated on SDS-PAGE gels, followed by electrotransferring onto polyvinylidene fluoride (PVDF) membranes. After blocking with 5% fat-free milk for 2 h at room temperature, the membranes were incubated with primary antibodies and subsequently incubated with secondary antibody. Information regarding the primary antibodies used is listed in **Supplementary Table S3**.

Colony Formation Assay

The cells (5000 cells/well) were seeded into 6-well plates. After overnight incubation, they were subjected to the indicated treatment and then cultured in a fresh medium for 2 weeks. Colonies were fixed in 4% paraformaldehyde and visualized with 0.1% crystalline violet.

Methylation Analyses

The association between GC and other common cancers with the degree of GSDME gene methylation was assessed using DiseaseMeth version 2.0 (http://biobigdata.hrbmu.edu.cn/diseasemeth/, accessed 30 August 2021). The database is used to provide information on abnormal DNA methylation in human diseases, especially cancer, in the most complete collection and annotations to date (Xiong et al., 2017).

Methylation-Specific PCR

The genomic DNA was extracted using a genomic DNA kit (Tiangen Biotech, Beijing, China) to determine the GSDME methylation status by MSP. Briefly, genomic DNA was bisulfite-treated using an EZ DNA Methylation-Gold Kit (Zymo Research, Cat. D5005). Bisulphite-treated DNA was amplified using primers specific for either methylated or unmethylated DNA, designed by Sangon Biotech (Shanghai, China). The methylated DNA-specific (M) and unmethylated DNA-specific (U) primer sequences for GSDME are shown in **Supplementary Table S5**.

Pyroptotic Cell Imaging

To observe the features of pyroptosis, the cells were plated in 24-well plates. The cytomembrane and the nucleus of cells post-treatment were stained with DIO (green fluorescence) and Hoechst 33342 (blue fluorescence), respectively. Fluorescence images were photographed using an inverted fluorescence microscope (Nikon Eclipse Ti, Tokyo, Japan).

In Vivo Experiments

All procedures involving animals were reviewed and approved by the Guizhou Medical University the Animal Care Welfare

Committee (approval number: 2001338). Five-week-old female immunodeficient BALB/c nude mice were purchased from the SLRC Laboratory Animal Center (Shanghai, China). MGC-803 cells w/wo Tet-on system for DOX-indicible GSDME were implanted subcutaneously in the right flanks of the mice to study the antitumor effects of SIM w/wo GSDME overexpression (mouse set 1) and w/wo the auxiliary therapy of 5-Aza-CdR (mouse set 2), respectively. When the tumours reached a volume of approximately 60 mm^3, the mice were randomly divided into four groups (n = 5 each). Groups in set 1 were DOX (-) vehicle control, DOX (+) GSDME overexpression, DOX (-) with SIM, and DOX (+) with SIM, as summarized in **Supplementary Figure S1A**. Groups in set 2 were vehicle control, 5-Aza-CdR, SIM and SIM+5-Aza-CdR group, as illustrated in **Supplementary Figure S1B**. Mice were weighed every 2–3 days. The tumour size was measured with digital callipers every 2 or 3 days. Tumour volume was calculated using the following equation: volume = (width^2 × length)/2. In each group, changes in the tumor sites were recorded every 7 days by the camera. The treatment lasted 18 days. At the end of the experiment, blood, tumours, livers, lungs, hearts, spleens, and kidneys of the mice were collected for subsequent experiments. Half of the tumour tissues and main organs were fixed in formalin and were paraffin-embedded for immunohistochemical (IHC) analysis, haematoxylin and eosin (H&E) staining and terminal deoxynucleotidyl transferase dUTP nick end labelling (TUNEL) assay (Roche, Cat. 1215679910). After TUNEL staining, the nucleus was counterstained with DAPI. The TUNEL-positive cells were photographed using an Ortho-Fluorescent Microscope (Nikon, Tokyo, Japan). The remaining tumour tissues were quickly frozen in liquid nitrogen and stored at −80°C for protein and nucleic acid detection. The blood was placed at room temperature for 2 h, centrifuged at 1,000 rpm for 20 min, and the separated serum was frozen at −80°C for subsequent experiments. The serum aspartate transaminase (AST), alanine transaminase (ALT), blood urea nitrogen (BUN), and creatinine (CRE) levels were analysed with an automated biochemical analyser, Chemray 240 (Lei Du Life Scientific and Technical Corporation, Shenzhen, China).

H&E Staining and Immunohistochemical

Xenograft tumour tissues and main organs of the mice as well as human GC tissues and paired adjacent non-cancerous tissues were dewaxed in xylene and rehydrated in a graded alcohol series. Tumour tissue and main organ morphology were observed using H&E staining. IHC was performed using antibodies against Ki67, GSDME, and cleaved (Cl)-caspase-3 using an immunohistochemical test kit (Boster, SA1020). Images were captured using a Nikon E100 upright microscope (Nikon, Tokyo, Japan). The source and dilution of the primary antibodies are listed in **Supplemenatry Table S2**. The mean analyses of integrated optical density (IOD) in IHC staining were calculated with Image-ProPlus6.0 (Media Cybernetics, Silver Spring, MD, United States). Protein expression levels were quantified by IOD in five random visual fields (×40) before calculating the average value. For animal experiments, from each group of mice, tissues of three mice were selected for statistical analysis.

Statistical Analysis

GraphPad Prism 7.04 (GraphPad, San Diego, CA, United States) was used for statistical analysis and graphics. The data are the mean ± SD of at least three independent experiments. Comparisons between two groups were analyzed by Student's t-test. Comparisons between multiple groups were made using one-way analysis of variance (ANOVA), and two-way ANOVA for comparisons between multiple groups with independent variables. A p-value < 0.05 was considered significant.

RESULTS

SIM Activates GSDME-Dependent Pyroptosis in GC Cells

Cell proliferation of the four different GC cell lines was inhibited to various degrees by treatment of SIM from 2.5 to 20 μM for 48 h (**Figure 1A**). Among them, MGC-803 cells were the most sensitive (IC_{50} = 4.623 μM), while HGC-27 cells were the most resistant (IC_{50} = 20.24 μM) to SIM (**Figure 1A; Table 1**). Consistently, membrane ballooning, a signature of pyroptosis, was revealed extensively in SIM-treated MGC-803 cells by microscopy, but sparse in HGC-27 cells (**Figure 1B**). The basal expression levels of GSDME protein and mRNA were low or undetectable in AGS and HGC-27 cells (**Figures 1C,D**), whereas the MGC-803 cells had the highest GSDME expression at both mRNA and protein levels. The different abundance of GSDME in the four cell lines displayed a positive correlation with cell sensitivity to SIM, which was not shown in GSDMD expression (**Figures 1C,E**). A dose-dependent increase in the LDH release rates in the culture medium of SIM-treated MGC-803 cells was detected (**Figure 1F**). SIM also induced the cleavage of caspase-3 (Cl-casp3) and GSDME (GSDME-N) in the MGC-803 cells in a dose-dependent manner, but not GSDMD (**Figure 1G**). Therefore, the involvement of GSDMD in SIM-induced pyroptosis is disproved. Treatment of SIM at 5 μM was chosen for all subsequent experiments in MGC-803 cells as the cells would retain half of the viability, plateaued LDH release and significant GSDME-N cleavage, representing an ideal induction of pyroptosis. Further observation of the morphological alterations by TEM showed that SIM-treated cells had typical pyroptosis features including membrane pore formation, membrane leakiness and organelle swelling, and low cytosol density (**Figure 1H**), confirming the microscopy results (**Figure 1B**). Collectively, these data indicate that SIM induces pyroptosis in GC cells by activating GSDME.

SIM-Induced Pyroptosis in GC cells Involves Caspase-3-Mediated Cleavage of GSDME

In MGC-803 cells with stable knock down of caspase-3 (CASP3) or GSDME by lentiviral shRNA (**Figures 2A–D**), SIM-induced

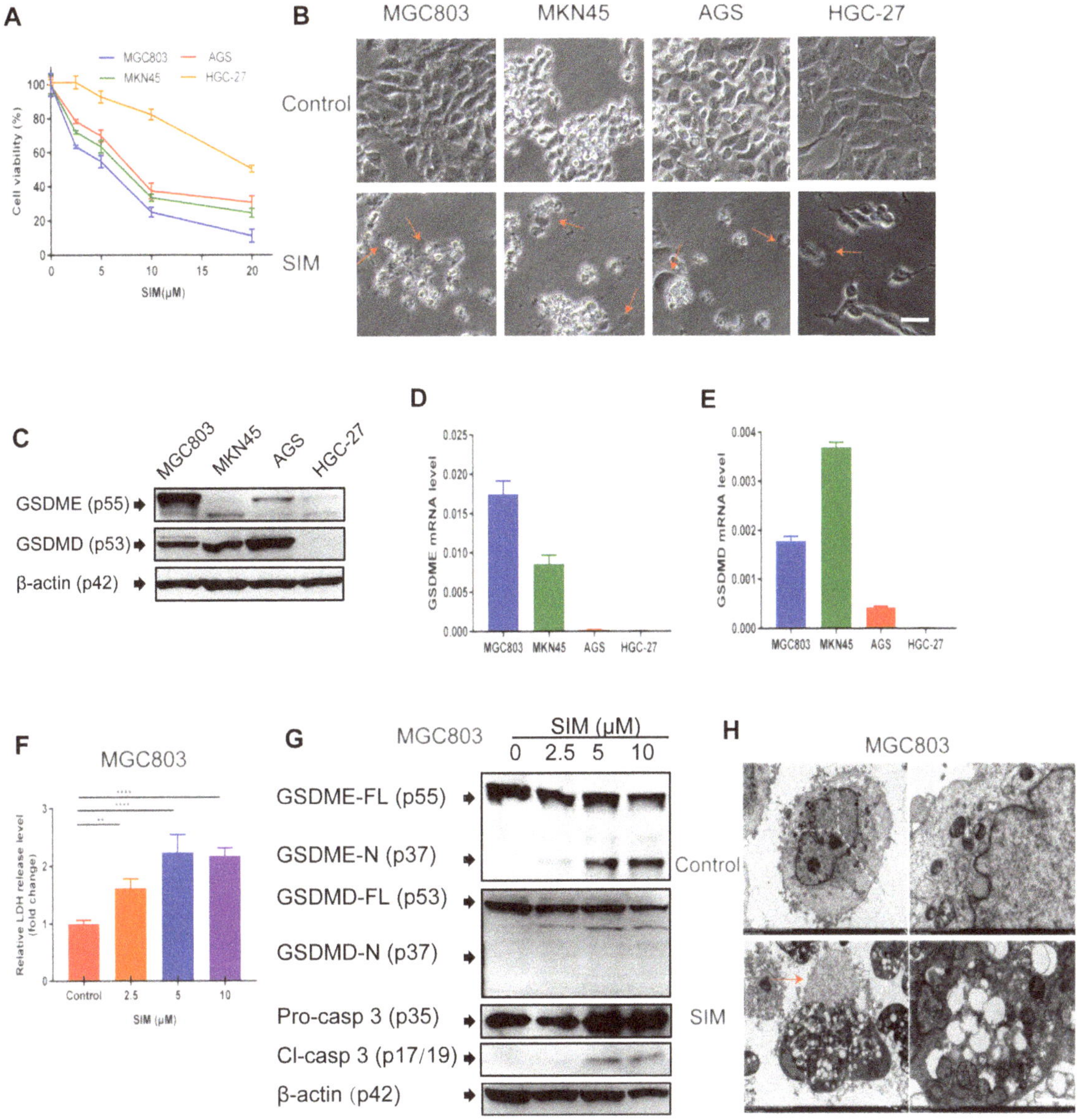

FIGURE 1 | SIM induces GSDME-dependent pyroptosis in GC cells. **(A)** Cell viability of four GC cell lines treated with different doses of SIM for 48 h, detected by CCK8 (n = 3). **(B)** Microscopic imaging of four GC cell lines treated with SIM. Red arrows indicate ballooned cell membrane, a characteristic of pyroptotic cells; scale bar = 50 μm. **(C)** Protein levels of GSDME and GSDMD in four GC cell lines, determined by Western blotting. **(D,E)** The mRNA expression of GSDME and GSDMD gene, detected by RT-qPCR. **(F)** Release of LDH into the culture supernatant, detected by LDH assay kit (n = 4). **(G)** Protein levels of full length (FL) or N-terminal of GSDME and GSDMD, pro-caspase 3 (pro-casp3) and cleaved caspase-3 (Cl-casp3) of SIM-treated MGC-803 cells. **(H)** Electron microscopic images of MGC-803 cells treated with 5 μM SIM for 48 h. Red arrows indicate ballooned cell membrane characteristic of pyroptotic cells; scale bar = 10 μm. Data are shown as mean ± SD or representatives of at least three independent experiments. β-actin was used as an internal control for Western blot. $^{**}p < 0.01$, and $^{****}p < 0.0001$.

TABLE 1 | IC_{50} values of SIM treatment on four GC cell lines.

Cell lines	IC_{50} (μM)	±SD
MGC-803	4.623	0.030
MKN45	6.630	0.026
AGS	8.376	0.033
HGC-27	20.240	0.016

SD, standard deviation.

proliferation inhibition (**Figure 2E**), LDH release (**Figure 2F**), cell swelling (**Figure 2G**), cleavage of GSDME-N and Cl-caspase 3 (**Figure 2H**) were all significantly blunted. Similar blocking effects were observed in the cells treated with caspase-3 inhibitor DMPD or DMLD, 6 h prior to SIM administration (**Figures 2I–K**). DMPD and DMLD bind directly to the catalytic domains of caspase-3 to specifically inhibit the activity of GSDME. The results indicated that caspase-3 and GSDME are necessary for SIM-induced pyroptosis.

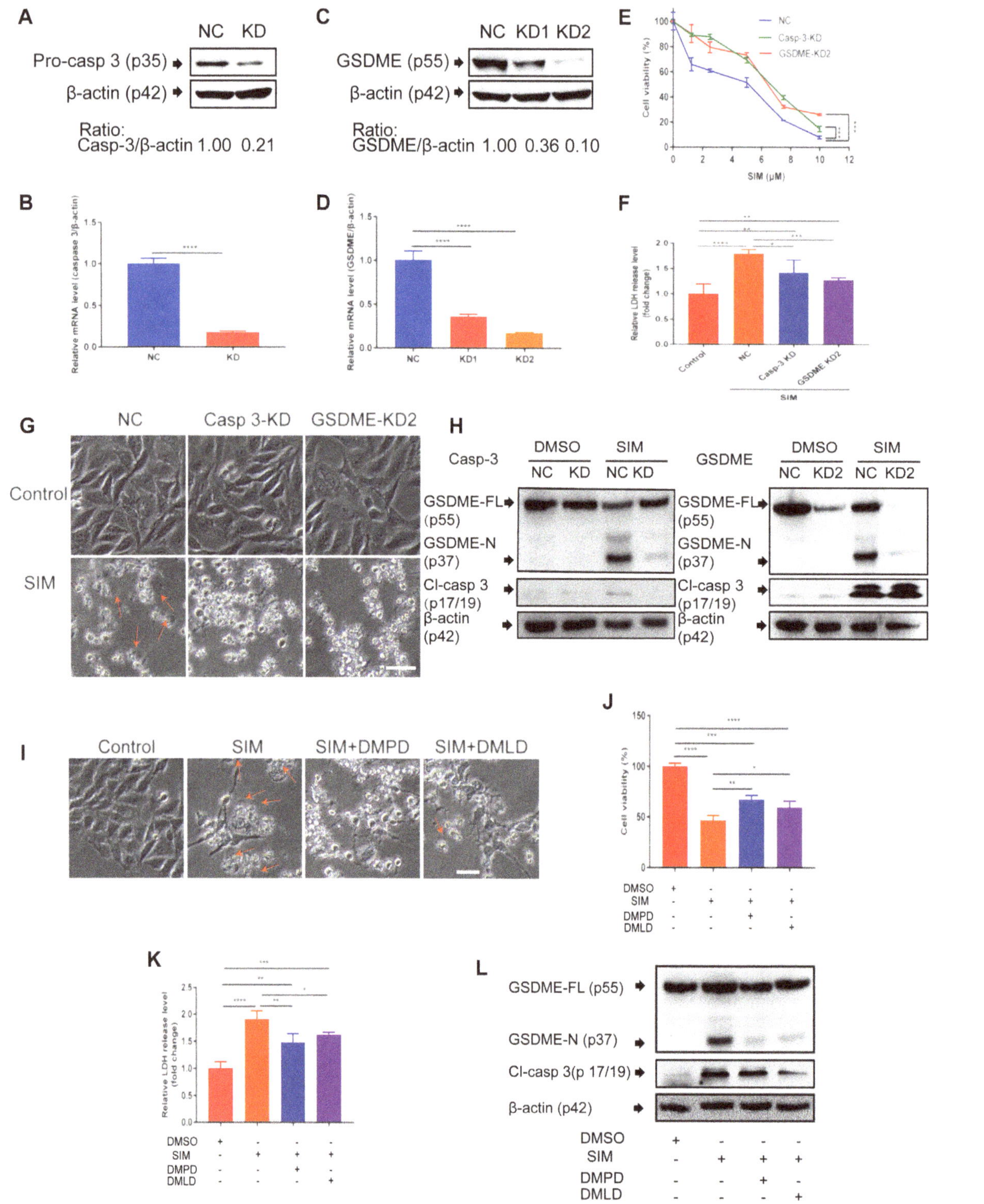

FIGURE 2 | Caspase-3 and GSDME are required in SIM-induced pyroptosis. **(A–D)** Validation of the shRNA knockdown of caspase 3 or GSDME in MGC-803 cells by Western blotting and RT-qPCR. After the treatment of SIM at concentrations ranging from 0 to 10 μM with caspase 3 or GSDME knockdown, scrambled NC as the control, **(E)** cell viability was detected by CCK8 ($n = 3$) and **(F)** release of LDH into the culture supernatant was detected by LDH assay kit ($n = 4$), **(G)** Microscopic imaging of the cells treated with 5 μM SIM for 48 h, w/wo caspase 3 or GSDME knockdown. Red arrows indicate ballooned cell membrane; scale bar = 50 μm ($n = 3$). **(H)** Representative immunoblotting analysis of GSDME and cl-casp3 of the cells treated with 5 μM SIM for 48 h, w/wo caspase 3 or GSDME knockdown. **(I–L)** Microscopic morphology, cell viability, LDH release and protein cleavage of GSDME and caspase-3 of MGC-803 cells treated with 5 μM SIM for 48 h, w/wo the caspase-3 inhibitor Ac-DMPD-CMK (DMPD) or Ac-DMLD-CMKR (DMLD). Data are shown as mean ± SD or representatives of at least three independent experiments. β-actin was used as an internal control for Western blot. $^{*}p < 0.05$, $^{**}p < 0.01$, $^{***}p < 0.001$ and $^{****}p < 0.0001$.

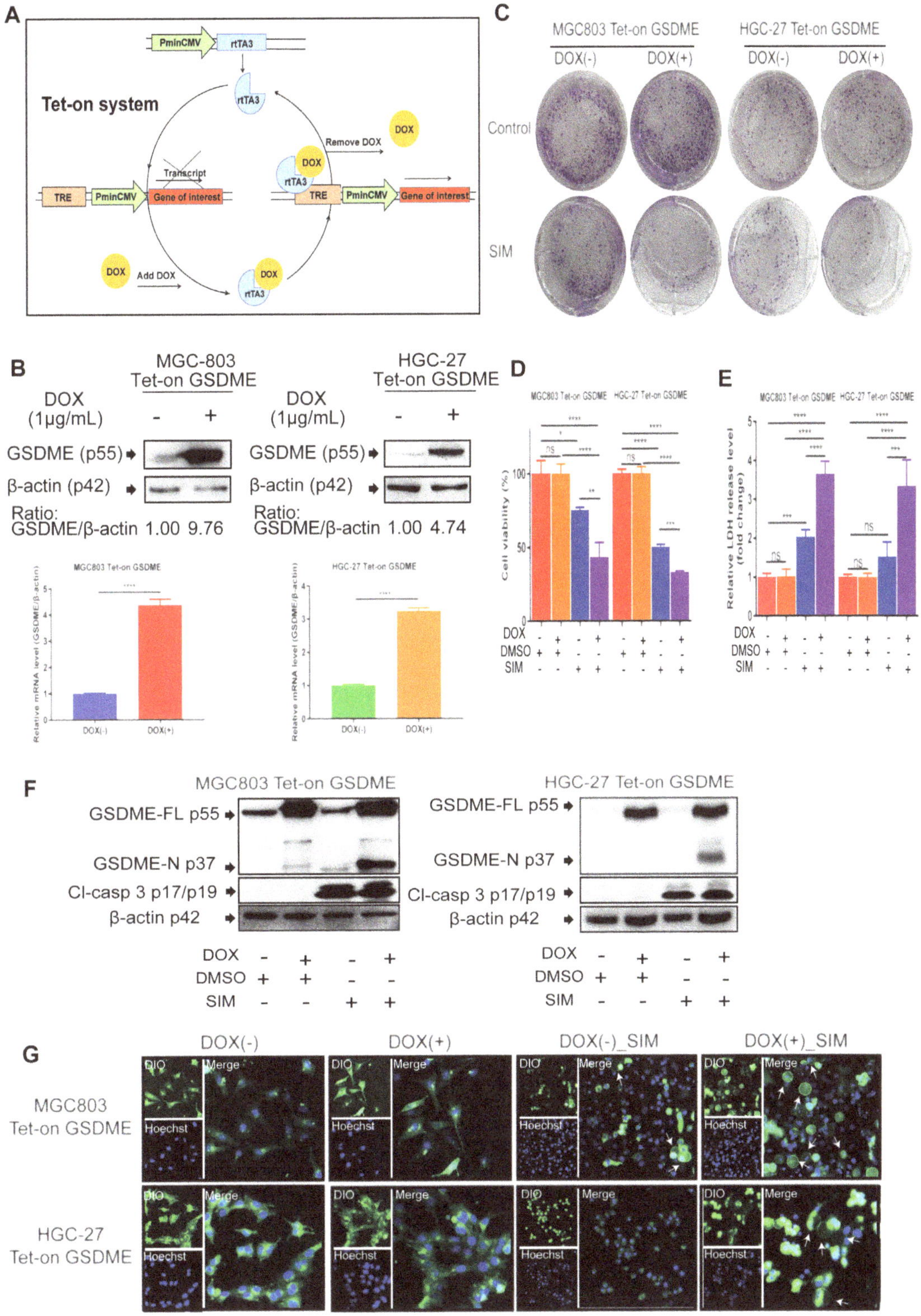

FIGURE 3 | Overexpression of GSDME enhanced SIM-induced cell pyroptosis. **(A)** Schematic representation of the DOX- controlled Tet-on system. **(B)** Validated of GSDME overexpression in MGC-803 or HGC-27 cells by Western blotting and RT-qPCR. Colony formation **(C)**, Cell viability **(D)**, LDH release **(E)** and protein cleavage of GSDME and caspase-3 **(F)** of GSDME-overexpressing MGC-803 and HGC-27 cells treated with SIM for 48 h. **(G)** Fluorescence microscopy imaging of GSDME-overexpressing MGC-803 and HGC-27 cells treated with SIM for 48 h, DIO (green fluorescence) was used to dye cell cytomembrane, and Hoechst 33342 (Blue fluorescence) the cell nucleus. White arrows indicate ballooned cell membrane; scale bar = 50 μm. Data are shown as mean ± SD or representatives of at least three independent experiments. β-actin was used as an internal control for Western blot. *$p < 0.05$, **$p < 0.01$, ***$p < 0.001$ and ****$p < 0.0001$.

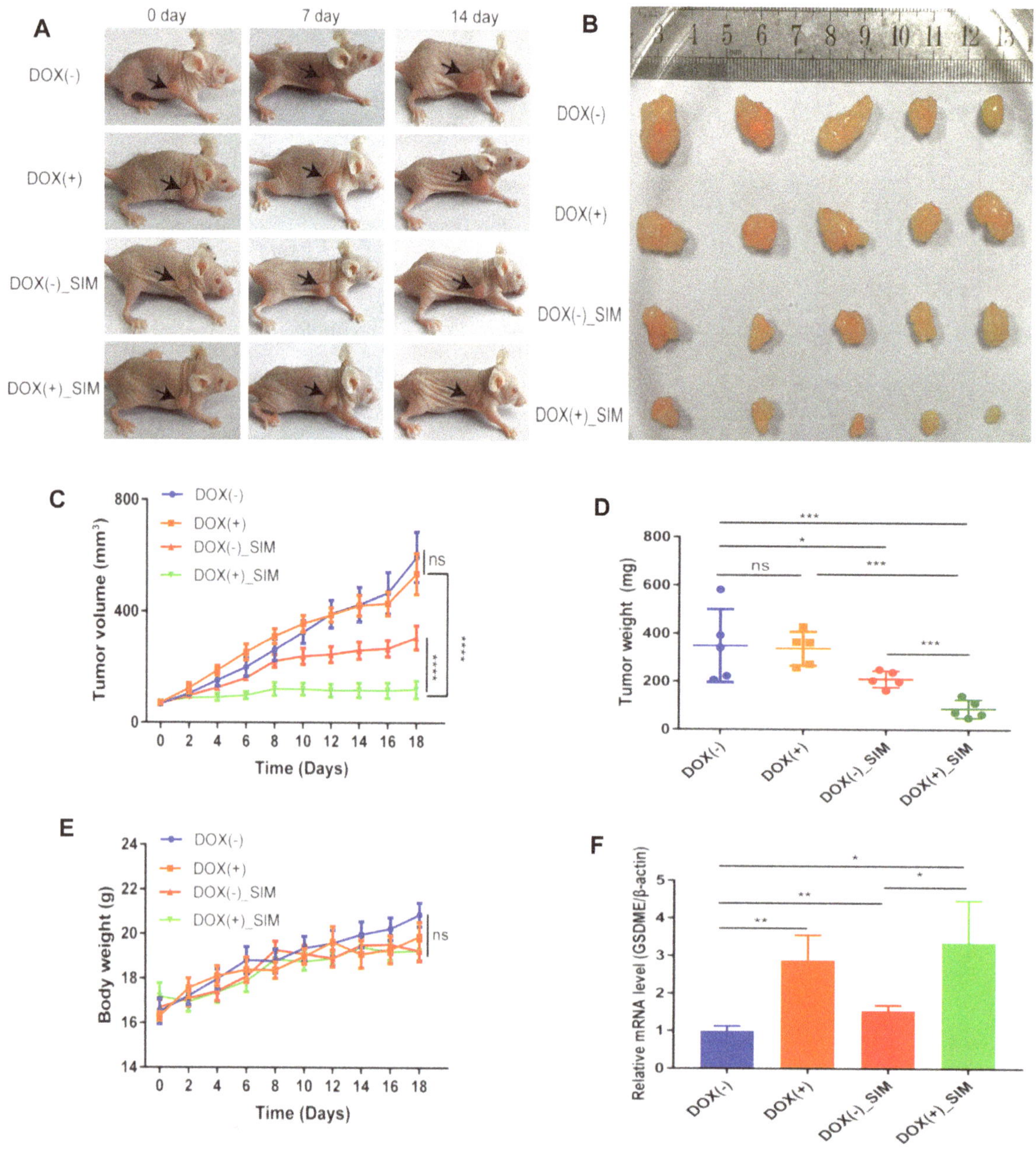

FIGURE 4 | SIM and GSDME overexpression additively inhibit tumour growth in mouse xenografts. **(A)** Photos of mice with xenograft tumours during the treatment. **(B)** Tumours dissected and imaged at the end point of experiment. **(C)** Tumour volumes during the treatment ($n = 5$). **(D)** Tumour weights at the end of the experiment ($n = 5$). **(E)** Average body weight of each group ($n = 5$) **(F)** The of GSDME gene expression in xenograft tumour tissues, detected by RT-qPCR ($n = 3$). $^{*}p < 0.05$, $^{**}p < 0.01$, $^{***}p < 0.001$, $^{****}p < 0.0001$ and $p > 0.05$ not significant (ns).

GSDME Overexpression Enhances SIM-Induced GC Cell Pyroptosis

To manipulate the gene expression of GSDME, we used the doxycycline (DOX)- inducible Tet-on system that allows reversibly switching on or off the GSDME gene by DOX (**Figure 3A**). The efficiency of the system was confirmed by successful induction of GSDME overexpression in MGC-803 and HGC-27 cells upon the addition of DOX to the culture medium (**Figure 3B**). While adding DOX alone had no impact on cell viability and colony formation, it synergistically enhanced the SIM-induced inhibition of proliferation and clonogenicity of these cells (**Figures 3C,D**). Moreover, LDH release (**Figure 3E**), GSDME cleavage (**Figure 3F**) and cell swelling (**Figure 3G**) were augmented with consistency, demonstrating an additive effect of GSDME overexpression on SIM-induced pyroptosis.

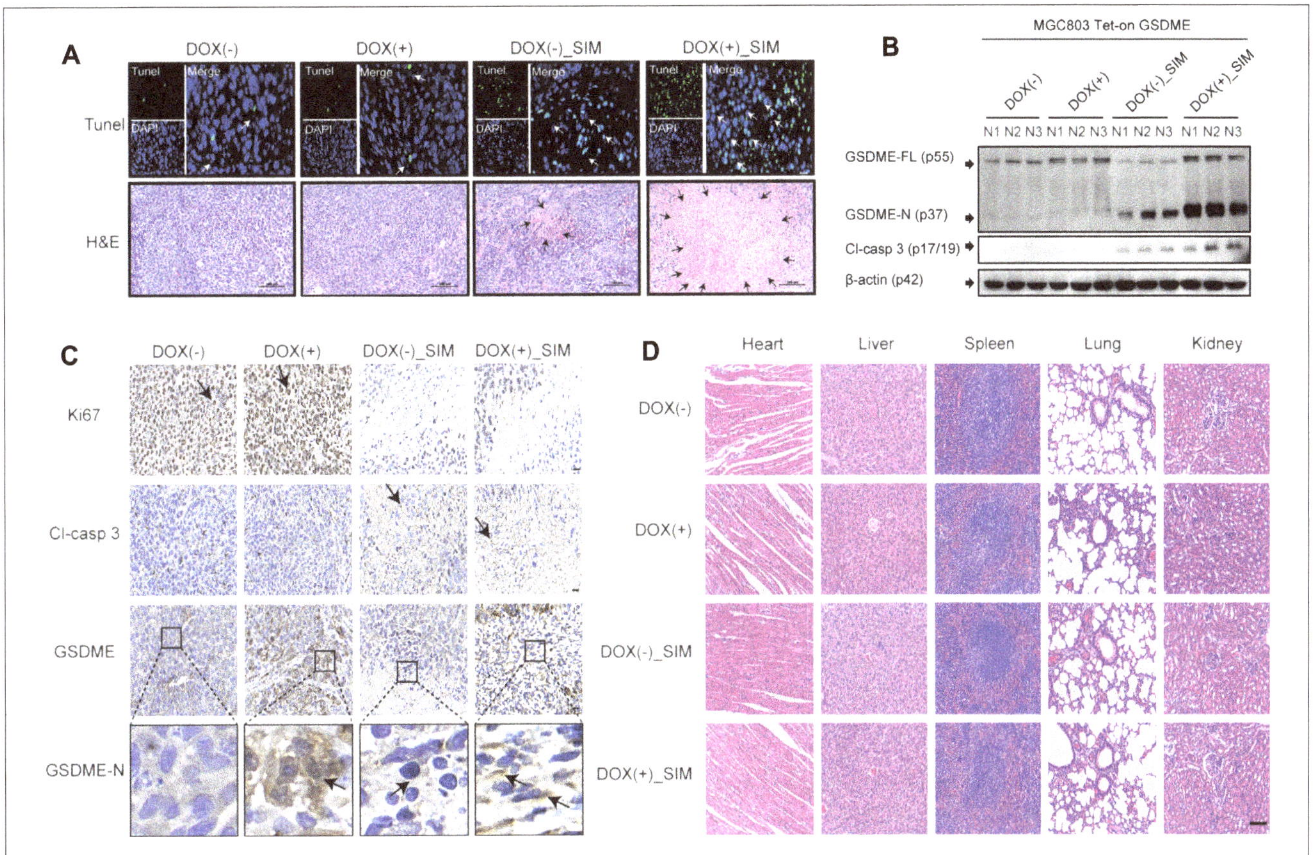

FIGURE 5 | SIM combined with overexpression-GSDME promotes the progression of GC pyroptosis *in vivo*. **(A)** TUNEL and H&E staining images for tumour slices after indicated treatment. White arrows indicate TUNEL positive cells. TUNEL scale bar: 20 μm; the areas of necrosis were indicated by black arrows in the figures. H&E scale bar: 100 μm. **(B)** Protein cleavage of GSDME and caspase-3 in tumour tissues, detected by Western blotting **(C)** Immunohistochemistry (IHC) images of Ki67, Cl-casp3, GSDME and GSDME-N for tumour tissues after indicated treatment; black arrows indicate the IHC staining-positive cells; scale bar: 20 μm. **(D)** HE staining of heart, liver, spleen, lung, and kidney tissues in each group; scale bar = 100 μm.

Combining SIM With GSDME Overexpression Potently Inhibits Tumour Growth *In Vivo*

To examine the *in vivo* GC tumorigenicity under influence of GSDME regulation, we established a xenograft model by injecting the DOX-inducible Tet-on MGC-803 cells into nude mice (**Supplementary Figure S1A**). During the 18-day treatment, the changes at tumour sites of each group were recorded every 7 days (**Figure 4A**). Both SIM group and DOX (+) _SIM group demonstrated significantly inhibited tumour growth (**Figure 4B**) and reduced tumour volume (**Figure 4C**) and tumour weight (**Figure 4D**), but no impact on body weight (**Figure 4E**). Compared to SIM alone, the extent of the inhibition was notably exaggerated when GSDME gene expression was promoted in the xenograft tissues by intake of DOX water by the mice (**Figures 4A–F**), whereas switching on the GSDME gene expression *per se* did not affect tumour development (**Figures 4C–E**). H&E and TUNEL staining indicated that GSDME overexpression combined with SIM induced more intensive DNA fragmentation and ultimately cell death in the tumour (**Figure 5A**), accompanied by decreased Ki67 expression, a cell proliferation marker (**Figure 5C; Supplementary Figure S2A**). The increased Cl-caspase-3 and GSDME-N abundance in the SIM group were evidently boosted by GSDME overexpression in DOX (+) SIM group, shown consistently by western blot (**Figure 5B**) and IHC (**Figure 5C; Supplementary Figures S2B,C**). Meanwhile, no damage was observed in the heart, spleen, lung, and kidney, compared between all groups (**Figure 5D**). The functionality of the liver and kidney remained intact, as suggested by the healthy serum levels of AST, ALT, BUN, and CRE in all groups ($p > 0.05$) (**Supplementary Table S5**). These *in vivo* data confirmed the previous finding that GSDME overexpression enhanced SIM-induced cell growth inhibition and pyroptosis by activating the caspase-3/GSDME pathway.

GSDME Demethylation Enhances SIM-Induced GC Cell Pyroptosis

The association between some common cancers and GSDME gene methylation was examined using DiseaseMeth version 2.0. Among all the malignancies examined, GC had the highest statistical significance of its positive association with GSDME

TABLE 2 | Association between disease and methylation of GSDME/DFNA5.

Disease name	Gene symbol	Mean methyl disease	Mean methyl normal	*p*-value	Methyl-type
Gastric cancer	GSDME/DFNA5	0.235	0.092	1.62E-12****	hyper-methyl
Breast neoplasms	GSDME/DFNA5	0.54	0.441	1.89E-05****	–
Esophageal cancer esophageal squamous cell carcinoma without metastasis	GSDME/DFNA5	0.392	0.308	3.22E-02*	–
Brain cancer ganglioneuroma	GSDME/DFNA5	0.03	0.022	1.98E-01	–
Lung cancer lung squamous cell carcinoma	GSDME/DFNA5	0.45	0.446	5.14E-01	–

*p < 0.05 and ****p < 0.0001.

hypermethylation (p = 1.62E-12, **Table 2**). The heatmap of methylation showed that GC tissues had a significantly higher degree of GSDME methylation than the normal tissues (**Figure 6A**). In the GC tissues, GSDME protein and mRNA levels were downregulated compared with the adjacent normal tissues, as determined by IHC and RT-qPCR (**Figures 6B,C; Supplementary Figure S2D**). However, no significant correlation was found between the clinicopathological parameters and GSDME expression levels in GC tissue of 20 patients with GC (**Supplementary Table S1**). MSP revealed partial methylation of GSDME at the promoter region in HGC-27 cells and to a lesser extent in MGC-803 cells (**Figure 6D**), which matched the superior resilience of HGC-27 cells to pyroptosis (**Figure 1**). Treatment of 5-Aza-CdR on MGC-803 and HGC-27 cells demethylated the GSDME gene (**Figure 6D**) and restored its mRNA transcription (**Figure 6E**). Cells pre-treated with 1 μM 5-Aza-CdR for 72 h were more responsive to SIM treatment than SIM alone, demonstrated by cell viability (**Figure 6F**), LDH release (**Figure 6G**), GSDME/caspase-3 cleavage (**Figure 6H**) and cell swelling (**Figure 6I**). These results implied that GSDME demethylation facilitated SIM-induced GC cell proliferation inhibition and pyroptosis.

5-Aza-CdR Amplifies the Antitumor Effects of SIM in a Xenograft Model

Mice bearing GC xenograft was generated by subcutaneous transplantation of MGC-803 cells into nude mice (**Supplementary Figure 1B**). Compared to the vehicle group, both the SIM and SIM+5-Aza-CdR combination group had significantly inhibited tumour growth (**Figures 7A,B**) and reduced tumour volume (**Figure 7C**) and tumour weight (**Figure 7D**). The delay in tumour growth was considerably more pronounced in the combination group compared with the SIM group (**Figures 7A–D**), which mirrored what we observed in the Tet-on GSDME overexpression mouse model. However, rather than continuous and undistinguishable bodyweight gain in all groups, as seen in the previous xenograft experiment, the bodyweight of the mice in the SIM+5-Aza-CdR combination group decreased during treatment and started to catch up at day 15 (**Figure 7E**). Compared with the vehicle, 5-Aza-CdR monotherapy promoted GSDME expression (**Figure 7F**) but did not affect tumour growth (**Figures 7C,D**). Furthermore, compared with the SIM group, the combination group induced more significant caspase-3-dependent cleavage of GSDME (**Figure 7F**). As expected, TUNEL and H&E staining showed more remarkable DNA breakdown and diminished Ki67 staining in tumour tissues, reflecting an increased vulnerability of cancer cells to pyroptosis triggered by the combined therapy (**Figure 8A**) than the SIM monotherapy. In addition to that, there was no detectable damage found in the heart, liver, spleen, lung, and kidney by H&E staining (**Figure 8B**), and the serum concentrations of AST, ALT, BUN, and CRE remained in the normal range throughout all groups (**Supplementary Table S6**). In summary, GSDME demethylation enhanced SIM-induced GC cell proliferation inhibition and pyroptosis by regulating the caspase-3/GSDME pathway, without damage to the main organs.

DISCUSSION

Beyond cardiovascular protection *via* interrupting the biosynthesis of cholesterol, statins merit great attention for their antineoplastic activity (Jiang et al., 2021a), evidenced in multiple clinical observations and experimental investigations. A recent South Korean prospective study pointed out that the use of statins could reduce GC mortality in the general population (Cho et al., 2021). In particular, pleiotropic mechanisms have been proposed to underlie the action of SIM against cancers (Chiu et al., 2011), such as inhibiting tumour cell proliferation, migration and invasion, and promoting apoptosis by simultaneously targeting YAP and β-catenin signalling (Liu et al., 2020). Adding to the extant knowledge, we found that SIM treatment for GC induces pyroptosis by activating caspase-3 to cleave GSDME.

Both GSDMD and GSDME could perforate cell membrane to initiate the pyroptosis process (Yu and He, 2017; Shi et al., 2015). GSDMD is abundantly present in GC cell lines except HGC-27. However, we found that the IC50 value of SIM on CG cells was negatively correlated with the baseline expression level of GSDME, not GSDMD (**Figure 1; Table 1**). The signs of pyroptosis including plasma membrane swelling and LDH release in SIM-treated MGC-803 cells were accompanied by the generation of GSDME-N, not GSDMD-N (**Figure 1**). Blocking the caspase-3/GSDME pathway by shRNA knockdown or inhibitors attenuated the SIM-induced pyroptosis, while conversely overexpressing GSDME encouraged GC cells to shift into pyroptotic death.

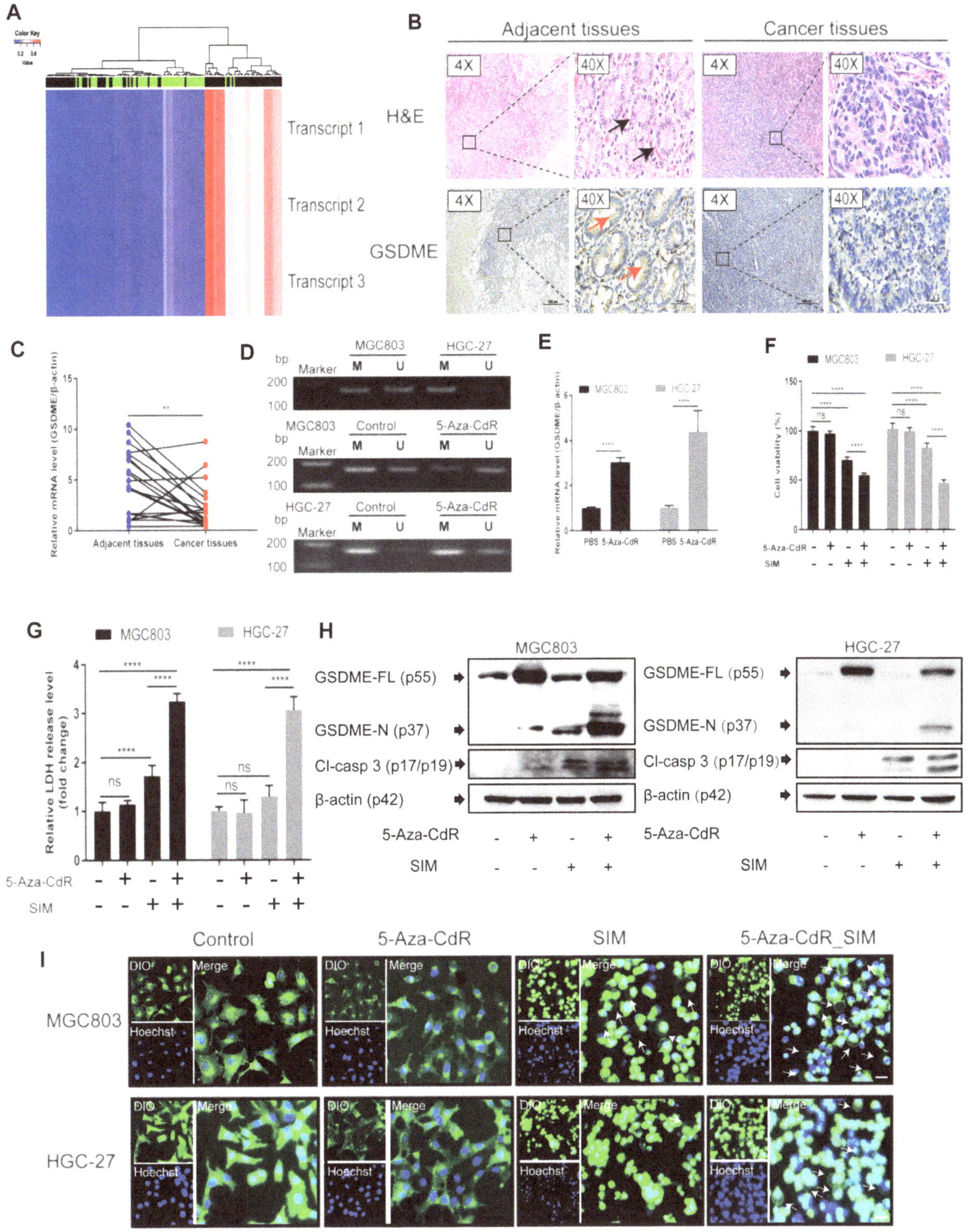

FIGURE 6 | Combination of SIM and 5-Aza-CdR enhances pyroptosis in GC. **(A)** The heatmap of GSDME methylation in GC. The heatmap contains methylation data of 3 transcripts from 141 samples of 27 k arrays. Rows represent transcripts and columns represent samples (green: normal profiles, black: disease profiles). **(B)** GSDME protein levels in human GC tissues and adjacent tissues, detected immunohistochemically using HE staining; black arrows indicate complete gastric gland; red arrows indicate the IHC staining-positive cells; scale bar = 50 μm. **(C)** Relative GSDME mRNA expression in human GC tissues and adjacent normal tissues, determined by RT-qPCR ($n = 20$). **(D)** MSP profiles of GSDME promoter methylation status in MGC-803 and HGC-27 cell before and after a daily dosing of 5-Aza-CdR for 72 h, M, methylated; U, unmethylated. After SIM treatment w/wo 5-Aza-CdR pre-dosing, **(E)** GSDME gene, **(F)** Cell viability, **(G)** LDH release, **(H)** protein cleavage of GSDME and caspase-3, and **(I)** fluorescence microscopy of theMGC-803 and HGC-27 cells examined. Data are shown as mean ± SD or representatives of at least three independent experiments. β-actin was used as an internal control for Western blot. $^{****}p < 0.0001$ and $p > 0.05$; ns, not significant.

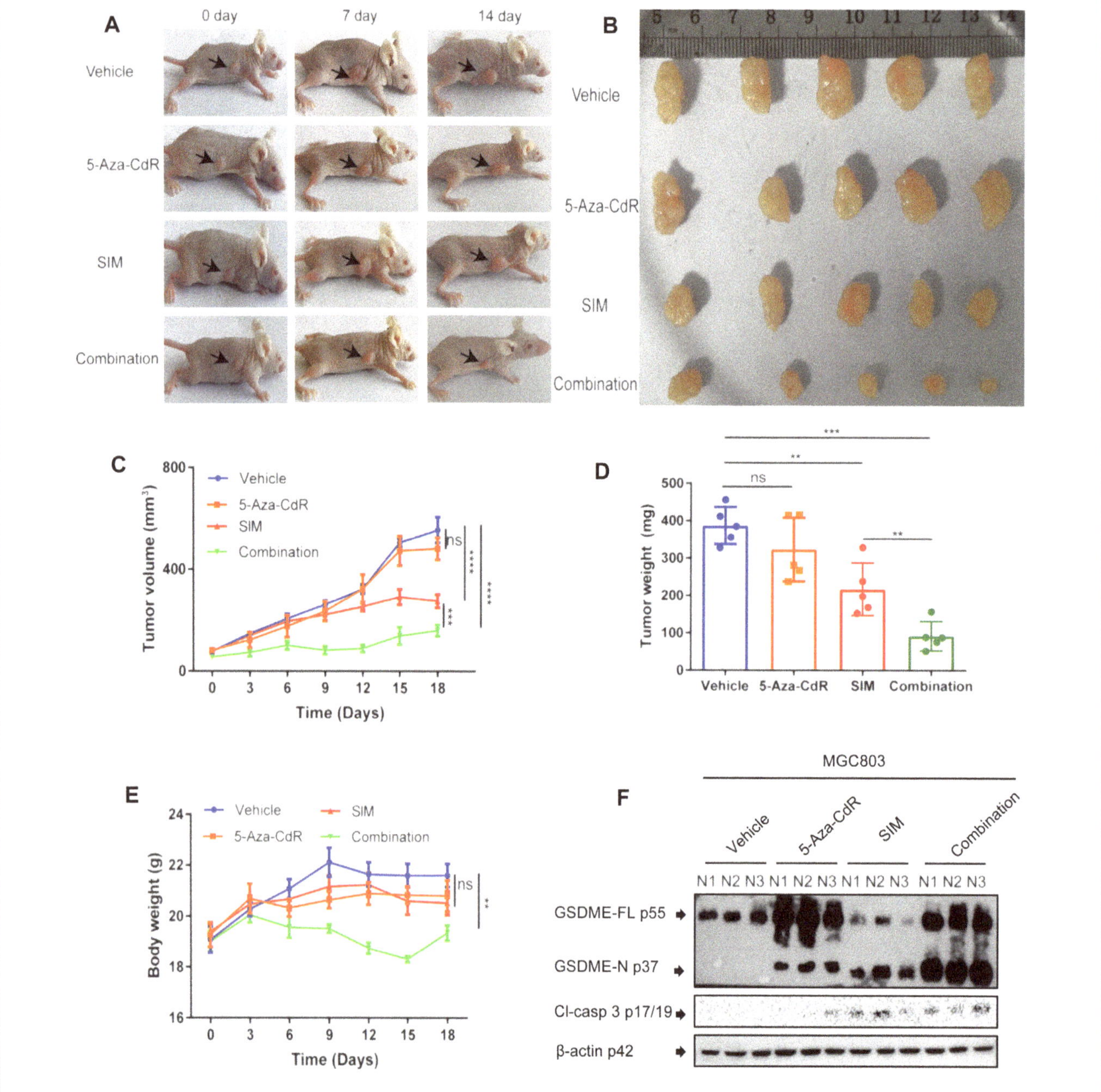

FIGURE 7 | Combination of SIM and 5-Aza-CdR potently inhibits tumour growth *in vivo*. **(A)** Photos of mice with xenograft tumours during the treatment. **(B)** Tumours dissected at the end point of the experiment. **(C)** Tumour volumes during the treatment ($n = 5$). **(D)** Tumour weights at the end of the experiment ($n = 5$). **(E)** Average body weight of each group during the treatment ($n = 5$). **(F)** Protein cleavage of GSDME and caspase-3 in tumour tissues, detected by Western blotting ($n = 3$). Data are shown as mean ± SD or representatives of at least three independent experiments. β-actin was used as an internal control for Western blot. $^{****}p < 0.0001$ and $p > 0.05$ not significant (ns).

These data demonstrate that GSDME, not GSDMD, is responsible for the pyroptosis in GC cells induced by SIM, corroborating the previous reports that GSDMD-dependent pyroptosis occurs mainly in non-cancerous cells (Ding et al., 2021; Han et al., 2021; Shi et al., 2021) and GSDME-dependent pyroptosis in cancer cells (Cai et al., 2021; Li et al., 2021; Shangguan et al., 2021).

Targeting pyroptosis is considered a novel enrichment to our cancer-fighting arsenal (Guo et al., 2021; Yuan et al., 2021) and GSDME is the newly recognized executor of pyroptosis (Xia et al., 2020). It has been reported that dihydroartemisinin (DHA), a conventional drug to kill malaria parasites, can induce pyroptosis of esophageal squamous cell carcinoma (ESCC) cells *via* PKM2 caspase-8/3-GSDME pathway, providing a potential therapeutic

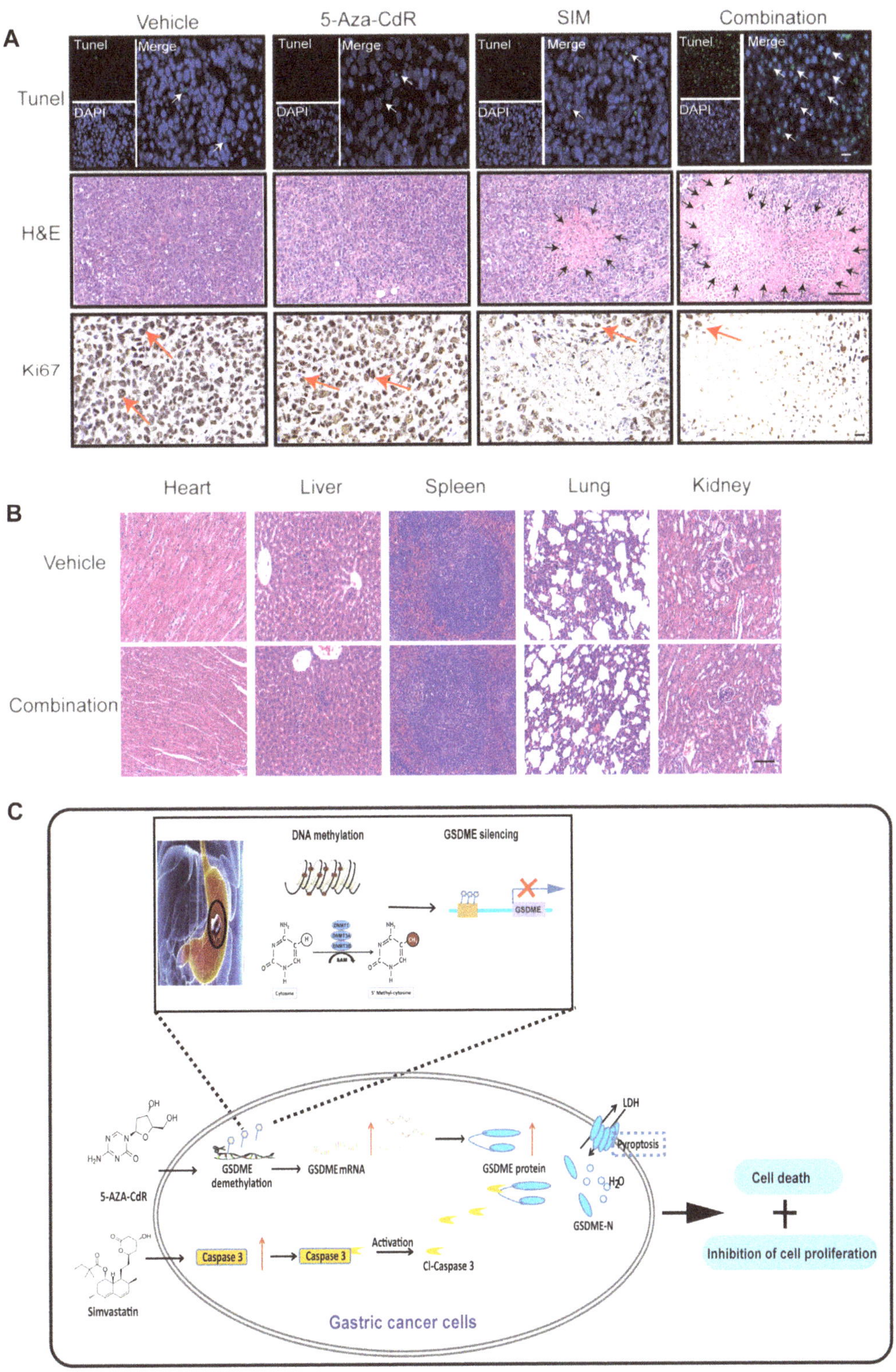

FIGURE 8 | 5-Aza-CdR promotes SIM-induced GC pyroptosis *via* caspase 3/GSDME pathway *in vivo*. **(A)** TUNEL, H&E staining and Ki67 IHC of xenograft tumour slices after indicated treatment. TUNEL scale bar: 20 μm. White arrows: TUNEL positive cells; H&E scale bar: 100 μm. Black arrows: the areas of necrosis; IHC scale bar: 20 μm. Red arrows: Ki67-positive cells. **(B)** HE staining of heart, liver, spleen, lung, and kidney tissues in each group; scale bar: 100 μm. **(C)** Schematic diagram to illustrate the mechanisms underlying the induction of pyroptosis in GC by a combined treatment of SIM with 5-Aza-CdR *via* caspase-3/GSDME activation.

agent for the treatment of ESCC (Jiang et al., 2021b). GSDME-dependent pyroptosis can also be triggered by chemotherapy (paclitaxel, cisplatin, lobaplatin, 5-fluorouracil (5-FU) and doxorubicin) or by targeted molecular drugs in malignant cells (Lu et al., 2018; Xia et al., 2020). As the GSDME gene is often silenced through hypermethylation in GC, either genetic tools or demethylating agents such as 5-Aza-CdR could restore the GSDME expression to facilitate a more efficient SIM therapy, as shown in our xenograft mice. As a potent methyltransferase inhibitor, 5-Aza-CdR is an FDA-approved epigenetic therapy to treat a wide array of cancers by reactivating multiple tumour suppressor genes (Christman, 2002). In our xenograft GC mice, combining SIM with GSDME overexpression demonstrated a tumour-specific targeting, and none of the main organs examined displayed observable damage. Nevertheless, effects of drug discontinuation and long-term administration, and potential adverse effects with a prolonged treatment duration, remain to be clarified by further investigation. Other vital tissues such as muscle and adipose would be included in future research too. In mice treated with both 5-Aza-CdR and SIM, we have seen a weight loss up to 37% to the initial value, which was rebounded promptly after treatment cessation. This side effect may be circumvented by an appropriate extension of the interval of the treatment cycle.

It must be stressed that SIM, the same as other statin medications, can exhibit anti-tumour effects from various aspects, such as metabolic reprogramming (Ni et al., 2021), immune regulation (Yu et al., 2022), and angiogenesis (Wesołowska et al., 2021), etc. that may not necessarily involve GSDME. Although the declined cell viability upon SIM treatment was attenuated significantly with disruption of caspase-3 or GSDME expression or function, the cytotoxicity of SIM was still profound, suggesting contributions of other mechanisms. How these different pathways crosstalk to each other is a burning question awaiting an answer.

In conclusion, SIM exerts an antitumor effect on GC *via* impaired cell proliferation and caspase-3/GSDME-mediated pyroptosis. Restorring GSDME expression by 5-Aza-CdR could be beneficial by sensitising GC cells to SIM.

LIMITATIONS OF THE STUDY

We noticed that SIM increased the transcription of the GSDME gene in MGC-803 cells and in the xenograft (**Figure 4F**; **Supplementary Figure S3**), and had to leave it unaddressed in the present work. Interestingly, statin has been hinted at as a DNA methyltransferase (DNMT) inhibitor. By suppressing DNMT, statins such as lovastatin and simvastatin could upregulate a couple of genes that were silenced by promoter hypermethylation, including BMP2, in colorectal cancer cells and xenograft mice. The outcome of this modulation by statin was a reversal of the malignant cells from the stem-like state into a more differentiated state (Kodach et al., 2011). We may speculate a similar epigenetic mechanism operating in our models.

AUTHOR CONTRIBUTIONS

YX and YJ performed the experiment, and was a major contributor in writing the manuscript. YX and XW analyzed and collected the patient data. DXC and CFS supervised the research of animal and provided facilities. HH and WLJ initiated the study. HH, WLJ and CFS revised the manuscript. All authors read and approved the final manuscript.

FUNDING

This study was supported by the research grants from the National Natural Science Foundation of China to HH (Grant No. 81760429 and 82060442), as well as the Research Funds for Guizhou Provincial Innovative Talents Team for 2019 (Grant No. 5610), the Science and Technology Project of Health and Family Planning Commission of Guizhou Province to YX (Grant No. gzwjkj 2018-1-072), the Science and Technology Project of Guizhou University of Traditional Chinese Medicine to YX [Grant No. (2018)101] and the Science and Technology Project of Guiyang City to YX [Grant No. (2019) 9-2].

ACKNOWLEDGMENTS

We thank Professor Li-Juan Cao for the gift of the caspase 3 inhibitors (Ac-DMPD-CMK and Ac-DMLD-CMK). The technical helps from Chang Yang, Hong Du, Wutong Zhou, and Shuqiang Chen are appreciated.

REFERENCES

Akino, K., Toyota, M., Suzuki, H., Imai, T., Maruyama, R., Kusano, M., et al. (2007). Identification of DFNA5 as a Target of Epigenetic Inactivation in Gastric Cancer. *Cancer Sci.* 98 (1), 88–95. doi:10.1111/j.1349-7006.2006.00351.x

Alhakamy, N. A., Fahmy, U. A., Ahmed, O. A. A., Caruso, G., Caraci, F., Asfour, H. Z., et al. (2020). Chitosan Coated Microparticles Enhance Simvastatin Colon Targeting and Pro-apoptotic Activity. *Mar. Drugs* 18 (4). doi:10.3390/md18040226

Cai, J., Yi, M., Tan, Y., Li, X., Li, G., Zeng, Z., et al. (2021). Natural Product Triptolide Induces GSDME-Mediated Pyroptosis in Head and Neck Cancer through Suppressing Mitochondrial Hexokinase-II. *J. Exp. Clin. Cancer Res.* 40 (1), 190. doi:10.1186/s13046-021-01995-7

Chiu, H. F., Ho, S. C., Chang, C. C., Wu, T. N., and Yang, C. Y. (2011). Statins Are Associated with a Reduced Risk of Gastric Cancer: a Population-Based Case-Control Study. *Am. J. Gastroenterol.* 106 (12), 2098–2103. doi:10.1038/ajg.2011.277

Cho, M. H., Yoo, T. G., Jeong, S. M., and Shin, D. W. (2021). Association of Aspirin, Metformin, and Statin Use with Gastric Cancer Incidence and Mortality: A Nationwide Cohort Study. *Cancer Prev. Res. (Phila)* 14 (1), 95–104. doi:10.1158/1940-6207.CAPR-20-0123

Christman, J. K. (2002). 5-Azacytidine and 5-Aza-2'-Deoxycytidine as Inhibitors of

DNA Methylation: Mechanistic Studies and Their Implications for Cancer Therapy. *Oncogene* 21 (35), 5483–5495. doi:10.1038/sj.onc.1205699

Croft, D. R., Crighton, D., Samuel, M. S., Lourenco, F. C., Munro, J., Wood, J., et al. (2011). p53-mediated Transcriptional Regulation and Activation of the Actin Cytoskeleton Regulatory RhoC to LIMK2 Signaling Pathway Promotes Cell Survival. *Cell Res* 21 (4), 666–682. doi:10.1038/cr.2010.154

Deng, J. L., Zhang, R., Zeng, Y., Zhu, Y. S., and Wang, G. (2019). Statins Induce Cell Apoptosis through a Modulation of AKT/FOXO1 Pathway in Prostate Cancer Cells. *Cancer Manag. Res.* 11, 7231–7242. doi:10.2147/CMAR.S212643

Ding, X., Kambara, H., Guo, R., Kanneganti, A., Acosta-Zaldívar, M., Li, J., et al. (2021). Inflammasome-mediated GSDMD Activation Facilitates Escape of Candida Albicans from Macrophages. *Nat. Commun.* 12 (1), 6699. doi:10.1038/s41467-021-27034-9

Fan, J. X., Deng, R. H., Wang, H., Liu, X. H., Wang, X. N., Qin, R., et al. (2019). Epigenetics-Based Tumor Cells Pyroptosis for Enhancing the Immunological Effect of Chemotherapeutic Nanocarriers. *Nano Lett.* 19 (11), 8049–8058. doi:10.1021/acs.nanolett.9b03245

Guo, J., Zheng, J., Mu, M., Chen, Z., Xu, Z., Zhao, C., et al. (2021). GW4064 Enhances the Chemosensitivity of Colorectal Cancer to Oxaliplatin by Inducing Pyroptosis. *Biochem. Biophys. Res. Commun.* 548, 60–66. doi:10.1016/j.bbrc.2021.02.043

Han, J., Zuo, Z., Shi, X., Zhang, Y., Peng, Z., Xing, Y., et al. (2021). Hirudin Ameliorates Diabetic Nephropathy by Inhibiting Gsdmd-Mediated Pyroptosis. *Cell Biol Toxicol.* doi:10.1007/s10565-021-09622-z

Hou, J., Hsu, J. M., and Hung, M. C. (2021). Molecular Mechanisms and Functions of Pyroptosis in Inflammation and Antitumor Immunity. *Mol. Cel* 81 (22), 4579–4590. doi:10.1016/j.molcel.2021.09.003

Huang, J., Fan, P., Liu, M., Weng, C., Fan, G., Zhang, T., et al. (2021). Famotidine Promotes Inflammation by Triggering Cell Pyroptosis in Gastric Cancer Cells. *BMC Pharmacol. Toxicol.* 22 (1), 62. doi:10.1186/s40360-021-00533-7

Jiang, M., Wu, Y., Qi, L., Li, L., Song, D., Gan, J., et al. (2021). Dihydroartemisinin Mediating PKM2-Caspase-8/3-GSDME axis for Pyroptosis in Esophageal Squamous Cell Carcinoma. *Chemico-Biological Interactions* 350, 109704. doi:10.1016/j.cbi.2021.109704

Jiang, W., Hu, J.-W., He, X.-R., Jin, W.-L., and He, X.-Y. (2021). Statins: a Repurposed Drug to Fight Cancer. *J. Exp. Clin. Cancer Res.* 40 (1), 241. doi:10.1186/s13046-021-02041-2

Jorgensen, I., and Miao, E. A. (2015). Pyroptotic Cell Death Defends against Intracellular Pathogens. *Immunol. Rev.* 265 (1), 130–142. doi:10.1111/imr.12287

Kim, M. S., Chang, X., Yamashita, K., Nagpal, J. K., Baek, J. H., Wu, G., et al. (2008). Aberrant Promoter Methylation and Tumor Suppressive Activity of the DFNA5 Gene in Colorectal Carcinoma. *Oncogene* 27 (25), 3624–3634. doi:10.1038/sj.onc.1211021

Kim, M. S., Lebron, C., Nagpal, J. K., Chae, Y. K., Chang, X., Huang, Y., et al. (2008). Methylation of the DFNA5 Increases Risk of Lymph Node Metastasis in Human Breast Cancer. *Biochem. Biophys. Res. Commun.* 370 (1), 38–43. doi:10.1016/j.bbrc.2008.03.026

Kodach, L. L., Jacobs, R. J., Voorneveld, P. W., Wildenberg, M. E., Verspaget, H. W., van Wezel, T., et al. (2011). Statins Augment the Chemosensitivity of Colorectal Cancer Cells Inducing Epigenetic Reprogramming and Reducing Colorectal Cancer Cell 'stemness' via the Bone Morphogenetic Protein Pathway. *Gut* 60 (11), 1544–1553. doi:10.1136/gut.2011.237495

Li, L., Song, D., Qi, L., Jiang, M., Wu, Y., Gan, J., et al. (2021). Photodynamic Therapy Induces Human Esophageal Carcinoma Cell Pyroptosis by Targeting the PKM2/caspase-8/caspase-3/GSDME axis. *Cancer Lett.* 520, 143–159. doi:10.1016/j.canlet.2021.07.014

Liu, Q., Xia, H., Zhou, S., Tang, Q., Zhou, J., Ren, M., et al. (2020). Simvastatin Inhibits the Malignant Behaviors of Gastric Cancer Cells by Simultaneously Suppressing YAP and β-Catenin Signaling. *Onco Targets Ther.* 13, 2057–2066. doi:10.2147/OTT.S237693

Lu, H., Zhang, S., Wu, J., Chen, M., Cai, M. C., Fu, Y., et al. (2018). Molecular Targeted Therapies Elicit Concurrent Apoptotic and GSDME-dependent Pyroptotic Tumor Cell Death. *Clin. Cancer Res.* 24 (23), 6066–6077. doi:10.1158/1078-0432.CCR-18-1478

Mattiuzzi, C., and Lippi, G. (2020). Cancer Statistics: a Comparison between World Health Organization (WHO) and Global Burden of Disease (GBD). *Eur. J. Public Health* 30 (5), 1026–1027. doi:10.1093/eurpub/ckz216

Ni, W., Mo, H., Liu, Y., Xu, Y., Qin, C., Zhou, Y., et al. (2021). Targeting Cholesterol Biosynthesis Promotes Anti-tumor Immunity by Inhibiting Long Noncoding RNA SNHG29-Mediated YAP Activation. *Mol. Ther.* 29 (10), 2995–3010. doi:10.1016/j.ymthe.2021.05.012

Op de Beeck, K., Van Camp, G., Thys, S., Cools, N., Callebaut, I., Vrijens, K., et al. (2011). The DFNA5 Gene, Responsible for Hearing Loss and Involved in Cancer, Encodes a Novel Apoptosis-Inducing Protein. *Eur. J. Hum. Genet.* 19 (9), 965–973. doi:10.1038/ejhg.2011.63

Peng, Z., Wang, P., Song, W., Yao, Q., Li, Y., Liu, L., et al. (2020). GSDME Enhances Cisplatin Sensitivity to Regress Non-small Cell Lung Carcinoma by Mediating Pyroptosis to Trigger Antitumor Immunocyte Infiltration. *Signal. Transduct Target. Ther.* 5 (1), 159. doi:10.1038/s41392-020-00274-9

Pushpakom, S., Iorio, F., Eyers, P. A., Escott, K. J., Hopper, S., Wells, A., et al. (2019). Drug Repurposing: Progress, Challenges and Recommendations. *Nat. Rev. Drug Discov.* 18 (1), 41–58. doi:10.1038/nrd.2018.168

Rogers, C., Fernandes-Alnemri, T., Mayes, L., Alnemri, D., Cingolani, G., and Alnemri, E. S. (2017). Cleavage of DFNA5 by Caspase-3 during Apoptosis Mediates Progression to Secondary Necrotic/pyroptotic Cell Death. *Nat. Commun.* 8, 14128. doi:10.1038/ncomms14128

Shangguan, F., Zhou, H., Ma, N., Wu, S., Huang, H., Jin, G., et al. (2021). A Novel Mechanism of Cannabidiol in Suppressing Hepatocellular Carcinoma by Inducing GSDME Dependent Pyroptosis. *Front Cel Dev Biol* 9, 697832. doi:10.3389/fcell.2021.697832

Shao, W., Yang, Z., Fu, Y., Zheng, L., Liu, F., Chai, L., et al. (2021). The Pyroptosis-Related Signature Predicts Prognosis and Indicates Immune Microenvironment Infiltration in Gastric Cancer. *Front. Cel Dev Biol* 9, 676485. doi:10.3389/fcell.2021.676485

Shi, H., Gao, Y., Dong, Z., Yang, J. e., Gao, R., Li, X., et al. (2021). GSDMD-mediated Cardiomyocyte Pyroptosis Promotes Myocardial I/R Injury. *Circ. Res.* 129 (3), 383–396. doi:10.1161/circresaha.120.318629

Shi, J., Zhao, Y., Wang, K., Shi, X., Wang, Y., Huang, H., et al. (2015). Cleavage of GSDMD by Inflammatory Caspases Determines Pyroptotic Cell Death. *Nature* 526 (7575), 660–665. doi:10.1038/nature15514

Sun, F. R., Wang, S. L., Wang, M., and Sun, L. M. (2020). Simvastatin Induces Apoptosis of Nasopharyngeal Carcinoma Cells through NF-Kb Signaling Pathway. *Eur. Rev. Med. Pharmacol. Sci.* 24 (12), 6726–6734. doi:10.26355/eurrev_202006_21660

Tan, G., Lin, C., Huang, C., Chen, B., Chen, J., Shi, Y., et al. (2021). Radiosensitivity of Colorectal Cancer and Radiation-Induced Gut Damages Are Regulated by Gasdermin. *E. Cancer Lett.* 529, 1–10. doi:10.1016/j.canlet.2021.12.034

Tan, Y., Chen, Q., Li, X., Zeng, Z., Xiong, W., Li, G., et al. (2021). Pyroptosis: a New Paradigm of Cell Death for Fighting against Cancer. *J. Exp. Clin. Cancer Res.* 40 (1), 153. doi:10.1186/s13046-021-01959-x

Van Laer, L., Huizing, E. H., Verstreken, M., van Zuijlen, D., Wauters, J. G., Bossuyt, P. J., et al. (1998). Nonsyndromic Hearing Impairment Is Associated with a Mutation in DFNA5. *Nat. Genet.* 20 (2), 194–197. doi:10.1038/2503

Wang, F., Liu, W., Ning, J., Wang, J., Lang, Y., Jin, X., et al. (2018). Simvastatin Suppresses Proliferation and Migration in Non-small Cell Lung Cancer via Pyroptosis. *Int. J. Biol. Sci.* 14 (4), 406–417. doi:10.7150/ijbs.23542

Wang, L., Zhang, C., Hong, Y., Li, X., Li, T., Gao, A., et al. (2021). Integrating Epigenetic Modulators in Nanofibers for Synergistic Gastric Cancer Therapy via Epigenetic Reprogramming. *Nano Lett.* 21 (1), 298–307. doi:10.1021/acs.nanolett.0c03665

Wang, Y., Gao, W., Shi, X., Ding, J., Liu, W., He, H., et al. (2017). Chemotherapy Drugs Induce Pyroptosis through Caspase-3 Cleavage of a Gasdermin. *Nature* 547 (7661), 99–103. doi:10.1038/nature22393

Wesołowska, A., Winiarska, H., Owoc, J., Borowska, M., Domagała, J., Mikołajczak, P. Ł., et al. (2021). Effects of Low-Dose Atorvastatin on the Peripheral Blood Mononuclear Cell Secretion of Angiogenic Factors in Type 2 Diabetes. *Biomolecules* 11 (12). doi:10.3390/biom11121885

Xia, S., Hollingsworth, L. R., and Wu, H. (2020). Mechanism and Regulation of Gasdermin-Mediated Cell Death. *Cold Spring Harb Perspect. Biol.* 12 (3), a036400. doi:10.1101/cshperspect.a036400

Xiong, Y., Wei, Y., Gu, Y., Zhang, S., Lyu, J., Zhang, B., et al. (2017). DiseaseMeth Version 2.0: a Major Expansion and Update of the Human Disease Methylation Database. *Nucleic Acids Res.* 45 (D1), D888–D895. doi:10.1093/nar/gkw1123

Xu, W. F., Zhang, Q., Ding, C. J., Sun, H. Y., Che, Y., Huang, H., et al. (2021). Gasdermin E-Derived Caspase-3 Inhibitors Effectively Protect Mice from Acute Hepatic Failure. *Acta Pharmacol. Sin* 42 (1), 68–76. doi:10.1038/s41401-020-0434-2

Yang, F., Sun, S. Y., Wang, S., Guo, J. T., Liu, X., Ge, N., et al. (2022). Molecular Regulatory Mechanism of Ferroptosis and its Role in Gastrointestinal Oncology: Progress and Updates. *World J. Gastrointest. Oncol.* 14 (1), 1–18. doi:10.4251/wjgo.v14.i1.1

Yanokura, M., Banno, K., and Aoki, D. (2020). MicroRNA-34b E-xpression E-nhances C-hemosensitivity of E-ndometrial C-ancer C-ells to P-aclitaxel. *Int. J. Oncol.* 57 (5), 1145–1156. doi:10.3892/ijo.2020.5127

Yokomizo, K., Harada, Y., Kijima, K., Shinmura, K., Sakata, M., Sakuraba, K., et al. (2012). Methylation of the DFNA5 Gene Is Frequently Detected in Colorectal Cancer. *Anticancer Res.* 32 (4), 1319–1322.

Yu, X., and He, S. (2017). GSDME as an Executioner of Chemotherapy-Induced Cell Death. *Sci. China Life Sci.* 60 (11), 1291–1294. doi:10.1007/s11427-017-9142-2

Yu, Z., Guo, J., Liu, Y., Wang, M., Liu, Z., Gao, Y., et al. (2022). Nano Delivery of Simvastatin Targets Liver Sinusoidal Endothelial Cells to Remodel Tumor Microenvironment for Hepatocellular Carcinoma. *J. Nanobiotechnology* 20 (1), 9. doi:10.1186/s12951-021-01205-8

Yuan, R., Zhao, W., Wang, Q. Q., He, J., Han, S., Gao, H., et al. (2021). Cucurbitacin B Inhibits Non-small Cell Lung Cancer *In Vivo* and *In Vitro* by Triggering TLR4/NLRP3/GSDMD-dependent Pyroptosis. *Pharmacol. Res.* 170, 105748. doi:10.1016/j.phrs.2021.105748

Zhou, C., Zhao, J., Liu, J., Wei, S., Xia, Y., Xia, W., et al. (2019). LncRNA SNHG16 Promotes Epithelial- Mesenchymal Transition via Down-Regulation of DKK3 in Gastric Cancer. *Cancer Biomark* 26 (4), 393–401. doi:10.3233/CBM-190497

Zhou, C. B., and Fang, J. Y. (2019). The Role of Pyroptosis in Gastrointestinal Cancer and Immune Responses to Intestinal Microbial Infection. *Biochim. Biophys. Acta Rev. Cancer* 1872 (1), 1–10. doi:10.1016/j.bbcan.2019.05.001

7

Anticancer Effects of Amlodipine Alone or in Combination with Gefitinib in Non-Small Cell Lung Cancer

Bingjie Fu[1†], Xiaojing Dou[1†], Miao Zou[1], Hao Lu[1], Kaixuan Wang[1], Qingxia Liu[1], Yao Liu[2], Wei Wang[2], Meihua Jin[1] and Dexin Kong[1*]*

[1]Tianjin Key Laboratory of Technologies Enabling Development of Clinical Therapeutics and Diagnostics, School of Pharmacy, Key Laboratory of Immune Microenvironment and Diseases (Ministry of Education), Tianjin Medical University, Tianjin, China, [2]Department of Otorhinolaryngology Head and Neck Surgery, Key Laboratory of Auditory Speech and Balance Medicine, Institute of Otolaryngology of Tianjin, Tianjin First Central Hospital, Tianjin, China

***Correspondence:**
Meihua Jin
jinmeihua@tmu.edu.cn
Dexin Kong
kongdexin@tmu.edu.cn

†These authors have contributed equally to this work

Amlodipine is a Ca^{2+} channel blocker commonly used to cardiovascular diseases such as hypertension and angina; however, its anticancer effects in lung cancer A549 cells remain unknown. In the present study, we explored the antitumor effects and molecular mechanisms underlying the action of amlodipine in non-small cell lung cancer (NSCLC) A549 cells *in vitro* and *in vivo*. We observed that amlodipine suppressed the proliferation of A549 lung cancer cells by arresting the tumor cell cycle. Mechanistically, our results revealed that amlodipine could attenuate the phosphoinositide 3 kinase (PI3K)/Akt and Raf/MEK/extracellular signal-regulated kinase (ERK) pathways through epidermal growth factor receptor (EGFR) and modulated cell cycle-related proteins such as cyclin D1, p-Rb, p27, and p21. Subsequently, amlodipine combined with gefitinib could synergistically inhibit cell proliferation by arresting the cell cycle. Moreover, amlodipine combined with gefitinib effectively attenuated the growth of A549 lung cancer xenografts when compared with monotherapy, affording an excellent therapeutic effect. Collectively, our results indicate that amlodipine alone or combined with the novel anticancer drug gefitinib might be a potential therapeutic strategy for NSCLC patients with wild-type EGFR.

Keywords: amlodipine, gefitinib, lung cancer, synergistic anticancer effect, cell cycle arrest

INTRODUCTION

Calcium channel blockers (CCBs) inhibit calcium flux through voltage-gated calcium channels (Wang et al., 2021) and are widely used to treat cardiovascular diseases such as angina, hypertension, and supraventricular arrhythmias (Sica, 2006). CCBs are classified as dihydropyridines or non-dihydropyridines. Dihydropyridines include nifedipine, nicardipine, felodipine, and amlodipine, while non-dihydropyridines include diltiazem and verapamil (Eisenberg et al., 2004). CCBs, such as diltiazem and verapamil, were shown to decrease tumor growth in a xenograft mouse meningioma tumor model (Jensen and Wurster, 2001), and verapamil could reversibly decrease human melanoma cell invasion and metastasis (Yohem et al., 1991). In addition, dihydropyridine derivatives, such as amlodipine, nicardipine, and nimodipine, reportedly suppressed the growth of human epidermoid carcinoma cells, whereas verapamil, diltiazem, and dihydropyridine nifedipine failed to inhibit human epidermoid carcinoma cell growth at the same concentration (Yoshida et al., 2003). However, the anticancer effect of amlodipine against non-small cell lung cancer (NSCLC) A549 cells remains unknown.

Lung cancer is the most frequent and leading cause of cancer-related deaths globally, and NSCLC constitutes approximately 75% of all lung cancers (Cersosimo, 2002; Hirsch et al., 2017). Epidermal growth factor receptor (EGFR) is a transmembrane protein with cytoplasmic kinase activity commonly overexpressed in various human cancers, including NSCLC (da Cunha Santos et al., 2011; Wee and Wang, 2017). EGFR tyrosine kinase inhibitors (TKIs), gefitinib and erlotinib, are targeted therapies, used as first-line treatments for patients with NSCLC harboring EGFR mutations (Shukuya et al., 2011; De Mello et al., 2016). EGFR-TKIs have demonstrated insufficient efficacy in patients with wild-type EGFR (Hirai et al., 2017). However, it has been reported that shikonin could enhance the anticancer efficacy of gefitinib/erlotinib in wild-type EGFR NSCLC cells (Li et al., 2018). And recently, we also reported that proton pump inhibitor, lansoprazole, in combination with gefitinib showed synergistic antitumor effect on NSCLC A549 cells and mouse xenograft models with wild-type EGFR (Zhao et al., 2021). Therefore, potential EGFR-TKI sensitizers and treatment strategies to improve the prognosis of lung cancer patients with wild-type EGFR are essential.

Combination therapy, rather than monotherapy, can afford synergistic clinical benefits. Amlodipine attenuates phosphorylation of EGFR in human epidermoid carcinoma A431 cells *in vitro* and *in vivo* (Yoshida et al., 2010). Therefore, we hypothesized that simultaneous treatment with amlodipine and gefitinib might have synergistic anticancer effects. In the present study, we investigated the anticancer effects and preliminary mechanisms of amlodipine alone or in combination with gefitinib in NSCLC A549 cells with wild-type EGFR. Our study provides a promising new therapeutic agent or combination treatment strategy for patients with NSCLC.

MATERIALS AND METHODS

Cell Culture

A549 cells were obtained from the Cell Resource Center of Peking Union Medical College (Beijing, China). This cell line has been authenticated using STR profiling within the last 3 years. In addition, A549 cells were confirmed to be free of *mycoplasma* contamination by PCR. Briefly, A549 cells were cultured in RPMI 1640 medium containing 10% fetal bovine serum (FBS), 100 U/ml penicillin, and 100 µg/ml streptomycin. The cell cultures were maintained in a humidified atmosphere containing 5% CO_2 at 37°C.

Reagents

Amlodipine and gefitinib were purchased from Selleck Chemicals (Houston, TX, United States) and TopScience (Shanghai, China), respectively. Propidium iodide (PI) was obtained from Sigma-Aldrich (St. Louis, MO, United States). The Annexin V/FITC-PI apoptosis detection kit was obtained from BD Biosciences (San Jose, CA, United States of America). RPMI 1640 and FBS were purchased from Biological Industries (Beit Haemek, Israel). The enhanced chemiluminescence (ECL) reagent was purchased from Thermo Fisher Scientific (Waltham, MA, United States). Antibodies against phospho-EGFR, phospho-PDK1 (Ser241), PDK1, phospho-Akt (Ser473), phospho-Akt (Thr308), Akt, phospho-mammalian target of rapamycin complex 1 (mTORC1) (Ser2448), mTOR, phospho-glycogen synthase kinase 3 (GSK-3) β, phospho-p70 S6K (Thr389), p27, cyclin D1, phospho-retinoblastoma protein (Rb), phospho-extracellular signal-regulated kinase (ERK) 1/2, phospho-c-Raf, β-actin, and horseradish peroxidase (HRP)-conjugated goat anti-rabbit and horse anti-mouse secondary antibodies were purchased from Cell Signaling Technology Inc. (Danvers, MA, United States). Antibody specific for p21 was obtained from Santa Cruz Biotechnology Inc. (Dallas, TX, United States).

Determination of Cell Viability

Cell viability was determined using an 3-(4,5-dimethylthiazol-2-yl)-2,5-diphenyltetrazolium bromide (MTT) assay. Briefly, A549 cells were seeded into 96-well plates at a density of 4×10^3 cells/well and then treated with amlodipine and/or gefitinib for 48 h, followed by the addition of 20 µl MTT (5 mg/ml) to each well and further incubation for 4 h. Dimethyl sulfoxide (DMSO) was used to dissolve purple crystals after incubation. Optical density was measured at 490 nm using an iMark microplate reader (Bio-Rad, Hercules, CA, United States).

Flow Cytometric Analysis

Briefly, A549 cells were plated in 6-well plates at a density of 2×10^5 cells/well and treated with amlodipine or gefitinib for 48 h. For cycle analysis, the cells were harvested with trypsin, washed with PBS, resuspended in 75% pre-chilled ethanol, and stored at 4 °C overnight. After 24 h, the fixed cells were collected and stained with PI. Then, 20,000 cells were collected for each sample and analyzed using a BD Accuri C6 flow cytometer (BD Biosciences, San Jose, CA, United States).

To analyze cell apoptosis, Annexin V-FITC/PI double staining was performed as previously reported, with minor modifications (Zhang et al., 2021). The drug-pretreated cells were harvested with trypsin, resuspended in Annexin V-FITC/PI (BD Biosciences, San Jose, CA, United States) mixture, and incubated in the dark for 15 min. Subsequently, cells were analyzed using a BD Accuri C6 flow cytometer (10,000 cells were analyzed for each sample).

Data were quantified with BD Accuri C6 Software.

Wound-Healing Assay

Briefly, A549 cells were seeded in 24-well plates at a density of 6×10^5 cells/well and a micropipette tip was used to create a vertical scratch (wound) in the cell monolayer. Subsequently, cells were treated with different concentrations of amlodipine for 48 h. Wound areas were imaged under a microscope.

Western Blotting

Western blot analysis was performed as previously described (Shao et al., 2021). Briefly, cells were lysed with RIPA lysis buffer, and the protein concentration of each sample was determined using a BCA protein assay kit. Protein extracts were separated by 10% sodium dodecyl sulfate-polyacrylamide gel electrophoresis (SDS-PAGE) and transferred to a PVDF membrane. Membranes were blocked with 5% non-fat milk, incubated with primary

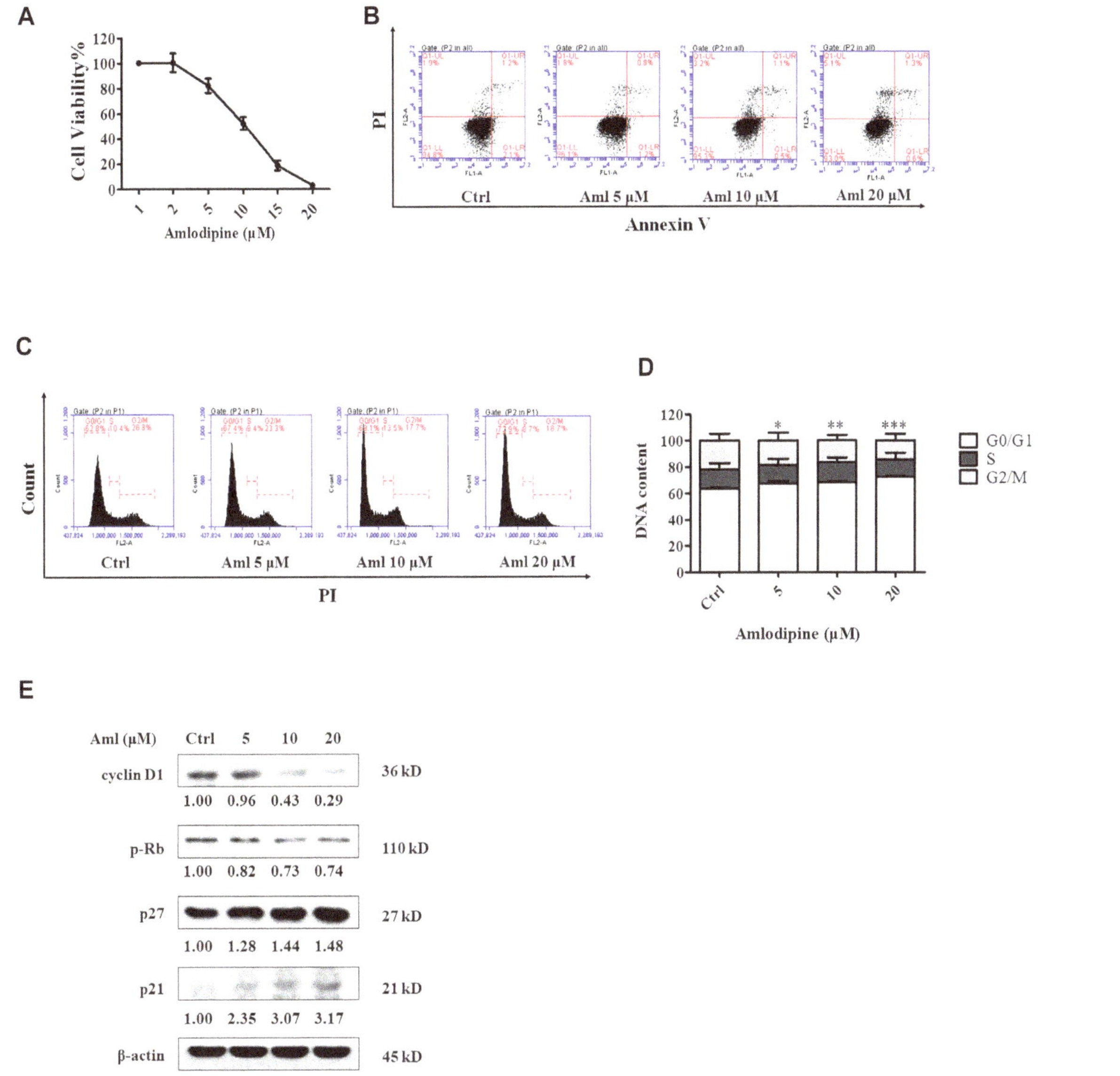

FIGURE 1 | Amlodipine inhibits A549 cell proliferation by blocking the cell cycle G0/G1 phase. **(A)** Incubation of A549 with various concentrations (1, 2, 5, 10, 15, and 20 μM) of amlodipine (Aml) for 48 h. The effects of amlodipine on A549 cell proliferation were determined by MTT assay. **(B)** A549 cells were harvested 48 h after treatment with indicated concentrations of amlodipine, and apoptotic cells were measured by flow cytometry analysis. **(C)** Cells were pre-incubated with different concentrations of amlodipine for 48 h, and the induction of cell cycle arrest was detected by flow cytometry analysis. **(D)** The percentage of total cells at G0/G1, S, and G2/M phases. **(E)** The expressions levels of cell cycle-related proteins were determined by Western blotting after treatment with amlodipine. Data are presented as mean ± SD of three independent experiments. $^{*}p < 0.05$, $^{**}p < 0.01$ and $^{***}p < 0.001$.

antibodies at 4 °C overnight, washed four times with Tris-buffered saline (TBS) containing Tween-20 (TBST), and incubated with the respective HRP-conjugated secondary antibody for 1 h. Protein bands were visualized using ECL reagents on a Bio-Rad ChemiDoc™ XRS + system (Bio-Rad, Hercules, CA, United States).

Nude Mouse Xenograft Tumor Experiments

All animal experiments were conducted at the Laboratory Animal Center of the Institute of Radiation Medicine, Chinese Academy of Medical Sciences, and were maintained in a pathogen-free environment. The experiments were performed under the Institutional Animal Care and Use Committee guidelines. Six-week-old male BALB/c nude mice were injected subcutaneously (s.c.) with 1×10^7 A549 cells, and then the sufficiently grown tumor tissue was divided into equal pieces, followed by subcutaneous implantation into the mice. Mice were randomly divided into four groups ($n = 4$) when tumors reached 20–30 mm^3, and then orally administered amlodipine (10 mg/kg) or gefitinib (50 mg/kg) alone or in combination every other day for 15 days. The growth of implanted tumors was monitored every other day, tumor volumes were measured using a caliper, and the tumor volume was calculated using the formula $V = 1/2 \times Length \times Width^2$.

Immunohistochemistry Analyses

At the end of the experimental period, animals were euthanized, and tumors were excised and fixed in paraformaldehyde for IHC analysis. Tumors were embedded in paraffin, sectioned at 5-µm thickness, and stained with hematoxylin and eosin (H&E) for morphological assessment. The formalin-fixed tissue was heated in an antigen retrieval solution before incubation with the antibody Ki67, and bound antibodies were detected with Bond Polymer (anti-rabbit poly-HRP-IgG) and visualized using diaminobenzidine (DAB) peroxidase substrate. Specimen images were examined using an Olympus BX51 microscope.

Statistical Analysis

Data values are expressed as the mean ± standard deviation (SD) of triplicate values. One-way ANOVA followed by Tukey's multiple comparison test was used to determine statistical significance using GraphPad Prism 5 (GraphPad, San Diego, CA, United States). Differences were considered statistically significant at $p < 0.05$.

RESULTS

Amlodipine Inhibits the Proliferation of NSCLC A549 Cells *Via* Cell Cycle Arrest at the G0/G1 Phase

The MTT assay was used to detect the inhibitory effect of amlodipine on A549 cell proliferation. A549 cells were treated with a series of amlodipine concentrations for 48 h. As shown in **Figure 1A**, amlodipine significantly suppressed the proliferation of A549 cells in a concentration-dependent manner, with an IC_{50} of 9.641 µM. Apoptosis is a common mechanism of cell death. We first determined whether amlodipine induces apoptosis in A549 cells. A flow cytometry assay with double staining using Annexin-V FITC/PI was performed to detect the percentage of apoptotic cells. A549 cells were treated with 5, 10, and 20 µM amlodipine for 48 h. As shown in **Figure 1B**, incubation with amlodipine showed no significant changes. To explore the effects of amlodipine on the cell cycle, flow cytometry was used to evaluate cell cycle phase distribution in A549 cells following amlodipine treatment for 48 h. As shown in **Figures 1C,D**, amlodipine-treated cells exhibited significantly enhanced cell cycle arrest at the G0/G1 phase when compared with the non-treated group. To further explore these findings, the levels of cyclin D1, p27, and p21, as well as the phosphorylation of their downstream protein Rb, were determined using Western blotting after treatment with 5, 10, and 20 µM amlodipine for 48 h. Cyclin D-cyclin dependent kinase (CDK) 4/6 complex phosphorylates Rb to facilitate cell cycle progression from G1 to S phase (Sherr, 1994; Shapiro, 2006). As shown in **Figure 1E**, the expression of cyclin D1 and level of p-Rb were decreased, while the expression levels of p27 and p21 (CDK inhibitors) were increased in a dose-dependent manner, compared with the non-treated group. These findings indicated that amlodipine inhibited A549 cell proliferation by inducing cell cycle arrest but did not significantly affect apoptosis.

Amlodipine Suppresses A549 Cell Migration

Metastasis is associated with poor prognosis, and cancer cell migration and invasion are recognized as the initial steps in metastasis. To examine the effects of amlodipine on A549 cell migration, a scratch-wound assay was performed using evenly space 24-well plates covered with A549 cells. Amlodipine was then administered at concentrations of 2, 5, and 10 µM (to avoid interference between cell proliferative activity and migration, we selected a concentration less than the IC_{50}), and scratches were examined after 48 h of culture. As shown in **Figures 2A,B**, cell migration was notably lower in the amlodipine group than in the untreated group, with amlodipine treatment exhibiting a concentration-dependent effect.

Amlodipine Inhibits PI3Ks/Akt and Raf/MEK/ERK MAPKs Pathways by Inhibiting EGFR Phosphorylation in A549 Cells

The phosphatidylinositol-3 kinase (PI3K) pathway plays an important role in regulating cell migration, proliferation, cell cycle progression, and apoptosis (Martini et al., 2014). Therefore, to explore the molecular mechanism underlying amlodipine-mediated inhibition of A549 cell proliferation and cell cycle arrest, cells were treated with 5, 10, and 20 µM amlodipine for 48 h, and Western blotting was performed to detect PI3Ks pathway proteins. As shown in **Figure 2C**, amlodipine treatment at 20 µM for 48 h significantly decreased phosphorylation levels of PDK1, Akt (both Ser473 and Thr308), mTOR, p70 S6K, and GSK-3β, without changes in total PDK1, Akt and mTOR levels.

The Ras/Raf/MEK/ERK pathway is the most pivotal signaling cascade among all MAPK signal transduction pathways and regulates the survival, growth, differentiation, and development of tumor cells (Degirmenci et al., 2020; Guo et al., 2020). In addition, to examine the role of MAPK signaling inhibition and the effects of amlodipine on proliferation and migration, A549 cells were pretreated with several amlodipine concentrations for 48 h. As shown in **Figure 2D**, phosphorylation levels of c-Raf and ERK were reduced in a concentration-dependent manner in cells treated with 10 and 20 µM amlodipine with no variation detected in total ERK, when compared with untreated cells.

EGFR is a receptor tyrosine kinase that plays a critical role in carcinogenesis, including cell proliferation, survival, and differentiation (da Cunha Santos et al., 2011). PI3K and MAPK signaling pathways are involved in EGFR signal transduction. To determine whether amlodipine affects the upstream regulator EGFR, we assessed EGFR phosphorylation after amlodipine treatment using Western blotting. As shown in **Figure 2C**, amlodipine significantly suppressed the level of p-EGFR when compared with the untreated control group, and the inhibitory effects were particularly significant following treatment with 10 and 20 µM amlodipine with no variation detected in total EGFR.

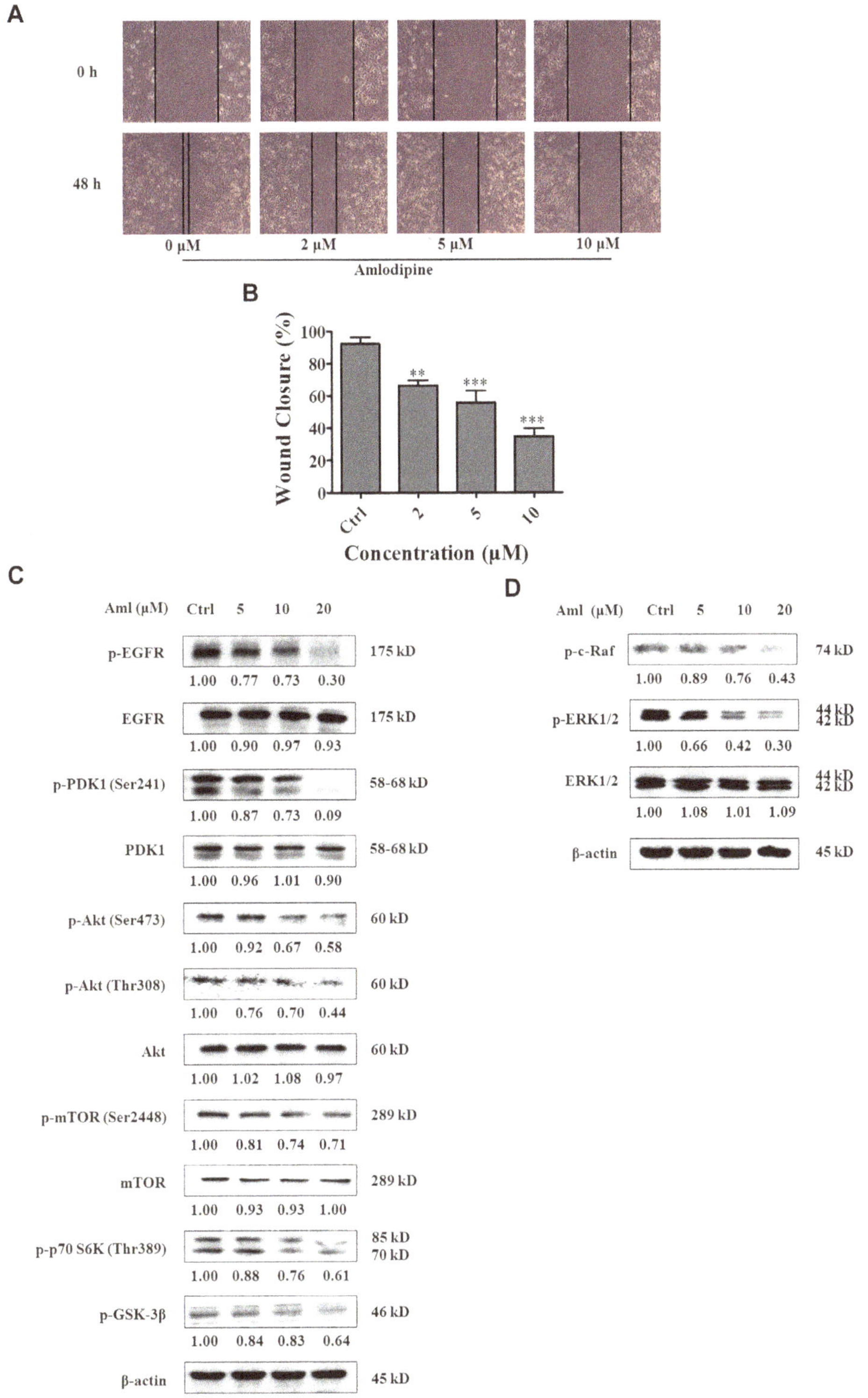

FIGURE 2 | Amlodipine suppresses A549 cells migration and PI3K/Akt and Raf/ERK MAPK pathways. **(A)** The effect of amlodipine on cell migration was detected by performing a wound-healing assay at 48 h. **(B)** Quantification of results in **(A)**. **(C)** The levels of Akt pathway proteins were analyzed by Western blotting after treatment with amlodipine. **(D)** The phosphorylation of Raf and phosphorylation and total ERK1/2 were analyzed by Western blotting after treatment with amlodipine. Data are presented as mean ± SD of three independent experiments. $^{**}p < 0.01$ and $^{***}p < 0.001$.

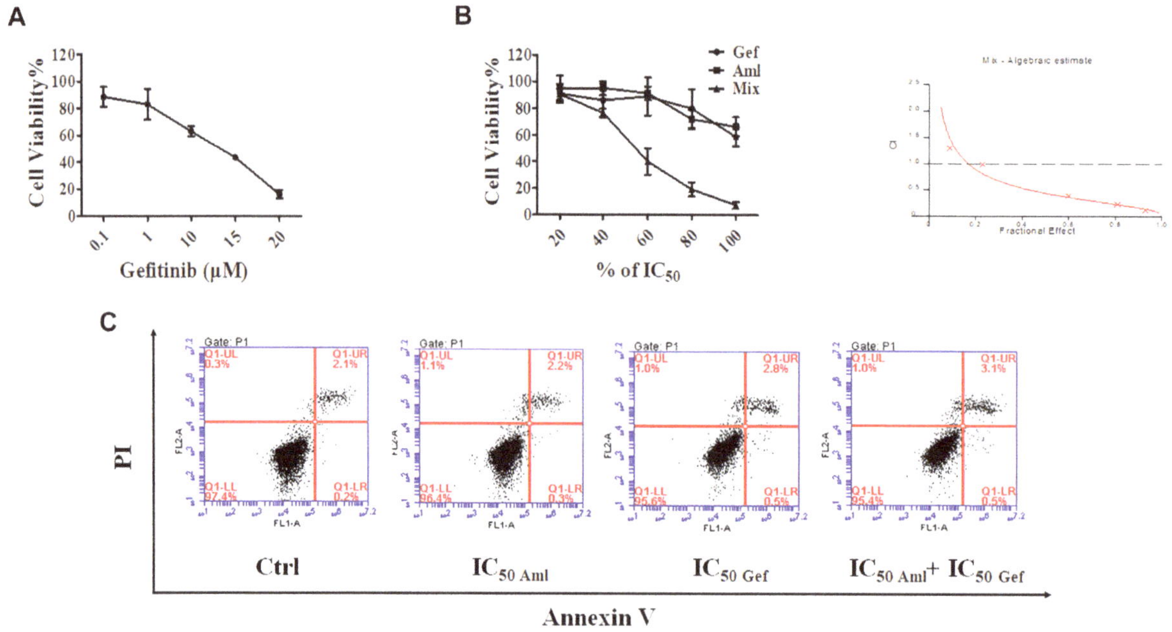

FIGURE 3 | Amlodipine combined with gefitinib led to a synergistic anti-proliferative effect on A549 cells. **(A)** MTT assay was used to detect the inhibitory effect of gefitinib (Gef) on cell proliferation. **(B)** A549 cells were treated with amlodipine, gefitinib, or a combination of these agents for 48 h. A549 cells were treated with amlodipine and gefitinib, with several percentages of IC_{50} value. **(C)** A549 cells were harvested 48 h after treatment with amlodipine, gefitinib, or a combination of these agents, and apoptotic cells were examined by flow cytometry analysis.

Amlodipine in Combination With Gefitinib Synergistically Reduces Cell Proliferation Through Cell Cycle Arrest at G0/G1 by Attenuating PI3K/Akt Signaling Pathway in A549 Cells

Several reports have shown that combination therapies afford synergistic antitumor effects when compared with the efficacy of either agent alone, such as a combination of cisplatin and vinorelbine, which is superior to cisplatin monotherapy in patients with advanced NSCLC (Wozniak et al., 1998). Therefore, gefitinib was selected and combined with amlodipine. First, the IC_{50} of gefitinib at 48 h was detected using the MTT assay, as shown in **Figure 3A**, notably inhibiting cell proliferation at an IC_{50} of 12.52 μM. To quantify the interaction between amlodipine and gefitinib, the multiple-drug effect evaluation introduced by Chou-Talalay was employed. The MTT assay was performed to measure the inhibitory activities of a series of drug concentration combinations (20, 40, 60, 80, and 100% of IC_{50} values of each drug) (**Figure 3B**). To detect the efficacy of the two-drug combination, combination index (CI) plots were generated using CalcuSyn software, and CI values were defined as follows; CI < 1, synergism; CI = 1, additive; and CI > 1, antagonism. The CI values for ED_{50}, ED_{75}, and ED_{90} were 0.43812, 0.26170, and 0.16192, respectively. Therefore, we fixed the ratio of $IC_{50\ amlodipine}$:$IC_{50\ gefitinib}$ (9.641 μM:12.52 μM) combination to perform a subsequent mechanistic study for examining the synergistic anti-proliferative effect.

We evaluated the effect of amlodipine combined with gefitinib on A549 cell apoptosis using Annexin V-FITC/PI staining. A549 cells were treated with amlodipine and gefitinib, either alone or in combination, for 48 h. The results revealed no significant changes following treatment with either amlodipine or a combination of amlodipine and gefitinib (**Figure 3C**). We further analyzed the effects of amlodipine in combination with gefitinib on the cell cycle. It has been reported that gefitinib, as well as amlodipine, can block the A549 cell cycle at the G0/G1 phase. Therefore, to clarify the combined anti-proliferation activity detected in the MTT assays, flow cytometry was performed to assess A549 cells treated with the two drugs alone or in combination for 48 h; the percentage of each cell cycle was determined by PI staining. As shown in **Figures 4A,B**, treatment of A549 cells with amlodipine combined with gefitinib significantly increased the proportion of cells in the G0/G1 phase (80.1%) when compared with amlodipine or gefitinib alone. A mechanistic assessment was performed using Western blotting, and the results indicated that the combined use of amlodipine and gefitinib significantly reduced levels of p-Rb and enhanced p27 when compared with amlodipine or gefitinib alone (**Figure 4C**).

In addition, the mechanism of action was investigated using Western blotting. Compared with amlodipine or gefitinib treatment alone, amlodipine combined with gefitinib could downregulate PI3K/Akt signaling pathway proteins, including phosphorylation of Akt (Ser473), Akt (Thr308), and mTOR (**Figure 4D**) with no variation detected in total Akt and mTOR levels. Furthermore, amlodipine combined with

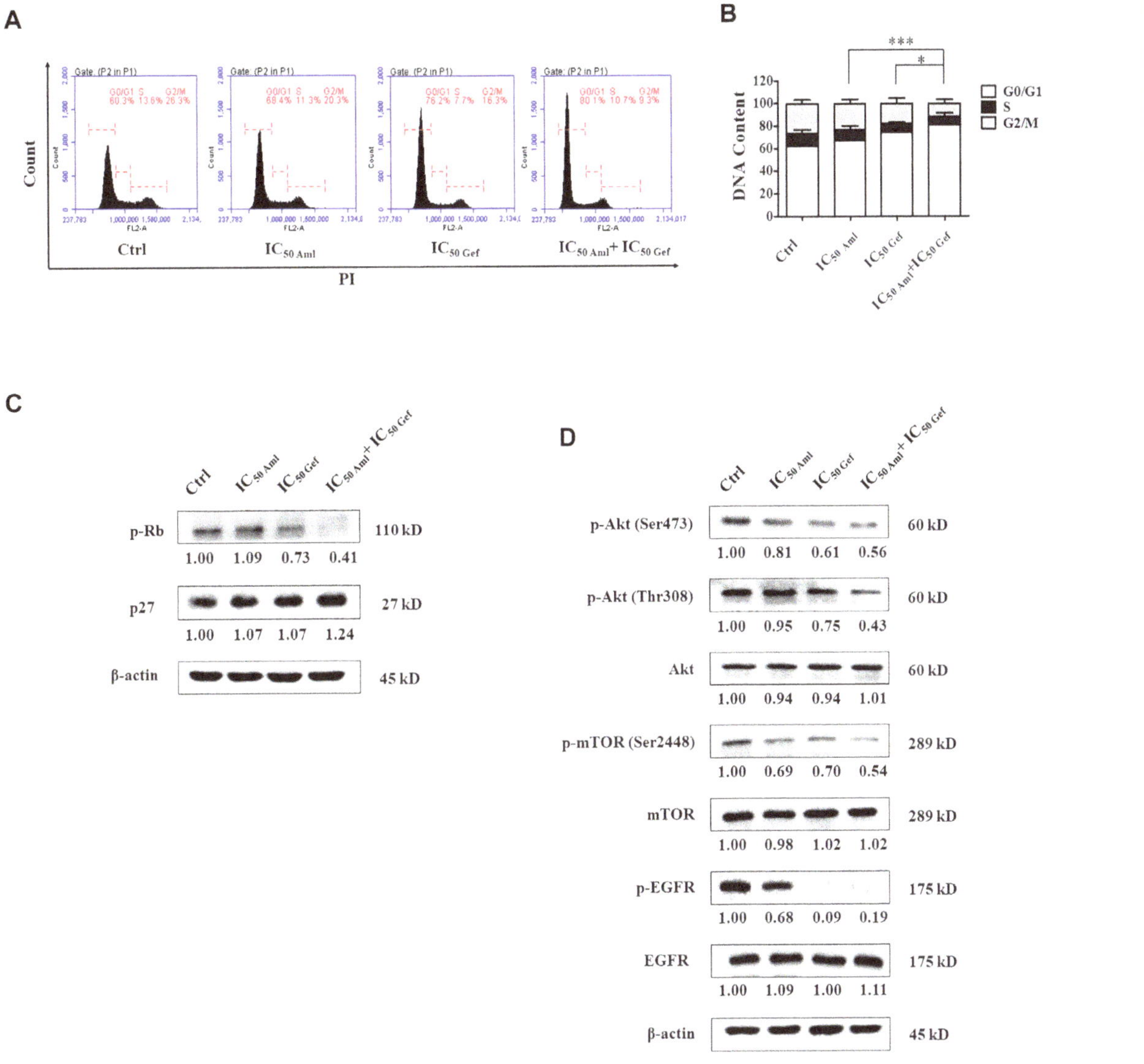

FIGURE 4 | Amlodipine combined with gefitinib induces cycle arrest in A549 cells. **(A)** Amlodipine combined with gefitinib increased the proportion of cells in the G0/G1 phase. **(B)** The percentage of total cells at G0/G1, S, and G2/M phases. **(C)** The levels of p-Rb and p27 were measured by Western blotting after treatment with amlodipine, gefitinib, or a combination of the two agents. **(D)** Phosphorylation and total levels of Akt, mTOR, and EGFR were analyzed by Western blotting after treatment with amlodipine, gefitinib, or a combination of the two agents. Data are presented as mean ± SD of three independent experiments. $^{*}p < 0.05$ and $^{***}p < 0.001$.

gefitinib decreased the phosphorylation of EGFR in A549 cells without any change in total EGFR when compared with the amlodipine alone group (**Figure 4D**).

Amlodipine Alone or in Combination With Gefitinib Suppresses A549 Xenograft Tumor Growth

Based on the aforementioned results from *in vitro* experiments, we speculated whether amlodipine or its combination with gefitinib could afford antitumor effects *in vivo*. Therefore, we examined the efficacy of amlodipine alone and in combination with gefitinib in an A549 xenograft mouse model. Tumor-bearing xenograft mice were orally administered amlodipine (10 mg/kg) or gefitinib (50 mg/kg), alone or in combination, every other day for 15 days. As shown in **Figures 5A,B**, amlodipine alone showed significant antitumor activity against A549 tumors, and this dose resulted in no significant weight loss when compared with the non-treated control group (**Figure 5C**). This result suggests that the test does not induce severe side effects. In addition, treatment with amlodipine combined with gefitinib markedly inhibited the growth of A549 tumors when compared with monotherapy with either agent, with no significant differences in body weight. Furthermore, we compared the histological findings following treatment with amlodipine alone or combined with gefitinib with the untreated group. H&E staining was used to confirm the tissue morphology (**Figure 5D**). Tumor tissue sections stained with the tumor cell proliferation marker Ki67 are shown in **Figure 5E**.

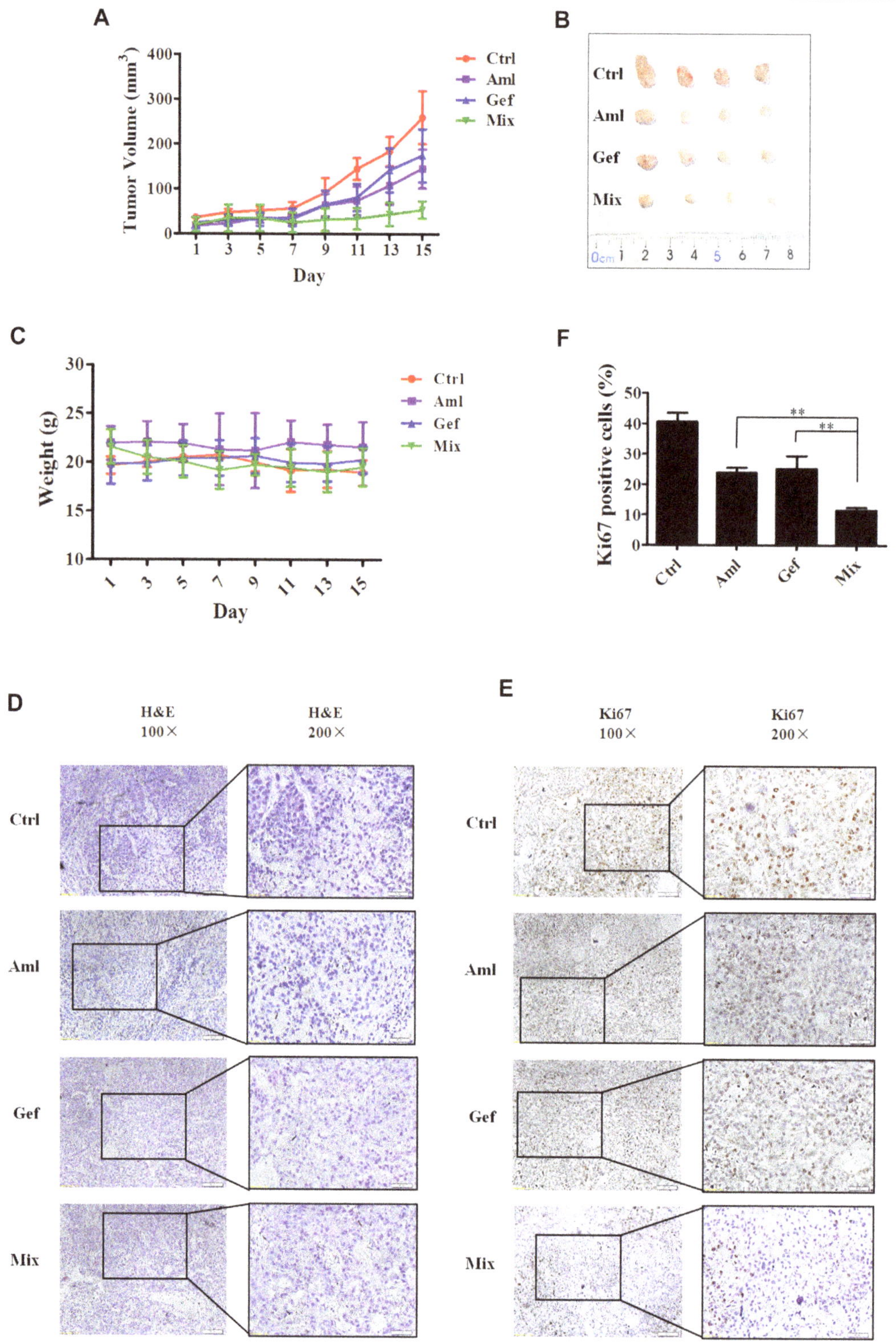

FIGURE 5 | Amlodipine combined with gefitinib inhibits tumor growth in nude mice bearing A549 xenograft. Tumor-bearing xenograft mice were orally administered amlodipine (10 mg/kg every other day) and gefitinib (50 mg/kg every other day), alone or in combination, for 15 days. **(A)** Tumor volumes were measured every alternate day. **(B)** Photographs of the isolated tumors in each group. **(C)** Representative body weights of mice in each group. **(D)** Tumor tissues were stained with H&E. **(E)** Tumor tissues were stained for the proliferation marker Ki67. **(F)** Quantitative analysis of the Ki67 positive cells in tumor sections from mice. Data are presented as mean ± SD obtained from at least 3 mice. $^{**}p < 0.01$.

Amlodipine combined with gefitinib reduced Ki67 positive brown cells when compared with either amlodipine or gefitinib alone (**Figure 5F**).

DISCUSSION

Amlodipine, a Ca^{2+} channel blocker, is frequently used to treat cardiovascular diseases, such as hypertension and angina (Sheraz et al., 2016). The efficacy and safety of long-term amlodipine combined with lisinopril were previously reported in patients with hypertension (Arslanagic et al., 2005). Recent studies have shown that amlodipine exhibits antitumor activity; for example Yoshida *et al.* have reported that amlodipine inhibits proliferation of human epidermoid carcinoma A431 cells, induces G1 phase A431 cell accumulation, retards tumor growth, and prolongs the survival of A431 tumor cell-bearing xenograft mice (Yoshida et al., 2003; 2004; 2007). However, the antitumor effects of amlodipine in NSCLC and its underlying antitumor effects have not been reported. In the present study, we found that amlodipine exhibited beneficial antitumor effects against lung A549 cancer cells both *in vitro* and *in vivo*, with no significant side effects. The mechanistic study revealed that amlodipine attenuated cell proliferation through cell cycle arrest at the G0/G1 phase without marked apoptosis induction. This result is consistent with that of Yoshida *et al.*, who reported that the anti-proliferative effect of amlodipine could not be attributed to cytotoxicity (Yoshida et al., 2003), and caused G1 cell cycle arrest and cell growth inhibition in human epidermoid carcinoma cells (Yoshida et al., 2007). In addition, we found that amlodipine arrested the cell cycle by regulating the cell cycle pathway. Western blot analysis revealed that cyclin D1 and p-Rb were significantly downregulated, while p27 and p21 were upregulated in amlodipine-treated A549 cells. There are three known D-type cyclins (D1, D2, and D3) that form active complexes with either CDK4 or CDK6, as well as cyclin E-CDK2 complexes, which phosphorylate Rb to facilitate the G1 to S phase transition (Shapiro, 2006; Qie and Diehl, 2016). CDK activity is negatively modulated by the INK4 and CIP/KIP families, which include p21 and p27 (Donjerkovic and Scott, 2000; Roskoski, 2019). In addition, reduced protein expression of p21 and p27 has been documented in breast, colon, and gastric tumors (Roskoski, 2019). Our present findings indicate that amlodipine could inhibit A549 cell proliferation by inducing cell cycle arrest *via* modulation of cyclin D1, p-Rb, p27, and p21.

Furthermore, we observed that amlodipine attenuated EGFR phosphorylation in A549 cells, and this finding is consistent with the report by Yoshida *et al.* who suggested that amlodipine suppresses the phosphorylation of EGFR in A431 cells (Yoshida et al., 2010). EGFR activation transduces multiple downstream pro-oncogenic signaling pathways, including the PI3K/Akt/mTOR and Ras/Raf/MEK/ERK pathways (Wee and Wang, 2017), which results in the progression of the G1/S cell cycle (Wee and Wang, 2017).

Subsequently, we noted that amlodipine could affect A549 cells by inhibiting the phosphorylation of PI3K/Akt pathway proteins such as PDK1, Akt (both Thr308 and Ser473), mTOR, p70 S6K, and GSK-3β. The PI3K/Akt/mTOR signaling pathway is one of the most frequently activated signal transduction pathways in human cancers (Martini et al., 2014; Alzahrani, 2019). PI3K phosphorylates phosphatidylinositol 4,5-bisphosphate (PIP2) and converts it to the secondary messenger, phosphatidylinositol 3,4,5-triphosphate (PIP3). PIP3 then recruits a subset of signaling proteins with pleckstrin homology domains, such as PDK1 and Akt, to the plasma membrane (Porta et al., 2014). PDK1 phosphorylates Akt in its activation loop at threonine 308 (Thr308), and full activation of Akt requires phosphorylation at serine 473 (Ser473) *via* mTORC2 activation (Martini et al., 2014; Alzahrani, 2019). Akt directly phosphorylates mTORC1 at Ser2448 (Navé et al., 1999), and activated mTORC1 regulates protein synthesis and cell survival by directly phosphorylating 4E-binding protein 1 and p70 S6K (Gibbons et al., 2009). Akt triggers a network that positively regulates G1/S cell cycle progression via GSK-3β inactivation, leading to increased cyclin D1 and decreased p27Kip1 (Liang and Slingerland, 2003). Dynamic regulated phosphorylation, which reduces the activity of GSK-3, occurs on Ser 9 of GSK-3β, and this N-terminal serine phosphorylation is mediated by Akt (Hermida et al., 2017).

Additionally, we observed that amlodipine effectively inhibited the phosphorylation of c-Raf and ERK, without impacting total ERK levels. The Ras/Raf/MEK/ERK pathway also plays an important role in cell proliferation and survival during several stages of cancer (Asati et al., 2016). Raf proteins are crucial components of the Ras/Raf/MEK/ERK signaling cascade and contain three isoforms; C-Raf (also called Raf-1), B-Raf, and A-Raf (Degirmenci et al., 2020). Activated C-Raf phosphorylates downstream MEK, which activates ERK by phosphorylating both Tyr and Thr regulatory sites (Vandamme et al., 2014; Muta et al., 2019; Guo et al., 2020). ERK1/2 are terminal kinases in MAPK signaling and are located in the cytoplasm when the signaling pathway is inactive. Once activated, ERK1/2 translocates to the nucleus and regulates the activity of several transcription factors, finally mediating cell growth, differentiation, and migration (Shin et al., 2018; Guo et al., 2020). In the present study, we found that amlodipine decreased A549 cell migration in a wound-healing assay. Thus, our results suggest that amlodipine suppresses A549 cell proliferation and migration by inhibiting EGFR-mediated PI3K/Akt and Raf/ERK pathways.

Several clinical studies have indicated that a single agent can present several limitations during the treatment of various cancers. Combination therapy involves the simultaneous administration of two or more therapeutic agents. Combination therapy has shown promising activity in cancer treatment; for example, sorafenib combined with other targeted agents, chemotherapy, and radiotherapy exhibits synergistic antitumor activity (Ibrahim et al., 2012), and gefitinib combined with carboplatin plus pemetrexed can improve progression-free survival when compared with gefitinib alone in patients with NSCLC (Hosomi et al., 2020). Our group has recently reported that combination therapy is beneficial in cancer treatment, such as biomimetic small-molecule self-assembly of the PI3K inhibitor, ZSTK474, integrated with the immunomodulator indomethacin to amplify anticancer efficacy (Zhang et al., 2022) and hydroxychloroquine combined with the PI3K inhibitor BKM120 to induce synergistic effects against tumor cells by manipulating reactive oxygen species clearance and homologous recombination repair processes independent of autophagy (Peng et al., 2021). Herein, we demonstrated that amlodipine acts synergistically with gefitinib by inducing cell cycle arrest in the G0/G1 phase of A549 cells. Compared with amlodipine or gefitinib treatment alone, combination therapy with amlodipine and gefitinib could significantly decrease p-Rb and increase p27 levels. In addition, amlodipine acts synergistically with gefitinib to downregulate the phosphorylation of Akt (Ser473), Akt (Thr308), and mTOR without impacting total Akt and mTOR levels, compared with either amlodipine or gefitinib alone, thus leading to the inhibition of cell cycle progression. Our results indicate that combined treatment with amlodipine and gefitinib exhibited a more potent antitumor effect than monotherapy suppressing A549 cell proliferation.

Furthermore, we investigated the tumor-inhibitory effect of amlodipine in combination with gefitinib in an *in vivo* mouse model. We found that combining amlodipine and gefitinib could enhance the antitumor effects without inducing evident toxicity. Tumors size was decreased, along with a reduction in Ki67-positive staining of the tumor tissue.

Collectively, these findings indicate that amlodipine is a distinct antitumor agent in combination with gefitinib against NSCLC proliferation both *in vivo* and *in vitro*. To the best of our knowledge, this is the first study to combine amlodipine with gefitinib. However, the precise molecular targets of amlodipine alone and in combination with gefitinib on anticancer effects in A549 cells remain elusive in the present study and will be investigated in our future work. Our findings support the potential utility of amlodipine treatment for NSCLC, and amlodipine in combination with gefitinib may be feasible for clinical use, potentially providing a new therapeutic strategy for NSCLC.

AUTHOR CONTRIBUTIONS

MJ and DK designed the experiments and acquired funding for the study; BF, XD, MZ, HL, KW, and QL performed the experiments; MJ, YL, and WW provided technical assistance; BF and MJ wrote the manuscript; DK edited the manuscript.

REFERENCES

Alzahrani, A. S. (2019). PI3K/Akt/mTOR Inhibitors in Cancer: At the Bench and Bedside. *Semin. Cancer Biol.* 59, 125–132. doi:10.1016/j.semcancer.2019.07.009

Arslanagic, A., Zulic, I., and Bajraktarevic, A. (2005). Clinical Study on Safety and Efficacy of the Administration of Amlodipine in a Combination with Lisinopril in Hypertensive Patients. *Med. Arh.* 59, 346–348.

Asati, V., Mahapatra, D. K., and Bharti, S. K. (2016). PI3K/Akt/mTOR and Ras/Raf/MEK/ERK Signaling Pathways Inhibitors as Anticancer Agents: Structural and Pharmacological Perspectives. *Eur. J. Med. Chem.* 109, 314–341. doi:10.1016/j.ejmech.2016.01.012

Cersosimo, R. J. (2002). Lung Cancer: a eview. *Am. J. Health Syst. Pharm.* 59, 611–642. doi:10.1093/ajhp/59.7.611

Da Cunha Santos, G., Shepherd, F. A., and Tsao, M. S. (2011). EGFR Mutations and Lung Cancer. *Annu. Rev. Pathol.* 6, 49–69. doi:10.1146/annurev-pathol-011110-130206

De Mello, R. A., Liu, D. J., Aguiar, P. N., and Tadokoro, H. (2016). EGFR and EML4-ALK Updated Therapies in Non-small Cell Lung Cancer. *Recent Pat. Anticancer Drug Discov.* 11, 393–400. doi:10.2174/1574892811666160803090944

Degirmenci, U., Wang, M., and Hu, J. (2020). Targeting Aberrant RAS/RAF/MEK/ERK Signaling for Cancer Therapy. *Cells* 9, 198. *Cells* 9. doi:10.3390/cells9010198

Donjerkovic, D., and Scott, D. W. (2000). Regulation of the G1 Phase of the Mammalian Cell Cycle. *Cell. Res.* 10, 1–16. doi:10.1038/sj.cr.7290031

Eisenberg, M. J., Brox, A., and Bestawros, A. N. (2004). Calcium Channel Blockers: an Update. *Am. J. Med.* 116, 35–43. doi:10.1016/j.amjmed.2003.08.027

Gibbons, J. J., Abraham, R. T., and Yu, K. (2009). Mammalian Target of Rapamycin: Discovery of Rapamycin Reveals a Signaling Pathway Important for Normal and Cancer Cell Growth. *Semin. Oncol.* 36 (Suppl. 3), S3–s17. doi:10.1053/j.seminoncol.2009.10.011

Guo, Y. J., Pan, W. W., Liu, S. B., Shen, Z. F., Xu, Y., and Hu, L. L. (2020). ERK/MAPK Signalling Pathway and Tumorigenesis. *Exp. Ther. Med.* 19, 1997–2007. doi:10.3892/etm.2020.8454

Hermida, M. A., Dinesh Kumar, J., and Leslie, N. R. (2017). GSK3 and its Interactions with the PI3K/AKT/mTOR Signalling Network. *Adv. Biol. Regul.* 65, 5–15. doi:10.1016/j.jbior.2017.06.003

Hirai, F., Edagawa, M., Shimamatsu, S., Toyozawa, R., Toyokawa, G., Nosaki, K., et al. (2017). Evaluation of Erlotinib for the Treatment of Patients with Non-small Cell Lung Cancer with Epidermal Growth Factor Receptor Wild Type. *Oncol. Lett.* 14, 306–312. doi:10.3892/ol.2017.6118

Hirsch, F. R., Scagliotti, G. V., Mulshine, J. L., Kwon, R., Curran, W. J., Jr., Wu, Y. L., et al. (2017). Lung Cancer: Current Therapies and New Targeted Treatments. *Lancet* 389, 299–311. doi:10.1016/s0140-6736(16)30958-8

Hosomi, Y., Morita, S., Sugawara, S., Kato, T., Fukuhara, T., Gemma, A., et al. (2020). Gefitinib Alone versus Gefitinib Plus Chemotherapy for Non-small-cell Lung Cancer with Mutated Epidermal Growth Factor Receptor: NEJ009 Study. *J. Clin. Oncol.* 38, 115–123. doi:10.1200/jco.19.01488

Ibrahim, N., Yu, Y., Walsh, W. R., and Yang, J. L. (2012). Molecular Targeted Therapies for Cancer: Sorafenib Mono-Therapy and its Combination with Other Therapies (Review). *Oncol. Rep.* 27, 1303–1311. doi:10.3892/or.2012.1675

Jensen, R. L., and Wurster, R. D. (2001). Calcium Channel Antagonists Inhibit Growth of Subcutaneous Xenograft Meningiomas in Nude Mice. *Surg. Neurol.* 55, 275–283. doi:10.1016/s0090-3019(01)00444-x

Li, Y. L., Hu, X., Li, Q. Y., Wang, F., Zhang, B., Ding, K., et al. (2018). Shikonin Sensitizes Wild-type EGFR NSCLC C-ells to E-rlotinib and G-efitinib T-herapy. *Mol. Med. Rep.* 18, 3882–3890. doi:10.3892/mmr.2018.9347

Liang, J., and Slingerland, J. M. (2003). Multiple Roles of the PI3K/PKB (Akt) Pathway in Cell Cycle Progression. *Cell. Cycle* 2, 339–345. doi:10.4161/cc.2.4.433

Martini, M., De Santis, M. C., Braccini, L., Gulluni, F., and Hirsch, E. (2014). PI3K/AKT Signaling Pathway and Cancer: an Updated Review. *Ann. Med.* 46, 372–383. doi:10.3109/07853890.2014.912836

Muta, Y., Matsuda, M., and Imajo, M. (2019). Divergent Dynamics and Functions of ERK MAP Kinase Signaling in Development, Homeostasis and Cancer: Lessons from Fluorescent Bioimaging. *Cancers (Basel)* 11, 513. doi:10.3390/cancers11040513

Navé, B. T., Ouwens, M., Withers, D. J., Alessi, D. R., and Shepherd, P. R. (1999). Mammalian Target of Rapamycin Is a Direct Target for Protein Kinase B: Identification of a Convergence Point for Opposing Effects of Insulin and Amino-Acid Deficiency on Protein Translation. *Biochem. J.* 344 Pt 2, 427–431.

Peng, X., Zhang, S., Jiao, W., Zhong, Z., Yang, Y., Claret, F. X., et al. (2021). Hydroxychloroquine Synergizes with the PI3K Inhibitor BKM120 to Exhibit Antitumor Efficacy Independent of Autophagy. *J. Exp. Clin. Cancer Res.* 40, 374. doi:10.1186/s13046-021-02176-2

Porta, C., Paglino, C., and Mosca, A. (2014). Targeting PI3K/Akt/mTOR Signaling in Cancer. *Front. Oncol.* 4, 64. doi:10.3389/fonc.2014.00064

Qie, S., and Diehl, J. A. (2016). Cyclin D1, Cancer Progression, and Opportunities in Cancer Treatment. *J. Mol. Med. Berl.* 94, 1313–1326. doi:10.1007/s00109-016-1475-3

Roskoski, R., Jr. (2019). Cyclin-dependent Protein Serine/threonine Kinase Inhibitors as Anticancer Drugs. *Pharmacol. Res.* 139, 471–488. doi:10.1016/j.phrs.2018.11.035

Shao, C., Huang, Y., Fu, B., Pan, S., Zhao, X., Zhang, N., et al. (2021). Targeting C-Jun in A549 Cancer Cells Exhibits Antiangiogenic Activity *In Vitro* and *In Vivo* through Exosome/miRNA-494-3p/PTEN Signal Pathway. *Front. Oncol.* 11, 663183. doi:10.3389/fonc.2021.663183

Shapiro, G. I. (2006). Cyclin-dependent Kinase Pathways as Targets for Cancer Treatment. *J. Clin. Oncol.* 24, 1770–1783. doi:10.1200/jco.2005.03.7689

Sheraz, M. A., Ahsan, S. F., Khan, M. F., Ahmed, S., and Ahmad, I. (2016). Formulations of Amlodipine: A Review. *J. Pharm. (Cairo)* 2016, 8961621. doi:10.1155/2016/8961621

Sherr, C. J. (1994). G1 Phase Progression: Cycling on Cue. *Cell.* 79, 551–555. doi:10.1016/0092-8674(94)90540-1

Shin, M., Franks, C. E., and Hsu, K. L. (2018). Isoform-selective Activity-Based Profiling of ERK Signaling. *Chem. Sci.* 9, 2419–2431. doi:10.1039/c8sc00043c

Shukuya, T., Takahashi, T., Kaira, R., Ono, A., Nakamura, Y., Tsuya, A., et al. (2011). Efficacy of Gefitinib for Non-adenocarcinoma Non-small-cell Lung Cancer Patients Harboring Epidermal Growth Factor Receptor Mutations: a Pooled Analysis of Published Reports. *Cancer Sci.* 102, 1032–1037. doi:10.1111/j.1349-7006.2011.01887.x

Sica, D. A. (2006). Pharmacotherapy Review: Calcium Channel Blockers. *J. Clin. Hypertens. (Greenwich)* 8, 53–56. doi:10.1111/j.1524-6175.2005.04140.x

Vandamme, D., Herrero, A., Al-Mulla, F., and Kolch, W. (2014). Regulation of the MAPK Pathway by Raf Kinase Inhibitory Protein. *Crit. Rev. Oncog.* 19, 405–415. doi:10.1615/critrevoncog.2014011922

Wang, J., Mcdonagh, D. L., and Meng, L. (2021). Calcium Channel Blockers in Acute Care: The Links and Missing Links between Hemodynamic Effects and Outcome Evidence. *Am. J. Cardiovasc. Drugs* 21, 35–49. doi:10.1007/s40256-020-00410-4

Wee, P., and Wang, Z. (2017). Epidermal Growth Factor Receptor Cell Proliferation Signaling Pathways. *Cancers (Basel)* 9. doi:10.3390/cancers9050052

Wozniak, A. J., Crowley, J. J., Balcerzak, S. P., Weiss, G. R., Spiridonidis, C. H., Baker, L. H., et al. (1998). Randomized Trial Comparing Cisplatin with Cisplatin Plus Vinorelbine in the Treatment of Advanced Non-small-cell Lung Cancer: a Southwest Oncology Group Study. *J. Clin. Oncol.* 16, 2459–2465. doi:10.1200/jco.1998.16.7.2459

Yohem, K. H., Clothier, J. L., Montague, S. L., Geary, R. J., Winters, A. L., 3rd, Hendrix, M. J., et al. (1991). Inhibition of Tumor Cell Invasion by Verapamil. *Pigment. Cell. Res.* 4, 225–233. doi:10.1111/j.1600-0749.1991.tb00445.x

Yoshida, J., Ishibashi, T., and Nishio, M. (2003). Antiproliferative Effect of Ca2+ Channel Blockers on Human Epidermoid Carcinoma A431 Cells. *Eur. J. Pharmacol.* 472, 23–31. doi:10.1016/s0014-2999(03)01831-4

Yoshida, J., Ishibashi, T., and Nishio, M. (2004). Antitumor Effects of Amlodipine, a Ca2+ Channel Blocker, on Human Epidermoid Carcinoma A431 Cells *In Vitro* and *In Vivo*. *Eur. J. Pharmacol.* 492, 103–112. doi:10.1016/j.ejphar.2004.04.006

Yoshida, J., Ishibashi, T., and Nishio, M. (2007). G1 Cell Cycle Arrest by Amlodipine, a Dihydropyridine Ca2+ Channel Blocker, in Human Epidermoid Carcinoma A431 Cells. *Biochem. Pharmacol.* 73, 943–953. doi:10.1016/j.bcp.2006.12.011

Yoshida, J., Ishibashi, T., Yang, M., and Nishio, M. (2010). Amlodipine, a Ca2+ Channel Blocker, Suppresses Phosphorylation of Epidermal Growth Factor Receptor in Human Epidermoid Carcinoma A431 Cells. *Life Sci.* 86, 124–132. doi:10.1016/j.lfs.2009.11.014

Zhang, S., Peng, X., Li, X., Liu, H., Zhao, B., Elkabets, M., et al. (2021). BKM120 Sensitizes Glioblastoma to the PARP Inhibitor Rucaparib by Suppressing Homologous Recombination Repair. *Cell. Death Dis.* 12, 546. doi:10.1038/s41419-021-03805-6

Zhang, Z., Hou, L., Yu, Z., Xu, Z., Li, S., Wang, Y., et al. (2022). Biomimetic Small-Molecule Self-Assembly of PI3K Inhibitor Integrated with Immunomodulator to Amplify Anticancer Efficacy. *Chem. Eng. J.* 433, 133747. doi:10.1016/j.cej.2021.133747

Zhao, X., Zhang, N., Huang, Y., Dou, X., Peng, X., Wang, W., et al. (2021). Lansoprazole Alone or in Combination with Gefitinib Shows Antitumor Activity against Non-small Cell Lung Cancer A549 Cells *In Vitro* and *In Vivo*. *Front. Cell. Dev. Biol.* 9, 655559. doi:10.3389/fcell.2021.655559

Hinokiflavone Inhibits Growth of Esophageal Squamous Cancer By Inducing Apoptosis via Regulation of the PI3K/AKT/mTOR Signaling Pathway

*Jida Guo†, Shengqiang Zhang†, Jun Wang, Pengfei Zhang, Tong Lu and Linyou Zhang**

Department of Thoracic Surgery, The Second Affiliated Hospital of Harbin Medical University, Harbin Medical University, Harbin, China

Correspondence:
Linyou Zhang
lyzhang@hrbmu.edu.cn

†These authors have contributed equally to this work

Background: Globally, esophageal cancer ranks as the seventh most common cancer. Esophageal squamous cell carcinoma (ESCC) is one of its major histological types. ESCC accounts for the vast majority of cases in China, and the mortality rate is high. Cisplatin, the standard adjuvant chemotherapy drug for ESCC, has a modest response rate due to the development of drug resistance. Hinokiflavone (HF) is a natural biflavonoid compound with anti-melanoma activity. However, its anti-tumor effect on ESCC and the underlying mechanisms remain largely unknown.

Methods: The ESCC cell lines KYSE150 and TE14 were used. The cell counting kit-8 assay and flow cytometry analysis, along with colony formation, EdU, wound healing, and Transwell migration assays, were performed to assess cell characteristics (viability, migration, invasion, and apoptosis) following treatment with HF. Gene Ontology (GO), Kyoto Encyclopedia of Genes and Genomes (KEGG), western blotting, and molecular docking were used to investigate the pathways potentially modulated by HF. *In vivo* anti-tumor effects of HF were also investigated using a mouse xenograft model.

Results: Our findings revealed that HF inhibited ESCC cell proliferation. Hoechst 33342 staining, annexin V-FITC/PI staining, and western blotting confirmed that HF causes caspase-dependent apoptosis. KEGG pathway enrichment analysis and western blotting indicated that the PI3K/AKT/mTOR pathway played an important role in the process of HF-induced apoptosis. Furthermore, HF effectively impaired the migration and invasion abilities of KYSE150 cells and downregulated the expression of the matrix metalloproteinases (MMP) MMP2 and MMP9. HF inhibited tumor growth and exhibited minimal toxicity in the organs of the KYSE150 xenograft model.

Conclusion: This is the first study to demonstrate the inhibition of ESCC growth and progression by HF. The underlying mechanism is through blocking the PI3K/AKT/mTOR signaling pathway, thereby inhibiting cell proliferation and inducing apoptosis. HF can be used as a complementary/alternative agent for ESCC therapy.

Keywords: esophageal cancer, hinokiflavone, apoptosis, KEGG analysis, molecular docking, PI3K/AKT/mTOR signal pathway

INTRODUCTION

Esophageal cancer is the sixth leading cause of cancer-related deaths and the seventh most common cancer worldwide (1). It is well known that there are two dominant histological types of esophageal cancer: esophageal adenocarcinoma and esophageal squamous cell carcinoma (ESCC). ESCC accounts for 90% of all esophageal cancer cases in Asia and Africa (1). In recent years, despite the development of multimodal treatment including surgery combined with chemoradiotherapy and targeted therapy, the prognosis of esophageal cancer patients remains poor due to the strong malignancy of this cancer (2, 3). Therefore, the development of novel therapeutic approaches for this disease is urgent and necessary.

Natural products have a long history of use for the treatment of human disease, which is of great value for drug discovery and development (4). Moreover, many common chemotherapeutic compounds have been derived from natural products (5, 6). Hinokiflavone (HF) (**Figure 1A**, $C_{30}H_{18}O_{10}$) has been extracted from several plants, including *Selaginella tamariscina, Juniperus phoenicea*, and *Rhus succedanea*, with high stability. It exhibits several biological activities including cytotoxicity (7), anti-HIV-1 reverse transcriptase activity (8), and antioxidant activity (9). Sui et al. (10) reported that the ethyl acetate extract of *Selaginella doederleinii* Hieron inhibits proliferation of A549 cell lines by inducing apoptosis. Magne et al. (11) also identified natural flavonoids in HF that are useful therapeutic agents for breast cancer. In addition, HF might also be a novel compound to treat melanoma by cell cycle arrest, inducing apoptosis and blocking cell migration and invasion (12). However, the antitumor effect of HF in ESCC and its specific targeted signaling pathways have not been investigated.

Multiple studies have demonstrated that phosphoinositides, the multiphosphorylated derivatives of phosphatidylinositol, are membrane-bound signaling molecules that play a crucial role in a variety of cellular biological processes (13–15). Under general physiological conditions, phosphatidylinositol-3-kinase (PI3K) activates AKT (protein kinase B) by phosphorylating Thr 308 and Ser 473 (p-AKT) (16, 17). p-Akt then phosphorylates several of its downstream effector proteins, such as tuberous sclerosis complex 2 (TSC2) and glycogen synthase kinase 3 (GSK3α/β), and these activated proteins subsequently regulate cell growth, survival, and apoptosis (18, 19). Whereas mammalian target of rapamycin (mTOR) was shown to be the major signaling molecule downstream of TSC2, targeting regulation of the PI3K/Akt/mTOR pathway has been proven effective in cancer therapies (20, 21). Accumulating evidence has also shown that the PI3K/Akt signaling pathway is activated in multiple tumor types and contributes to tumor progression by promoting tumor cell proliferation, apoptosis resistance, and distant metastasis (22, 23). Moreover, the PI3K/AKT signaling pathway plays a vital role in ESCC growth and metastasis (24, 25).

In the current study, we extensively explored the anti-tumor effects of HF on human esophageal cancer cells *in vitro* and *in vivo* as well as the underlying molecular mechanisms. We found that HF exhibited a strong growth inhibitory effect on two ESCC cell lines (KYSE150 and TE14) and the PI3K/AKT/mTOR signaling pathway plays a crucial role in HF-induced apoptosis in these cells. These results indicate that HF has potential anti-tumor activity, which can be exploited to develop effective therapeutic strategies for ESCC.

MATERIALS AND METHODS

Reagents, Antibodies and Kits

HF of 98% purity was purchased from Chengdu Biopurify Phytochemicals, Ltd. (Chengdu, China). Dimethylsulfoxide (DMSO), RPMI 1640 medium, and fetal bovine serum (FBS) were purchased from Sigma Chemical Co. (St Louis, MO, USA). Antibodies against β-actin, phosphorylated PI3K [p-PI3K (Tyr458 and Tyr199)], PI3K, phosphorylated AKT [p-AKT (Ser473 and Thr308)], AKT, cleaved Caspase 3 (c-Caspase 3), phosphorylated mTOR [p-mTOR (Ser2448)], mTOR, matrix metalloproteinase-2 (MMP2), and MMP9 were purchased from Cell Signaling Technology, Inc. (Danvers, MA, USA). Antibodies against Bcl-2 and Bax were purchased from Proteintech Group, Inc. (Chicago, IL, USA). RIPA lysis buffer, phenylmethanesulfonyl fluoride (PMSF), and the bicinchoninic acid (BCA) protein assay kit were from Beyotime (Nanjing, China). Enhanced chemiluminescence detection reagent was obtained from GE Healthcare Life Sciences Inc. (Marlborough, MA, USA). SC-79 (AKT activator) was purchased from MedChemExpress (Shanghai, China). Cell Counting Kit-8 (CCK-8) was obtained from Dojindo Laboratories (Kumamoto, Japan). Hoechst33342 and BeyoClick™ EdU Cell Proliferation Kit with Alexa Fluor 594 and the Annexin V-fluorescein isothiocyanate (FITC)/propidium iodide (PI) apoptosis detection kit were purchased from Beyotime Biotechnology (Jiangsu, China).

A stock solution of HF dissolved in DMSO (40 mM) was stored at -20°C and diluted with medium for experimental applications.

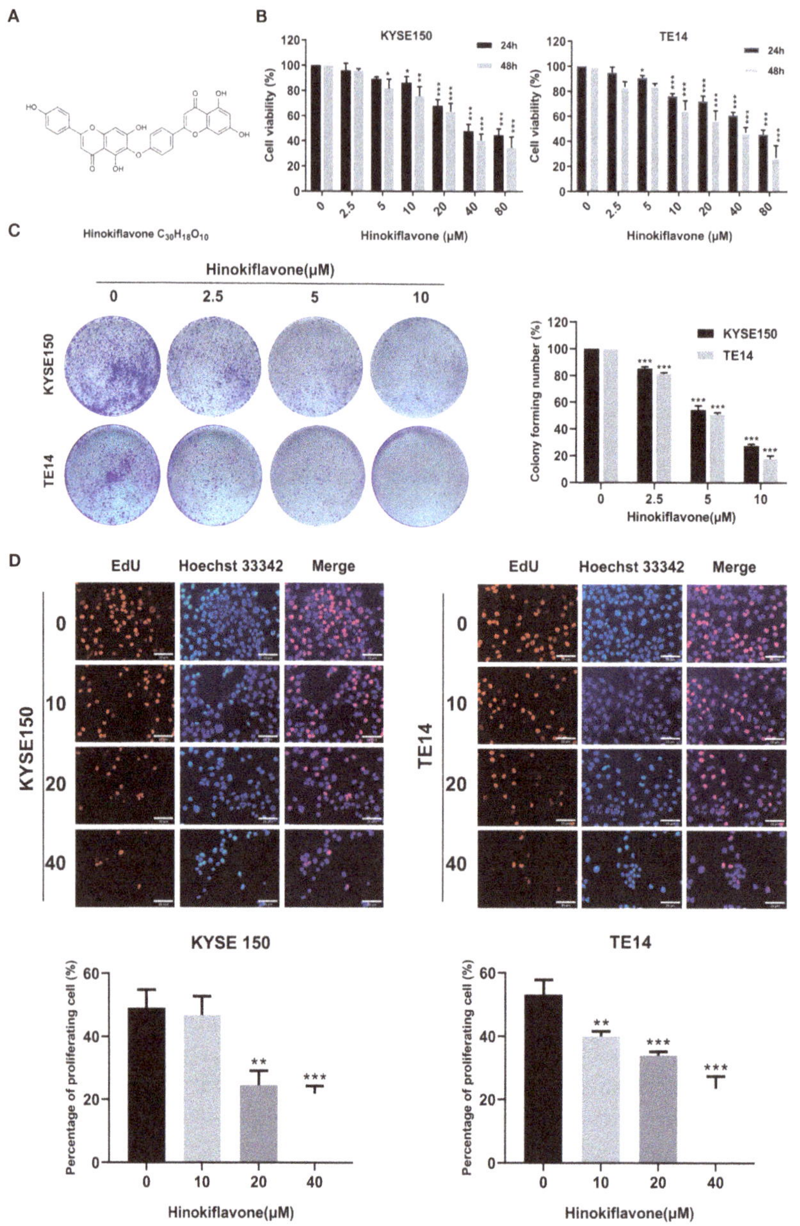

FIGURE 1 | Effect of hinokiflavone (HF) on the proliferation of esophageal squamous cell carcinoma (ESCC) cells. **(A)** Two-dimensional chemical structure of HF ($C_{30}H_{18}O_{10}$). **(B)** KYSE150 and TE14 cell lines were incubated with different concentrations of HF for 24 and 48 h Cell viability was evaluated using the CCK-8 assay. **(C)** HF reduced colony formation of ESCC cells. KYSE150 and TE14 cells were treated with 0, 2.5, 5, and 10 μM of HF and cultured for 9 days to form colonies. Colonies were stained with crystal violet and counted. **(D)** EdU assay analyzed the antiproliferative effect of HF on ESCC cells. Hoechst 33342 cell nuclei dye presented as blue fluorescence cells represent total cells, and EdU positive cells presented as red fluorescence represent proliferating cells. Magnification, ×200; scale bars = 25 μm. All the above experimental data are presented as the mean ± SD of three independent experiments. *P < 0.05; **P < 0.01; ***P < 0.001 compared to vehicle control (0 μM) group.

Cell Culture

KYSE150 and TE14 cell lines were purchased from the Cell Bank of the Chinese Academy of Sciences. Cells were cultured in RPMI 1640 medium with 10% FBS and 1% penicillin-streptomycin at 37°C in a humidified incubator with 5% CO_2 and 95% humidity.

Cell Proliferation Assay

Cell viability was determined using the CCK-8 assay. KYSE150 and TE14 cells were seeded at a density of 1×10^4 cells/well in 96-well plates. After 24 h of incubation, the cells were treated with 0, 2.5, 5, 10, 20, 40, and 80 μM of HF. Controls were treated with

RPMI medium containing DMSO only. After 24 h and 48 h, old medium was aspirated and 100 μL of CCK-8 working solution, diluted to 10% in culture medium, was added to each well and further incubated for 4 h at 37°C in a humidified incubator. The absorbance at 450 nm was measured using a microplate reader. IC_{50} values were calculated with Graphpad Prism 8 using data obtained from three independent experiments.

Colony Formation Assay

KYSE150 and TE14 cells were plated in 6-well plates (1.0×10^3 cells/well). After 24 h of incubation, the cells were incubated with various concentrations (0, 2.5, 5, and 10 μM) of HF for 9 days. Cells were fixed with 4% paraformaldehyde and then stained with 0.5% crystal violet for 15 min, after which a dissecting microscope was used to count colonies (> 50 cells).

EdU Assay

The EdU assay was performed to analyze proliferating cells by evaluating the incorporation of fluorescent labeled EdU into replicating DNA in the S phase of cell cycle. The BeyoClick™ EdU Cell Proliferation Kit with Alexa Fluor 594 was used for this purpose, according to the manufacturer's instructions. The maximum excitation wavelength of Alexa 594 is 590 nm, and the maximum emission wavelength is 615 nm. Briefly, KYSE150 and TE14 cells were seeded in 96-well plates at a cell density of 5.0×10^3 cells/well and treated with different concentrations of HF for 24 h. Edu was added to the culture medium and brought to a final concentration of 10 μM, and the cells were cultured for an additional 2.5 h at 37°C. Afterwards, cells were washed twice using phosphate-buffered saline (PBS) and fixed by 4% paraformaldehyde for 15 min at approximately 25°C. After co-staining with Hoechst 33342, the cells were imaged using a fluorescence microscope (Leica, Wetzlar, Germany).

Morphological Analysis by Hoechst 33342 Staining

Alterations in cell morphology, including cell shrinkage and apoptotic body formation, were analyzed after Hoechst 33342 staining to identify apoptotic cells. KYSE150 and TE14 cells were seeded in 96-well plates at a density of 5.0×10^3 cells/well and cultured for 24 h. After treatment with different concentrations of HF (0, 10, 20, and 40 μM) for 24 h, the cells were washed twice using PBS and fixed in 4% paraformaldehyde for 15 min. Then, the cells were stained using Hoechst 33342 working solution diluted well according to the instructions for 15 min at 25°C and analyzed under a fluorescence microscope (Zeiss, Axiovert 200, Oberkochen, Germany).

Quantification of Apoptosis

Further verification of HF-induced apoptosis was carried out using the Annexin V-FITC/PI apoptosis detection kit. After treatment with HF (0, 10, 20, and 40 μM) for 24 h, KYSE150 and TE14 cells at a cell density of 1.0×10^6 cells/well were trypsinized, collected by centrifugation, and washed twice with ice-cold PBS. The cells were then co-stained with 5 μL FITC-Annexin V and 5 μL PI for 15 min at 20–25 °C in the dark. The apoptosis rate was measured by flow cytometry (CytoFLEX, Beckman Coulter, Brea, CA, USA).

Gene Ontology and Kyoto Encyclopedia of Genes and Genomes Pathway Enrichment Analyses

A total of 355 and 100 potential targets for HF were searched from the Pharma Mapper (http://www.lilab-ecust.cn/pharmmapper/) and Swiss target prediction (http://www.swisstargetprediction.ch/) databases, respectively. GO and KEGG pathway enrichment analyses was performed using the DAVID database (26, 27).

Molecular Docking

The 3D structures of PI3K (code 6pys) and AKT1 (code 4ejn) were downloaded from the Protein Data Bank (https://www.rcsb.org/). Chemical structure data of HF was obtained from PubChem (http://pubchem.ncbi.nlm.nih.gov/). Molecular docking was implemented using the LibDock module of the Discovery Studio 2016, and the results were evaluated using the LibDock score. A higher libdock score indicates a higher activity of the small molecule (such as HF) binding to the target protein.

Western Blot Analysis

KYSE150 and TE14 cells at a cell density of 5.0×10^6 cells/well were treated with various concentrations of HF (0, 10, 20, and 40 μM) for 24 h. Cells were washed twice using PBS and lysed by adding RIPA cell lysis buffer containing PMSF. The cell lysate was centrifuged at 12,000 × *g* for 20 min at 4°C, after which the supernatant was gently aspirated using a pipette. The total protein content in the supernatant was measured using the BCA protein assay kit. Equal amounts of protein (20 μg) were separated by SDS-PAGE (8%–12%). The separated proteins were then transferred onto a PVDF membrane. The membranes were blocked with Quickblock blocking buffer (Beyotime Biotechnology, China) for 0.5 h and incubated with specific primary antibodies overnight at 4°C on a shaker. Membranes were washed three times for 10 min each with Tris-buffered saline-Tween 20 (TBST), completed by incubation with horseradish peroxidase (HRP)-conjugated secondary antibody for 1 h at approximately 25°C. Our study used the following primary antibodies: β-actin (1:1,000), phosphorylated PI3K (p-PI3K) (Tyr458, 1:1,000 and Tyr199, 1:1,000), PI3K (1:1,000), phosphorylated AKT (p-AKT) (Ser473, 1:1,000; Thr308, 1:1,000), AKT (1:1,000), c-Caspase 3 (1:1,000), p-mTOR (Ser2448, 1:1,000), mTOR (1:1,000), matrix metalloproteinase-2 (MMP2) (1:1,000), MMP9 (1:1,000), Bcl-2 (1:2,000), and Bax (1:1,000). The secondary antibody was HRP-conjugated goat anti-rabbit antibody (1:10,000; Cell Signaling Technology, Inc.). After three 10 min washes with TBST, the protein band was visualized using enhanced chemiluminescence detection reagent (GE Healthcare Life Sciences). Finally, protein bands were quantified by densitometric analysis using ImageJ software, and the protein amounts were expressed relative to the corresponding reference protein.

Wound-Healing Migration Assay

KYSE150 cells were grown to a density of approximately 80-90% in 6-well plates, after which the cell monolayer was scraped using a sterile 100-μL pipette tip to create "wounds". Reduced serum medium (1 mL) containing HF (0, 10, 20, or 40 μM) was gently added to the wells along the lateral wall to ensure that it covered the entire bottom. After incubation for 24 h in an incubator, the cells were washed and fixed with 4% paraformaldehyde (1 mL/well), and images were acquired under a microscope (Zeiss, Jena, Germany). Cell movement distances were measured by ImageJ (v1.8.0).

Cell Migration and Invasion Assay

Transwell migration and invasion assays were implemented by using Boyden chamber (8 μm pore size, Corning, NY, USA). For migration assay, KYSE150 cells (2.0×10^4 cells in 100 μL serum-free medium) were added into the upper chamber, and 600 μL of medium with 10% FBS was added into the lower chamber. For invasion assay, the upper surface of the Transwell membrane was coated with Matrigel (BD Biosciences, Franklin lakes, NJ, USA) diluted 1:8 with serum-free medium before adding cells. For both assays, various concentrations of HF (0, 10, 20, and 40 μM) were added into the lower chamber. After incubation for 24 h, the medium was discarded, the cells were gently removed from the upper surface of the Transwell membrane with a cotton swab, and the migrated or invaded cells on the lower surface were fixed with 4% paraformaldehyde, after which they were stained with 0.5% crystal violet. Using microscopy, the number of stained cells on the lower surface was counted in five random fields per Transwell membrane (×100 magnification), and the Image J software was used to enumerate the migrated/invaded cells.

Mouse Xenograft Model

All experimental procedures and manipulations involving animals were performed in compliance with the guidelines of the National Institutes of Health Guide for the Care and Use of Laboratory Animals. Moreover, all animal experiments were approved by the Institutional Animal Care and Use Committee of the Second Affiliated Hospital of Harbin Medical University (SYDW2021-046). Female BALB/c-nu athymic mice, at 6 weeks and weighing 14-17 g, were purchased from Beijing Vital River Laboratory Animal Technology Co., Ltd. (Beijing, China). Mice were maintained in a specific pathogen-free (SPF) grade rearing environment using sterile water and food feeding. KYSE150 cells (1.0×10^7 cells in 100 μL PBS) were injected subcutaneously into the right shoulders of the mice (n=18). Tumor size was measured every 3 days using a caliper. The formula for calculating tumor volume was as follows: $V = 0.5 \times L \times W^2$ (L, tumor longest diameter; W, tumor shortest diameter). When the tumor volume reached 50 mm^3, mice were randomized into three groups (n=6/group; control, 25 mg/kg HF, and 50 mg/kg HF). Next, HF (25 mg/kg and 50 mg/kg in 200 μL saline) was administered by intraperitoneal injection to the two treatment group mice daily for 21 days. The control mice received saline alone. The body weight and tumor volume of mice were measured every 3 days. After completion of drug administration, all animals were fed normal diet for another 3 days, after which they were euthanized by cervical dislocation. The tumors were excised, weighed, and immunohistochemical staining was performed. The internal organs were collected for hematoxylin and eosin (H&E) staining.

Immunohistochemistry

Tumor tissues from mice were formalin fixed, then embedded in paraffin and sectioned at 4 μm thin sections were used for examination. For staining, tissue sections were deparaffinized and rehydrated following standard protocols. Antigen retrieval of tissues in our study was performed by boiling in sodium citrate buffer (10 mM, pH 6.0) for 10 min, after which the samples were treated with 3% H_2O_2 for an additional 10 min. Each section was blocked with 10% goat serum albumin in a humidified chamber for 1 h at approximately 20–25°C. Then, tissue sections were incubated with specific primary antibodies (p-AKT, p-mTOR, Bax, and c-Caspase 3) overnight at 4°C in a humidified chamber. After further washing, the sections were incubated with secondary antibody for 30 min at approximately 25°C, followed by incubation with 3,3'-diaminobenzidine and counterstaining with hematoxylin. Stained sections were imaged under a microscope (Leica, DM4000B).

H&E Staining

Mouse organs (heart, liver, spleen, lung, and kidney) were fixed in formaldehyde, embedded in paraffin, and sectioned at 4 μm thickness. After deparaffinization and rehydration, tissue sections were stained with hematoxylin for 10 min, 1% ethanol-hydrochloric acid for 30 s, and eosin solution for 3 min. The sections were dehydrated in graded alcohol, after which they were cleared with xylene and finally mounted using neutral balsam.

Statistical Analysis

All data are presented using the mean ± SD of three independent experiments. Statistical analysis was performed using GraphPad Prism version 8 (GraphPad Software, San Diego, CA, USA). Student's *t*-test was used to compare two groups, and one-way analysis of variance was used for multiple comparisons. Statistically significant *P*-values are labeled as follows: $^*P < 0.05$, $^{**}P < 0.01$, $^{***}P < 0.001$.

RESULTS

HF Inhibits the Proliferation of ESCC Cells

The chemical structure of HF was drawn with ChemDraw software as shown in **Figure 1A**. KYSE150 and TE14 cell lines were treated with HF at different concentrations (0, 2.5, 5, 10, 20, 40, or 80 μM) for 24 or 48 h, and cell proliferation was assessed by CCK-8 assay, as described in the Methods. As shown in **Figure 1B**, HF significantly inhibited the cell viability of both ESCC cell lines in a concentration- and time-dependent manner. Furthermore, the IC_{50} values for KYSE150 cells treated with HF for 24 h and 48 h were 27.92 μM and 24.91 μM, respectively, while the respective values for TE14 cells were 26.21 μM and 22.07 μM. Long-term cell viability assays (colony formation assays) showed that KYSE150 and TE14 cells formed significantly fewer colonies with increasing HF concentrations. (**Figure 1C**). The anti-proliferative activity of HF was further verified using an EdU assay. As shown in **Figure 1D**, the proportion of proliferating KYSE150 and TE14 cells decreased from 49.1% and 53.2% to 21.9% and 23.6%, respectively, after 40 μM HF treatment for 24 h. Taken together, these results indicate that HF effectively inhibits ESCC cell proliferation.

HF Induces Apoptosis in ESCC Cells

We next explored whether HF induces apoptosis in ESCC cells. Induction of apoptosis by HF was first evaluated by Hoechst

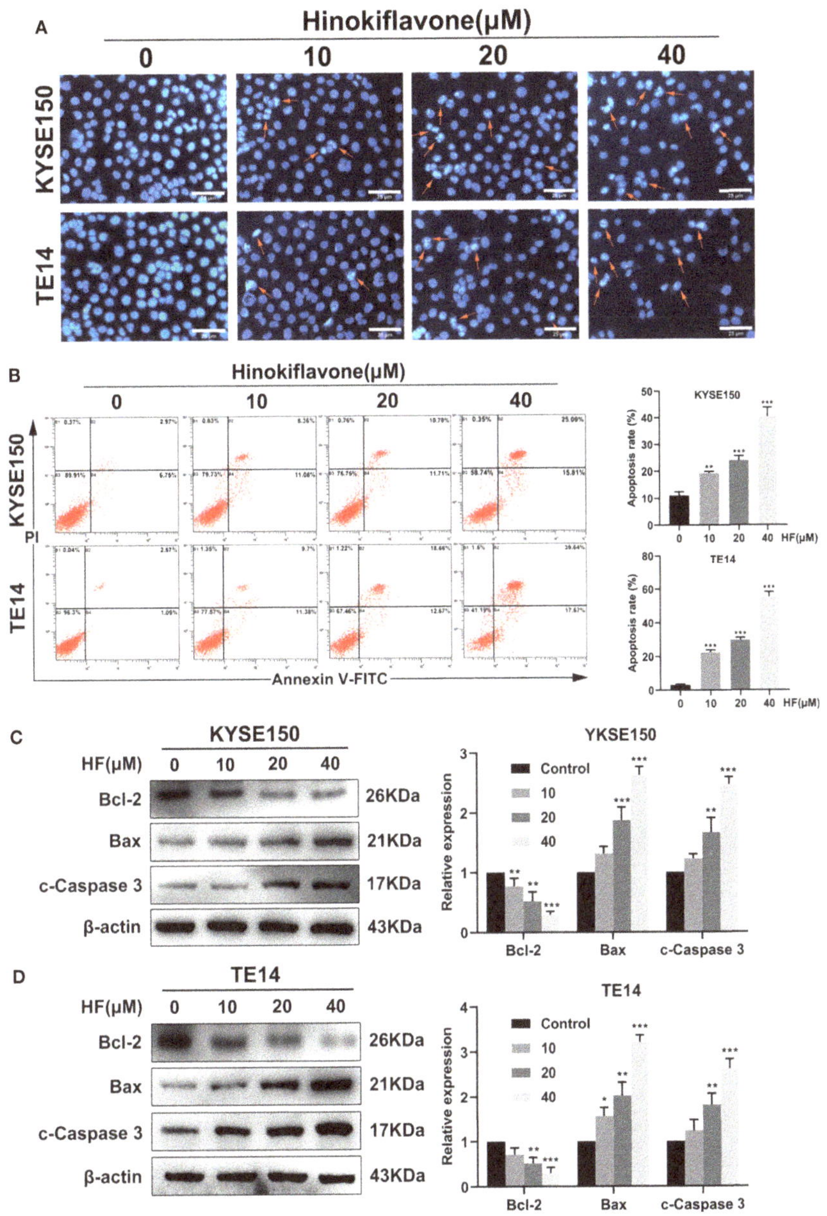

FIGURE 2 | Induction of apoptosis in ESCC cells by HF. **(A)** Hoechst 33342 nuclear dye was used to stain the KYSE150 and TE14 cells and utilized fluorescence microscopy to detect HF induced apoptotic nuclear morphological alterations (indicated by red arrows). Magnification, ×200; scale bars = 25 μm. **(B)** Percentage of KYSE150 and TE14 cells apoptosis after HF treatment was measured using Annexin V-fluorescein isothiocyanate (FITC)/propidium iodide (PI) double staining and analyzed by flow cytometry. **(C, D)** Expression levels of Bcl-2, Bax, and c-Caspase 3 were detected by western blot and quantitated *via* densitometric analysis using ImageJ software, while the expression level of β-actin was used as an internal control. The relative expression of experimental histones was calculated according to the protein scale set to 1 for 0 μM control group. All the above experimental data are presented as the mean ± SD of three independent experiments. $^{*}P < 0.05$; $^{**}P < 0.01$; $^{***}P < 0.001$ compared to vehicle (0 μM) group.

33342 staining assay. As shown in **Figure 2A**, HF-treated KYSE150 and TE14 cell cultures contained dense and heavily stained apoptotic cells, suggesting that HF might cause various degrees of cell shrinkage, nuclear fragmentation, and condensed nuclei formation. Furthermore, flow cytometric analysis of Annexin V-FITC and PI staining revealed that the ratio of early and late apoptotic cells increased in a dose-dependent manner after treatment with HF for 24 h. As shown in **Figure 2B**, the mean apoptosis ratios (from three independent experiments) were 11.0% (0 μM), 19.2% (10 μM), 24.2% (20 μM), 40.6% (40 μM) for KYSE150 cells; 3.3% (0 μM), 22.3% (10 μM), 29.9% (20 μM), and 55.6% (40 μM group) for TE14 cells.

Next, apoptosis-related proteins Bcl-2 (anti-apoptotic) and Bax (pro-apoptotic) were analyzed by western blot. Caspase-3, which is a member of the caspase family and is cleaved during apoptosis (28–30), was also analyzed by western blot. Treatment of KYSE150 and TE14 cells with HF significantly reduced the protein level of Bcl-2, while increasing the protein levels of Bax and c-Caspase 3 in a dose-dependent manner (**Figures 2C, D**). These results indicate that HF induced apoptosis of ESCC cells involves the mitochondrial pathway.

GO and KEGG Pathway Enrichment Analyses

GO enrichment analysis of HF was performed on the 355 putative targets of HF that were collected from the Pharma Mapper database to determine the relative significance with regards to biological processes, cell components, and molecular functions. The top 20 significantly enriched GO terms are listed in **Figures 3A–C** and **Table S1**. KEGG pathway enrichment analysis of HF was performed, and the top 20 targets are listed in **Figure 3D** and **Table S2**. The results show pathway enrichment for the GO and KEGG terms "negative regulation of apoptotic process," "pathways in cancer," and "PI3K-AKT signaling pathway," based on the Pharma Mapper database. Similarly, we obtained 100 putative targets of HF from the Swiss database. The GO enrichment analysis of the Swiss database is shown in **Figures S1A–C** and **Table S3**, and the KEGG pathway enrichment analysis is shown in **Figure S1D** and **Table S4**. Interestingly, the results analyzed according to the Swiss database were similar to those analyzed by the Pharma Mapper database. In summary, the analysis results of both databases indicate that HF might target the PI3K-AKT signaling pathway, leading to induction of apoptosis.

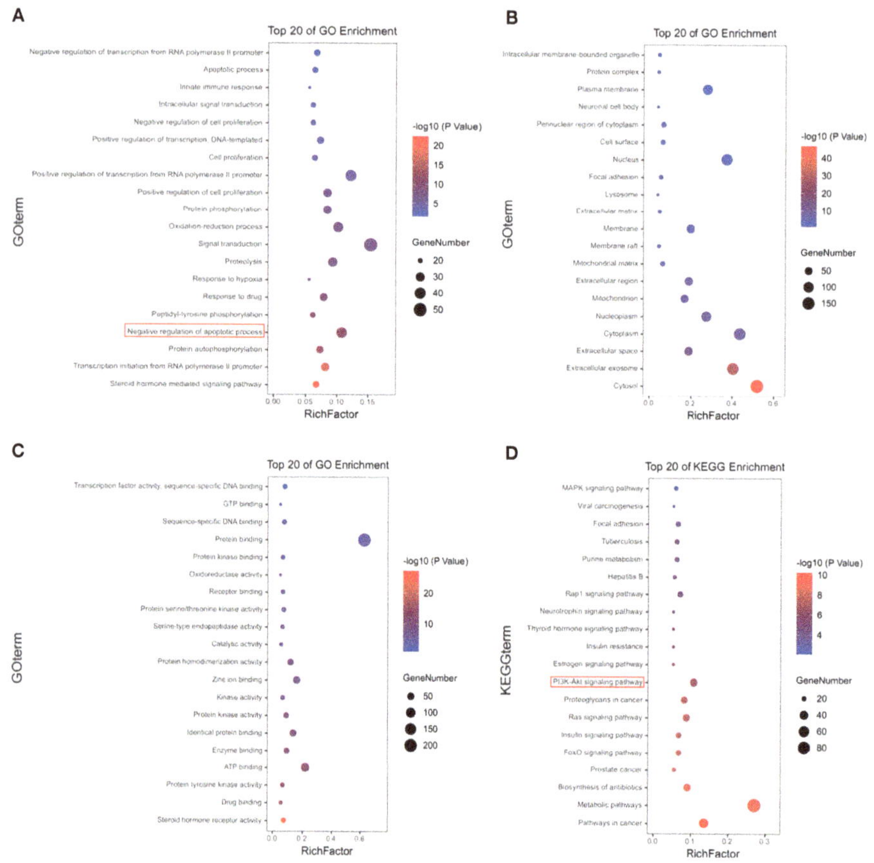

FIGURE 3 | Gene Ontology (GO) and Kyoto Encyclopedia of Genes and Genomes (KEGG) pathway analyses of HF. Top 20 signaling pathways of HF in **(A)** GO-BP pathway analysis, **(B)** GO-CC pathway analysis, and **(C)** GO-MF pathway analysis. **(D)** Top 20 signaling pathways of HF in KEGG enrichment pathway analysis.

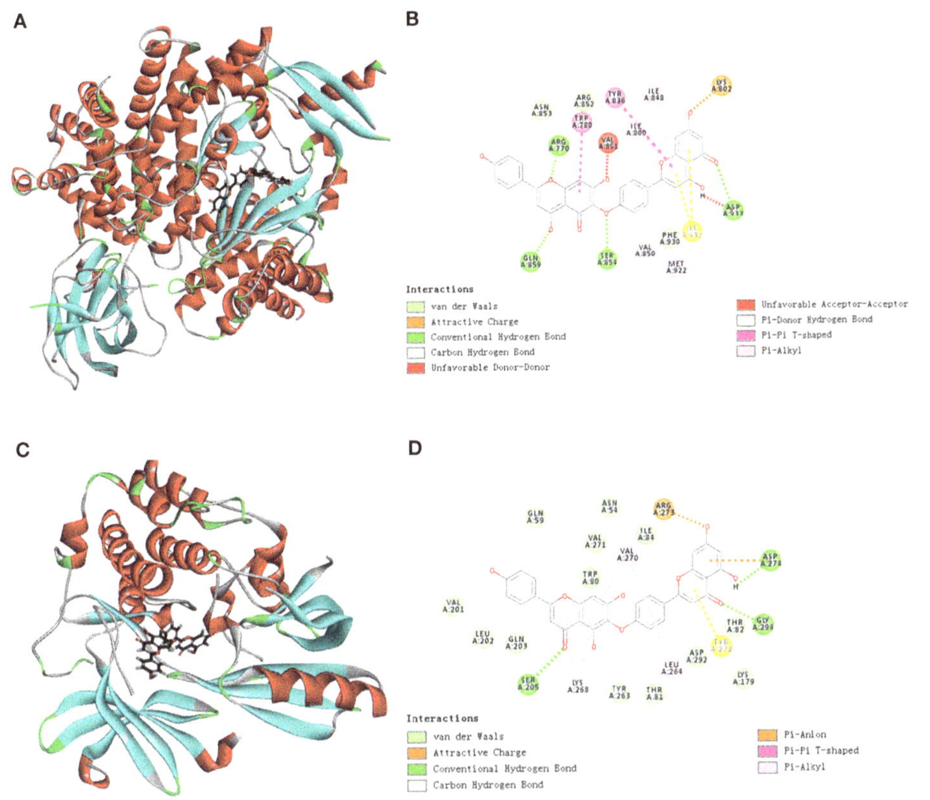

FIGURE 4 | Schematic representation of three- and two-dimensional molecular docking models. **(A)** Three-dimensional view of HF and PI3K docking scenario. **(B)** Two-dimensional view of HF and PI3K docking scenario. **(C)** Three-dimensional view of HF and AKT1 docking scenario. **(D)** Two-dimensional view of HF and AKT1 docking scenario.

HF Is Predicted to Have Direct Interaction With PI3K and AKT1

To predict the possible mutual binding mode of HF with PI3K and Akt, we further used molecular docking analysis. As shown in **Figure 4A**, HF was predicted to have a strong interaction with PI3K (LibDock score 115.982). The molecular docking of other conformations of HF with the protein PI3K is shown in **Figures S2A, B**. The binding affinity was attributed to the following: hydrogen bonding with the ARG-770, GLN-895, SER-854, and ASP-933 residues; the pi-pi T-shaped interaction with the TRP-780 and TYR-836 residues; the pi-alkyl interactions with the ILE-800, ILE-848, VAL-850, and MET-922 residues of PI3K (**Figure 4B**). Moreover, the analysis results show that HF could also interact strongly with protein AKT1 (LibDock score 143.752, **Figure 4C**). Molecular docking of other conformations of HF with AKT1 is shown in **Figures S2C, D**. The binding affinity was attributed to the following: hydrogen bonding with the SER-205, GLY-294, and ASP-274 residues; the pi-alkyl interactions with the LYS-268, VAL-270, and LEU-264 residues, and pi-anion interactions with the ARG-273 and ASP-274 residues of AKT1 (**Figure 4D**). Therefore, in common with the results of KEGG pathway enrichment analysis, HF showed high binding activity with PI3K and AKT in this study.

HF Inhibits the PI3K/AKT/mTOR Pathway in ESCC Cells

To verify the interaction of HF with PI3K/AKT, we analyzed HF-treated KYSE150 and TE14 cells *via* western blotting. Our results showed that the protein levels of p-PI3K, p-AKT, and p-mTOR in KYSE150 and TE14 cells were significantly reduced by HF treatment at 10, 20, and 40 μM, whereas total expression levels of PI3K, AKT, and mTOR were not significantly changed (**Figures 5A–C**). To verify whether HF induces apoptosis through the inhibition of PI3K/AKT/mTOR pathway, KYSE150 cells were treated with HF in the presence or absence of SC-79, a specific AKT activator (31). As shown in **Figures 5D, E**, SC-79 effectively enhanced the levels of phosphorylated proteins including p-AKT and p-mTOR. Meanwhile, pretreatment with SC-79 improved the inhibitory effect of HF on the protein expression of p-AKT, p-mTOR, and Bcl-2. Furthermore, the effect of HF to increase the expression amounts of apoptosis-related proteins (Bax and c-Caspase 3) could be reversed by pretreatment with SC-79 as well. We also found an increased viability of KYSE150 cells in the HF and SC-79 co-treatment group compared with HF alone treatment (**Figure 5F**), suggesting that activation of AKT attenuated the ability of HF to inhibit cell proliferation. These results indicate

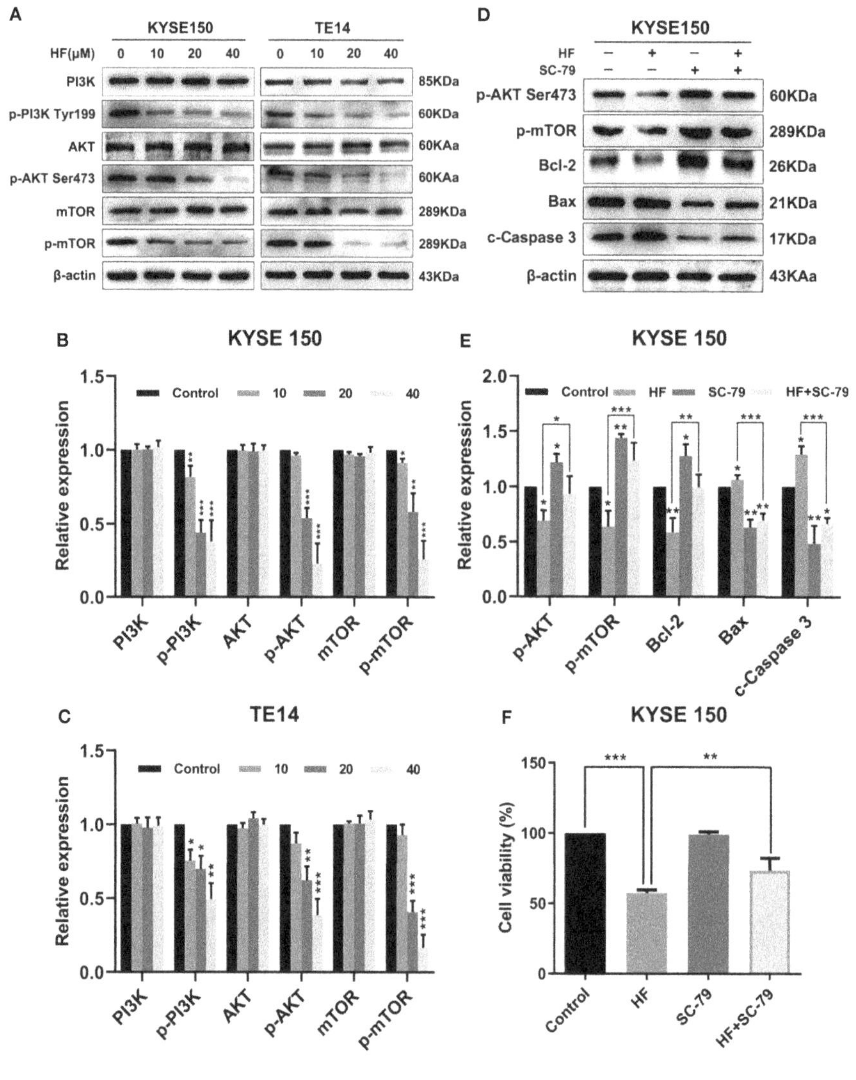

FIGURE 5 | HF induces apoptosis of ESCC cells by negatively regulating the PI3K/Akt/mTOR pathway. **(A–C)** KYSE150 and TE14 cells received various concentrations of HF intervention for 24 h, and the expression of pathway related proteins PI3K, p-PI3k, Akt, p-Akt, mTOR, and p-mTOR was detected by western blotting and quantified *via* densitometric analysis. **(D, E)** KYSE150 cells were pretreated with SC-79 (10 μM) for 24 h, and the expression of apoptosis related proteins Bcl-2, Bax and c-caspase 3 was determined by western blotting. **(F)** KYSE150 cells were first cultured with HF with or without addition of SC-79 (10 μM) for 24 h, and cell viability was detected using CCK-8 assays. The above experimental data are presented as the mean ± SD of three independent experiments. **P* < 0.05; ***P* < 0.01; ****P* < 0.001 compared to the control group.

that the anticancer effect of HF on ESCC involves regulation of PI3K/AKT/mTOR pathway.

HF Suppresses Migration and Invasion in ESCC Cells

Esophageal cancer patients with distant metastases have a very poor prognosis (32), and the migration and invasion abilities of tumor cells are vital factors affecting the process of tumor metastasis (33). Therefore, we evaluated whether HF could inhibit the migration and invasion of ESCC cells. As revealed by wound-healing assay (**Figure 6A**), the migratory ability of KYSE150 cells gradually became weaker with higher HF concentrations. Moreover, compared with the control group, HF treatment significantly inhibited the Transwell migration and invasion of ESCC cells in a dose-dependent manner (**Figure 6B**). Studies have shown that MMP family proteins play an important role in the regulation of cell migration and invasion abilities, and that MMPs are always upregulated in invasive epithelial cancers (34, 35). Therefore, we explored whether the protein levels of MMP2 and MMP9 are associated with alterations in ESCC cell migration and invasion following treatment with HF. As shown in **Figures 6C, D**, we found that HF significantly downregulated the expression of MMP2 and MMP9 in ESCC cells. Altogether, these results suggest that HF possesses an effective ability to inhibit ESCC cell migration and invasion.

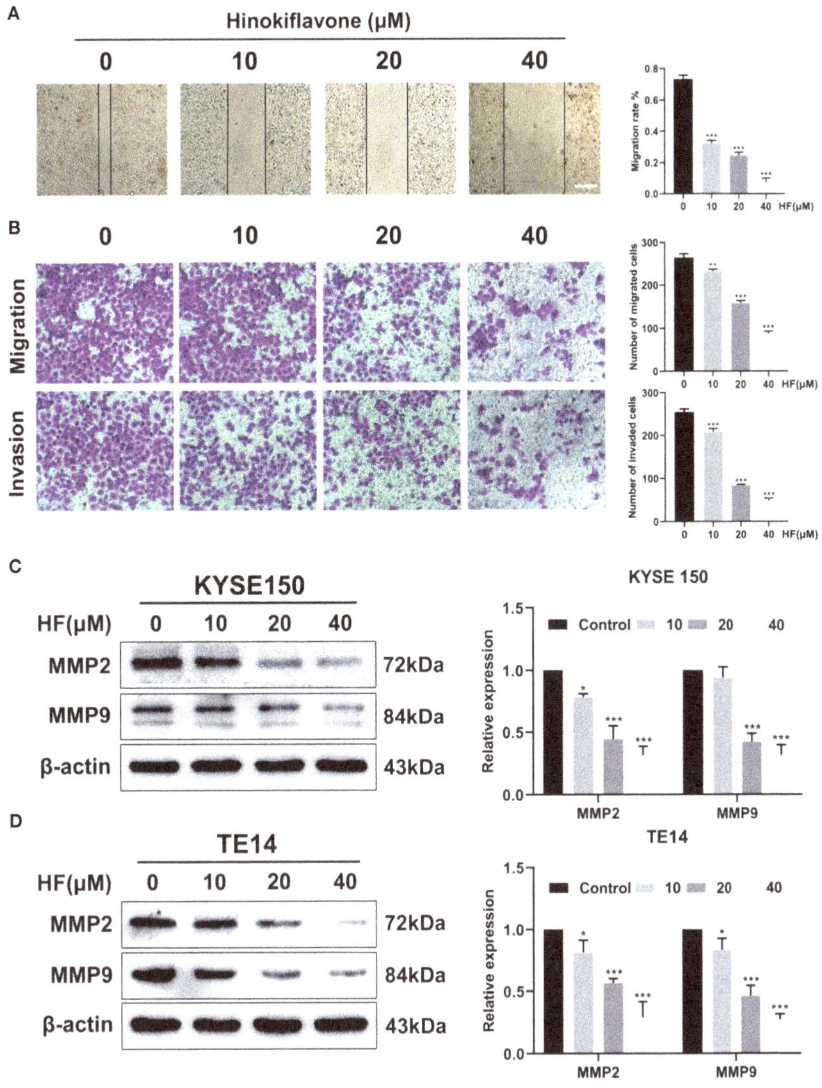

FIGURE 6 | HF inhibits ESCC cell migration and invasion. **(A)** Cell migration was measured in a scratch-wound assay. KYSE150 cells were cultured until reaching approximately 80-90% cell density, the culture was scratched as described in Methods, and further cultured with various concentrations of HF (0, 10, 20, and 40 μM) for 24 h, after which the cells were fixed and photographed. Magnification, ×100; scale bars = 100 μm. The distance of cell migration from the same region was quantified using ImageJ. **(B)** KYSE150 cells were placed in the top chamber on the Transwell membrane with serum-free medium and the upper surface of the Transwell membrane was coated with/without Matrigel. Cells were treated using HF with a concentration gradient for 24 h, and then the cells were fixed and photographed using a microscope after crystal violet staining. Magnification, ×100; scale bars = 100 μm. Migrated and invaded cells were counted as described in the Methods. **(C, D)** KYSE150 cells and TE14 cells were treated with various concentrations of HF for 24 h, and then the cells were collected for protein extraction. The extracted proteins were later used for western blot analysis to determine the protein expression levels of MMP2 and MMP9. All the above experimental data are presented as the mean ± SD of three independent experiments. $^{*}P < 0.05$; $^{***}P < 0.001$ compared to 0 μM vehicle group.

Antitumor Effect of HF in Mouse Xenograft Model of ESCC

To investigate whether the antitumor effect of HF *in vivo* is consistent with its *in vitro* effects, ESCC xenografts were established by subcutaneously transplantation of KYSE150 cells into BALB/c-nu mice, followed by treatment with HF (saline control, 25 mg/kg HF, 50 mg/kg HF) for 3 weeks, as described in the Methods (**Figure 7A**). Results from the animal experiments showed that transplanted tumors in the HF intervention groups grew much slower than those in the control group (**Figures 7B–D**). The mean size (or weight) of the tumors in HF 25 mg/kg, and HF 50 mg/kg group was reduced to 348.9 mm^3 (or 0.315 g) and 126.9 mm^3 (or 0.08 g), compared with 738.9 mm^3 (or 0.525 g) in the control group (**Figures 7B, D**). As a crucial indicator of health, the average body weights of the control and HF-treated mice were not significantly different at all time points (**Figure 7E**). Moreover, immunohistochemical analysis showed that HF suppressed the protein expression levels of p-AKT and p-mTOR, while upregulating those of Bax and c-Caspase 3 (**Figure 7F**). As shown in **Figure 7G**, the results of H&E staining experiments

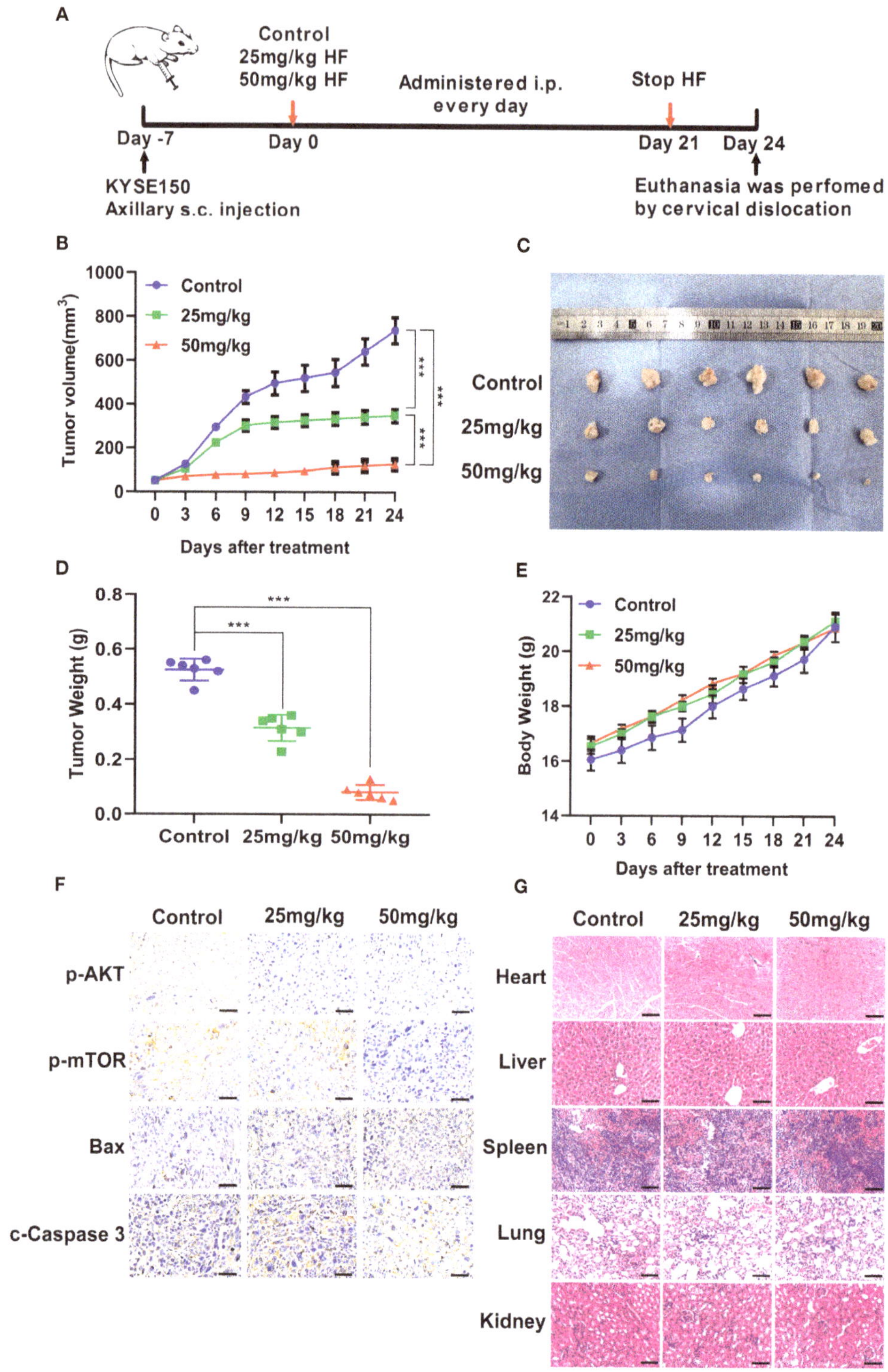

FIGURE 7 | HF suppresses the growth of mouse ESCC xenograft tumors. **(A)** BALB/c-nu mice implanted with KYSE150 xenograft tumors were treated daily with an equal volume of saline (control group) or HF (25 or 50 mg/kg) by intraperitoneal injection for total 21 days. **(B)** The tumor volume was measured every 3 days, and the difference in tumor volume between HF treated and control mice is shown. ***$P < 0.001$. **(C)** After euthanasia of mice, subcutaneous xenografts were removed and photographed. **(D)** The removed xenograft tumors were weighed and graphed for statistical analysis. ***$P < 0.001$ vs the control group. **(E)** Body weights of tumor-bearing mice were measured every 3 days in the HF-treated and control groups. **(F)** Expression levels of p-AKT, p-mTOR, Bax, and cleaved-Caspase 3 were detected by immunohistochemistry in the xenograft tumors. Magnification, ×400; scale bars = 50 μm. **(G)** H&E staining of the heart, liver, spleen, lung, and kidney of experimental mice shows no pathological changes in the organ tissues of any group. Magnification, ×200; scale bars = 100 μm.

on the heart, liver, spleen, lung, and kidney of mice exhibited no obvious pathological changes, such as necrosis, edema, or hemorrhage, indicating that HF possessed no major organ-related toxicity. Consistent with the experimental results *in vitro*, these data suggest that HF inhibits tumor growth by inducing apoptosis and does not have apparent adverse effects at the dose tested.

DISCUSSION

Despite progressive advances in the treatment of esophageal cancer, its mortality rate remains high worldwide. Currently, surgery and chemotherapy remain the main treatment modalities for esophageal cancer patients. However, since chemotherapeutics have their own disadvantages, such as drug resistance and systemic toxicity, more effective therapeutic strategies with fewer side-effects are urgently needed. Many studies have demonstrated the promising antitumor activity of some naturally active compounds (36). Our study is the first to indicate that HF inhibits the growth of ESCC cells. Furthermore, we comprehensively and profoundly explored the detailed molecular mechanisms underlying the antitumor effects of HF on ESCC *in vitro* and *in vivo* experiments.

In this study, the CCK-8 and colony formation assays demonstrated that HF had an effective anti-proliferative effect on KYSE150 and TE14 cells, which was validated by the EdU assay results. To investigate the anti-proliferation mechanism of HF in ESCC cells, we used Hoechst 33342 staining assay to identify apoptotic features of cell shrinkage, nuclear fragmentation, and condensed nuclei formation in HF-treated KYSE150 and TE14 cells. Flow cytometric analysis further illustrated induction of apoptosis in ESCC cells by HF in a concentration-dependent manner. Apoptosis is an orderly enzymatic cascade that induces DNA fragmentation into characteristic nucleosome fragments and culminates in cell death (30, 37, 38). Previous study has shown that apoptosis *via* the mitochondrial pathway is commonly regulated by Bcl-2 family proteins, with representative proteins such as the anti-apoptotic protein Bcl-2 and the pro-apoptotic protein Bax (39). In this context, our experimental results proved that HF intervention can cause a decreased expression of Bcl-2 protein and an increase in Bax and c-Caspase 3 expression, suggesting that HF induced apoptosis of ESCC cells occurs through the mitochondrial pathway.

We next used two databases, the Pharma Mapper and Swiss database, to screen the putative molecular targets of HF. The GO functional enrichment analysis showed that the predicted potential targets of HF were significantly enriched in "negative regulation of apoptotic process." Furthermore, KEGG pathway analysis revealed that HF might affect the PI3K-AKT signaling pathway. Our molecular docking analysis further indicated that HF can dock with PI3K and AKT1. Western blot analysis demonstrated a progressive decrease in p-PI3K, p-AKT, and p-mTOR protein levels with increasing concentrations of HF in KYSE150 and TE14 cells (**Figure 5A**). Interestingly, western blot analysis showed that the activation (phosphorylation) of PI3K, as indicated by levels of p-PI3K, was inhibited by HF, whereas expression of PI3K protein itself was not significantly altered. This suggested that HF can regulate post-translational modification of PI3K by physically interacting with the protein, as shown by the results of the GO enrichment, KEGG pathway, and molecular docking analyses. It is plausible that HF may directly attenuate the phosphorylation of PI3K at tyrosine 199, as reported in another study (40). The PI3K/Akt/mTOR pathway is a crucial signaling cascade in living organisms that has to be activated in a variety of cancers and to regulate cell proliferation, invasion, and migration (20, 41). We observed (**Figures 5D–F**) that SC-79 usage could activate the PI3K/AKT/mTOR pathway and partially counteract the pro-apoptotic and anti-proliferative effects of HF in ESCC cells. Overall, our results clearly show that the PI3K/AKT/mTOR pathway was inhibited by HF, which induced apoptosis in ESCC cells.

Metastasis is known to be a multistep biological process wherein subsets of cancer cells spread from the primary tumor to distant tissues or other organs to form metastases affects the body's normal physiological functions, which is the leading cause of cancer-related death (42). Moreover, for esophageal cancer patients, approximately 50% have already developed distant metastasis by the time of initial diagnosis (43, 44). Members of the MMP family of proteins, particularly MMP2 and MMP9, play a crucial role in cancer metastasis (34, 45, 46). The results of the migration and invasion assay we performed showed HF exhibited an obvious inhibitory effect on the metastatic potential of ESCC cells. We also found that HF significantly reduced MMP2 and MMP9 expression in KYSE150 and TE14 cells. These results suggest that HF can significantly hinder the metastasis of ESCC cells.

Finally, to verify the antitumor effect of HF *in vivo*, an esophageal cancer cell xenograft model was used in our study. Our experimental results showed that HF treatment significantly inhibited xenograft tumor growth in mice. In addition, the body weight of the experimental group mice receiving HF treatment was not significantly different from that of the control group mice. H&E staining also revealed no significant histopathological alterations in the heart, liver, lung, and kidney tissues of HF treated BALB/c-nu mice, indicating that HF did not induce significant systemic toxicity at the tested doses.

CONCLUSION

Data from our *in vitro*, in silico, and *in vivo* experiments showed that HF exerts antitumor effects against ESCC by inhibiting tumor growth and promoting apoptosis through the PI3K/AKT/mTOR signaling pathway. HF may also possibly inhibit metastasis by regulating MMPs. Overall, these findings reveal the underlying mechanisms by which HF inhibits the growth of human ESCC and provide new evidence supporting therapeutic potential of HF in ESCC.

AUTHOR CONTRIBUTIONS

JG, SZ, and LZ contributed to the conception and design of this research. JG and SZ performed the experiments. JG and SZ analyzed the results. JG, SZ, JW, PZ, TL, and LZ wrote the paper. All authors contributed to the article and approved the submitted version.

REFERENCES

Sung H, Ferlay J, Siegel RL, Laversanne M, Soerjomataram I, Jemal A, et al. Global Cancer Statistics 2020: GLOBOCAN Estimates of Incidence and Mortality Worldwide for 36 Cancers in 185 Countries. *CA Cancer J Clin* (2021) 71(3):209–49. doi: 10.3322/caac.21660

Bang YJ, Van Cutsem E, Feyereislova A, Chung HC, Shen L, Sawaki A, et al. Trastuzumab in Combination With Chemotherapy Versus Chemotherapy Alone for Treatment of HER2-Positive Advanced Gastric or Gastro-Oesophageal Junction Cancer (Toga): A Phase 3, Open-Label, Randomised Controlled Trial. *Lancet* (2010) 376(9742):687–97. doi: 10.1016/S0140-6736(10)61121-X

Yang H, Liu H, Chen Y, Zhu C, Fang W, Yu Z, et al. Neoadjuvant Chemor-Adiotherapy Followed by Surgery Versus Surgery Alone for Locally Advanced Squamous Cell Carcinoma of the Esophagus (NEOCRTEC5010): A Phase III Multi-Center, Randomized, Open-Label Clinical Trial. *J Clin Oncol* (2018) 36 (27):2796–803. doi: 10.1200/JCO.2018.79.1483

Newman DJ, Cragg GM. Natural Products as Sources of New Drugs Over the 30 Years From 1981 to 2010. *J Nat Prod* (2012) 75(3):311–35. doi: 10.1021/np200906s

Rane R, Karpoormath R. "Discovery and Development of New Anticancer Drugs Inspired From Natural Product Leads" Part 1. *Anticancer Agents Med Chem* (2015) 15(5):536. doi: 10.2174/187152061505150514130306

Rane R, Karpoormath R. "Discovery and Development of New Anticancer Drugs Inspired From Natural Product Leads" Part 2. *Anticancer Agents Med Chem* (2015) 15(8):932. doi: 10.2174/187152061508150817112012

Lin YM, Chen FC, Lee KH. Hinokiflavone, a Cytotoxic Principle From Rhus Succedanea and the Cytotoxicity of the Related Biflavonoids. *Planta Med* (1989) 55(2):166–8. doi: 10.1055/s-2006-961914

Lin YM, Anderson H, Flavin MT, Pai YH, Mata-Greenwood E, Pengsuparp T, et al. *In Vitro* Anti-HIV Activity of Biflavonoids Isolated From Rhus Succedanea and Garcinia Multiflora. *J Nat Prod* (1997) 60(9):884–8. doi: 10.1021/np9700275

Wang G, Yao S, Zhang XX, Song H. Rapid Screening and Structural Characterization of Antioxidants From the Extract of Selaginella Doederleinii Hieron With DPPH-UPLC-Q-TOF/MS Method. *Int J Anal Chem* (2015) 2015(undefined):849769. doi: 10.1155/2015/849769

Sui Y, Li S, Shi P, Wu Y, Li Y, Chen W, et al. Ethyl Acetate Extract From Selaginella Doederleinii Hieron Inhibits the Growth of Human Lung Cancer Cells A549 *via* Caspase-Dependent Apoptosis Pathway. *J Ethnopharmacol* (2016) 190(undefined):261–71. doi: 10.1016/j.jep.2016.06.029

Magne Nde CB, Zingue S, Winter E, Creczynski-Pasa TB, Michel T, Fernandez X, et al. Flavonoids, Breast Cancer Chemopreventive and/or Chemotherapeutic Agents. *Curr Med Chem* (2015) 22(30):3434–46. doi: 10.2174/0929867322666150729115321

Yang S, Zhang Y, Luo Y, Xu B, Yao Y, Deng Y, et al. Hinokiflavone Induces Apoptosis in Melanoma Cells Through the ROS-Mitochondrial Apoptotic Pathway and Impairs Cell Migration and Invasion. *BioMed Pharmacother* (2018) 103(undefined):101–10. doi: 10.1016/j.biopha.2018.02.076

Boss WF, Im YJ. Phosphoinositide Signaling. *Annu Rev Plant Biol* (2012) 63 (undefined):409–29. doi: 10.1146/annurev-arplant-042110-103840

Wymann MP, Schneiter R. Lipid Signalling in Disease. *Nat Rev Mol Cell Biol* (2008) 9(2):162–76. doi: 10.1038/nrm2335

Engelman JA, Luo J, Cantley LC. The Evolution of Phosphatidylinositol 3- Kinases as Regulators of Growth and Metabolism. *Nat Rev Genet* (2006) 7 (8):606–19. doi: 10.1038/nrg1879

Vanhaesebroeck B, Stephens L, Hawkins P. PI3K Signalling: The Path to Discovery and Understanding. *Nat Rev Mol Cell Biol* (2012) 13(3):195–203. doi: 10.1038/nrm3290

Vicinanza M, D'Angelo G, Di Campli A, De Matteis MA. Phosphoinositides as Regulators of Membrane Trafficking in Health and Disease. *Cell Mol Life Sci* (2008) 65(18):2833–41. doi: 10.1007/s00018-008-8353-2

Inoki K, Li Y, Zhu T, Wu J, Guan KL. TSC2 is Phosphorylated and Inhibited by Akt and Suppresses Mtor Signalling. *Nat Cell Biol* (2002) 4(9):648–57. doi: 10.1038/ncb839

Cross DA, Alessi DR, Cohen P, Andjelkovich M, Hemmings BA. Inhibition of Glycogen Synthase Kinase-3 by Insulin Mediated by Protein Kinase B. *Nature* (1995) 378(6559):785–9. doi: 10.1038/378785a0

Serra V, Markman B, Scaltriti M, Eichhorn PJ, Valero V, Guzman M, et al. NVP-BEZ235, a Dual PI3K/Mtor Inhibitor, Prevents PI3K Signaling and Inhibits the Growth of Cancer Cells With Activating PI3K Mutations. *Cancer Res* (2008) 68(19):8022–30. doi: 10.1158/0008-5472.CAN-08-1385

Roulin D, Waselle L, Dormond-Meuwly A, Dufour M, Demartines N, Dormond O. Targeting Renal Cell Carcinoma With NVP-BEZ235, a Dual PI3K/Mtor Inhibitor, in Combination With Sorafenib. *Mol Cancer* (2011) 10 (undefined):90. doi: 10.1186/1476-4598-10-90

Ko FC, Chan LK, Tung EK, Lowe SW, Ng IO, Yam JW. Akt Phosphorylation of Deleted in Liver Cancer 1 Abrogates Its Suppression of Liver Cancer Tumorigenesis and Metastasis. *Gastroenterology* (2010) 139(4):1397–407. doi: 10.1053/j.gastro.2010.06.051

Vivanco I, Sawyers CL. The Phosphatidylinositol 3-Kinase AKT Pathway in Human Cancer. *Nat Rev Cancer* (2002) 2(7):489–501. doi: 10.1038/nrc839

Li B, Tsao SW, Li YY, Wang X, Ling MT, Wong YC, et al. Id-1 Promotes Tumorigenicity and Metastasis of Human Esophageal Cancer Cells Through Activation of PI3K/AKT Signaling Pathway. *Int J Cancer* (2009) 125 (11):2576–85. doi: 10.1002/ijc.24675

Hong P, Liu QW, Xie Y, Zhang QH, Liao L, He QY, et al. Echinatin Suppresses Esophageal Cancer Tumor Growth and Invasion Through Inducing AKT/Mtor-Dependent Autophagy and Apoptosis. *Cell Death Dis* (2020) 11(7):524. doi: 10.1038/s41419-020-2730-7

Huang DW, Sherman BT, Lempicki RA. Systematic and Integrative Analysis of Large Gene Lists Using DAVID Bioinformatics Resources. *Nat Protoc* (2009) 4(1):44–57. doi: 10.1038/nprot.2008.211

Huang DW, Sherman BT, Lempicki RA. Bioinformatics Enrichment Tools: Paths Toward the Comprehensive Functional Analysis of Large Gene Lists. *Nucleic Acids Res* (2009) 37(1):1–13. doi: 10.1093/nar/gkn923

Pawlowski J, Kraft AS. Bax-Induced Apoptotic Cell Death. *Proc Natl Acad Sci USA* (2000) 97(2):529–31. doi: 10.1073/pnas.97.2.529

Kirsch DG, Doseff A, Chau BN, Lim DS, de Souza-Pinto NC, Hansford R, et al. Caspase-3-Dependent Cleavage of Bcl-2 Promotes Release of Cytochrome C. *J Biol Chem* (1999) 274(30):21155–61. doi: 10.1074/ jbc.274.30.21155

Dolka I, Krol M, Sapierzynski R. Evaluation of Apoptosis-Associated Protein (Bcl-2, Bax, Cleaved Caspase-3 and P53) Expression in Canine Mammary Tumors: An Immunohistochemical and Prognostic Study. *Res Vet Sci* (2016) 105:124–33. doi: 10.1016/j.rvsc.2016.02.004

Jo H, Mondal S, Tan D, Nagata E, Takizawa S, Sharma AK, et al. Small Molecule-Induced Cytosolic Activation of Protein Kinase Akt Rescues Ischemia-Elicited Neuronal Death. *Proc Natl Acad Sci USA* (2012) 109 (26):10581–6. doi: 10.1073/pnas.1202810109

Tanaka T, Fujita H, Matono S, Nagano T, Nishimura K, Murata K, et al. Outcomes of Multimodalitytherapy for Stage IVB Esophageal Cancer With Distant Organ Metastasis (M1-Org). *Dis Esophagus* (2010) 23(8):646–51. doi: 10.1111/j.1442-2050.2010.01069.x

Friedl P, Wolf K. Tumour-Cell Invasion and Migration: Diversity and Escape Mechanisms. *Nat Rev Cancer* (2003) 3(5):362–74. doi: 10.1038/nrc1075

Chang C, Werb Z. The Many Faces of Metalloproteases: Cell Growth, Invasion, Angiogenesis and Metastasis. *Trends Cell Biol* (2001) 11(11):37– 43. doi: 10.1016/s0962-8924(01)02122-5

Huang W, Dong Z, Wang F, Peng H, Liu JY, Zhang JT. A Small Molecule Compound Targeting STAT3 DNA-Binding Domain Inhibits Cancer Cell Proliferation, Migration, and Invasion. *ACS Chem Biol* (2014) 9(5):1188–96. doi: 10.1021/cb500071v

Atanasov AG, Waltenberger B, Pferschy-Wenzig EM, Linder T, Wawrosch C, Uhrin P, et al. Discovery and Resupply of Pharmacologically Active Plant-Derived Natural Products: A Review. *Biotechnol Adv* (2015) 33(8):1582–614. doi: 10.1016/j.biotechadv.2015.08.001

Ou L, Lin S, Song B, Liu J, Lai R, Shao L. The Mechanisms of Graphene-Based Materials-Induced Programmed Cell Death: A Review of Apoptosis, Autophagy, and Programmed Necrosis. *Int J Nanomed* (2017) 12 (undefined):6633–46. doi: 10.2147/IJN.S140526

Elmore S. Apoptosis: A Review of Programmed Cell Death. *Toxicol Pathol* (2007)

35(4):495–516. doi: 10.1080/01926230701320337

Cory S, Adams JM. The Bcl 2 Family: Regulators of the Cellular Life-or-Death Switch. *Nat Rev Cancer* (2002) 2(9):647–56. doi: 10.1038/nrc883

Katase N, Nishimatsu SI, Yamauchi A, Yamamura M, Fujita S. DKK3 Knockdown Confers Negative Effects on the Malignant Potency of Head and Neck Squamous Cell Carcinoma Cells *via* the PI3K/Akt and MAPK Signaling Pathways. *Int J Oncol* (2019) 54(3):1021–32. doi: 10.3892/ijo.2018.4667

Mi Y, Xiao C, Du Q, Wu W, Qi G, Liu X. Momordin Ic Couples Apoptosis With Autophagy in Human Hepatoblastoma Cancer Cells by Reactive Oxygen Species (ROS)-Mediated PI3K/Akt and MAPK Signaling Pathways. *Free Radic Biol Med* (2016) 90(undefined):230–42. doi: 10.1016/j.freeradbiomed.2015.11.022

Chen YQ. Cancer and Metastasis Reviews. Introduction. *Cancer Metastasis Rev* (2013) 32(null):3–4. doi: 10.1007/s10555-012-9411-7

Enzinger PC, Mayer RJ. Esophageal Cancer. *N Engl J Med* (2003) 349 (23):2241–52. doi: 10.1056/NEJMra035010

Horner MJ, Ries LAG, Krapcho M, Aminou R, Howlader N, Altekruse SF, et al. *Seer Cancer Statistics Review, 1975–2006*. Bethesda, MD: National Cancer Institute (2009). Available at: http://seer.cancer.gov/csr/ 1975_2006/.

Liu F, Cao J, Wu J, Sullivan K, Shen J, Ryu B, et al. Stat3-Targeted Therapies Overcome the Acquired Resistance to Vemurafenib in Melanomas. *J Invest Dermatol* (2013) 133(8):2041–9. doi: 10.1038/jid.2013.32

Xia Y, Lei Q, Zhu Y, Ye T, Wang N, Li G, et al. SKLB316, a Novel Small- Molecule Inhibitor of Cell-Cycle Progression, Induces G2/M Phase Arrest and Apoptosis *In Vitro* and Inhibits Tumor Growth *In Vivo*. *Cancer Lett* (2014) 355(2):297–309. doi: 10.1016/j.canlet.2014.09.042

9

VRK1 Predicts Poor Prognosis and Promotes Bladder Cancer Growth and Metastasis In Vitro and In Vivo

Jiacheng Wu[1†], Tao Li[2†], Hao Ji[1], Zhi Chen[3] and Baoqian Zhai[4*]*

[1]Department of Urology, The Affiliated Tumor Hospital of Nantong University, Nantong, China, [2]Department of Medical Oncology, The Affiliated Tumor Hospital of Nantong University, Nantong, China, [3]Department of Pathology, The First People's Hospital of Longquanyi District, Chengdu, China, [4]Department of Oncology Radiotherapy, Yancheng No. 1 People's Hospital, Yancheng, China

***Correspondence:**
Baoqian Zhai
baoqzhai2018@163.com
Zhi Chen
459509409@163.com

[†]These authors have contributed equally to this work

Bladder cancer (BC) is one of the most common malignant tumors in the urinary system with growing morbidity and diagnostic rate in recent years. Therefore, identifying new molecular biomarkers that inhibit the progression of bladder cancer is needed for developing further therapeutics. This study found a new potential treatment target: vaccinia-related kinase 1 (VRK1) and explored the function and mechanism of VRK1 in the development of bladder cancer. First, TCGA database and tissue microarray analysis showed that VRK1 was significantly upregulated in bladder cancer. Kaplan–Meier survival analysis indicates that the OS and PFS of the VRK1 high expression group were significantly lower than the VRK1 low expression group ($p = 0.002$, $p = 0.005$). Cox multi-factor analysis results show that VRK1 expression is an independent risk factor affecting tumor progress. The maximum tumor diameter, staging, and adjuvant chemotherapy also have a certain impact on tumor progression ($p < 0.05$). In internal validation, the column C index is 0.841 (95% CI, 0.803–0.880). In addition, cell functional studies have shown that VRK1 can significantly inhibit the proliferation, migration, and invasiveness of bladder cancer cells. *In vivo*, nude mice transplanted tumors further prove that low VRK1 can significantly inhibit the proliferation capacity of bladder cancer cells. In summary, VRK1 expression is significantly related to the staging, grade, and poor prognosis of patients with bladder cancer. At the same time, *in vivo* and *in vitro* experiments have shown that downregulation of VRK1 can significantly inhibit the proliferation of bladder cancer cells. These findings provide a basis for using VRK1 as a potential therapeutic target for patients with bladder cancer.

Keywords: VRK1, bladder cancer, growth and metastasis, nomogram, TCGA (the cancer genome atlas program), GEO, GSEA

INTRODUCTION

Bladder cancer (BC) is one of the most common malignant tumors in the urinary system, and is the 11th most common cancer in the world (Torre et al., 20122015). More than 430,000 patients have been diagnosed with bladder cancer (Rajwa et al., 2018) every year, and about 165,000 people will die. Although considerable progress has been made in surgical techniques, its 5-year survival rate remains at a relatively low level (Li et al., 2017; Peng et al., 2017). Postoperative tumor recurrence and progress are the major clinical events affecting the prognosis of these patients (Wang et al., 2019). Recent research studies show that relative parameters such as postoperative pathological staging of the tumor can predict the survival and prognosis of bladder cancer patients, but the effectiveness is not reliable. Thus, new prognosis indicators and possible targets for bladder cancer are crucial.

VRK1 is a member of the vaccinia-related kinase (VRK) family of serine/threonine protein kinases. It is a Ser–Thr kinase with atypical activity (Campillo-Marcos et al., 2021), and a nucleosome kinase or chromatin kinase (Kang et al., 2007). It can interact directly and stably with different chromatin proteins, and is related to cell cycle entry, apoptosis, and autophagy control (Kim et al., 2012). It regulates a variety of transcription factors, including ATF2 (Sevilla et al., 2004), p53 (Lopez-Borges and Lazo, 2000), and c-Jun (Liu et al., 2017). All of them are highly involved in tumorigenesis. Studies have indicated that VRK1 is highly expressed in many human tumors and affects the prognosis of patients. For example, VRK1 increases the number of G1-arrested cells by reducing cyclin D1 and p-Rb while upregulating p21 and p27. Its consumption downregulates the phosphorylation of CREB to participate in the tumorigenesis and development of liver cancer (Huang et al., 2016). VRK1 relates to poor prognosis of glioma by participating in the PI3K/AKT pathway (Ben et al., 2018); studies have also shown that ginsenoside Rg3 affects DNA damage and causes VRK1 upregulation and P53BP1 foci formation, thereby inhibiting lung cancer cell viability (Liu et al., 2019). VRK1 overexpression can promote breast cancer cell mesenchymal transition (MET) by regulating the transcriptional repressor snail, slug, and twist (Mon et al., 2018). At the same time, there are related research reports on rectal adenocarcinoma (Del Puerto-Nevado et al., 2016) and other tumors. However, there is no relevant research on VRK1 and bladder cancer. Therefore, the purpose of this study is to evaluate the role of VRK1 in the prognosis of bladder cancer. In addition, our research hopes to further explore the specific biological functions of VRK1 in bladder cancer through *in vivo* and *in vitro* experiments.

MATERIALS AND METHODS

Classification of Differentially Expressed Genes in TCGA and GEO Database

We used the GEO query package to download two RNA expression data sets GSE13507 and GSE65635 (containing tumor tissue and normal tissue) from the GEO database (https://www.ncbi.nlm.nih.gov/geo/query/acc.cgi). GEO online GEO2R tool was used to analyze the differential genes. The parameters for screening DEG are selected if the log2FC is greater than 0 and p value is less than 0.02. The data set of differentially expressed genes of bladder cancer is downloaded from the TCGA database (https://tcga-data.nci.nih.gov/), and the parameters for screening DEG are determined if the log2FC is greater than 0 and p value is less than 0.0001 (Diboun et al., 2006; Davis and Meltzer, 2007; Gu et al., 2016). Finally, the intersection of the three data sets is showed in a Venn diagram to obtain the common upregulated differentially expressed genes.

Data Analysis Using the TCGA Database

In order to study the expression of VRK1 in bladder cancer, we used the TCGA database (https://tcga-data.nci.nih.gov/) for analysis. Among them, 414 cases of cancer tissues and 19 paracancerous tissues were included in the study. R 3.6.3 software is used to collect and analyze the data. The expression of VRK1 gene in bladder cancer tissue and paracancerous tissue was compared according to the standard calculation method as described previously.

Gene Enrichment of VRK1

We used gene enrichment methods to further explore the possible signaling pathways VRK1 may participate in the poor prognosis of bladder cancer. GSEA analysis is mainly performed using GSEA software version 2.2.2.0 (Mootha et al., 2003), which uses a predefined gene set from the molecular signature database (MSigDB v5.0) (Subramanian et al., 2005). A gene set is a group of genes that share pathways, functions, chromosomal locations, or other characteristics. In this study, we used all the C sets for GSEA analysis (i.e., C1–C7 sets in MsigDB), and listed the ranking genes based on the score of -log10 of the p value multiplied by the fraction of multiple change of the expression. The gene sets collected according to the minimum and maximum selection criteria were 10 and 500 genes, respectively.

Clinical Data Selection

The clinical data of 101 patients with bladder cancer who underwent surgical resection in the Department of Urology, Nantong Cancer Hospital from May 2013 to May 2015 were selected. Among them, 30 cases of bladder cancer were accompanied by corresponding paracancerous tissues. The inclusion criteria were: ① all patients who were diagnosed with bladder cancer for the first time and only had bladder cancer as tumor diagnosis and surgery; ② clinical staging was stage I–III; ③ postoperative pathology was confirmed to be bladder cancer (urothelial carcinoma); ④ have complete clinical data and follow-up data; ⑤ have no other antitumor therapy before admission (neoadjuvant chemoradiation or other antitumor therapies); and ⑥ good patient compliance. The exclusion criteria were: ① received radiotherapy, chemotherapy, hormone therapy, etc., before surgery; ② combined with other serious diseases, such as severe hypertension; ③ combined with certain acute-stage diseases, such as infection; and ④ refused to follow-up. The age range of the patients included in this study was 34–81 years old, with an average age of (63.0 ± 9.5) years. There are 82 males and 19 females. All samples were collected under the written informed consent of the participants, and the experiment was approved by the Ethics Committee of Nantong Cancer Hospital. Follow-up is carried out by outpatient review or telephone follow-up. The outpatient follow-up was conducted every 3 months in the first year after surgery, every 6 months in the second year, and once a year after 2 years until May 2020. Follow-up examination: cystoscopy, abdominal MRI, CT or color Doppler ultrasound, tumor markers, urinalysis, etc., (additional examinations might be added depending on the patient's condition). Observation indicators: OS is defined as the time from the diagnosis of the disease to death from any cause or the cut-off time of follow-up. PFS is defined as the time from the beginning of treatment to any follow-up examination that indicates disease progression. At the end of the follow-up, if the subject was still alive but lost to the follow-up, the data from the final cut-off time will be used for statistical analysis.

Cell Source

The five bladder cancer cell lines (J82, SW780, T24, 5637, and UM-UC-3) and a normal human bladder normal epithelial cell (SV-HUC-1) used in this study were mainly purchased from Chinese Academy of Sciences Cell bank, Shanghai.

Tissue Microarray Construction, Immunohistochemistry, and Its Correlation With Survival Prognosis and Clinical Data Parameters

The tissue microarray was constructed by the Department of Pathology, Nantong Cancer Hospital. Hematoxylin–eosin was used to stain the paraffin embedded tissue blocks of 101 cases of bladder cancer. The most typical features were selected and marked at fixed points under the microscope. Each dot array contains less than 160 dots. A 3-micron-thick section was cut from the paraffin embedded tissue block and transferred to a glass slide using tape transfer system for UV cross-linking. IHC staining was performed according to the previously described protocol (Laurberg et al., 2014). Anti-VRK1 antibody [5D1]-N-terminal mouse monoclonal antibody (1:500, abcam ab171933) was used. The tissue sections were examined through two experienced pathologists under double-blind condition. The immunohistochemistry results were scored considering two factors: the proportion of positive cells and the intensity of cell staining. We found that VRK1 is mainly located in the nucleus. The score according to the proportion of positive staining cells: 0 (negative), 1 (< 25%), 2 (25–50%), 3 (51–75%), and 4 (>75%), and staining intensity: 0 (negative or no staining), 1 (weak positive), 2 (central type), and 3 (strong positive). The value obtained by multiplying these two scores is the final score corresponding to each specimen. After calculating the arithmetic mean of these scores, the specimen with a score lower than 6 is finally defined as a low expression of VRK1. According to the expression of VRK1 under immunohistochemistry, the 101 bladder cancer patients included in the study were divided into two groups: high and low expression of VRK1. SPSS software was used to compare the correlation between the expression of VRK1 in these two groups and the survival prognosis and clinical parameters of the patients. Meanwhile, the independent prognostic factors that are meaningful for the prognosis of bladder cancer patients were further screened through uni- and multi-variate analysis.

Reverse Transcription Quantitative PCR Method to Detect the mRNA Encoding VRK1

Take 100 mg sample of both the tumor tissue and paracancerous tissue of the patients included in the study and mill these samples into powder by the liquid nitrogen grinding method. Add 1 ml Trizol lysis solution, and extract the total RNA according to the instructions. The primers are: 5′-CTTCAGAGTCAGTTGGCA GTG-3′, 5′-CTTCAGCTTACGGGTACGAAT-3′; GAPDH is 5′-CAT GGG TGT GAA CCA TGA GAA GTA-3′. Use the reverse transcription kit to reverse transcribe RNA to obtain cDNA. Perform real-time fluorescent quantitative PCR on a fluorescent quantitative PCR machine. Calculate the relative expression of the target molecule's mRNA by the $2^{-\triangle\triangle ct}$ method. Therefore, we obtained the expression of VRK1 in cancer and paracancerous tissue.

In vitro Cytology Experiment Verification

CCK8-Detection Cell Activity

1) Screen five bladder cancer cell lines (J82, SW780, T24, 5637, and UM-UC-3) with high VRK1 expression. Construct VRK1 knockdown bladder cancer cell lines by using small interfering RNA knockdown techniques. Digest the T24 and 5637 cells transfected with these siRNA and the negative control cells separately. Centrifuge at low speed, then resuspend the target cells using complete medium.
2) Use a cell counter to adjust all sample cells to the same number (about 4^*10^3 cells in each well in a 96-well plate). Add 100 uL of culture medium per well.
3) Set up three replicate wells for each experimental group. Set complete medium as the blank control group at the same time. Shake well and then observe the cell distribution under the microscope to ensure that the cells are evenly distributed without accumulation or overlap. Transfer to 37°C, 5% CO_2 cell incubator for overnight culture.
4) After overnight incubation, add CCK-8 reagent to each well, usually 10 ul, and then move it again into a 37°C, 5% CO_2 cell incubator for incubation for 2 h.
5) Determine the absorbance value at 450 nm according to the instruction manual of the microplate reader. Record the OD value, and draw the proliferation curve according to the data.

Cloning Formation Assay

1) Prepare a suspension of the target cells. Adjust the cell density of the stock solution by cell counter. Dilute slowly till the cell density decreased to about 300 cells in each well of the 6-well plate. Cultivate for about 14 days without replacing complete medium.
2) After the incubation, absorb the original medium as much as possible. Add paraformaldehyde (4%) to fix the cells for about 20 min.
3) Rinse with pre-cooled PBS (1x) 2–3 times. After the last PBS buffer rinsing, add crystal violet staining solution (0.1%) for about 30 min to stain the cell.
4) Use pre-cooled PBS (1x) to wash 2–3 times to wash off the excess crystal violet staining solution as much as possible and calculate the number of clone groups.

Transwell Migration Experiment

1) Digest the selected target cells, centrifuge, and then resuspend the target cells with PBS (1x) to wash. Centrifuge and then remove the upper layer of the liquid. Resuspend the cells with serum-free medium.

2) Take the serum-free minimal medium cell stock solution for cell count. Adjust the cell density with serum-free minimal medium to reach the target cell number, about $3*10^5$.
3) Put 500 ml of complete culture (containing 10% fetal bovine serum) in the lower chamber of the sterile 24-well plate. Put the small chamber into the corresponding 24-well plate.
4) Add the cell suspension stock solution to the upper chamber of the 24-well plate; the volume is about 200 ul. Shake slightly. Incubate in cell incubator for 24 h.
5) After incubation, add about 600 ml 4% paraformaldehyde dropwise to the blank wells. Rinse the small chamber with PBS and put it back in for fixation for 20 min.
6) Generally, use PBS to rinse slowly after the fixation. After letting it air dry for a proper amount of time, stain with crystal violet staining solution (0.1%) for 30 min.
7) Gently take out the small chamber and wash it with PBS 2–3 times. Then, use a cotton swab to clean the cells that have not migrated in the upper small chamber. After drying, observe and take pictures with a microscope.

Transwell Invasion Experiment

Transwell Chamber Preparation

i) Matrigel-Free Transwell Cell Preparation

① Coating basement membrane: Coat the upper chamber surface of the bottom membrane of the Transwell chamber with 50 mg/L Matrigel 1:8 dilution. Air-dry at 4°C.

Preparation of Cell Suspension

① Before preparing the cell suspension, the cells can be de-serum-starved for 12–24 h to further remove the influence of the serum, but this step is not necessary.

② Digest the cells: centrifuge and discard the culture medium after terminating the digestion. Wash 1–2 times with PBS, and resuspend in serum-free medium containing BSA. Adjust the cell density to $1–10 \times 10^5$.

Inoculation of the Cells

① Take 200 μl of cell suspension into the Transwell chamber.

② Generally, 500 μl of medium containing FBS is added to the lower chamber of the 24-well plate. Please refer to the instructions for details. Special attention should be paid to the fact that there are often bubbles between the lower culture medium and the chamber. Once bubbles are generated, the chemotaxis of the lower culture medium is weakened or even disappeared. Pay special attention when planting plates. Lift the chamber to remove air bubbles, and then put the chamber into the culture plate.

③ Cultivate cells: conventionally culture for 12–48 h (mainly depending on the invasiveness of the cancer cells). In addition to the invasiveness of cells, when selecting the incubation time, the influence of each process on the number of cells cannot be ignored.

"Adherent" Cell Count

① By staining the cells, the cells can be counted under the microscope.

② Wipe off the Matrigel and the cells in the upper chamber with a cotton swab.

③ Dyeing: The commonly used dyeing methods include crystal violet dyeing.

Western Blot Detection

1) Electrophoresis process: Choose a constant voltage of 80 V for the upper layer of compression gel. After the protein sample runs to the lower layer of the separation gel and the protein marker layer can be observed with the naked eye, change the voltage to 120–150 V. End the electrophoresis when the sample runs to a distance of about 0.5 cm from the bottom edge of the separation gel.
2) Transfer: Pour the 1x transfer membrane solution prepared 1 day in advance from the refrigerator into the iron pan used in the operation. Immerse the required PVDF membrane in methanol to activate (about 15–30 s) in advance, and then transfer the PVDF membrane so that it is completely immersed in ddH_2O for depolarization. Place the PVDF membrane in the pre-cooled transfer buffer. Soak the black sponge pad and filter paper larger than the size of the PVDF membrane into the transfer fluid (1x) in advance. Gently lift one end of the short glass plate to leave the gel, and then cut out the upper layer glue and the excess part of the lower layer glue and move the gel to the black side of the transfer membrane clamp. The black side of the transfer membrane is the bottom and the white side is the top. It is placed layer by layer in the order of sponge pad, two layers of filter paper, gel, PVDF membrane, two layers of filter paper, sponge pad, etc., from bottom to top. Slowly clamp the transfer membrane and immerse into the electrophoresis tank containing the transfer buffer. It must be ensured that a suitable ice box has been placed outside the transfer tank. Add the transfer buffer to the silver wire on the upper edge of the transfer membrane clamp. Tighten the lid and put it in an ice–water mixed bath and turn on the power. Generally, the transfer uses a constant current of 300 mA for 90 min.
3) Blocking: After transfer time, immerse the PVDF membrane faceup in the pre-prepared skimmed milk blocking solution (5%), and place it in a room temperature slow-speed shaker for about 2 h.
4) Incubate the primary antibody: Prepare the wet box and the incubation tank. Dilute with the special primary antibody diluent according to the instructions of the primary antibody. Put it into the corresponding incubation tank. Wash the completely blocked PVDF membrane using TBST (1x) 2–3 times. Use filter paper to remove excess liquid. Completely soak the membrane containing the target protein facedown in the primary antibody incubation solution. Put it in the refrigerator at 4° overnight.
5) Wash the membrane: Take out the wet box from the refrigerator and let it stand for 20–30 min at room temperature. Recover the primary antibody and note the relevant information of the antibody. Put the membrane faceup in TBST (1x) to wash 3–4 times with gentle but quick shaking for cleaning. Each cleaning period should last for about 4–5 min.

6) Incubate the secondary antibody: Following the instructions of the secondary antibody, use TBST (1x) to dilute the corresponding secondary antibody to the corresponding concentration. Use filter paper to absorb the excess solution on the membrane. Turn the membrane containing the target protein facedown to ensure that it is completely immersed in the secondary antibody. Normally, it should be incubated at room temperature for about 2 h.
7) Wash the membrane again: After secondary antibody incubation, place the membrane containing the target protein faceup. Wash it in TBST (1x) 3–4 times, with gentle but quick shaking for cleaning. Each cleaning period should last for about 20 min. Soak the membrane in the last cleaning solution to prepare for Chemiluminescent.
8) Chemiluminescent: Fully mix ECL developer A and B at equal volume. Add sufficient amount of mixed liquid on the front of the membrane. Perform the chemiluminesent according to the instructions of the instrument and save the picture.

In Vivo Nude Mice Experimental

For animal experiments, male NOD-SCID nude mice, 6–7 weeks old (weight 18–20 g), were purchased from the Animal Center of the Chinese Academy of Sciences. All mice are raised in the SPF animal room of the Key Laboratory of the Ministry of Health in accordance with the NIH animal experiment guidelines in the United States. In this project, we used a total of eight animals, with four animals in each group. 1) T24 bladder tumor cell lines (shVRK1-NC and shVRK1-2) at exponential growth phase were selected. Cell line was digested using Trypsin and neutralized with complete medium. Transfer it to a 50 ml sterile centrifuge tube with a pipette, centrifuge at 1000 rpm for 5 min, and then discard the supernatant. Mix the cells thoroughly with appropriate complete medium and count the cells. 2) Dilute the cells to 5×10^7/ml, according to the calculated cell concentration. 3) Randomly divide the mice into an experimental group and a control group: each nude mouse is subcutaneously injected into the lower abdominal wall under the axillary region with 100 μL of 5 × 106 cells per mice with a syringe. 4) After 1 week of subcutaneous injection, measure the tumor on the abdominal wall of nude mice every 2–3 days to calculate the volume of the tumor (cm3) = width (cm) x width (cm) x length (cm)/2; 5). After 6 weeks, the nude mice of the experimental group and the control group were sacrificed using cervical dislocation. The tumors formed under the skin were collected, the size and weight were measured, and the relationship between the growth of tumor tissue and the proliferation ability of bladder cancer cells in the body were analyzed, followed by the follow-up immunohistochemistry experiment.

Statistical Analysis

Use software R (version 3.6.3) for statistical analysis and visualization; R package: DESeq2 (version 1.26.0) (Love MI et al., 2014) for data download; limma package (version 3.42.2) for difference analysis. Use the ggplot2 package (version 3.3.3) for image visualization. Through gene set enrichment analysis (GSEA), use R package: mainly clusterProfiler package (3.14.3 version) (for GSEA analysis) to explore the possible cellular mechanism of VRK1. Use SPSS version 22.0 (IBM) software for statistical analysis. The chi-square test was used to compare and analyze the clinicopathological conditions of the two groups of patients. The Kaplan–Meier method was used to evaluate the survival of patients, and the log rank statistical method was used for significance testing. The Cox proportional hazard regression model is used to clarify the independent prognostic factors that are meaningful for the prognosis of bladder cancer patients. On this basis, the R language is used to draw a nomogram to construct a predictive model: nomogram drawing is composed of survival and rms software packages in R. The main steps for creating a nomogram model are as follows: 1) Select a research model: According to the research data and corresponding results, different models can be selected for the nomogram. This study is the survival analysis of 101 patients with bladder cancer undergoing surgical resection, so COX risk ratio model is ideal. 2) Selection of predictors: The COX risk ratio model can be used to obtain the independent risk factors and risk ratios (HR) of 101 bladder cancer patients undergoing surgical resection. R gives the impact score of each risk factor according to the degree of contribution of different risk factors to the result, and finally obtains the corresponding survival rate of the individual patient based on the total score. The difference was statistically significant with $p < 0.05$.

RESULTS

Selection of Differentially Expressed Genes, Their Expression in the TCGA Database, and Using GSEA, GO, and KEGG for Gene Enrichment Analysis

We used the GEO query package to download two RNA expression data sets GSE13507 and GSE65635 (containing tumor tissue and normal tissue) from the GEO database (https://www.ncbi.nlm.nih.gov/geo/query/acc.cgi). We used the GEO online GEO2R tool to analyze the differential genes. The parameters for screening DEG were selected if the log2FC is greater than 0 and *p* value is less than 0.02. Then, the data set of differentially expressed genes for bladder cancer from the TCGA database was downloaded (https://tcga-data.nci.nih.gov/). The parameters for screening DEG were selected if the log2FC is greater than 0 and *p* value is less than 0.0001 (**Figure 1A**). The differentially expressed gene is screened and confirmed to be VRK1. In order to confirm the expression level of VRK1 in bladder cancer tissues, we used the TCGA database (https://tcga-data.nci.nih.gov/) to search and analyze the mRNA expression level of VRK1. Meanwhile, we found that compared with the paracancerous tissues in the TCGA database, the mRNA expression of VRK1 in tumor tissues is upregulated (**Figures 1B,C**).

In order to further explore the possible role of the differentially expressed genes screened in bladder cancer, we first predicted the possible related molecular mechanisms through GSEA. We found that VRK1 may participate in DNA repair, cell cycle checkpoints, NOTCH signaling pathways, WNT signal pathway, and the

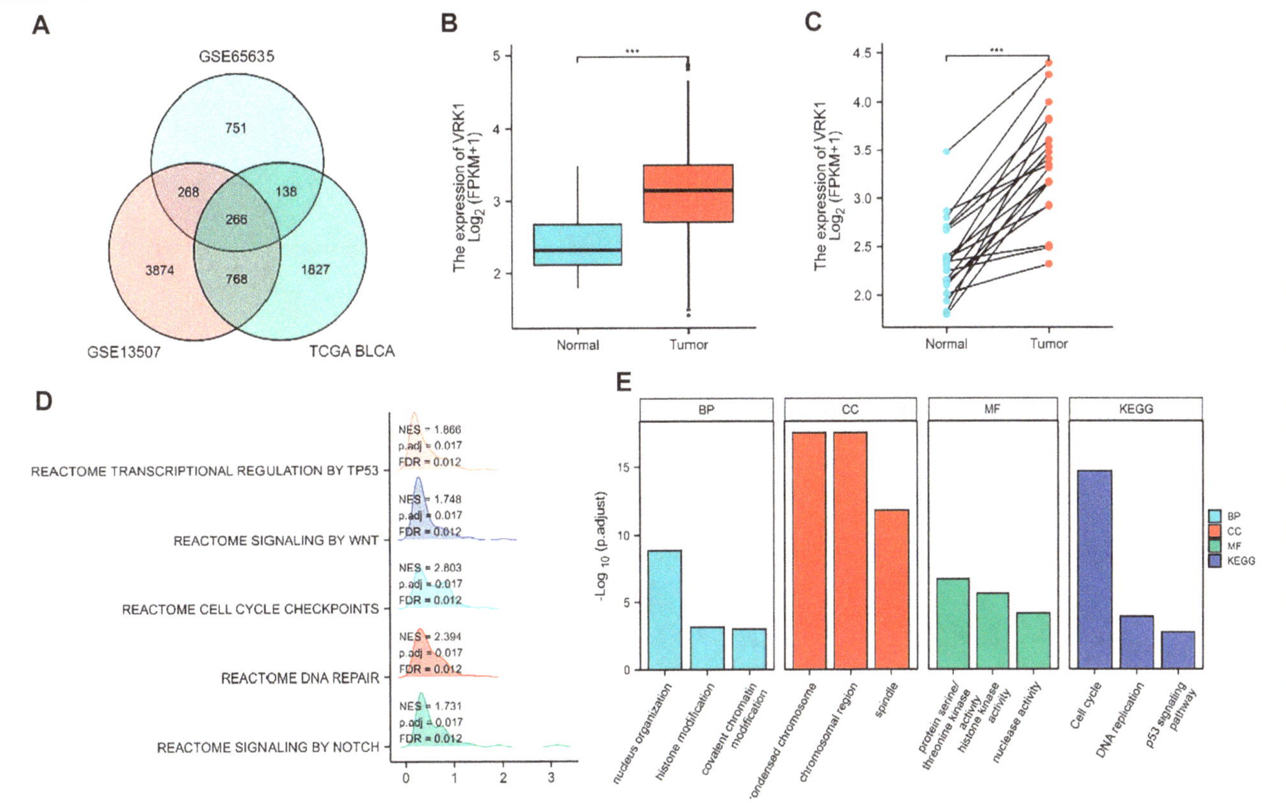

FIGURE 1 | Differentially expressed genes (DEGs) and their expression in the TCGA database and gene enrichment analysis results of VRK1. **(A)** Venn diagrams of upregulated genes in three data sets. **(B)** VRK1 in unmatched bladder cancer tissues (n = 414) and paracancerous tissues (n = 19) in the TCGA database is highly expressed in tumor tissues. **(C)** VRK1 in the matched bladder cancer tissues (n = 19) and paracancerous tissues (n = 19) in the TCGA database is highly expressed in tumor tissues. **(D)** GSEA analysis results for VRK1. **(E)** Functional analysis results of GO and KEGG. Note: ***<0.001, the difference is statistically significant.

transcription and regulation of TP53 to affect the biological process of bladder cancer, leading to different prognosis of bladder cancer (**Figure 1D**). We also used Metascape for online functional analysis. The differential genes were added to Metascape for functional analysis of GO and KEGG. GO-BP analysis showed that nucleus organization, histone modification, and covalent chromatin modification are possible cytological behaviors involved. GO-CC analysis found that condensed chromosome, chromosomal region, and spindle are possible sites involved. GO-MF analysis found that protein serine/threonine kinase activity, histone kinase activity, and nuclease activity are the molecular functions that may be affected. KEGG analysis found that cell cycle, DNA replication, and p53 signaling pathway are signaling pathways that may be affected (**Figure 1E**).

Expression of VRK1 in Bladder Cancer Tissue and VRK1 Knockdown can Significantly Inhibit the Proliferation and Clonal Formation Assay of Bladder Cancer Cells

The tumor tissues and paracancerous tissues of the patients included in the study were taken to compare the VRK1 expression. Using reverse transcription quantitative PCR (**Figure 2A**) and Western blotting (**Figure 2B**), we found that VRK1 expression in cancer tissues is higher than that in adjacent tissues ($p < 0.05$). The Human Protein Atlas (https://www.proteinatlas.org/) database indicates that VRK1 has a higher expression in cancerous tissues than in paracancerous tissues. Moreover, the gene is mainly located in the nucleus, with a small amount expressed in the cytoplasm (**Figure 2C**). We used immunohistochemistry to check the expression of VRK1 in the pathological tissues studied in this project. We found that VRK1 is also mainly expressed in the nucleus (**Figure 2D**), which is consistent with the expression in the database. Moreover, VRK1 was low expressed in 43 bladder cancer tissue samples (42.6%), and highly expressed in 58 bladder cancer tissue samples (57.4%).

The aforementioned results indicate that VRK1 is highly expressed in bladder cancer tissues. Therefore, in order to study the specific biological function of this gene in bladder cancer, it is planned to use bladder cancer cell lines for further functional research. qRT-PCR was used to detect the expression level of VRK1 in 5 bladder cancer cell lines (J82, SW780, T24, 5637, and UM-UC-3) and a normal human bladder normal epithelial cell (SV-HUC-1). The results of fluorescence qPCR and Western blot showed that the expression levels of VRK1 in various bladder cancer cell lines are quite different, with the highest expression levels in T24 and 5637

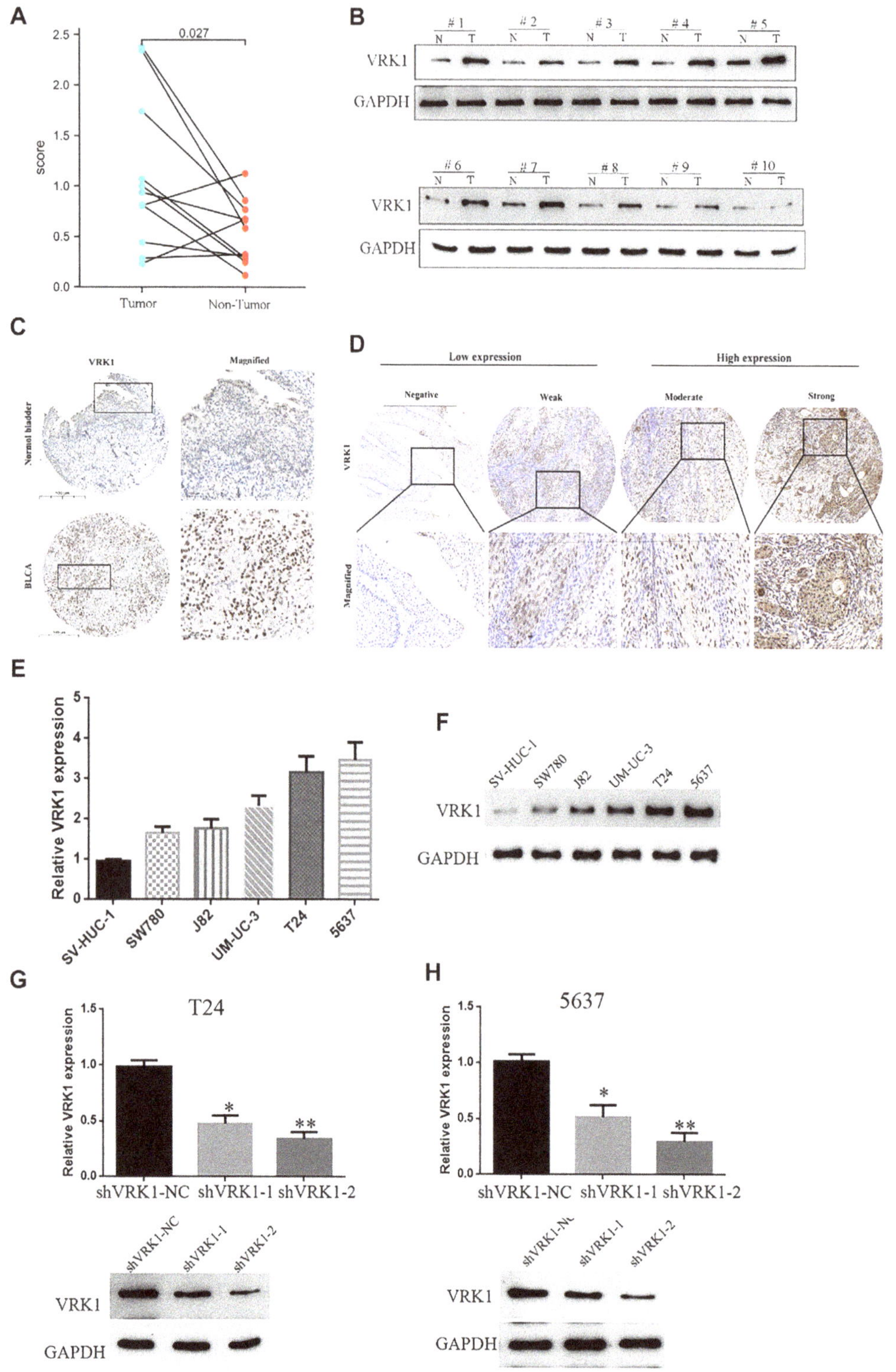

FIGURE 2 | High expression of VRK1 in bladder cancer tissues and bladder cancer cell lines. **(A)** Reverse transcription quantitative PCR showed that the expression of VRK1 in cancer tissues was higher than that in paracancerous tissues at the mRNA level ($p < 0.05$). **(B)** Western blot experiments showed that the expression of VRK1 in cancer tissues was higher than that in paracancerous tissues at the protein level ($p < 0.05$). **(C)** In The Human Protein Atlas database, VRK1 is higher expressed in cancerous tissues than in paracancerous tissues, and is mainly expressed in the nucleus. **(D)** Immunohistochemistry showed that VRK1 was mainly expressed in the nucleus. **(E)** Fluorescence qPCR to detect the expression of VRK1 in bladder cancer cell lines and normal human bladder normal epithelial cells. The experiments were repeated three times. **(F)** Western blot to detect the expression of VRK1 in bladder cancer cell lines and normal human bladder normal epithelial cells. **(G,H)** Fluorescence qPCR and Western blot to detect the expression in bladder cancer T24 and 5637 cells after knocking down VRK1, $^{*}p < 0.05$, $^{**}p < 0.01$.

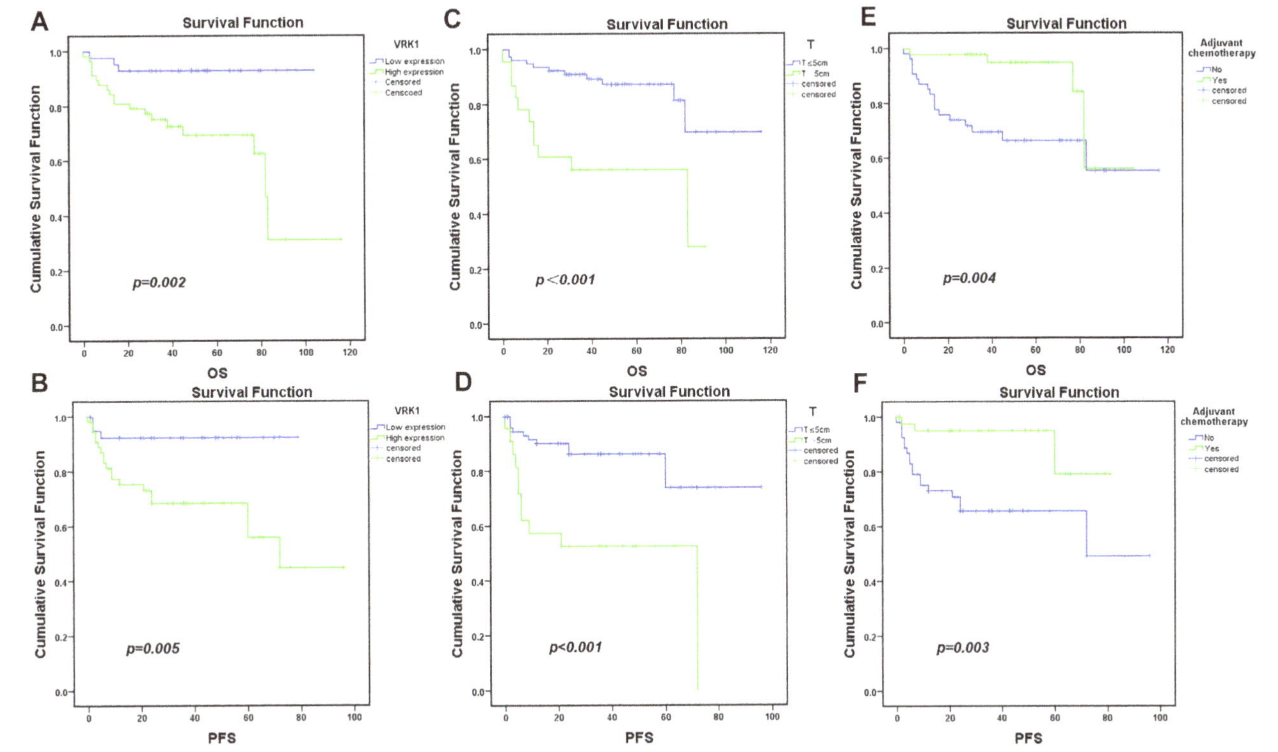

FIGURE 3 | Survival and prognosis of patients included in the study. **(A,B)**: OS and PFS of patients in the VRK1 low expression group are better than those in the VRK1 high expression group. **(C,D)**: OS and PFS of patients with tumor diameter ≤5 cm are better than those in the group with tumor diameter >5 cm. **(E,F)**: OS and PFS of patients that have undergone adjuvant chemotherapy are better than those of those who have not undergone adjuvant chemotherapy.

cells, followed by UM-UC-3, J82, and SW780 cells (**Figures 2E,F**). Therefore, in the follow-up cell function research, we selected VRK1 highly expressing T24 and 5637 cells as the research objects to conduct in-depth cell function and molecular mechanism research. First, we constructed two lentiviral-mediated RNA interference vectors targeting VRK1 gene (shVRK1-1 and shVRK1-2) and shVRK1-control (shVRK1-NC) in T24 and 5637 cells, respectively, and then detected knockdown by fluorescent qPCR and Western blot. The results suggested: compared with the blank control group (shVRK1-NC), shVRK1-1 and shVRK1-2 can significantly knockdown the expression level of VRK1 in bladder cancer cells after transfection, and shVRK1-2 has a higher knockdown efficiency (**Figures 2G,H**). The aforementioned results indicate that the bladder cancer cell line with VRK1 knockdown is successfully constructed, providing experimental materials for subsequent functional studies.

Survival and Prognosis of Patients Included in This Study

All patients were followed up for 5 years. A total of 79 patients survived, with a survival rate of 78.2%, and 22 patients died, with a mortality rate of 21.8%. Kaplan–Meier survival analysis results showed that the OS and PFS of patients in the VRK1 high expression group were significantly lower than those in the VRK1 low expression group (p = 0.002, p = 0.005) (**Figures 3A,B**). Meanwhile, further stratified analysis also reveals that patients with tumor diameters ≤5 cm and undergoing adjuvant chemotherapy had better OS and PFS (**Figures 3C–F**).

Relationship Between VRK1 and Clinicopathological Data of Patients With Bladder Cancer

Among the 101 bladder cancer patients included, 43 cases (42.6%) were in the VRK1 low expression group, and 58 cases (57.4%) were in the VRK1 high expression group. The difference between two groups of patients in terms of gender, age, recurrence, surgical methods, adjuvant chemotherapy, invasion of the bladder triangle, tumor invasion, vascular tumor thrombus, T stage, grade, lymph node metastasis, and presence or absence of distant metastasis was not statistically significant ($p > 0.05$), but the difference in tumor size was statistically significant ($p < 0.05$) (**Table 1**). This also provides some reference for our follow-up experiments to explore the role of VRK1 in the tumorigenesis and development of bladder cancer.

Results of Univariate Analysis and Multi-Factor Analysis

In order to further determine the risk factors associated with OS in patients with bladder cancer, we conducted univariate and

TABLE 1 | Relationship between the expression of VRK1 and clinicopathological data.

Variable	Total	Low expression	High expression	p
	n (%)	n (%)	n (%)	
Gender				
Male	82 (81.2)	37 (36.6)	45 (44.6)	0.282
Female	19 (18.8)	6 (5.9)	13 (12.9)	
Age				
≤65	56 (55.4)	21 (20.8)	35 (34.7)	0.250
> 65	45 (44.6)	22 (21.8)	23 (22.8)	
Recurrence				
Yes	23 (22.8)	11 (10.9)	12 (11.9)	0.562
No	78 (77.2)	32 (31.7)	46 (45.5)	
Tumor size (cm)				
≤5	78 (77.2)	38 (37.6)	40 (39.6)	0.021[a]
> 5	23 (22.8)	5 (5.0)	18 (17.8)	
Operation mode				
Transurethral resection	50 (49.5)	23 (22.8)	27 (26.7)	0.491
Radical cystectomy	51 (50.5)	20 (19.8)	31 (30.7)	
Adjuvant chemotherapy				
Yes	47 (46.5)	24 (23.8)	23 (22.8)	0.107
No	54 (53.5)	19 (18.8)	35 (34.7)	
Bladder triangle involvement				
Yes	36 (35.6)	15 (14.9)	21 (20.8)	0.891
No	65 (64.4)	28 (27.7)	37 (36.6)	
External invasion				
Yes	13 (12.9)	6 (5.9)	78 (6.9)	0.780
No	88 (87.1)	37 (36.6)	51 (50.5)	
Vascular tumor thrombus				
Yes	2 (2.0)	0 (0.0)	2 (2.0)	0.219
No	99 (98.0)	43 (42.6)	56 (55.4)	
T stage				
T1	22 (21.8)	9 (8.9)	13 (12.9)	0.858
T2+T3	79 (78.2)	34 (33.7)	45 (44.6)	
Grade				
G1+G2	53 (52.5)	26 (25.7)	27 (26.7)	0.166
G3	48 (47.5)	17 (16.8)	31 (30.7)	
Lymph node metastasis				
Yes	32 (31.7)	14 (13.9)	18 (17.8)	0.871
No	69 (68.3)	29 (28.7)	40 (39.6)	
Other site metastasis				
Yes	10 (9.9)	3 (3.0)	7 (6.9)	0.397
No	91 (90.1)	40 (39.6)	51 (50.5)	

[a]<0.05, the difference is statistically significant.

multivariate analysis to confirm whether VRK1 is an independent risk factor for poor prognosis. Univariate analysis showed that the maximum pathological diameter of the tumor, whether adjuvant chemotherapy, the presence or absence of vascular tumor thrombus, T stage, and VRK1 expression are factors that affect the patient's OS ($p < 0.05$). The results of Cox multivariate analysis showed that the expression of VRK1 is an independent risk factor affecting tumor progression. The pathological maximum diameter, staging, and adjuvant chemotherapy also have a certain impact on tumor progression ($p < 0.05$) (**Table 2**).

Nomogram Construction

Predicting the 2-, 4-, and 6-year survival rates of patients with bladder cancer has a certain guiding effect to improve the prognosis of patients with poor prognostic characteristics in the clinical practice. Compared with the nomogram constructed using a single prognostic factor, the nomogram constructed by a combined model might be the bettter nomogram for predicting short-term survival rates (2, 4, and 6 years). We constructed a nomogram based on Cox regression analysis. The model successfully included 4 independent prognostic factors, including tumor diameter, adjuvant chemotherapy, T stage, and VRK1 expression. Predictive models were contracted with internal validation. In internal validation, the nomogram C-index was 0.841 (95% CI, 0.803–0.880) (**Figure 4**). Therefore, the prediction model has better accuracy.

Knockdown of VRK1 Significantly Inhibits the Invasion and Migration of Bladder Cancer Cells

The results showed that compared with the blank control group (shVRK1-NC), shVRK1-1 and shVRK1-2 began to significantly

TABLE 2 | Univariate analysis and multivariate analysis of clinical factors on 101 patients with OS.

Variable	Univariate analysis			Multivariate analysis		
	HR	(95%CI)	p	HR	(95%CI)	P
Gender						
Male	1.019	(0.344–3.021)	0.972			
Female	1					
Age						
≤65	1	(0.953–5.427)	0.064			
> 65	2.274					
Recurrence						
Yes	0.896	(0.332–2.417)	0.829			
No	1					
Tumor size (cm)						
≤5	1	(1.834–9.875)	0.001[a]	1	(1.182–6.719)	0.019[a]
> 5	4.256			2.818		
Operation mode						
Transurethral resection	1	(0.704–4.075)	0.240			
Radical cystectomy	1.693					
Adjuvant chemotherapy						
Yes	0.230	(0.078–0.684)	0.008[a]	0.275	(0.088–0.858)	0.026[a]
No	1			1		
Bladder triangle involvement						
Yes	2.271	(0.965–5.347)	0.060			
No	1					
External invasion						
Yes	1.469	(0.493–4.374)	0.490			
No	1					
Vascular tumor thrombus						
Yes	11.994	(2.633–54.642)	0.001[a]			
No	1					
T stage						
T1	1	(1.164–78.517)	0.036[a]	1	(1.241–147.896)	0.033[a]
T2+T3	9.561			13.547		
Grade						
G1+G2	1	(0.792–4.527)	0.151			
G3	1.893					
Lymph node metastasis						
Yes	0.949	(0.383–2.347)	0.909			
No	1					
Other site metastasis						
Yes	2.319	(0.779–6.897)	0.131			
No	1					
Expression of VRK1						
Low expression	1	(1.672–19.238)	0.005[a]	1	(1.114–13.338)	0.033[a]
High expression	5.671			3.854		

Note: [a]<0.05, the difference is statistically significant.

inhibit cell proliferation at 48 h. The inhibition phenomenon is particularly significant when cultured to 72 h (**Figure 5A**). The results of the clone formation assay showed that compared with the blank control group (shVRK1-NC), shVRK1-1 and shVRK1-2 could significantly inhibit the number of T24 and 5637 clones (**Figure 5B**). This indicates that knocking down VRK1 can significantly inhibit the proliferation of bladder cells (T24 and 5637).

In order to further study the role of VRK1 in the invasion and migration of bladder cancer cells, Transwell was used to detect the invasion and migration ability of T24 and 5637 cells after knocking down VRK1. The test results showed that compared with the blank control group (shVRK1-NC), knocking down VRK1 (shVRK1-1 and shVRK1-2) can significantly inhibit the invasion and migration of T24 and 5637 cells (**Figure 5C**).

Knockdown of VRK1 Significantly Inhibits the Expression of Proliferation- and Invasion-Related Molecules in Bladder Cancer Cells

The aforementioned results indicate that knockdown of VRK1 can significantly inhibit the proliferation and invasion of bladder cancer cells. To further detect whether knockdown of VRK1 affects the proliferation- (Ki-67, PCNA, and p21) and invasion- (E-cadherin, N-cadherin, vimentin, and fibronectin) related molecules of bladder cancer T24 cells, Western blot was

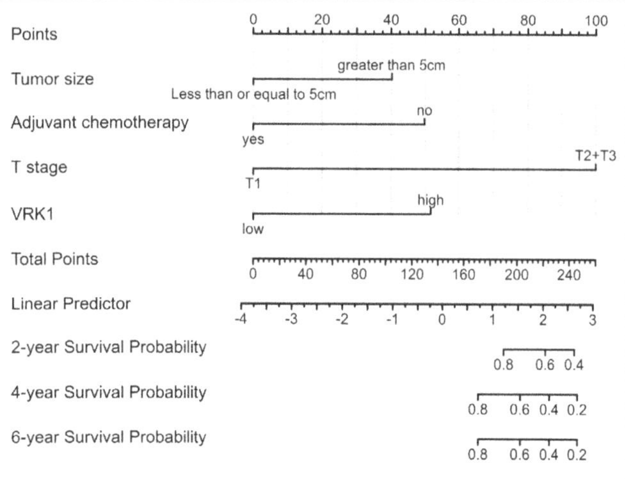

FIGURE 4 | Nomogram predicts the overall survival of bladder cancer patients. For each patient, draw four lines up to determine the points received from the four predictors in the nomogram. The sum of these points is on the "Total Points" axis. Then, draw a line down to determine the probability of 2-, 4-, and 6-year overall survival for bladder cancer. * The C-index is 0.841 (95% CI is 0.803–0.880).

performed. Results suggested that compared with the blank control group (shVRK1-NC), knocking down VRK1 can significantly affect the expression of proliferating cell nuclear antigen Ki-67 and PCNA, and promote the expression of cell cycle inhibitory protein p21 (**Figure 6A**). In addition, knocking down VRK1 can significantly promote the expression of E-cadherin and inhibit the expression of N-cadherin, vimentin, and fibronectin (**Figure 6C**). The abovementioned results indicate that knocking down VRK1 can significantly inhibit the expression of proliferation and invasion-related molecules in T24 cells. Moreover, we found that VRK1 gene was positively correlated with Ki-67 (MKI67), PCNA, N-cadherin (CDH2), and Fibronectin (FN1), and negatively correlated with P21(CDKN1A) in TCGA database (**Figures 6B,D**).

Knockdown of VRK1 Significantly Inhibits the Proliferation of Bladder Cancer Cells *in vivo*

In order to further study the effect of knocking down VRK1 on the proliferation of bladder cancer cells *in vivo*, the shVRK1-NC and shVRK1-2 bladder cancer T24 cells transfected with lentivirus were collected, and then injected into nude mice under the skin. The growth of tumor-bearing tissues was observed and recorded. After 30 days, the nude mice were sacrificed, and the tumor-bearing tissue was taken out for photographing and measurement. The results manifest that compared with the blank control group (shVRK1-NC), knocking down VRK1-2 can significantly inhibit the growth of bladder cancer cell T24 *in vivo* (**Figures 7A,B**). Then, the stripped tumor-bearing tissue was weighed, and the results imply that compared with the blank control group (shVRK1-NC), the proliferation ability of bladder cancer cell T24 *in vivo* was significantly reduced after knocking down VRK1-2 (**Figure 7C**). The aforementioned results show that knocking down VRK1 significantly inhibits the proliferation of bladder cancer cells *in vivo*.

In order to further detect the expression of VRK1 and proliferation-related proteins in tumor-bearing tissues, after fixing the tumor-bearing tissues, immunohistochemistry was used to detect the expression of VRK1 and Ki-67 proteins in the tumor-bearing tissues. The results suggest, compared with the blank control group (shVRK1-NC) tumor-bearing tissue, the expression of VRK1 in the tumor-bearing tissue of the knockdown group (shVRK1-2) was significantly reduced. Similarly, compared with the blank control group (shVRK1-NC) tumor-bearing tissue, the expression level of Ki-67 in the knockdown group (shVRK1-2) tumor-bearing tissue was significantly reduced (**Figures 7D,E**).

DISCUSSION

In this study, we first screened the differential genes of bladder cancer from GEO and TCGA data, and screened the differentially expressed molecules VRK1 from the differential genes. Further data analysis found that the expression differences of VRK1 is not only in between the cancer and paracancerous tissues as described in the database but also in the clinical data we included, which related to the prognosis of patients. The expression level of VRK is an independent risk factor for the prognosis of bladder cancer. We found that patients with low expression of the VRK1 molecule have a better prognosis. Then, we verified from the cytology and the nude mouse level that the reduction of VRK1 expression can inhibit the proliferation and invasion of bladder cancer cells. These results also consistently reflect the potential importance of using VRK1 to assess the prognosis of bladder cancer.

At the beginning of this study, we downloaded two RNA expression data sets GSE13507 and GSE65635 (containing tumor tissue and normal tissue) through GEO database (https://www.ncbi.nlm.nih.gov/geo/query/acc.cgi) *via* GEO query pack. The GEO online GEO2R tool was used to analyze the differential genes, using log2FC greater than 0 and p value less than 0.02 as the parameters to determine the screening DEG. Then, the data set of differentially expressed genes for bladder cancer was downloaded from the TCGA database (https://tcga-data.nci.nih.gov/), and the parameters for screening DEG according to log_2FC greater than 0 and p value less than 0.0001 were determined. Finally, the intersection of the three data sets is mapped in a Venn diagram to obtain the common upregulated differentially expressed genes. Thus, we determined our research molecule VRK1, and verified in the TCGA database that the expression of VRK1 in cancer tissues is higher than that in paracancerous tissues. The current clinical treatment of bladder cancer is now in the era of immunotherapy, and previous analysis has shown that tumor infiltrating lymphocytes are an independent predictor of the sentinel lymph node status and survival rate in cancer patients (Azimi et al., 2012). We also used the established computing resource

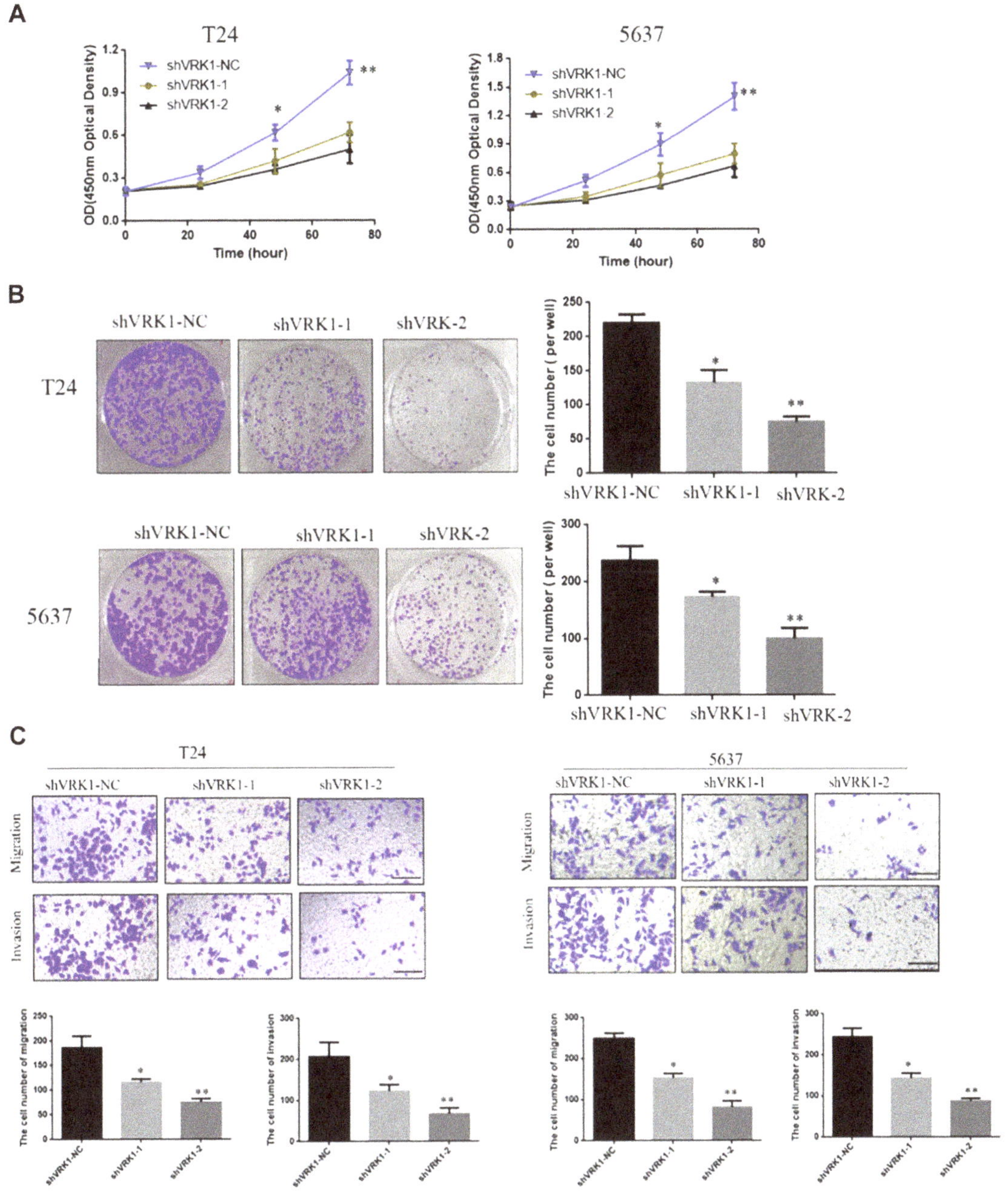

FIGURE 5 | Knockout of VRK1 inhibited the proliferation, clonal capacity, migration, and invasion of bladder cancer T24 and 5637 cells. **(A)** CCK-8 detects the effect of knocking down VRK1 on the proliferation of bladder cancer T24 and 5637 cells. **(B)** Clone formation assay: The effect of knocking down VRK1 on the cloning ability of bladder cancer T24 and 5637 cells. **(C)** The effect of knocking down VRK1 on the migration and invasion of bladder cancer T24 and 5637 cells. $^{*}p < 0.05$, $^{**}p < 0.01$; the scale is 100 μm.

(CIBERSORT) (http://cibersort.stanford.edu/) to explore the gene expression profile of the downloaded sample (Gentles et al., 2015; Ali et al., 2016; Bense et al., 2017). A total of 24 types of TIIC immune response in bladder cancer are detected to evaluate their correlation with survival and molecular subgroups. We tried to find out whether the expression of VRK1 is related to the immune infiltration of bladder cancer. We were surprised to find that pDC, NK cells, Th2 cells, Tgd, T-helper cells, NK CD56 bright cells, and mast cells are the main immune cells affected by the expression of VRK1 ($p < 0.001$). Therefore, the expression of VRK1 may also have a certain relationship with the immune infiltration of bladder cancer (**Supplementary Figure S1**). We used the string database to analyze related genes that interact with VRK1 from the perspectives of protein–protein, protein–DNA and genetic interactions, pathways, physiological and biochemical reactions, gene and protein expression, protein domains, and phenotype screening to construct a protein–protein interaction (PPI) network. Based on the

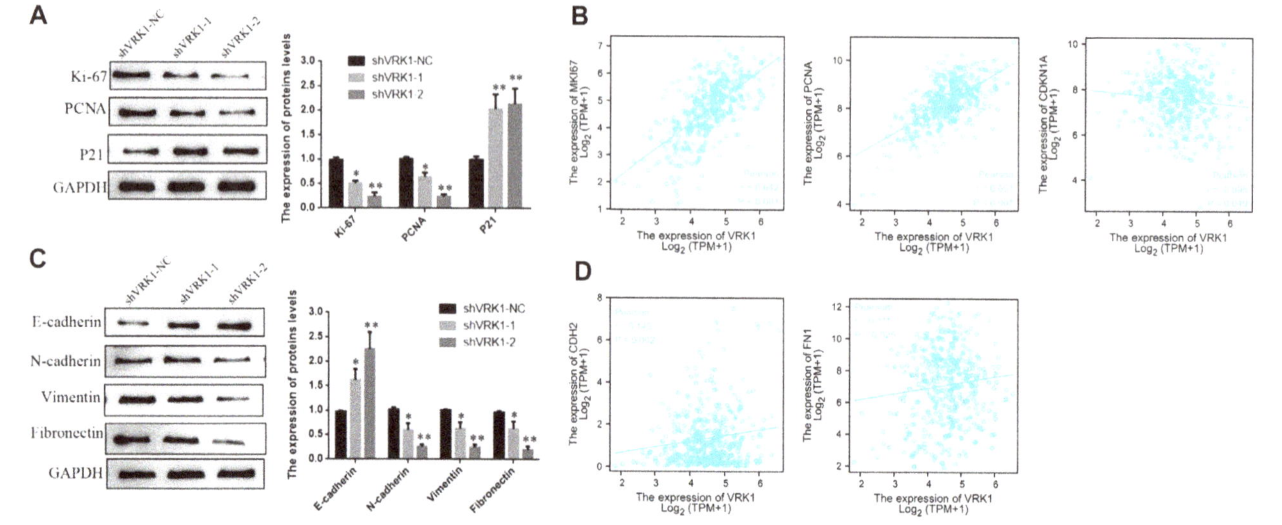

FIGURE 6 | Knockdown of VRK1 inhibited proliferation and invasion in BLCA cells. **(A)** A significant reduction of Ki-67 and PCNA but increase P21 was detected in shVRK1 cells compared to shNC cells by Western blotting. GAPDH was used as an internal control. Data are presented as means ± SD of three independent experiments. **(B)** The correlation between VRK1 and Ki67, PCNA, P21 (CDNK1A) at the mRNA level was detected in the TCGA database **(C)** A significant reduction of N-cadherin, vimentin and Fibronectin but increase E-cadherin was detected in shVRK1 cells compared to shNC cells by Western blotting. GAPDH was used as an internal control. Data are presented as means ± SD of three independent experiments. **(B,D)** The correlation between VRK1 and N-cadherin (CDH2) and Fibronectin (FN1) at the mRNA level was detected in the TCGA database $^{*}p < 0.05$, $^{**}p < 0.01$.

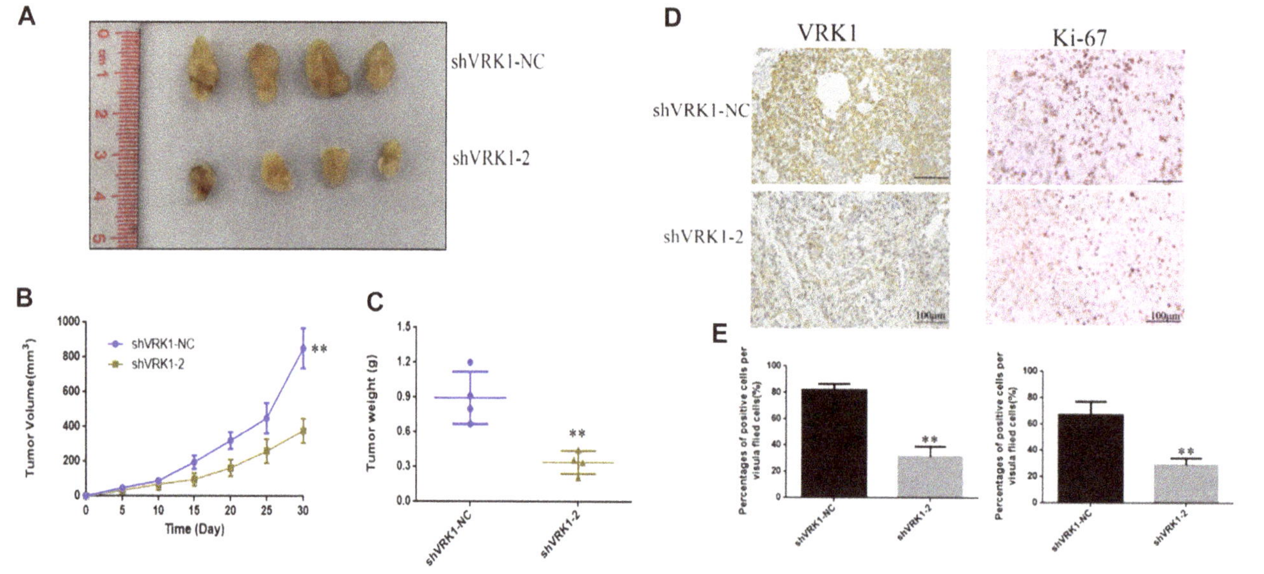

FIGURE 7 | Knockdown of VRK1 significantly inhibits the proliferation of bladder cancer cells *in vivo*. **(A)** Pictures after stripping the tumor-bearing tissue from nude mice. **(B)** Measure the tumor-bearing tissue every 5 days. **(C)** Weigh the tumor-bearing tissue. **(D,E)** Immunohistochemistry to detect the expression of VRK1 and Ki-67 in tumor-bearing tissues. $^{*}p < 0.05$, $^{**}p < 0.01$.

strength of the interaction, we selected the top 100 genes from this database (**Supplementary Figure S2**). We also used GSEA to predict possible related molecular mechanisms. We found that VRK1 may affect the biological processes of bladder cancer by participating in DNA repair, cell cycle checkpoints, NOTCH signaling pathway, WNT signaling pathway, and transcription and regulation of TP53, eventually leading to different prognosis of bladder cancer. We also used Metascape for online functional analysis. The differential genes were added to Metascape for functional analysis of GO and KEGG. GO-BP analysis found that nucleus organization, histone modification, and covalent chromatin modification are possible cytological behaviors involved. GO-CC analysis found that condensed chromosome, chromosomal region, and spindle are possible sites involved. GO-MF analysis found that protein serine/threonine kinase activity, histone kinase activity, and nuclease activity are the molecular functions that may be affected. KEGG analysis found that cell cycle, DNA replication, and p53 signaling pathway may be affected. Studies have found that VRK1 has regulatory effects on transcription factors such as p53 (Yokobori et al., 2020), ATF2 (Sevilla et al., 2004), CREB (Kim et al., 2014), c-Jun (Martín-Doncel et al., 2019), and p300 acetyltransferase (Valbuena et al., 2008). Moreover, these transcription factors have a regulatory effect on both the progression and evolution of tumors.

Studies have also pointed out that VRK1 promotes cisplatin resistance by upregulating c-MYC through c-Jun activation and serves as a therapeutic target for esophageal squamous cell carcinoma (Liu et al., 2017). The mutual influence of VRK1 and NOTCH pathways is related to the prognosis of laryngeal cancer (de Miguel-Luken et al., 2016). VRK1 may provide new potential biomarkers for improving the prognosis and treatment of Wilms tumor (WT) patients by showing the WNT signaling pathway (Liu et al., 2021). At the same time, the WNT pathway is also a crucial pathway for regulating epithelial mesenchymal EMT. VRK1 is a member of the VRK family, which also includes VRK2 and VRK3. These members have also been reported to be mostly related to the poor prognosis of tumors. For example, VRK1 is highly expressed in many human tumors and affects the prognosis of patients. For example, the consumption of VRK1 can delay cell cycle progression and reduce the proliferation of liver cancer cells, that is, the high expression of VRK1 contributes to the cell proliferation and survival of hepatocellular carcinoma (Huang et al., 2016). VRK2 regulates tumor cell invasion through the over-activation of NFAT1 and the expression of cyclooxygenase 2 (Vázquez-Cedeira and Lazo, 2012). VRK3 is involved in the cell cycle regulation, DNA repair, and neuronal differentiation of diffuse pontine gliomas, which are the essential genes for tumor cell survival (Silva-Evangelista et al., 2019). These mature research studies also provide better help for follow-up research on the role of VRK1 in bladder cancer.

The key factors in predicting outcomes and discovering the biological mechanisms leading to poor prognosis are two important parts in cancer research (Quan et al., 2015). We verified the bladder cancer tissue of the patients we included in the study by reverse transcription qPCR, and found that the expression of VRK1 in cancer tissues was significantly higher than that in paracancerous tissues. The immunohistochemistry results also confirmed that VRK1 is highly expressed in bladder cancer tissues and mainly expressed in the nucleus. These results are also consistent with the expression of VRK1 in the database. We further analyzed the expression of VRK1 with the patient's prognosis and clinical parameters. The results reveal that the OS and PFS of patients in the VRK1 high expression group were significantly lower than those in the VRK1 low expression group ($p < 0.05$), which was also comparable to the immunohistochemistry results that patients with high VRK1 expression had worse tumor differentiation than patients with low VRK1 expression. In the analysis of clinical data, among 101 bladder cancer patients included, 43 cases (42.6%) were in the VRK1 low expression group, and 58 cases (57.4%) were in the VRK1 high expression group. The difference in tumor size between the two groups of patients was statistically significant ($p < 0.05$). This also provides some reference for our follow-up experiments to explore the role of VRK1 in the biological process of the tumorigenesis and development of bladder cancer. Further COX regression analysis indicated that the expression of VRK1 is an independent risk factor affecting tumor progression. The pathological maximum diameter, staging, and adjuvant chemotherapy also have a certain impact on tumor progression ($p < 0.05$). Based on the results of Cox regression analysis, we constructed a nomogram through a combined model and conducted internal verification, so as to have a more accurate judgment on the prediction of the 2-, 4-, and 6-year survival rate of bladder cancer patients. This is useful for the development of clinical practice. In internal verification, the C-index of the nomogram is 0.841 (95% CI is 0.803–0.880), so this prediction model also has good accuracy. Our analysis of health information and clinical data have reflected that the high expression of VRK1 is related to the poor prognosis of patients with bladder cancer, which has also aroused our interest in further research and exploration at the level of cytology and nude mice.

At the cytological level, we first used qRT-PCR to detect the expression level of VRK1 in five bladder cancer cell lines (J82, SW780, T24, 5637, and UM-UC-3) and a normal human bladder normal epithelial cell (SV-HUC- 1). The T24 and 5637 cells with high expression of VRK1 were selected as the research objects through fluorescence qPCR and Western blot. We constructed VRK knockdown cell line through lentivirus-mediated RNA interference vector for subsequent functional studies. Both CCK-8 and clone formation assay showed that knocking down VRK1 can significantly inhibit the proliferation of bladder cells (T24 and 5637). Transwell experiment results show that knocking down VRK1 can also significantly inhibit the invasion and migration ability of T24 and 5637 cells. To our surprise, further experimental studies found that knocking down VRK1 can significantly affect the expression of proliferating cell nuclear antigen Ki-67 and PNCA and promote the expression of cell cycle inhibitory protein p21. This is also consistent with the study reported by Huang et al. (2016) that the low expression of VRK1 in hepatocellular carcinoma can stabilize p53, thereby promoting the expression of P21, causing necessary cell cycle arrest and leading to a better prognosis. Knockdown of VRK1 can significantly promote the expression of E-cadherin and inhibit the expression of N-cadherin, vimentin, and fibronectin. This is also consistent with the abovementioned prediction and analysis results of GSEA that VRK1 may participate in the proliferation and metastasis of bladder cancer through certain pathways. The results of *in vitro* cytology experiments all show that VRK1 exhibits a kind of "oncogene" performance in bladder cancer cell lines. In order to better study the possible mechanism of VRK1 in the biology of bladder cancer, we conducted *in vivo* experiments. We collected shVRK1-NC and shVRK1-2 T24 bladder cancer cells transfected with lentivirus, and then injected them under the skin of nude mice to observe and record the growth of tumor-bearing tissues. By comparing the weight of tumor-bearing tissues, we found that VRK1 knockdown can significantly inhibit the proliferation of bladder cancer cells in the body. Further immunohistochemistry results of tumor-bearing tissues suggested that the expression of VRK1 in tumor-bearing tissues of the knockdown group (shVRK1-2) was significantly lower than that of the blank control group (shVRK1-NC). Compared with the blank control group (shVRK1-NC), the expression level of Ki-67 in the knockdown group (shVRK1-2) tumor-bearing tissue was significantly reduced. *In vivo* experimental results also indicate that VRK1 has the expression status of "oncogenes" in the bladder cancer tissue.

CONCLUSION

Our research results range from bioinformatics data analysis to patient clinical data comparison and from *in vitro* cytology experiments to *in vivo* nude mouse experiments. All research results consistently reflect the positive relationship between low VRK1 expression and better prognosis of bladder cancer. Therefore, further research is necessary to clarify more specific molecular mechanisms, which will also be helpful for the development of new drug candidates for targeted therapies for bladder cancer.

AUTHOR CONTRIBUTIONS

JCW, TL, and BQZ developed the project. JCW, HJ, and BQZ performed experiments and wrote the manuscript. TL and ZC supervised the work. All authors contributed to the article and approved the submitted version.

REFERENCES

Ali, H. R., Chlon, L., Pharoah, P. D., Markowetz, F., and Caldas, C. (2016). Patterns of Immune Infiltration in Breast Cancer and Their Clinical Implications: A Gene-Expression-Based Retrospective Study. *Plos Med.* 13 (12), e1002194. doi:10.1371/journal.pmed.1002194

Azimi, F., Scolyer, R. A., Rumcheva, P., Moncrieff, M., Murali, R., McCarthy, S. W., et al. (2012). Tumor-infiltrating Lymphocyte Grade Is an Independent Predictor of sentinel Lymph Node Status and Survival in Patients with Cutaneous Melanoma. *J. Clin. Oncol.* 30 (21), 2678–2683. doi:10.1200/JCO.2011.37.8539

Ben, Z., Gong, L., and Qiu, Y. (2018). High Expression of VRK1 Is Related to Poor Prognosis in Glioma. *Pathol. Res. Pract.* 214 (1), 112–118. doi:10.1016/j.prp.2017.10.014

Bense, R. D., Sotiriou, C., Piccart-Gebhart, M. J., Haanen, J. B. A. G., van Vugt, M. A. T. M., de Vries, E. G. E., et al. (2017). Relevance of Tumor-Infiltrating Immune Cell Composition and Functionality for Disease Outcome in Breast Cancer. *J. Natl. Cancer Inst.* 109 (1). doi:10.1093/jnci/djw192

Campillo-Marcos, I., García-González, R., Navarro-Carrasco, E., and Lazo, P. A. (2021). The Human VRK1 Chromatin Kinase in Cancer Biology. *Cancer Lett.* 503, 117–128. doi:10.1016/j.canlet.2020.12.032

Davis, S., and Meltzer, P. S. (2007). GEOquery: a Bridge between the Gene Expression Omnibus (GEO) and BioConductor. *Bioinformatics* 23 (14), 1846–1847. doi:10.1093/bioinformatics/btm254

de Miguel-Luken, M. J., Chaves-Conde, M., and Carnero, A. (2016). A Genetic View of Laryngeal Cancer Heterogeneity. *Cell Cycle* 15 (9), 1202–1212. doi:10.1080/15384101.2016.1156275

Del Puerto-Nevado, L., Marin-Arango, J. P., Fernandez-Aceñero, M. J., Arroyo-Manzano, D., Martinez-Useros, J., Borrero-Palacios, A., et al. (2016). Predictive Value of Vrk 1 and 2 for Rectal Adenocarcinoma Response to Neoadjuvant Chemoradiation Therapy: a Retrospective Observational Cohort Study. *BMC Cancer* 16, 519. doi:10.1186/s12885-016-2574-9

Diboun, I., Wernisch, L., Orengo, C. A., and Koltzenburg, M. (2006). Microarray Analysis after RNA Amplification Can Detect Pronounced Differences in Gene Expression Using Limma. *BMC Genomics* 7, 252. doi:10.1186/1471-2164-7-252

Gentles, A. J., Newman, A. M., Liu, C. L., Bratman, S. V., Feng, W., Kim, D., et al. (2015). The Prognostic Landscape of Genes and Infiltrating Immune Cells across Human Cancers. *Nat. Med.* 21 (8), 938–945. doi:10.1038/nm.3909

Gu, Z., Eils, R., and Schlesner, M. (2016). Complex Heatmaps Reveal Patterns and Correlations in Multidimensional Genomic Data. *Bioinformatics* 32 (18), 2847–2849. doi:10.1093/bioinformatics/btw313

Huang, W., Cui, X., Chen, Y., Shao, M., Shao, X., Shen, Y., et al. (2016). High VRK1 Expression Contributes to Cell Proliferation and Survival in Hepatocellular Carcinoma. *Pathol. Res. Pract.* 212 (3), 171–178. doi:10.1016/j.prp.2015.11.015

Kang, T. H., Park, D. Y., Choi, Y. H., Kim, K. J., Yoon, H. S., and Kim, K. T. (2007). Mitotic Histone H3 Phosphorylation by Vaccinia-Related Kinase 1 in Mammalian Cells. *Mol. Cel Biol* 27 (24), 8533–8546. doi:10.1128/MCB.00018-07

Kim, W., Chakraborty, G., Kim, S., Shin, J., Park, C. H., Jeong, M. W., et al. (2012). Macro Histone H2A1.2 (macroH2A1) Protein Suppresses Mitotic Kinase VRK1 during Interphase. *J. Biol. Chem.* 287 (8), 5278–5289. doi:10.1074/jbc.M111.281709

Kim, Y. S., Kim, S. H., Shin, J., Harikishore, A., Lim, J. K., Jung, Y., et al. (2014). Luteolin Suppresses Cancer Cell Proliferation by Targeting Vaccinia-Related Kinase 1. *PLoS One* 9 (10), e109655. doi:10.1371/journal.pone.0109655

Laurberg, J. R., Jensen, J. B., Schepeler, T., Borre, M., Ørntoft, T. F., and Dyrskjøt, L. (2014). High Expression of GEM and EDNRA Is Associated with Metastasis and Poor Outcome in Patients with Advanced Bladder Cancer. *BMC Cancer* 14, 638. doi:10.1186/1471-2407-14-638

Li, B., Xie, F., Zheng, F. X., Jiang, G. S., Zeng, F. Q., and Xiao, X. Y. (2017). Overexpression of CircRNA BCRC4 Regulates Cell Apoptosis and MicroRNA-101/EZH2 Signaling in Bladder Cancer. *J. Huazhong Univ. Sci. Technolog Med. Sci.* 37 (6), 886–890. doi:10.1007/s11596-017-1822-9

Liu, H., Zhang, M., Shi, M., Zhang, T., Zhang, Z., Cui, Q., et al. (2021). A Survival-Related Competitive Endogenous RNA Network of Prognostic lncRNAs, miRNAs, and mRNAs in Wilms Tumor. *Front. Oncol.* 11, 608433. doi:10.3389/fonc.2021.608433

Liu, T., Zuo, L., Guo, D., Chai, X., Xu, J., Cui, Z., et al. (2019). Ginsenoside Rg3 Regulates DNA Damage in Non-small Cell Lung Cancer Cells by Activating VRK1/P53BP1 Pathway. *Biomed. Pharmacother.* 120, 109483. doi:10.1016/j.biopha.2019.109483

Liu, Z. C., Cao, K., Xiao, Z. H., Qiao, L., Wang, X. Q., Shang, B., et al. (2017). VRK1 Promotes Cisplatin Resistance by Up-Regulating C-MYC via C-Jun Activation and Serves as a Therapeutic Target in Esophageal Squamous Cell Carcinoma. *Oncotarget* 8 (39), 65642–65658. doi:10.18632/oncotarget.20020

Lopez-Borges, S., and Lazo, P. A. (2000). The Human Vaccinia-Related Kinase 1 (VRK1) Phosphorylates Threonine-18 within the Mdm-2 Binding Site of the P53 Tumour Suppressor Protein. *Oncogene* 19 (32), 3656–3664. doi:10.1038/sj.onc.1203709

Martín-Doncel, E., Rojas, A. M., Cantarero, L., and Lazo, P. A. (2019). VRK1 Functional Insufficiency Due to Alterations in Protein Stability or Kinase Activity of Human VRK1 Pathogenic Variants Implicated in Neuromotor Syndromes. *Sci. Rep.* 9 (1), 13381. doi:10.1038/s41598-019-49821-7

Mon, A. M., MacKinnon, A. C., Jr., and Traktman, P. (2018). Overexpression of the VRK1 Kinase, Which Is Associated with Breast Cancer, Induces a Mesenchymal to Epithelial Transition in Mammary Epithelial Cells. *PLoS One* 13 (9), e0203397. doi:10.1371/journal.pone.0203397

Mootha, V. K., Lindgren, C. M., Eriksson, K. F., Subramanian, A., Sihag, S., Lehar, J., et al. (2003). PGC-1alpha-responsive Genes Involved in Oxidative Phosphorylation Are Coordinately Downregulated in Human Diabetes. *Nat. Genet.* 34 (3), 267–273. doi:10.1038/ng1180

Peng, D., Gong, Y. Q., Hao, H., He, Z. S., Li, X. S., Zhang, C. J., et al. (2017). Preoperative Prognostic Nutritional Index Is a Significant Predictor of Survival with Bladder Cancer after Radical Cystectomy: a Retrospective Study. *BMC Cancer* 17 (1), 391. doi:10.1186/s12885-017-3372-8

Quan, Y., Xu, M., Cui, P., Ye, M., Zhuang, B., and Min, Z. (2015). Grainyhead-like 2 Promotes Tumor Growth and Is Associated with Poor Prognosis in Colorectal Cancer. *J. Cancer* 6 (4), 342–350. doi:10.7150/jca.10969

Rajwa, P., Życzkowski, M., Paradysz, A., Bujak, K., and Bryniarski, P. (2018). Evaluation of the Prognostic Value of LMR, PLR, NLR, and dNLR in Urothelial Bladder Cancer Patients Treated with Radical Cystectomy. *Eur. Rev. Med. Pharmacol. Sci.* 22 (10), 3027–3037. doi:10.26355/eurrev_201805_15060

Sevilla, A., Santos, C. R., Vega, F. M., and Lazo, P. A. (2004). Human Vaccinia-Related Kinase 1 (VRK1) Activates the ATF2 Transcriptional Activity by Novel Phosphorylation on Thr-73 and Ser-62 and Cooperates with JNK. *J. Biol. Chem.* 279 (26), 27458–27465. doi:10.1074/jbc.M401009200

Silva-Evangelista, C., Barret, E., Ménez, V., Merlevede, J., Kergrohen, T., Saccasyn, A., et al. (2019). A Kinome-wide shRNA Screen Uncovers Vaccinia-Related Kinase 3 (VRK3) as an Essential Gene for Diffuse Intrinsic Pontine Glioma Survival. *Oncogene* 38 (38), 6479–6490. doi:10.1038/s41388-019-0884-5

Subramanian, A., Tamayo, P., Mootha, V. K., Mukherjee, S., Ebert, B. L., Gillette, M. A., et al. (2005). Gene Set Enrichment Analysis: a Knowledge-Based Approach for Interpreting Genome-wide Expression Profiles. *Proc. Natl. Acad. Sci. U S A.* 102 (43), 15545–15550. doi:10.1073/pnas.0506580102

Torre, L. A., Bray, F., Siegel, R. L., Ferlay, J., Lortet-Tieulent, J., and Jemal, A. (20122015). Global Cancer Statistics, 2012. *CA Cancer J. Clin.* 65 (2), 87–108. doi:10.3322/caac.21262

Valbuena, A., Blanco, S., Vega, F. M., and Lazo, P. A. (2008). The C/H3 Domain of P300 Is Required to Protect VRK1 and VRK2 from Their Downregulation Induced by P53. *PLoS One* 3 (7), e2649. doi:10.1371/journal.pone.0002649

Vázquez-Cedeira, M., and Lazo, P. A. (2012). Human VRK2 (Vaccinia-related Kinase 2) Modulates Tumor Cell Invasion by Hyperactivation of NFAT1 and Expression of Cyclooxygenase-2. *J. Biol. Chem.* 287 (51), 42739–42750. doi:10.1074/jbc.M112.404285

Wang, Q. H., Ji, J. L., Li, H., He, P. L., Song, L. X., Zhao, Y., et al. (2019). Preoperative Lymphocyte-To-Monocyte Ratio Predicts Prognosis in Patients with Stage T1 Non-muscle Invasive Bladder Cancer. *Zhongguo Yi Xue Ke Xue Yuan Xue Bao* 41 (5), 622–629. doi:10.3881/j.issn.1000-503X.11227

Wang, Y., and Zheng, T. (2014). Screening of Hub Genes and Pathways in Colorectal Cancer with Microarray Technology. *Pathol. Oncol. Res.* 20 (3), 611–618. doi:10.1007/s12253-013-9739-5

Yokobori, K., Miyauchi, Y., Williams, J. G., and Negishi, M. (2020). Phosphorylation of Vaccinia-Related Kinase 1 at Threonine 386 Transduces Glucose Stress Signal in Human Liver Cells. *Biosci. Rep.* 40 (4). doi:10.1042/BSR20200498

10

Nucleic Acid Sensing Pathways in DNA Repair Targeted Cancer Therapy

Bingteng Xie[1,2]* *and Aiqin Luo*[1,2]*

[1]*School of Life Science, Beijing Institute of Technology, Beijing, China,* [2]*Key Laboratory of Molecular Medicine and Biological Diagnosis and Treatment, Beijing Institute of Technology, Ministry of Industry and Information Technology, Beijing, China*

***Correspondence:**
Bingteng Xie
xiebingteng@bit.edu.cn
Aiqin Luo
aqluobit@163.com

The repair of DNA damage is a complex process, which helps to maintain genome fidelity, and the ability of cancer cells to repair therapeutically DNA damage induced by clinical treatments will affect the therapeutic efficacy. In the past decade, great success has been achieved by targeting the DNA repair network in tumors. Recent studies suggest that DNA damage impacts cellular innate and adaptive immune responses through nucleic acid-sensing pathways, which play essential roles in the efficacy of DNA repair targeted therapy. In this review, we summarize the current understanding of the molecular mechanism of innate immune response triggered by DNA damage through nucleic acid-sensing pathways, including DNA sensing *via* the cyclic GMP-AMP synthase (cGAS), Toll-like receptor 9 (TLR9), absent in melanoma 2 (AIM2), DNA-dependent protein kinase (DNA-PK), and Mre11-Rad50-Nbs1 complex (MRN) complex, and RNA sensing *via* the TLR3/7/8 and retinoic acid-inducible gene I (RIG-I)-like receptors (RLRs). Furthermore, we will focus on the recent developments in the impacts of nucleic acid-sensing pathways on the DNA damage response (DDR). Elucidating the DDR-immune response interplay will be critical to harness immunomodulatory effects to improve the efficacy of antitumor immunity therapeutic strategies and build future therapeutic approaches.

Keywords: DNA damage and repair, DDR inhibitors, nucleic acid-sensing pathways, innate immunity, immunotherapy

OVERVIEW OF DNA DAMAGE AND REPAIR NETWORK

Up until now, chemotherapy and radiotherapy have remained the important treatment options for a variety of cancers (Hellmann et al., 2016; Chu et al., 2018; Qin et al., 2018; De Ruysscher et al., 2019; Grassberger et al., 2019; Galluzzi et al., 2020; Huang and Zhou, 2020; McLaughlin et al., 2020). The key mechanism of tumor cell death induced by standard chemotherapy and radiotherapy is DNA damage, leading to cell-cycle arrest and death directly or after S-phase DNA replication in the cell cycle. On the other hand, to deal with possible DNA lesions, tumors cells have evolved intricate repair mechanisms, and the ability to repair therapy-induced DNA damage would influence the therapeutic efficacy (Bouwman and Jonkers, 2012; Gavande et al., 2016). Here, we first overview the various types of DNA damage caused by radiotherapy and chemotherapy and the corresponding DNA damage repair pathways (see previous reviews for details) (Ciccia and Elledge, 2010; Giglia-Mari et al., 2011; Pinder et al., 2013; Chatterjee and Walker, 2017; Cussiol et al., 2019; Souliotis et al., 2020).

Some commonly used potent chemotherapy compounds (cyclophosphamide, dacarbazine, cisplatin, etc.) act by adding the alkyl groups to specific bases of DNA, yielding alkylated products such as O2-alkylthymine, O4-alkylthymine, O6-methylguanine, and O6-ethylguanine (Serrone et al., 2000; Emadi et al., 2009; Dasari and Tchounwou, 2014). Monofunctional alkylating agents have one active moiety and can only modify a single base, while bifunctional alkylating agents have two reaction sites, which can crosslink DNA to protein or another DNA base resulting in intra-strand crosslinks or inter-strand crosslinks. Radiotherapy by ionizing radiation (IR) can attack DNA directly by breaking the phosphodiester bond and the deoxyribose, and other indirect means have also been confirmed, for example, highly reactive oxygen species (ROS) produced from water radiolysis could result in the oxidization of the DNA desoxyribose moiety and the four nitrogenous bases (Henner et al., 1982; Desouky et al., 2015). Thereby, chemotherapy and radiotherapy can result in various kinds of DNA damage including base damage, single-strand breaks (SSBs), and double-strand breaks (DSBs). Among them, DSBs are thought to be the most harmful to cell survival and are the main mechanism to promote the therapeutic effect.

To remedy various DNA damage types, there has developed a complex DNA damage response (DDR) network (Giglia-Mari et al., 2011). The pathways involved in DNA damage repair mainly include direct reversal, base excision repair (BER), nucleotide excision repair (NER), non-homologous end joining (NHEJ), and homologous recombination (HR) pathway. Direct reversal, the simplest DNA repair pathway, depends primarily on a single protein and does not involve nucleotide removal, resynthesis, or ligation. For example, the O6-alkyl group of guanines can be removed by O6-methylguanine DNA methyltransferase (MGMT). BER and NER pathways take part in the DNA SSBs repairment. BER often participates in the repair of the small but highly mutagenic DNA lesions, which usually significantly undermine genomic fidelity and stability (Dianov and Hübscher, 2013). The BER pathway is initiated with the excision of the damaged base by any of 11 DNA glycosylases (Krokan et al., 1997), after which the exposed gap will be filled by a different set of proteins, among which the repair of single-base gaps require the short-patch pathway while polybasic gaps are in need of the long-patch pathway (Woodrick et al., 2017; Biau et al., 2019; Caldecott 2020). The NER pathway involves multiple steps requiring more than 30 proteins and is the main pathway used by mammals to remove bulky DNA lesions, including numerous chemical adducts, intra-strand crosslinking of DNA, and some forms of oxidative damage. In the NER pathway, the damaged bases are first recognized, then the DNA double-strand is unwound, and then the excision repair complex will remove the damaged bases followed by filling and ligating of the gap (Gillet and Schärer, 2006; Shuck et al., 2008).

DSB is a highly toxic gene damage that seriously threatens cellular homeostasis by affecting the transcription of genes, DNA replication, and chromosome segregation. Failure in repairing DSBs can lead to devastating chromosomal instabilities, and result in the dysregulation of gene expression and an increased hazard of carcinogenesis (Kryston et al., 2011). In human cells, two pathways, HDR and NHEJ, take part in DNA DSBs repair (Chang et al., 2017). HDR is generally considered to be participated in DSBs repair only during the S and G2 phases of the cell cycle given that it needs a homologous template to replace the damaged DNA segment in the genome, but it has been shown that centromeric DSBs in the G1 phase can activate the HDR pathway to maintain centromeric integrity recently (Yilmaz et al., 2021). The canonical HDR pathway is relatively slow but error-free, which needs numerous factors involved in homology search, Holliday junction formation, DNA synthesis, and the final DNA ligation (San Filippo et al., 2008; Krejci et al., 2012). Unlike the HR pathway, the NHEJ pathway does not need a DNA template and is active throughout the whole cell cycle, therefore it responds relatively quickly but is error-prone (Chang et al., 2017). In NHEJ pathway, four specific steps are involved including DNA termini recognition, bridging of the DNA ends, DNA end processing, and DNA ligation.

DNA REPAIR TARGETED THERAPY

Given that tumor cells could repair DNA damage induced by chemotherapy and radiotherapy in order to survive, the use of inhibitors of specific DNA repair pathways combined with DNA-damaging treatment can be efficacious. Some DNA repair inhibitors have been exploited as clinical agents targeting the proteins involved in sensing and conducting DNA damage signals as well as other proteins in DNA repair pathways (Mateo et al., 2019; Cheng et al., 2022).

DNA damage sensor proteins are key functional proteins to initiate repair and can sense multiple DNA damage signals, in which poly (ADP-ribosyl) polymerase-1 (PARP-1) is widely recognized to be the primary responder to SSBs while it could also bind and signal DSBs (Li and Yu 2013; Ceccaldi et al., 2015; Mateos-Gomez et al., 2015; Pandey and Black, 2021). After rapidly detecting the DNA damage, PARP-1 synthesizes of poly (ADP-ribose) (PAR) chains on itself and many different proteins near the damage site initiating recruitment of DNA repair complexes. The formation of the PAR chain can promote the release of PARP-1 from the position where it binds to the damaged DNA so that the other repair proteins could contact with the damaged site. Inhibition of PARP will reduce the synthesis of PAR chains, making PARP unable to dissociate from damaged DNA, thus preventing the recruitment of other repair proteins (Zandarashvili et al., 2020). The failure of PAR chain formation and the release of PARP from damaged DNA will lead to the enrichment of SSBs, which can be transformed into single-sided DSBs during DNA replication (Bixel and Hays, 2015). However, in the cells with the absence of intact DSBs repair pathways, such as in BRCA1 and BRCA2 mutated cells, the persistent DSBs are toxic and even deadly. Many small molecule PARP inhibitors (PARPi) targeting the catalytic activity of PARP-1 are now approved and clinically used in patients with breast, ovarian, prostate, and pancreatic cancers deficient in other DDR components, and the expanded utilities of small molecule PARP inhibitors in other cancer types are under consideration (Ramakrishnan Geethakumari et al., 2017; Zimmer et al., 2018; Hammel et al., 2020; Xie et al., 2020).

For DSBs, lupus Ku autoantigen protein (Ku) and the Mre11-Rad50-Nbs1 complex (MRN) play important roles. Ku is a protein heterodimer composed of Ku70/Ku80, which takes part in the NHEJ pathway and binds to DNA DSBs (Chen et al., 2021). Upon recognition and binding of DSBs, Ku recruits the DNA-dependent protein kinase catalytic subunit (DNA-PKcs) that assists in classical NHEJ repair. A class of compounds has been developed that abrogates the Ku-DNA end binding activity, inhibits cellular NHEJ, and enhances the cellular activity of radiomimetic agents and IR (Gavande et al., 2020). The MRN complex has nuclease activity and can bind DNA, so it can participate in the initial detection and processing of DSB (Rupnik et al., 2008), which is dependent on the nuclease activity of Mre11, the central factor of the MRN complex with endonuclease activity and 3′–5′ exonuclease activity (Stracker and Petrini, 2011). Upon bound to the damaged position, MRN recruits the DNA-damage signaling kinase ataxia-telangiectasia mutated (ATM), activates it, and triggers a series of signaling events that drive HR repair (Uziel et al., 2003). A class of inhibitors has been developed to selectively block the nuclease activity of Mre11 and prevent DNA damage repair (Dupré et al., 2008).

DNA damage signaling proteins trigger multiple post-translational modifications and the assembly of protein complexes, which amplify and diversify the DNA damage signals. Initially, one of three phosphatidylinositol-3 kinase-related kinases (PIKKs): DNA-PKcs, ATM, or ATM- and Rad3-Related (ATR) is activated by phosphorylation in response to DNA damage (Woods and Turchi, 2013). DNA-PKcs, forming a heterotrimeric complex with Ku, are required for proper DSBs repair by NHEJ. Using its activated kinase activity after being bound to the DNA terminus, it will phosphorylate itself and other target proteins to coordinates the NHEJ pathway (Falck et al., 2005; Uematsu et al., 2007). Following the appearance of DSB, the MRN complex activates ATM, which then phosphorylates histone H2AX as the main kinase (Burma et al., 2001). ATM could also phosphorylate checkpoint kinase 2 (Chk2) and p53 to impact cell cycle regulation and cytotoxicity (Cheng and Chen, 2010; Smith et al., 2010). ATR participates in HR, NER, long-patch BER, postreplication repair, interstrand cross-link repair, and replication fork restart after its activation by replication protein A (RPA)-coated ssDNA (Cimprich and Cortez, 2008). Several small molecules targeting three PIKKs such as VX-984 and CC-115 for DNA-PKcs, AZD0156 for ATM, VX-970, and AZD6738 for ATR are currently in different stages of clinical trials (Munster et al., 2016; Foote et al., 2018; Pike et al., 2018; Timme et al., 2018; Gorecki et al., 2020). In addition, checkpoint kinase 1 (Chk1) and Chk2, protein kinases that lie downstream of ATR and ATM, have also been utilized as therapeutic targets for drug development (Jobson et al., 2009; King et al., 2014).

NUCLEIC ACID-SENSING PATHWAYS CONNECT DNA DAMAGE TO INNATE IMMUNITY

Cancer chemotherapy and radiotherapy aim to induce catastrophic DNA damage such as DSBs to cause cancer cell apoptosis, which can further aggravate the degree of DNA damage and promote the therapeutic effect when combined with DNA damage repair inhibitors. According to the severity of the DNA damage, some cancer cells directly initiate programmed cell death to clear the damaged genome beyond endurance. Besides, nucleic acid released from dying cells can activate the innate immune response of surrounding cells (Wang et al., 2021b). Even if DNA damage does not directly kill cells, increasing evidence indicates that the accumulation of nucleic acids in the cytoplasm caused by DNA damage can also trigger an inflammatory response within the cells (Nastasi et al., 2020). DNA damage-induced cytosolic nucleic acid shares common receptors (pattern recognition receptors, PRRs) and downstream effectors with those induced by viral or bacterial infections (Takeuchi and Akira, 2010; Taffoni et al., 2021), which are summarized below (**Figure 1**). And some agonists of these nucleic acid-sensing pathways are already in clinical trials (**Table 1**). Strikingly, recent research has indicated that the proteins that participated in DNA repair also play active roles in innate immune signaling.

DNA Sensing Pathways

Cyclic GMP-AMP Synthase

Normally, DNA is trapped in the nucleus and mitochondria and rapidly degraded by nucleases in the cytoplasm and endolysosomes. DNA-sensing receptors could detect increased amounts of intracellular DNA. Currently, cyclic GMP-AMP synthase (cGAS), a nucleotidyltransferase (NTase), is the most widely accepted dsDNA sensor that acts followed by stimulator of interferon genes (STING) performing multiple functions (Kuchta et al., 2009; Sun et al., 2013; Wu et al., 2013). cGAS normally resides to be inactive. Initial studies considered cGAS as a cytoplasmic protein, in which cGAS could not interact with nuclear or mitochondrial DNA, but some recent works indicate that cGAS also resides in the nucleus constitutively (Gentili et al., 2019; Jiang et al., 2019; Volkman et al., 2019). cGAS can be activated not only by viral or bacterial infection-related DNA entering the cytoplasm but also by endogenous self-DNA, including cytosolic DNA from nucleus and mitochondria, DNA in cytoplasmic micronucleus, and chromatin in the nucleus (Li X.-D. et al., 2013; West et al., 2015; Dou et al., 2017; Glück et al., 2017; Harding et al., 2017; Mackenzie et al., 2017; Gratia et al., 2019). Upon binding to DNA, cGAS assembles into a dimer at an active state and converts ATP and GTP into the second messenger cyclic GMP-AMP (cGAMP) (Ablasser et al., 2013; Diner et al., 2013; Gao et al., 2013; Zhang et al., 2013). The complete activation and stabilization of cGAS-DNA complexes require DNA lengths to exceed a certain threshold, allowing two or more cGAS molecules to bind to the same DNA to form oligomeric structures or condensates (Li X. et al., 2013; Zhang J.-Z. et al., 2014; Andreeva et al., 2017; Luecke et al., 2017; Du and Chen, 2018; Hooy and Sohn, 2018). The cyclic-dinucleotide sensor STING, an ~40 kDa dimeric transmembrane protein located in the endoplasmic reticulum (ER), could detect and bind to cGAMP to make a conformational change, which results in its translocation from the ER to the Golgi apparatus and the activation of TANK-binding kinase 1 (TBK1) (Ishikawa and Barber, 2008; Burdette et al., 2011; Liu et al., 2015; Ergun et al., 2019; Shang et al., 2019; Zhang et al., 2019; Zhao et al., 2019). The activated TBK1 phosphorylates itself, STING, and the interferon regulatory factor 3 (IRF3), after which the active IRF3 dimer is transported to the nucleus to activate the expression of type I interferon genes. The cGAS-STING signaling can also lead to the transcription of pro-inflammatory cytokines-related genes

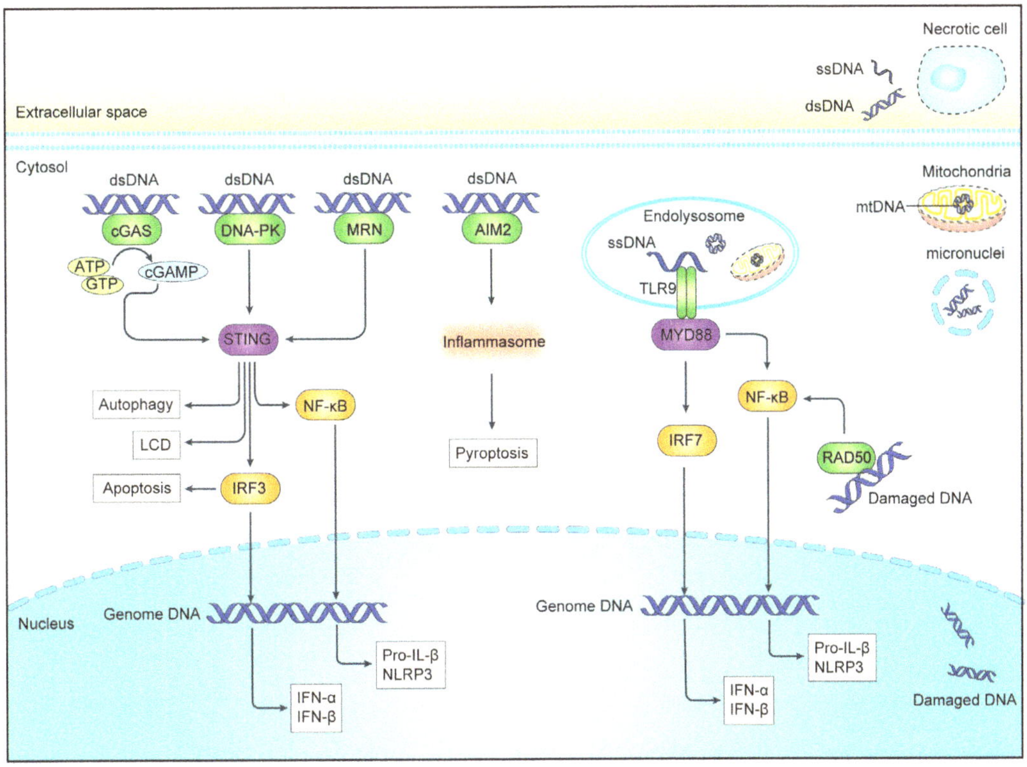

FIGURE 1 | DNA sensing pathways triggered by DNA damage. An abnormal increase of intracellular DNA could come from the nucleus, micronuclei, or mitochondria after chemotherapy or radiation. DNA in endosomal may be from extracellular DNA of necrotic cells through endocytosis or cytoplasmic DNA through autophagy. Sensors for DNA are shown in green, including cGAS, DNA-PK, MRN, AIM2, and RAD50 in the cytoplasm, and TLR9 in the endolysosome. Adaptor molecules are shown in pink and downstream signaling molecules are shown in yellow. Activation of these pathways may result in the production of interferon (IFN) and other cytokines, apoptosis, pyroptosis, autophagy, etc., cGAS, cyclic GMP-AMP synthase; DNA-PK, DNA-dependent protein kinase complex; MRN, Mre11-Rad50-Nbs1 complex; AIM2, absent in melanoma 2; TLR9, Toll-like receptor 9; cGAMP, cyclic GMP-AMP; STING, stimulator of interferon genes; MYD88, myeloid differentiation primary response protein 88; IRF3/7, interferon regulatory factor 3/7; NF-κB, nuclear factor-κB; NLRP3, NOD-, LRR- and pyrin domain-containing 3; LCD, a lytic cell death program; dsDNA, double stranded DNA; ssDNA, single stranded DNA; mtDNA, mitochondrial DNA.

via nuclear factor-κB (NF-κB) (de Oliveira Mann et al., 2019). In addition, STING is related to autophagy induction, however, its functional mechanism still remains to be elucidated (Watson et al., 2012). Growing studies suggest that the activation of STING can trigger cell death by various means. For example, STING could facilitate respective programmed cell death by inducing the production of many pro-apoptotic and pro-necroptotic molecules (Paludan et al., 2019). Furthermore, the accumulation of lysosomal STING could trigger lysosome membrane permeabilization, leading to the release of lysosomal hydrolases with cell death as a result (Gaidt et al., 2017). Besides, phosphorylated IRF3 downstream of STING can stimulate apoptosis by reducing the Bcl-xL-dependent suppression of the permeability of mitochondrial outer membrane in mitotic cells (Zierhut et al., 2019; Xie et al., 2021).

Toll-Like Receptors 9

Toll-like receptors (TLRs) are important components of innate immune responses induced by pathogenic microorganisms or tissue injury (Moresco et al., 2011). TLR, a highly conserved intracellular transmembrane protein, has emerged as a key PRR in the past 20 years. It exists in multiple types of cells, such as T cells, B cells, APC, epithelial cells, and endothelial cells (Chang 2010). All TLRs possess a leucine-rich-repeat (LRR) domain binding ligand extracellularly, a transmembrane domain, and a cytosolic Toll/IL-1 receptor (TIR) homology domain (Delneste et al., 2007). In all TLRs, TLR9 is found specifically in the endosomes and can be activated by single-stranded DNA containing unmethylated cytidine-phosphate-guanosine (CpG) dinucleotides escaping from the digestion of nucleases such as DNase II (Kumagai et al., 2008). TLR9 must undergo proteolytic processing in the endosomal compartments to complete ligand-mediated dimerization and activation (Majer et al., 2017). TLR9 not only triggers plasmacytoid dendritic cells to produce type I IFN and activate the polyclonal B cells through the myeloid differentiation primary response protein 88 (MYD88) and interferon-regulatory factor 7 (IRF7) signaling pathway, but also induces the production of inflammasome-related factors pro-interleukin-1β (pro-IL-1β) and NOD-, LRR- and pyrin domain-containing 3 (NLRP3) *via* NF-κB (Honda et al., 2005; Zhang X. et al., 2014). According to a recent study, TLR9 can sense mitochondrial DNA during mitophagy, and induce C-X-C motif chemokine ligand 10 (CXCL10) expression and $CD8^+$ T cell recruitment, which reveals a novel role of chemotherapy in the innate immune response (Limagne et al., 2022).

TABLE 1 | Summary of clinical trials of nucleic acid-sensing pathways-related agonists.

PRR	ClinicalTrials.gov Identifier	Agent(s)	Route of administration	Cancer type(s)	Clinical phase of development
STING	NCT04144140	E7766	Intratumoral	Lymphoma; advanced solid tumors	Phase 1/1b
STING	NCT04609579	SNX281 (or in combination with pembrolizumab)	Intravenous	Advanced solid tumor; advanced lymphoma	Phase 1
STING	NCT05070247	TAK-500 (or in combination with pembrolizumab)	Intravenous	Select locally advanced; metastatic solid tumors	Phase 1
TLR	NCT00960752	R848 gel (in combination with gp100 and MAGE-3 peptide vaccine)	Intradermally and subcutaneously	Melanoma	Phase 2
TLR	NCT02668770	MGN1703 (in combination with ipilimumab)	Subcutaneously and intratumoral injection	Advanced cancers; melanoma	Phase 1
TLR3	NCT03734692	Rintatolimod (in combination with cisplatin and pembrolizumab)	Intraperitoneal	Ovarian cancer recurrent	Phase 1; Phase 2
TLR7	NCT00899574	Imiquimod	Cream	Breast cancer; breast neoplasms	Phase 2
TLR7	NCT00941811	Imiquimod	Cream	HPV	Phase 2
TLR7	NCT01421017	Imiquimod (in combination with cyclophosphamide or radiotherapy)	Cream	Breast cancer; metastatic breast cancer; recurrent breast cancer	Phase 1; Phase 2
TLR7	NCT03416335	DSP-0509 (or in combination with pembrolizumab)	Intravenous	Neoplasms	Phase 1; Phase 2
TLR7	NCT04101357	BNT411 (or in combination with atezolizumab, carboplatin and etoposide)	Intravenous	Solid tumor; extensive-stage small cell lung cancer	Phase 1; Phase 2
TLR7	NCT04338685	RO7119929 (in combination with Tocilizumab)	Oral	Carcinoma; hepatocellular; biliary tract cancer; secondary liver cancer; liver metastases	Phase 1
TLR7	NCT04588324	SHR2150 (or in combination with chemotherapy plus PD-1 or CD47 antibody)	Oral	Solid tumor	Phase 1; Phase 2
TLR7/8	NCT00821652	Resiquimod (in combination with NY-ESO-1 protein vaccination)	Subcutaneously	Tumors	Phase 1
TLR7/8	NCT04278144	BDC-1001 (or in combination with nivolumabe)	Intravenous	HER2 positive solid tumors	Phase 1; Phase 2
TLR7/8	NCT04799054	TransCon (or in combination with pembrolizumab)	Intratumoral	Advanced solid tumor; locally advanced solid tumor; metastatic solid tumor	Phase 1; Phase 2
TLR7/8	NCT04840394	BDB018 (or in combination with pembrolizumab)	Intravenous	Advanced solid tumors	Phase 1
TLR8	NCT01294293	VTX-2337 (in combination with pegylated liposomal doxorubicin hydrochloride or paclitaxel)	Subcutaneously	Ovarian epithelial; fallopian tube; peritoneal cavity cancer	Phase 1
TLR8	NCT01334177	VTX-2337 (in combination with cetuximab)	Subcutaneously	Locally advanced; recurrent; metastatic squamous cell cancer of head and neck	Phase 1
TLR8	NCT01666444	VTX-2337 (in combination with pegylated liposomal doxorubicin)	Intravenous	Epithelial ovarian cancer; fallopian tube cancer; primary peritoneal cancer	Phase 2
TLR8	NCT01836029	VTX-2337 (in combination with chemotherapy and cetuximab)	Intravenous	Carcinoma; squamous cell of head and neck	Phase 2
TLR8	NCT03906526	VTX-2337 (or in combination with nivolumabe)	Subcutaneously or intratumoral injection	Carcinoma; squamous cell	Phase 1
TLR9	NCT00185965	CPG 7909 (in combination with radiation therapy)	Intratumoral	Recurrent low-grade lymphomas	Phase 1; Phase 2
TLR9	NCT02254772	SD-101 (in combination with ipilimumab and radiation therapy)	Intratumoral	Recurrent low-grade B-cell lymphoma	Phase 1; Phase 2
TLR9	NCT02927964	SD-101 (in combination with Ibrutinib and radiation therapy)	Intratumoral	Relapsed or refractory grade 1–3A follicular lymphoma	Phase 1; Phase 2
TLR9	NCT03410901	SD-101 (in combination with anti-OX40 antibody BMS 986178 and radiation therapy)	Intratumoral	Low-grade B-cell non-hodgkin lymphomas	Phase 1
TLR9	NCT03618641	CMP-001 (in combination with nivolumab)	Intravenous	Melanomal; lymph node cancer	Phase 2
TLR9	NCT03831295	SD-101 (in combination with anti-OX40 antibody BMS 986178)	Intratumoral	Advanced malignant solid neoplasm; extracranial solid neoplasm; metastatic malignant solid neoplasm	Phase 1
TLR9	NCT04050085	SD-101 (in combination with nivolumab and radiation therapy)	Intratumoral	Chemotherapy-refractory metastatic pancreatic cancer	Phase 1
TLR9	NCT04270864	Tilsotolimod (in combination with ipilimumab and nivolumab)	Intratumoral	Advanced cancer	Phase 1
TLR9	NCT04387071	CMP-001 (in combination with INCAGN01949)	Intratumoral	Stage IV pancreatic; other cancers except melanoma	Phase 1; Phase 2

(Continued on following page)

TABLE 1 | *(Continued)* Summary of clinical trials of nucleic acid-sensing pathways-related agonists.

PRR	ClinicalTrials.gov Identifier	Agent(s)	Route of administration	Cancer type(s)	Clinical phase of development
TLR9	NCT04401995	Vidutolimod (in combination with nivolumab)	Subcutaneously and intratumoral injection	Melanoma	Phase 2
TLR9	NCT04708418	CMP-001 (in combination with pembrolizumab)	Subcutaneously and intratumoral injection	Operable melanoma	Phase 2
TLR9	NCT04935229	SD-101 (or in combination with nivolumab or ipilimumab)	Pressure-enabled hepatic artery infusion	Metastatic uveal melanoma in the liver	Phase 1
TLR9	NCT05220722	SD-101 (in combination with checkpoint blockade)	Pressure-enabled hepatic artery infusion	Hepatocellular carcinoma; intrahepatic cholangiocarcinoma	Phase 1; Phase 2

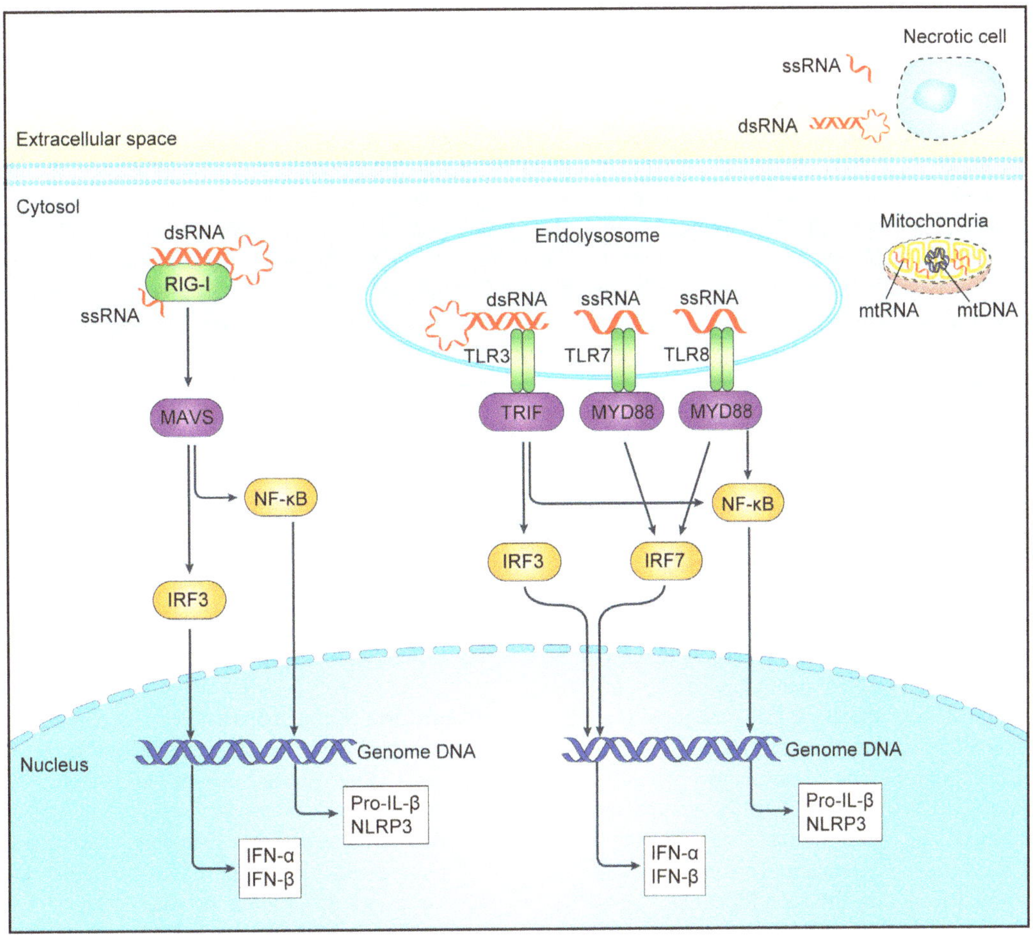

FIGURE 2 | RNA sensing pathways triggered by DNA damage. Aberrant increase of intracellular RNA could be from mitochondria after chemotherapy or radiation. RNA in endosomal may be from extracellular RNA of necrotic cells through endocytosis or cytoplasmic RNA through autophagy. Sensors for RNA are shown in green, including RIG-1 in the cytoplasm, and TLR3/7/8 in the endolysosome. Adaptor molecules are shown in pink and downstream signaling molecules are shown in yellow. Activation of these pathways may result in the production of interferon (IFN) and other cytokines, etc. RIG-I, a retinoic acid-inducible gene I; TLR3/7/8, Toll-like receptor 3/7/8; MAVS, mitochondrial antiviral signaling protein; TRIF, Toll-like receptor adaptor molecule 1; MYD88, myeloid differentiation primary response protein 88; IRF3/7, interferon regulatory factor 3/7; NF-κB, nuclear factor-κB; dsRNA, double stranded RNA; ssRNA, single stranded RNA; mtRNA, mitochondrial RNA; mtDNA, mitochondrial DNA.

Absent in Melanoma 2

The absent in melanoma 2 (AIM2), containing pyrin and HIN domains, takes an important part in inflammasome activation as the dsDNA-sensing receptor in the cytoplasm of cells (Fernandes-Alnemri et al., 2009; Hornung et al., 2009). The N-terminal pyrin domain (PYD) of AIM2 could interact with apoptosis-associated speck-like protein (ASC), which possesses a caspase recruitment domain (CARD) and a C-terminal HIN domain sensing cytoplasmic DNA (Hornung et al., 2009; Wang and Yin, 2017). The recruitment of ASC leads to the generation of fibrilar super-structures, to which Caspase-1 is bound by CARD-CARD interactions (Miao et al., 2011; Lugrin and Martinon, 2018). The oligomerization of ASC leads to the activation of some proteins such as the conversion of pro-IL-1β into the biologically active IL-1β. The inflammasome can also trigger pro-inflammatory pyroptosis (Liang et al., 2020). Gasdermins family proteins are the important factors mediating inflammatory cell death (Kovacs and Miao, 2017), in which Gasdermin D (GSDMD) can be cleaved by Caspase-1 to release the N-terminal of Gasdermin so that it can polymerize and cause perforation of the plasma membrane, allowing the intracellular substance to leak out, causing cell death (Lammert et al., 2020). It is well known that AIM2 can detect dsDNA in the cytosol, but recent studies have found that AIM2 can also sense DSBs directly within the nucleus to induce intestinal epithelial cells and bone marrow cells to initiate the caspase-1-dependent death (Hu et al., 2016).

DNA-PK Complex

Recent findings reveal that some proteins in DNA repair also take part in the sense of foreign DNA in the cytosol. DNA-dependent protein kinase (DNA-PK) complex assembled from Ku70/Ku80 heterodimer and the kinase subunit (DNA-PKcs) can sense DNA DSBs in response to repair the DNA damage in the NHEJ pathway, and Ku has also been reported to detect viral DNA in human cells as a PRR to induce type I and type III interferons or pro-inflammatory cytokines (Abe et al., 2019). DNA stimulates the Ku complex to translocate into the cytoplasm and bind to the dsDNA terminals using its middle domain independent of DNA sequence (Sui et al., 2021a; Sui et al., 2021b). Numerous studies have reported that STING is the downstream adaptor of Ku to induce type I/III interferons and inflammatory cytokines *via* phosphorylation of IRF3 (Sui et al., 2017). Ku complex is abundantly expressed in aged human and mouse $CD4^+$ T cells, and it recognizes accumulating cytoplasmic DNA in the cytoplasm, which facilitates the recruitment of DNA-PKcs and phosphorylation of the kinase ZAK, ultimately promoting the proliferation and activation of $CD4^+$ T cells (Wang et al., 2021a).

Mre11-Rad50-Nbs1 Complex

MRN complex consisting of two MRE11 subunits, two RAD50 units, and two NBS1 subunits, can sense and respond to DNA damage firstly in DDR to orchestrate DDR response in DSBs and replication fork collapse (Zhu et al., 2018; Tisi et al., 2020). The hetero-hexamers MRN complex could conduct ATP hydrolysis of RAD50, bind multiple DNA molecules, and link DNA molecules with exonuclease and endonuclease (Kondo et al., 2013). RAD50 could recognize cytosolic dsDNA and bind caspase-recruitment domain (CARD9), a pro-inflammatory signaling adaptor, to its zinc-hook region, which tends to recruit Bcl-10, leading to the activation of NF-κB and the generation of pro-inflammatory cytokine IL-1β (Roth et al., 2014).

RNA Sensing Pathways

Toll-Like Receptor 3/7/8

In mammalian cells, both single-stranded and double-stranded RNA can be recognized by PRR as pathogen-associated molecular patterns (PAMPs) or damage-associated molecular patterns (DAMPs) (**Figure 2**). RNA from necrotic cells may be internalized by cells *via* clathrin-dependent endocytosis, or it can enter cells after complexation with peptides or within immune complexes (Lövgren et al., 2004; Barrat et al., 2005; Itoh et al., 2008; Ganguly et al., 2009). The activation of TLR, a type I transmembrane protein, is required for inducing innate and adaptive immune responses, among which TLR3 can recognize double-stranded RNA and structured RNA containing a partial stem in secondary structures of single-stranded RNA, and TLR7/8 can recognize the fragments of single-stranded RNA (Alexopoulou et al., 2001; Karikó et al., 2004; Cavassani et al., 2008; Tatematsu et al., 2013). Depending on the intracellular compartments to recognize ligands, discriminate self-and non-self-derived nucleic acids, TLRs activate the downstream signaling pathways (Gay et al., 2014). Upon ligand binding, the dimers of TLRs will emerge after binding ligands to recruit the cytosolic adaptor proteins with TIR domain, such as MyD88 and Toll-like receptor adaptor molecule 1 (TRIF) (Yamamoto et al., 2003; Vyncke et al., 2016). The recruitment of MyD88 could activate NF-κB through type I interferon induction by IRF7 and tumor necrosis factor receptor-associated factor 6 (TRAF6). Intriguingly, among the TLRs, only TLR3 could signal to induce the generation of type I interferon and proinflammatory cytokines by the recruitment of TRIF rather than depending on MyD88 (Oshiumi et al., 2003).

(RIG-I)-Like Receptors

RLRs are composed of retinoic acid-inducible gene I (RIG-I), melanoma differentiation-associated protein 5 (MDA5), and laboratory of genetics and physiology2 (LGP2), which can help the innate immune system sense cytosolic RNA (Kang et al., 2004; Yoneyama et al., 2004; Yoneyama et al., 2005; Ori et al., 2017). RIG-I and MDA5 contain two CARDs at the N-terminus, a DExD/H box RNA helicase domain in the central and a C-terminal domain (CTD), which mediate downstream signaling by sensing RNA. MDA5 preferentially recognizes dsRNA longer than 1 kb unlike RIG-I, which could bind relatively short dsRNA (Kato et al., 2008; Goubau et al., 2014). The CARD domains of RIG-I and MDA5 oligomerize after binding to dsRNA and tend to interact with the CARD of mitochondrial antiviral signaling protein (MAVS) (Kawai et al., 2005; Seth et al., 2005). Then the oligomerization of MAVS occurs after binding to RIG-I or MDA5 to form prion-like aggregates, upon which the downstream signaling pathways can be activated (Hou et al., 2011). Besides, MAVS could trigger the transcription of type I IFNs *via* IRF3 or IRF7 by activating TBK1, and the transcription of inflammatory cytokines *via* NF-κB by activating the IKK complex (IKKα, IKKβ, NEMO) (Goubau et al., 2013; Ori et al., 2017).

Recent research has found that the DNA fragments released from ionizing radiation-induced double-strand DNA breaks could activate both the cGAS/STING-dependent DNA-sensing pathway and the MAVS-dependent RNA sensing pathway (Feng et al., 2020). Interestingly, chemotherapeutic agents and ionizing radiation can also lead to mitochondrial DNA double-strand breaks (mtDSBs). After mtDNA breaks, BAX and BAK mediate herniation, then the mitochondrial RNA will be released into the cytoplasm, triggering the RIG-I-MAVS-dependent immune response (Tigano et al., 2021). These studies suggest that DNA damage can also activate innate immune responses through RNA sensing pathways.

THE IMPACTS OF NUCLEIC ACID-SENSING PATHWAYS ON DNA REPAIR

Cyclic GMP-AMP Synthase-Stimulator of Interferon Genes

As mentioned above, several DDR proteins, such as DNA-PK and MRN complex, can not only can participate in the DNA repair, but also take part in the onset of inflammatory responses. Conversely, PRRs, first discovered to sense immune-stimulatory nucleic acids, have also been found to take part in the regulation of DDR. Previously, cGAS-STING signaling was simply identified as a response pathway to cytosol dsDNA, however, they have recently been found to function in DNA repair, independent of interferon response. cGAS could inhibit the repair of DNA DSBs by HR without relying on STING and the catalytic activity of cGAS (Hopfner and Hornung, 2020). There are two mechanisms for cGAS-dependent HR inhibition. In one of them, because it has been found at the sites of chromosomal damage marked by PARP1 and γ-H2AX, cGAS could prevent the recruitment of proteins necessary for the HR process by interacting with γ-H2AX and PAR (Liu et al., 2018). On the other hand, subsequent work suggested that cGAS could prevent RAD51-DNA filaments to pair and the broken DNA strand from invading into the homologous strand by binding the homologous dsDNA template to form oligomeric clusters (Jiang et al., 2019). However, the detailed mechanism remains to be investigated further.

STING has been confirmed to promote DDR and enable cell survival without cGAS, though they are partners (Cheradame et al., 2021). Downregulation of STING increases cell death and makes breast cancer cells more sensitive to genotoxic treatment. Following chemotherapy regimens, some STINGs are found to be located at the inner nuclear membrane and bind the NHEJ proteins DNA-PKcs, Ku70, and Ku80, suggesting that STING may control NHEJ-mediated DNA repair by cooperating with DNA-PK (Ferguson et al., 2012; Morchikh et al., 2017; Sui et al., 2017; Cheradame et al., 2021). Regrettably, its specific mechanism remains unclear.

Recent research has proposed a novel mechanism that IR-induced DNA damages would trigger the phosphorylation and activation of phosphoribosyl pyrophosphate synthetases PRPS1/2 *via* ATM and cGAS/STING/TBK1, which could promote the synthesis of deoxyribonucleotide given that the PRPSs are the rate-limiting enzymes. Then the increased deoxyribonucleotide will help for DNA repair. Nevertheless, it remains to be clarified how the cells respond to DNA damage *via* the cGAS-STING pathway under different contexts (Kornberg et al., 1955; Hove-Jensen, 1988; Liu et al., 2021).

Toll-Like Receptors

TLRs are the key members of the innate immune system, functioning as the first line of defense against multiple injurious substances (Trinchieri and Sher, 2007; Barton and Kagan, 2009; Kawai and Akira, 2011). Recent literature has shown that activation of TLRs could also promote DNA repair by upregulating the expression of DNA repair genes, apart from upregulating cellular defense systems. Upon TLR9 stimulation, there is a significant increase of mRNAs to participate in adjusting cell cycles and DNA repair after CpG DNA is injected into the abdominal cavity (Zheng et al., 2008; Klaschik et al., 2010; Sommariva et al., 2011). And NER gene expression is increased by treating bone marrow-derived cell lines with the TLR7/8 agonist (Imiquimod) *in vitro* (Fishelevich et al., 2011). It has been deduced that TLR signaling pathways may result in transcriptional activation of DNA repair machinery through direct and indirect mechanisms. The promoter regions of many genes involved in DNA repair contain the binding sites of activator protein-1 (AP-1) (Xiao et al., 1993; Zhong et al., 2000). The transcriptional control of DNA repair might be linked to TLR agonist treatment through the transcriptional activation function of the AP-1. On the other hand, DNA repair can be promoted because the activated TLR could induce the generation of cytokines. The cytokines such as IL-12 may be sensed by their appropriate cytokine receptor, leading to the increased transcription levels of DNA repair genes (Majewski et al., 2010). However, increased DNA repair is detrimental for cancer treatment. The previous study has found that TLR9 agonist treatment upregulates the genes associated with DNA repair in immune cells but downregulates them in tumor cells, which is contributed to the death of cancer cells (Sommariva et al., 2011). Those conflicting data highlight the need for further research into how immune versus stromal cells, and normal versus cancerous cells respond to TLR agonists, as well as related DNA repair and cell survival.

AIM2-Like Receptors

AIM2-like receptors (ALRs) are a large family of structurally related proteins that are generally considered to act as intracellular DNA sensors alerting the innate immune system. Recent studies reveal that ALRs perform different functions outside the immune system. It has been demonstrated that DNA breaks are repaired more efficiently in mice and cells lacking ALRs ($ALR^{-/-}$ mice lack the entire ALR locus containing all 13 ALR genes on Chromosome 13), resulting in the stronger resistance to the genotoxic effects of irradiation and chemotherapy (Brunette et al., 2012; Gray et al., 2016; Jiang et al., 2021). Mechanistically, nuclear ALRs limit DNA repair machinery access to damaged sites by binding the chromatin, and self-oligomerization promoted chromatin compaction. These findings reveal that ALRs could be the possible target for new interventions against genotoxic tissue injury, but more research into the different members of the ALR family is needed.

CONCLUSION AND FUTURE PERSPECTIVE

Targeting DDR factors in tumors has achieved outstanding success over the last decade, especially PARP inhibitors for cancer therapy. Recently, we have gained an improved understanding of the molecular mechanism of how DNA damage is interconnected to cellular innate immunity, which plays essential roles in the therapeutic efficacy of DNA repair targeted treatments (Pantelidou et al., 2019). Damaged nucleic acids also shape adaptive immune responses by activating innate immune cells. Accumulation of nucleic acids from necrotic cells can induce type I IFNs and other immune-regulatory cytokines production from bystander cells [e.g., dendritic cells (DCs)] to promote antitumor immunity through nucleic acid-sensing pathways. The DCs activated by the type I IFNs secretion will be transported to tumor-draining lymph nodes and cross-prime naïve $CD8^+$ T lymphocytes (Ellermeier et al., 2013; Duewell et al., 2014; Klarquist et al., 2014; Woo et al., 2014). The cancer-induced host response and tumor rejection relies heavily on the immunological responses to danger DAMPs signals.

Immune checkpoint blockade (ICB), as a promising therapeutic strategy, has made tremendous strides in recent years providing an alternative to irradiation therapy or traditional chemotherapies. Unfortunately, the efficacy of ICB is limited to only a subgroup of cancer patients (depending on the type of the tumor), with an overall response rate of about 20% for all malignancies to date (Hargadon et al., 2018; Chowell et al., 2021). ICB is effective in "hot" tumors with T cell infiltration rather than in "cold" tumors lacking T cell infiltration (Petitprez et al., 2020). Novel strategies for activating innate immunity within the TME to promote the antitumor immune responses have emerged in recent years, with the goal of eradicating the disease in "cold" tumors (Iurescia et al., 2018). Agonists of the nucleic acid-sensing pathways (such as cGAMP, agonists of STING) have been applied to eradicate tumor mass and induce a durable anti-tumor immune response (Chin et al., 2020; Pan et al., 2020). However, since some PRRs are involved in DDR and tumorigenesis, the impact of nucleic acid-sensing pathways on DNA repair cannot be ignored in therapeutic strategies aiming at promoting the activation of nucleic acid-sensing pathways.

As DDR inhibitors can trigger innate immune responses, DDR inhibition could be effective in combination with ICBs. The DDR inhibitors that target PARP have been investigated the most in anticancer immunotherapies. PARP inhibition could increase $CD8^+$ T-cell infiltration and IFN-γ generation in tumors, and promote the tumor regression when used accompanied with anti-PD-1 antibody (Pantelidou et al., 2019; Shen et al., 2019). Recently, many other regents inhibiting DDR components have been developed and used preclinically (Cleary et al., 2020). DDR inhibition strategies combined with other therapeutic strategies possess tremendous potential to improve the effectiveness of cancer treatment because of their immunomodulatory effect on radiation and chemotherapies and immune checkpoint blocking. Furthermore, in order to kill tumor cells more precisely, innovative approaches (such as nanoparticles, viral particles, and targeted deliveries) beneficial to the precise delivery of a chemotherapeutic drug, DDR inhibitors, or nucleic acid-sensing pathways agonists to tumors can be used to induce local specific antitumor immune responses, which could significantly expand the therapeutic window for their use in cancer immunotherapies (Gentili et al., 2015; Wilson et al., 2018; Wang et al., 2020; Xu et al., 2021).

AUTHOR CONTRIBUTIONS

BX and AL drafted the manuscript. All authors contributed to the article and approved the submitted version.

REFERENCES

Abe, T., Marutani, Y., and Shoji, I. (2019). Cytosolic DNA-Sensing Immune Response and Viral Infection. *Microbiol. Immunol.* 63, 51–64. doi:10.1111/1348-0421.12669

Ablasser, A., Goldeck, M., Cavlar, T., Deimling, T., Witte, G., Röhl, I., et al. (2013). cGAS Produces a 2′-5′-linked Cyclic Dinucleotide Second Messenger that Activates STING. *Nature* 498, 380–384. doi:10.1038/nature12306

Alexopoulou, L., Holt, A. C., Medzhitov, R., and Flavell, R. A. (2001). Recognition of Double-Stranded RNA and Activation of NF-Kb by Toll-like Receptor 3. *Nature* 413, 732–738. doi:10.1038/35099560

Andreeva, L., Hiller, B., Kostrewa, D., Lässig, C., de Oliveira Mann, C. C., Jan Drexler, D., et al. (2017). cGAS Senses Long and HMGB/TFAM-bound U-Turn DNA by Forming Protein-DNA Ladders. *Nature* 549, 394–398. doi:10.1038/nature23890

Barrat, F. J., Meeker, T., Gregorio, J., Chan, J. H., Uematsu, S., Akira, S., et al. (2005). Nucleic Acids of Mammalian Origin Can Act as Endogenous Ligands for Toll-like Receptors and May Promote Systemic Lupus Erythematosus. *J. Exp. Med.* 202, 1131–1139. doi:10.1084/jem.20050914

Barton, G. M., and Kagan, J. C. (2009). A Cell Biological View of Toll-like Receptor Function: Regulation through Compartmentalization. *Nat. Rev. Immunol.* 9, 535–542. doi:10.1038/nri2587

Biau, J., Chautard, E., Verrelle, P., and Dutreix, M. (2019). Altering DNA Repair to Improve Radiation Therapy: Specific and Multiple Pathway Targeting. *Front. Oncol.* 9, 1009. Epub 2019/10/28. doi:10.3389/fonc.2019.01009

Bixel, K., and Hays, J. (2015). Olaparib in the Management of Ovarian Cancer. *Pgpm* 8, 127–135. Epub 2015/08/27. doi:10.2147/pgpm.s62809

Bouwman, P., and Jonkers, J. (2012). The Effects of Deregulated DNA Damage Signalling on Cancer Chemotherapy Response and Resistance. *Nat. Rev. Cancer* 12, 587–598. Epub 2012/08/25. doi:10.1038/nrc3342

Brunette, R. L., Young, J. M., Whitley, D. G., Brodsky, I. E., Malik, H. S., and Stetson, D. B. (2012). Extensive Evolutionary and Functional Diversity Among Mammalian AIM2-like Receptors. *J. Exp. Med.* 209, 1969–1983. doi:10.1084/jem.20121960

Burdette, D. L., Monroe, K. M., Sotelo-Troha, K., Iwig, J. S., Eckert, B., Hyodo, M., et al. (2011). STING Is a Direct Innate Immune Sensor of Cyclic Di-GMP. *Nature* 478, 515–518. doi:10.1038/nature10429

Burma, S., Chen, B. P., Murphy, M., Kurimasa, A., and Chen, D. J. (2001). ATM Phosphorylates Histone H2AX in Response to DNA Double-Strand Breaks. *J. Biol. Chem.* 276, 42462–42467. Epub 2001/09/26. doi:10.1074/jbc.c100466200

Caldecott, K. W. (2020). Mammalian DNA Base Excision Repair: Dancing in the Moonlight. *DNA Repair* 93, 102921. Epub 2020/10/23. doi:10.1016/j.dnarep.2020.102921

Cavassani, K. A., Ishii, M., Wen, H., Schaller, M. A., Lincoln, P. M., Lukacs, N. W., et al. (2008). TLR3 Is an Endogenous Sensor of Tissue Necrosis during Acute Inflammatory Events. *J. Exp. Med.* 205, 2609–2621. doi:10.1084/jem.20081370

Ceccaldi, R., Liu, J. C., Amunugama, R., Hajdu, I., Primack, B., O'Connor, M. I. R., et al. (2015). Homologous-recombination-deficient Tumours Are Dependent on Polθ-Mediated Repair. *Nature* 518, 258–262. doi:10.1038/nature14184

Chang, H. H. Y., Pannunzio, N. R., Adachi, N., and Lieber, M. R. (2017). Non-homologous DNA End Joining and Alternative Pathways to Double-Strand Break Repair. *Nat. Rev. Mol. Cell Biol* 18, 495–506. Epub 2017/05/18. doi:10.1038/nrm.2017.48

Chang, Z. L. (2010). Important Aspects of Toll-like Receptors, Ligands and Their Signaling Pathways. *Inflamm. Res.* 59, 791–808. doi:10.1007/s00011-010-0208-2

Chatterjee, N., and Walker, G. C. (2017). Mechanisms of DNA Damage, Repair, and Mutagenesis. *Environ. Mol. Mutagen.* 58, 235–263. Epub 2017/05/10. doi:10.1002/em.22087

Chen, X., Xu, X., Chen, Y., Cheung, J. C., Wang, H., Jiang, J., et al. (2021). Structure of an Activated DNA-PK and its Implications for NHEJ. *Mol. Cell* 81, 801–810. e803Epub 2021/01/02. doi:10.1016/j.molcel.2020.12.015

Cheng, B., Pan, W., Xing, Y., Xiao, Y., Chen, J., and Xu, Z. (2022). Recent Advances in DDR (DNA Damage Response) Inhibitors for Cancer Therapy. *Eur. J. Med. Chem.* 230, 114109. Epub 2022/01/21. doi:10.1016/j.ejmech.2022.114109

Cheng, Q., and Chen, J. (2010). Mechanism of P53 Stabilization by ATM after DNA Damage. *Cell Cycle* 9, 472–478. Feb 1Epub 2010/01/19. doi:10.4161/cc.9.3.10556

Cheradame, L., Guerrera, I. C., Gaston, J., Schmitt, A., Jung, V., Goudin, N., et al. (2021). STING Protects Breast Cancer Cells from Intrinsic and Genotoxic-Induced DNA Instability via a Non-canonical, Cell-Autonomous Pathway. *Oncogene* 40, 6627–6640. Epub 2021/10/10. doi:10.1038/s41388-021-02037-4

Chin, E. N., Yu, C., Vartabedian, V. F., Jia, Y., Kumar, M., Gamo, A. M., et al. (2020). Antitumor Activity of a Systemic STING-Activating Non-nucleotide cGAMP Mimetic. *Science* 369, 993–999. Epub 2020/08/21. doi:10.1126/science.abb4255

Chowell, D., Yoo, S.-K., Valero, C., Pastore, A., Krishna, C., Lee, M., et al. (2021). Improved Prediction of Immune Checkpoint Blockade Efficacy across Multiple Cancer Types. *Nat. Biotechnol.* 1, 1–8. Epub 2021/11/03. doi:10.1038/s41587-021-01070-8

Chu, W., Jin, W., Liu, D., Wang, J., Geng, C., Chen, L., et al. (2018). Diffusion-weighted Imaging in Identifying Breast Cancer Pathological Response to Neoadjuvant Chemotherapy: A Meta-Analysis. *Oncotarget* 9, 7088–7100. Epub 2018/02/23. doi:10.18632/oncotarget.23195

Ciccia, A., and Elledge, S. J. (2010). The DNA Damage Response: Making it Safe to Play with Knives. *Mol. Cell* 40, 179–204. Epub 2010/10/23. doi:10.1016/j.molcel.2010.09.019

Cimprich, K. A., and Cortez, D. (2008). ATR: an Essential Regulator of Genome Integrity. *Nat. Rev. Mol. Cell Biol* 9, 616–627. Epub 2008/07/03. doi:10.1038/nrm2450

Cleary, J. M., Aguirre, A. J., Shapiro, G. I., and D'Andrea, A. D. (2020). Biomarker-Guided Development of DNA Repair Inhibitors. *Mol. Cell* 78, 1070–1085. Jun 18Epub 2020/05/28. doi:10.1016/j.molcel.2020.04.035

Cussiol, J. R. R., Soares, B. L., and Oliveira, F. M. B. (2019). From Yeast to Humans: Understanding the Biology of DNA Damage Response (DDR) Kinases. *Genet. Mol. Biol.* 43, e20190071. Epub 2020/01/14. doi:10.1590/1678-4685-GMB-2019-0071

Dasari, S., and Tchounwou, P. B. (2014). Cisplatin in Cancer Therapy: Molecular Mechanisms of Action. *Eur. J. Pharmacol.* 740, 364–378. Epub 2014/07/25. doi:10.1016/j.ejphar.2014.07.025

de Oliveira Mann, C. C., Orzalli, M. H., King, D. S., Kagan, J. C., Lee, A. S. Y., and Kranzusch, P. J. (2019). Modular Architecture of the STING C-Terminal Tail Allows Interferon and NF-Kb Signaling Adaptation. *Cell Rep.* 27, 1165–1175. e1165. doi:10.1016/j.celrep.2019.03.098

De Ruysscher, D., Niedermann, G., Burnet, N. G., Siva, S., Lee, A. W. M., and Hegi-Johnson, F. (2019). Radiotherapy Toxicity. *Nat. Rev. Dis. Primers* 5, 13–20. doi:10.1038/s41572-019-0064-5

Delneste, Y., Beauvillain, C., and Jeannin, P. (2007). Immunité Naturelle. *Med. Sci. (Paris)* 23, 67–74. Epub 2007/01/11. doi:10.1051/medsci/200723167

Desouky, O., Ding, N., and Zhou, G. (2015). Targeted and Non-targeted Effects of Ionizing Radiation. *J. Radiat. Res. Appl. Sci.* 8, 247–254. doi:10.1016/j.jrras.2015.03.003

Dianov, G. L., and Hübscher, U. (2013). Mammalian Base Excision Repair: the Forgotten Archangel. *Nucleic Acids Res.* 41, 3483–3490. Apr 1Epub 2013/02/15. doi:10.1093/nar/gkt076

Diner, E. J., Burdette, D. L., Wilson, S. C., Monroe, K. M., Kellenberger, C. A., Hyodo, M., et al. (2013). The Innate Immune DNA Sensor cGAS Produces a Noncanonical Cyclic Dinucleotide that Activates Human STING. *Cell Rep.* 3, 1355–1361. doi:10.1016/j.celrep.2013.05.009

Dou, Z., Ghosh, K., Vizioli, M. G., Zhu, J., Sen, P., Wangensteen, K. J., et al. (2017). Cytoplasmic Chromatin Triggers Inflammation in Senescence and Cancer. *Nature* 550, 402–406. Epub 2017/10/05. doi:10.1038/nature24050

Du, M., and Chen, Z. J. (2018). DNA-induced Liquid Phase Condensation of cGAS Activates Innate Immune Signaling. *Science* 361, 704–709. Epub 2018/07/07. doi:10.1126/science.aat1022

Duewell, P., Steger, A., Lohr, H., Bourhis, H., Hoelz, H., Kirchleitner, S. V., et al. (2014). RIG-I-like Helicases Induce Immunogenic Cell Death of Pancreatic Cancer Cells and Sensitize Tumors toward Killing by CD8+ T Cells. *Cell Death Differ* 21, 1825–1837. Epub 2014/07/12. doi:10.1038/cdd.2014.96

Dupré, A., Boyer-Chatenet, L., Sattler, R. M., Modi, A. P., Lee, J. H., Nicolette, M. L., et al. (2008). A Forward Chemical Genetic Screen Reveals an Inhibitor of the Mre11-Rad50-Nbs1 Complex. *Nat. Chem. Biol.* 4, 119–125. doi:10.1038/nchembio.63

Ellermeier, J., Wei, J., Duewell, P., Hoves, S., Stieg, M. R., Adunka, T., et al. (2013). Therapeutic Efficacy of Bifunctional siRNA Combining TGF-B1 Silencing with RIG-I Activation in Pancreatic Cancer. *Cancer Res.* 73, 1709–1720. doi:10.1158/0008-5472.can-11-3850

Emadi, A., Jones, R. J., and Brodsky, R. A. (2009). Cyclophosphamide and Cancer: golden Anniversary. *Nat. Rev. Clin. Oncol.* 6, 638–647. Epub 2009/09/30. doi:10.1038/nrclinonc.2009.146

Ergun, S. L., Fernandez, D., Weiss, T. M., and Li, L. (2019). STING Polymer Structure Reveals Mechanisms for Activation, Hyperactivation, and Inhibition. *Cell* 178, 290–301. Epub 2019/06/25. doi:10.1016/j.cell.2019.05.036

Falck, J., Coates, J., and Jackson, S. P. (2005). Conserved Modes of Recruitment of ATM, ATR and DNA-PKcs to Sites of DNA Damage. *Nature* 434, 605–611. Epub 2005/03/11. doi:10.1038/nature03442

Feng, X., Tubbs, A., Zhang, C., Tang, M., Sridharan, S., Wang, C., et al. (2020). ATR Inhibition Potentiates Ionizing Radiation-Induced Interferon Response via Cytosolic Nucleic Acid-Sensing Pathways. *EMBO J.* 39, e104036. doi:10.15252/embj.2019104036

Ferguson, B. J., Mansur, D. S., Peters, N. E., Ren, H., and Smith, G. L. (2012). DNA-PK Is a DNA Sensor for IRF-3-dependent Innate Immunity. *elife* 1, e00047. doi:10.7554/eLife.00047

Fernandes-Alnemri, T., Yu, J.-W., Datta, P., Wu, J., and Alnemri, E. S. (2009). AIM2 Activates the Inflammasome and Cell Death in Response to Cytoplasmic DNA. *Nature* 458, 509–513. Epub 2009/01/23. doi:10.1038/nature07710

Fishelevich, R., Zhao, Y., Tuchinda, P., Liu, H., Nakazono, A., Tammaro, A., et al. (2011). Imiquimod-induced TLR7 Signaling Enhances Repair of DNA Damage Induced by Ultraviolet Light in Bone Marrow-Derived Cells. *J.I.* 187, 1664–1673. Epub 2011/07/19. doi:10.4049/jimmunol.1100755

Foote, K. M., Nissink, J. W. M., McGuire, T., Turner, P., Guichard, S., Yates, J. W. T., et al. (2018). Discovery and Characterization of AZD6738, a Potent Inhibitor of Ataxia Telangiectasia Mutated and Rad3 Related (ATR) Kinase with Application as an Anticancer Agent. *J. Med. Chem.* 61, 9889–9907. doi:10.1021/acs.jmedchem.8b01187

Gaidt, M. M., Ebert, T. S., Chauhan, D., Ramshorn, K., Pinci, F., Zuber, S., et al. (2017). The DNA Inflammasome in Human Myeloid Cells Is Initiated by a STING-Cell Death Program Upstream of NLRP3. *Cell* 171, 1110–1124. e1118. doi:10.1016/j.cell.2017.09.039

Galluzzi, L., Humeau, J., Buqué, A., Zitvogel, L., and Kroemer, G. (2020). Immunostimulation with Chemotherapy in the Era of Immune Checkpoint Inhibitors. *Nat. Rev. Clin. Oncol.* 17, 725–741. Epub 2020/08/08. doi:10.1038/s41571-020-0413-z

Ganguly, D., Chamilos, G., Lande, R., Gregorio, J., Meller, S., Facchinetti, V., et al. (2009). Self-RNA-antimicrobial Peptide Complexes Activate Human Dendritic Cells through TLR7 and TLR8. *J. Exp. Med.* 206, 1983–1994. doi:10.1084/jem.20090480

Gao, P., Ascano, M., Wu, Y., Barchet, W., Gaffney, B. L., Zillinger, T., et al. (2013). Cyclic [G(2′,5′)pA(3′,5′)p] Is the Metazoan Second Messenger Produced by DNA-Activated Cyclic GMP-AMP Synthase. *Cell* 153, 1094–1107. doi:10.1016/j.cell.2013.04.046

Gavande, N. S., VanderVere-Carozza, P. S., Hinshaw, H. D., Jalal, S. I., Sears, C. R., Pawelczak, K. S., et al. (2016). DNA Repair Targeted Therapy: The Past or Future of Cancer Treatment? *Pharmacol. Ther.* 160, 65–83. Epub 2016/02/21. doi:10.1016/j.pharmthera.2016.02.003

Gavande, N. S., VanderVere-Carozza, P. S., Pawelczak, K. S., Mendoza-Munoz, P., Vernon, T. L., Hanakahi, L. A., et al. (2020). Discovery and Development of Novel DNA-PK Inhibitors by Targeting the Unique Ku-DNA Interaction. *Nucleic Acids Res.* 48, 11536–11550. doi:10.1093/nar/gkaa934

Gay, N. J., Symmons, M. F., Gangloff, M., and Bryant, C. E. (2014). Assembly and Localization of Toll-like Receptor Signalling Complexes. *Nat. Rev. Immunol.* 14, 546–558. Epub 2014/07/26. doi:10.1038/nri3713

Gentili, M., Kowal, J., Tkach, M., Satoh, T., Lahaye, X., Conrad, C., et al. (2015). Transmission of Innate Immune Signaling by Packaging of cGAMP in Viral Particles. *Science* 349, 1232–1236. Epub 2015/08/01. doi:10.1126/science.aab3628

Gentili, M., Lahaye, X., Nadalin, F., Nader, G. P. F., Puig Lombardi, E., Herve, S., et al. (2019). The N-Terminal Domain of cGAS Determines Preferential Association with Centromeric DNA and Innate Immune Activation in the Nucleus. *Cell Rep.* 26, 2377–2393. e2313. doi:10.1016/j.celrep.2019.01.105

Giglia-Mari, G., Zotter, A., and Vermeulen, W. (2011). DNA Damage Response. *Cold Spring Harbor Perspect. Biol.* 3, a000745. Epub 2010/10/29. doi:10.1101/cshperspect.a000745

Gillet, L. C. J., and Schärer, O. D. (2006). Molecular Mechanisms of Mammalian Global Genome Nucleotide Excision Repair. *Chem. Rev.* 106, 253–276. Epub 2006/02/09. doi:10.1021/cr040483f

Glück, S., Guey, B., Gulen, M. F., Wolter, K., Kang, T. W., Schmacke, N. A., et al. (2017). Innate Immune Sensing of Cytosolic Chromatin Fragments through cGAS Promotes Senescence. *Nat. Cell Biol* 19, 1061–1070. doi:10.1038/ncb3586

Gorecki, L., Andrs, M., Rezacova, M., and Korabecny, J. (2020). Discovery of ATR Kinase Inhibitor Berzosertib (VX-970, M6620): Clinical Candidate for Cancer Therapy. *Pharmacol. Ther.* 210, 107518. Epub 2020/02/29. doi:10.1016/j.pharmthera.2020.107518

Goubau, D., Deddouche, S., and Reis e Sousa, C. (2013). Cytosolic Sensing of Viruses. *Immunity* 38, 855–869. Epub 2013/05/28. doi:10.1016/j.immuni.2013.05.007

Goubau, D., Schlee, M., Deddouche, S., Pruijssers, A. J., Zillinger, T., Goldeck, M., et al. (2014). Antiviral Immunity via RIG-I-Mediated Recognition of RNA Bearing 5′-diphosphates. *Nature* 514, 372–375. doi:10.1038/nature13590

Grassberger, C., Ellsworth, S. G., Wilks, M. Q., Keane, F. K., and Loeffler, J. S. (2019). Assessing the Interactions between Radiotherapy and Antitumour Immunity. *Nat. Rev. Clin. Oncol.* 16, 729–745. doi:10.1038/s41571-019-0238-9

Gratia, M., Rodero, M. P., Conrad, C., Bou Samra, E., Maurin, M., Rice, G. I., et al. (2019). Bloom Syndrome Protein Restrains Innate Immune Sensing of Micronuclei by cGAS. *J. Exp. Med.* 216, 1199–1213. Epub 2019/04/03. doi:10.1084/jem.20181329

Gray, E. E., Winship, D., Snyder, J. M., Child, S. J., Geballe, A. P., and Stetson, D. B. (2016). The AIM2-like Receptors Are Dispensable for the Interferon Response to Intracellular DNA. *Immunity* 45, 255–266. Aug 16Epub 2016/08/09. doi:10.1016/j.immuni.2016.06.015

Hammel, P., Zhang, C., Matile, J., Colle, E., Hadj-Naceur, I., Gagaille, M.-P., et al. (2020). PARP Inhibition in Treatment of Pancreatic Cancer. *Expert Rev. Anticancer Ther.* 20, 939–945. Epub 2020/09/17. doi:10.1080/14737140.2020.1820330

Harding, S. M., Benci, J. L., Irianto, J., Discher, D. E., Minn, A. J., and Greenberg, R. A. (2017). Mitotic Progression Following DNA Damage Enables Pattern Recognition within Micronuclei. *Nature* 548, 466–470. doi:10.1038/nature23470

Hargadon, K. M., Johnson, C. E., and Williams, C. J. (2018). Immune Checkpoint Blockade Therapy for Cancer: An Overview of FDA-Approved Immune Checkpoint Inhibitors. *Int. Immunopharmacology* 62, 29–39. Epub 2018/07/11. doi:10.1016/j.intimp.2018.06.001

Hellmann, M. D., Li, B. T., Chaft, J. E., and Kris, M. G. (2016). Chemotherapy Remains an Essential Element of Personalized Care for Persons with Lung Cancers. *Ann. Oncol.* 27, 1829–1835. Epub 2016/07/28. doi:10.1093/annonc/mdw271

Henner, W. D., Grunberg, S. M., and Haseltine, W. A. (1982). Sites and Structure of Gamma Radiation-Induced DNA Strand Breaks. *J. Biol. Chem.* 257, 11750–11754. Epub 1982/10/10. doi:10.1016/s0021-9258(18)33827-4

Honda, K., Ohba, Y., Yanai, H., Negishi, H., Mizutani, T., Takaoka, A., et al. (2005). Spatiotemporal Regulation of MyD88-IRF-7 Signalling for Robust Type-I Interferon Induction. *Nature* 434, 1035–1040. doi:10.1038/nature03547

Hooy, R. M., and Sohn, J. (2018). The Allosteric Activation of cGAS Underpins its Dynamic Signaling Landscape. *Elife* 7, e39984. Epub 2018/10/09. doi:10.7554/eLife.39984

Hopfner, K.-P., and Hornung, V. (2020). Molecular Mechanisms and Cellular Functions of cGAS-STING Signalling. *Nat. Rev. Mol. Cell Biol* 21, 501–521. doi:10.1038/s41580-020-0244-x

Hornung, V., Ablasser, A., Charrel-Dennis, M., Bauernfeind, F., Horvath, G., Caffrey, D. R., et al. (2009). AIM2 Recognizes Cytosolic dsDNA and Forms a Caspase-1-Activating Inflammasome with ASC. *Nature* 458, 514–518. doi:10.1038/nature07725

Hou, F., Sun, L., Zheng, H., Skaug, B., Jiang, Q.-X., and Chen, Z. J. (2011). MAVS Forms Functional Prion-like Aggregates to Activate and Propagate Antiviral Innate Immune Response. *Cell* 146, 448–461. Epub 2011/07/26. doi:10.1016/j.cell.2011.06.041

Hove-Jensen, B. (1988). Mutation in the Phosphoribosylpyrophosphate Synthetase Gene (Prs) that Results in Simultaneous Requirements for Purine and Pyrimidine Nucleosides, Nicotinamide Nucleotide, Histidine, and Tryptophan in *Escherichia coli*. *J. Bacteriol.* 170, 1148–1152. doi:10.1128/jb.170.3.1148-1152.1988

Hu, B., Jin, C., Li, H.-B., Tong, J., Ouyang, X., Cetinbas, N. M., et al. (2016). The DNA-Sensing AIM2 Inflammasome Controls Radiation-Induced Cell Death and Tissue Injury. *Science* 354, 765–768. Epub 2016/11/16. doi:10.1126/science.aaf7532

Huang, R.-X., and Zhou, P.-K. (2020). DNA Damage Response Signaling Pathways and Targets for Radiotherapy Sensitization in Cancer. *Sig Transduct Target. Ther.* 5, 60. Epub 2020/05/02. doi:10.1038/s41392-020-0150-x

Ishikawa, H., and Barber, G. N. (2008). STING Is an Endoplasmic Reticulum Adaptor that Facilitates Innate Immune Signalling. *Nature* 455, 674–678. doi:10.1038/nature07317

Itoh, K., Watanabe, A., Funami, K., Seya, T., and Matsumoto, M. (2008). The Clathrin-Mediated Endocytic Pathway Participates in dsRNA-Induced IFN-β Production. *J. Immunol.* 181, 5522–5529. doi:10.4049/jimmunol.181.8.5522

Iurescia, S., Fioretti, D., and Rinaldi, M. (2018). Targeting Cytosolic Nucleic Acid-Sensing Pathways for Cancer Immunotherapies. *Front. Immunol.* 9, 711. Epub 2018/04/25. doi:10.3389/fimmu.2018.00711

Jiang, H., Xue, X., Panda, S., Kawale, A., Hooy, R. M., Liang, F., et al. (2019). Chromatin-bound cGAS Is an Inhibitor of DNA Repair and Hence Accelerates Genome Destabilization and Cell Death. *EMBO J.* 38, e102718. doi:10.15252/embj.2019102718

Jiang, H., Swacha, P., and Gekara, N. O. (2021). Nuclear AIM2-Like Receptors Drive Genotoxic Tissue Injury by Inhibiting DNA Repair. *Adv. Sci.* 8, 2102534. doi:10.1002/advs.202102534

Jobson, A. G., Lountos, G. T., Lorenzi, P. L., Llamas, J., Connelly, J., Cerna, D., et al. (2009). Cellular Inhibition of Checkpoint Kinase 2 (Chk2) and Potentiation of Camptothecins and Radiation by the Novel Chk2 Inhibitor PV1019 [7-nitro-1H-indole-2-carboxylic Acid {4-[1-(guanidinohydrazone)-Ethyl]-Phenyl}-Amide]. *J. Pharmacol. Exp. Ther.* 331, 816–826. Epub 2009/09/11. doi:10.1124/jpet.109.154997

Kang, D.-c., Gopalkrishnan, R. V., Lin, L., Randolph, A., Valerie, K., Pestka, S., et al. (2004). Expression Analysis and Genomic Characterization of Human Melanoma Differentiation Associated Gene-5, Mda-5: a Novel Type I Interferon-Responsive Apoptosis-Inducing Gene. *Oncogene* 23, 1789–1800. Epub 2003/12/17. doi:10.1038/sj.onc.1207300

Karikó, K., Ni, H., Capodici, J., Lamphier, M., and Weissman, D. (2004). mRNA Is an Endogenous Ligand for Toll-like Receptor 3. *J. Biol. Chem.* 279, 12542–12550. doi:10.1074/jbc.M310175200

Kato, H., Takeuchi, O., Mikamo-Satoh, E., Hirai, R., Kawai, T., Matsushita, K., et al. (2008). Length-dependent Recognition of Double-Stranded Ribonucleic Acids

by Retinoic Acid-Inducible Gene-I and Melanoma Differentiation-Associated Gene 5. *J. Exp. Med.* 205, 1601–1610. doi:10.1084/jem.20080091
Kawai, T., and Akira, S. (2011). Toll-like Receptors and Their Crosstalk with Other Innate Receptors in Infection and Immunity. *Immunity* 34, 637–650. doi:10.1016/j.immuni.2011.05.006
Kawai, T., Takahashi, K., Sato, S., Coban, C., Kumar, H., Kato, H., et al. (2005). IPS-1, an Adaptor Triggering RIG-I- and Mda5-Mediated Type I Interferon Induction. *Nat. Immunol.* 6, 981–988. doi:10.1038/ni1243
King, C., Diaz, H., Barnard, D., Barda, D., Clawson, D., Blosser, W., et al. (2014). Characterization and Preclinical Development of LY2603618: a Selective and Potent Chk1 Inhibitor. *Invest. New Drugs* 32, 213–226. Epub 2013/10/12. doi:10.1007/s10637-013-0036-7
Klarquist, J., Hennies, C. M., Lehn, M. A., Reboulet, R. A., Feau, S., and Janssen, E. M. (2014). STING-mediated DNA Sensing Promotes Antitumor and Autoimmune Responses to Dying Cells. *J.I.* 193, 6124–6134. Epub 2014/11/12. doi:10.4049/jimmunol.1401869
Klaschik, S., Tross, D., Shirota, H., and Klinman, D. M. (2010). Short- and Long-Term Changes in Gene Expression Mediated by the Activation of TLR9. *Mol. Immunol.* 47, 1317–1324. Epub 2009/12/17. doi:10.1016/j.molimm.2009.11.014
Kondo, T., Kobayashi, J., Saitoh, T., Maruyama, K., Ishii, K. J., Barber, G. N., et al. (2013). DNA Damage Sensor MRE11 Recognizes Cytosolic Double-Stranded DNA and Induces Type I Interferon by Regulating STING Trafficking. *Proc. Natl. Acad. Sci. U.S.A.* 110, 2969–2974. Epub 2013/02/08. doi:10.1073/pnas.1222694110
Kornberg, A., Lieberman, I., and Simms, E. S. (1955). Enzymatic Synthesis and Properties of 5-phosphoribosylpyrophosphate. *J. Biol. Chem.* 215, 389–402. Epub 1955/07/01. doi:10.1016/s0021-9258(18)66047-8
Kovacs, S. B., and Miao, E. A. (2017). Gasdermins: Effectors of Pyroptosis. *Trends Cell Biol.* 27, 673–684. Epub 2017/06/18. doi:10.1016/j.tcb.2017.05.005
Krejci, L., Altmannova, V., Spirek, M., and Zhao, X. (2012). Homologous Recombination and its Regulation. *Nucleic Acids Res.* 40, 5795–5818. Epub 2012/04/03. doi:10.1093/nar/gks270
Krokan, H. E., Standal, R., and Slupphaug, G. (1997). DNA Glycosylases in the Base Excision Repair of DNA. *Biochem. J.* 325 (Pt 1), 1–16. Epub 1997/07/01. doi:10.1042/bj3250001
Kryston, T. B., Georgiev, A. B., Pissis, P., and Georgakilas, A. G. (2011). Role of Oxidative Stress and DNA Damage in Human Carcinogenesis. *Mutat. Research/Fundamental Mol. Mech. Mutagenesis* 711, 193–201. Epub 2011/01/11. doi:10.1016/j.mrfmmm.2010.12.016
Kuchta, K., Knizewski, L., Wyrwicz, L. S., Rychlewski, L., and Ginalski, K. (2009). Comprehensive Classification of Nucleotidyltransferase Fold Proteins: Identification of Novel Families and Their Representatives in Human. *Nucleic Acids Res.* 37, 7701–7714. doi:10.1093/nar/gkp854
Kumagai, Y., Takeuchi, O., and Akira, S. (2008). TLR9 as a Key Receptor for the Recognition of DNA☆. *Adv. Drug Deliv. Rev.* 60, 795–804. doi:10.1016/j.addr.2007.12.004
Lammert, C. R., Frost, E. L., Bellinger, C. E., Bolte, A. C., McKee, C. A., Hurt, M. E., et al. (2020). AIM2 Inflammasome Surveillance of DNA Damage Shapes Neurodevelopment. *Nature* 580, 647–652. Epub 2020/05/01. doi:10.1038/s41586-020-2174-3
Li, M., and Yu, X. (2013). Function of BRCA1 in the DNA Damage Response Is Mediated by ADP-Ribosylation. *Cancer cell* 23, 693–704. doi:10.1016/j.ccr.2013.03.025
Li, X.-D., Wu, J., Gao, D., Wang, H., Sun, L., and Chen, Z. J. (2013b). Pivotal Roles of cGAS-cGAMP Signaling in Antiviral Defense and Immune Adjuvant Effects. *Science* 341, 1390–1394. Epub 2013/08/31. doi:10.1126/science.1244040
Li, X., Shu, C., Yi, G., Chaton, C. T., Shelton, C. L., Diao, J., et al. (2013a). Cyclic GMP-AMP Synthase Is Activated by Double-Stranded DNA-Induced Oligomerization. *Immunity* 39, 1019–1031. doi:10.1016/j.immuni.2013.10.019
Liang, F., Zhang, F., Zhang, L., and Wei, W. (2020). The Advances in Pyroptosis Initiated by Inflammasome in Inflammatory and Immune Diseases. *Inflamm. Res.* 69, 159–166. Epub 2020/01/15. doi:10.1007/s00011-020-01315-3
Limagne, E., Nuttin, L., Thibaudin, M., Jacquin, E., Aucagne, R., Bon, M., et al. (2022). MEK Inhibition Overcomes Chemoimmunotherapy Resistance by Inducing CXCL10 in Cancer Cells. *Cancer cell* 40, 136–152. Feb 14e112Epub 2022/01/21. doi:10.1016/j.ccell.2021.12.009
Liu, H., Zhang, H., Wu, X., Ma, D., Wu, J., Wang, L., et al. (2018). Nuclear cGAS Suppresses DNA Repair and Promotes Tumorigenesis. *Nature* 563, 131–136. Epub 2018/10/26. doi:10.1038/s41586-018-0629-6
Liu, R., Li, J., Shao, J., Lee, J.-H., Qiu, X., Xiao, Y., et al. (2021). Innate Immune Response Orchestrates Phosphoribosyl Pyrophosphate Synthetases to Support DNA Repair. *Cell Metab.* 33, 2076–2089. Epub 2021/08/04. doi:10.1016/j.cmet.2021.07.009
Liu, S., Cai, X., Wu, J., Cong, Q., Chen, X., Li, T., et al. (2015). Phosphorylation of Innate Immune Adaptor Proteins MAVS, STING, and TRIF Induces IRF3 Activation. *Science* 347, aaa2630. Epub 2015/02/01. doi:10.1126/science.aaa2630
Lövgren, T., Eloranta, M. L., Båve, U., Alm, G. V., Rönnblom, L. J. A., and Rheumatology, R. O. (2004). Induction of Interferon-α Production in Plasmacytoid Dendritic Cells by Immune Complexes Containing Nucleic Acid Released by Necrotic or Late Apoptotic Cells and Lupus IgG. *Arthritis Rheum.* 50, 1861–1872. doi:10.1002/art.20254
Luecke, S., Holleufer, A., Christensen, M. H., Jønsson, K. L., Boni, G. A., Sørensen, L. K., et al. (2017). cGAS Is Activated by DNA in a Length-dependent Manner. *EMBO Rep.* 18, 1707–1715. doi:10.15252/embr.201744017
Lugrin, J., and Martinon, F. (2018). The AIM2 Inflammasome: Sensor of Pathogens and Cellular Perturbations. *Immunol. Rev.* 281, 99–114. doi:10.1111/imr.12618
Mackenzie, K. J., Carroll, P., Martin, C.-A., Murina, O., Fluteau, A., Simpson, D. J., et al. (2017). cGAS Surveillance of Micronuclei Links Genome Instability to Innate Immunity. *Nature* 548, 461–465. Epub 2017/07/25. doi:10.1038/nature23449
Majer, O., Liu, B., and Barton, G. M. (2017). Nucleic Acid-Sensing TLRs: Trafficking and Regulation. *Curr. Opin. Immunol.* 44, 26–33. Epub 2016/12/03. doi:10.1016/j.coi.2016.10.003
Majewski, S., Jantschitsch, C., Maeda, A., Schwarz, T., and Schwarz, A. (2010). IL-23 Antagonizes UVR-Induced Immunosuppression through Two Mechanisms: Reduction of UVR-Induced DNA Damage and Inhibition of UVR-Induced Regulatory T Cells. *J. Invest. Dermatol.* 130, 554–562. doi:10.1038/jid.2009.274
Mateo, J., Lord, C. J., Serra, V., Tutt, A., Balmaña, J., Castroviejo-Bermejo, M., et al. (2019). A Decade of Clinical Development of PARP Inhibitors in Perspective. *Ann. Oncol.* 30, 1437–1447. Epub 2019/06/21. doi:10.1093/annonc/mdz192
Mateos-Gomez, P. A., Gong, F., Nair, N., Miller, K. M., Lazzerini-Denchi, E., and Sfeir, A. (2015). Mammalian Polymerase θ Promotes Alternative NHEJ and Suppresses Recombination. *Nature* 518, 254–257. doi:10.1038/nature14157
McLaughlin, M., Patin, E. C., Pedersen, M., Wilkins, A., Dillon, M. T., Melcher, A. A., et al. (2020). Inflammatory Microenvironment Remodelling by Tumour Cells after Radiotherapy. *Nat. Rev. Cancer* 20, 203–217. AprEpub 2020/03/13. doi:10.1038/s41568-020-0246-1
Miao, E. A., Rajan, J. V., and Aderem, A. (2011). Caspase-1-induced Pyroptotic Cell Death. *Immunological Rev.* 243, 206–214. doi:10.1111/j.1600-065x.2011.01044.x
Morchikh, M., Cribier, A., Raffel, R., Amraoui, S., Cau, J., Severac, D., et al. (2017). HEXIM1 and NEAT1 Long Non-coding RNA Form a Multi-Subunit Complex that Regulates DNA-Mediated Innate Immune Response. *Mol. Cel.* 67, 387–399. e385. doi:10.1016/j.molcel.2017.06.020
Moresco, E. M. Y., LaVine, D., and Beutler, B. (2011). Toll-like Receptors. *Curr. Biol.* 21, R488–R493. Epub 2011/07/12. doi:10.1016/j.cub.2011.05.039
Munster, P. N., Mahipal, A., Nemunaitis, J. J., Mita, M. M., Paz-Ares, L. G., Massard, C., et al. (2016). Phase I Trial of a Dual TOR Kinase and DNA-PK Inhibitor (CC-115) in Advanced Solid and Hematologic Cancers. *J. Clin. Oncol.* 34–2505. doi:10.1200/jco.2016.34.15_suppl.2505
Nastasi, C., Mannarino, L., and D'Incalci, M. (2020). DNA Damage Response and Immune Defense. *Ijms* 21, 7504. Epub 2020/10/16. doi:10.3390/ijms21207504
Ori, D., Murase, M., and Kawai, T. (2017). Cytosolic Nucleic Acid Sensors and Innate Immune Regulation. *Int. Rev. Immunol.* 36, 74–88. Epub 2017/03/24. doi:10.1080/08830185.2017.1298749
Oshiumi, H., Matsumoto, M., Funami, K., Akazawa, T., and Seya, T. (2003). TICAM-1, an Adaptor Molecule that Participates in Toll-like Receptor 3-mediated Interferon-β Induction. *Nat. Immunol.* 4, 161–167. doi:10.1038/ni886
Paludan, S. R., Reinert, L. S., and Hornung, V. (2019). DNA-stimulated Cell Death: Implications for Host Defence, Inflammatory Diseases and Cancer. *Nat. Rev. Immunol.* 19, 141–153. Epub 2019/01/16. doi:10.1038/s41577-018-0117-0
Pan, B. S., Perera, S. A., Piesvaux, J. A., Presland, J. P., Schroeder, G. K., Cumming, J. N., et al. (2020). An Orally Available Non-nucleotide STING Agonist with Antitumor Activity. *Science* 369, eaba6098. Epub 2020/08/21. doi:10.1126/science.aba6098
Pandey, N., and Black, B. E. (2021). Rapid Detection and Signaling of DNA Damage by PARP-1. *Trends Biochem. Sci.* 46, 744–757. Epub 2021/03/07. doi:10.1016/j.tibs.2021.01.014

Pantelidou, C., Sonzogni, O., De Oliveria Taveira, M., Mehta, A. K., Kothari, A., Wang, D., et al. (2019). PARP Inhibitor Efficacy Depends on CD8+ T-Cell Recruitment via Intratumoral STING Pathway Activation in BRCA-Deficient Models of Triple-Negative Breast Cancer. *Cancer Discov.* 9, 722–737. Epub 2019/04/25. doi:10.1158/2159-8290.cd-18-1218

Petitprez, F., Meylan, M., de Reyniès, A., Sautès-Fridman, C., and Fridman, W. H. (2020). The Tumor Microenvironment in the Response to Immune Checkpoint Blockade Therapies. *Front. Immunol.* 11, 784. Epub 2020/05/28. doi:10.3389/fimmu.2020.00784

Pike, K. G., Barlaam, B., Cadogan, E., Campbell, A., Chen, Y., Colclough, N., et al. (2018). The Identification of Potent, Selective, and Orally Available Inhibitors of Ataxia Telangiectasia Mutated (ATM) Kinase: the Discovery of AZD0156 (8-{6-[3-(Dimethylamino) Propoxy] Pyridin-3-Yl}-3-Methyl-1-(tetrahydro-2 H-Pyran-4-Yl)-1, 3-dihydro-2 H-Imidazo [4, 5-c] Quinolin-2-One). *J. Med. Chem.* 61, 3823–3841. doi:10.1021/acs.jmedchem.7b01896

Pinder, J. B., Attwood, K. M., and Dellaire, G. (2013). Reading, Writing, and Repair: the Role of Ubiquitin and the Ubiquitin-like Proteins in DNA Damage Signaling and Repair. *Front. Genet.* 4, 45. Epub 2013/04/05. doi:10.3389/fgene.2013.00045

Qin, S.-Y., Cheng, Y.-J., Lei, Q., Zhang, A.-Q., and Zhang, X.-Z. (2018). Combinational Strategy for High-Performance Cancer Chemotherapy. *Biomaterials* 171, 178–197. Epub 2018/04/27. doi:10.1016/j.biomaterials.2018.04.027

Ramakrishnan Geethakumari, P., Schiewer, M. J., Knudsen, K. E., and Kelly, W. K. (2017). PARP Inhibitors in Prostate Cancer. *Curr. Treat. Options. Oncol.* 18, 37. Epub 2017/05/26. doi:10.1007/s11864-017-0480-2

Roth, S., Rottach, A., Lotz-Havla, A. S., Laux, V., Muschaweckh, A., Gersting, S. W., et al. (2014). Rad50-CARD9 Interactions Link Cytosolic DNA Sensing to IL-1β Production. *Nat. Immunol.* 15, 538–545. doi:10.1038/ni.2888

Rupnik, A., Grenon, M., and Lowndes, N. (2008). The MRN Complex. *Curr. Biol.* 18, R455–R457. Epub 2008/06/05. doi:10.1016/j.cub.2008.03.040

San Filippo, J., Sung, P., and Klein, H. (2008). Mechanism of Eukaryotic Homologous Recombination. *Annu. Rev. Biochem.* 77, 229–257. Epub 2008/02/16. doi:10.1146/annurev.biochem.77.061306.125255

Serrone, L., Zeuli, M., Sega, F. M., and Cognetti, F. (2000). Dacarbazine-based Chemotherapy for Metastatic Melanoma: Thirty-Year Experience Overview. *J. Exp. Clin. Cancer Res.* 19, 21–34. Epub 2000/06/07.

Seth, R. B., Sun, L., Ea, C.-K., and Chen, Z. J. (2005). Identification and Characterization of MAVS, a Mitochondrial Antiviral Signaling Protein that Activates NF-Kb and IRF3. *Cell* 122, 669–682. doi:10.1016/j.cell.2005.08.012

Shang, G., Zhang, C., Chen, Z. J., Bai, X.-c., and Zhang, X. (2019). Cryo-EM Structures of STING Reveal its Mechanism of Activation by Cyclic GMP-AMP. *Nature* 567, 389–393. doi:10.1038/s41586-019-0998-5

Shen, J., Zhao, W., Ju, Z., Wang, L., Peng, Y., Labrie, M., et al. (2019). PARPi Triggers the STING-dependent Immune Response and Enhances the Therapeutic Efficacy of Immune Checkpoint Blockade Independent of BRCAness. *Cancer Res.* 79, 311–319. Epub 2018/11/30. doi:10.1158/0008-5472.can-18-1003

Shuck, S. C., Short, E. A., and Turchi, J. J. (2008). Eukaryotic Nucleotide Excision Repair: from Understanding Mechanisms to Influencing Biology. *Cell Res* 18, 64–72. Epub 2008/01/02. doi:10.1038/cr.2008.2

Smith, J., Mun Tho, L., Xu, N., and Gillespie, D. A. (2010). The ATM-Chk2 and ATR-Chk1 Pathways in DNA Damage Signaling and Cancer. *Adv. Cancer Res.* 108, 73–112. doi:10.1016/b978-0-12-380888-2.00003-0

Sommariva, M., De Cecco, L., De Cesare, M., Sfondrini, L., Ménard, S., Melani, C., et al. (2011). TLR9 Agonists Oppositely Modulate DNA Repair Genes in Tumor versus Immune Cells and Enhance Chemotherapy Effects. *Cancer Res.* 71, 6382–6390. Epub 2011/09/01. doi:10.1158/0008-5472.can-11-1285

Souliotis, V. L., Vlachogiannis, N. I., Pappa, M., Argyriou, A., Ntouros, P. A., and Sfikakis, P. P. (2020). DNA Damage Response and Oxidative Stress in Systemic Autoimmunity. *Int. J. Mol. Sci.* 21, 55. doi:10.3390/ijms21010055

Stracker, T. H., and Petrini, J. H. J. (2011). The MRE11 Complex: Starting from the Ends. *Nat. Rev. Mol. Cell Biol* 12, 90–103. Epub 2011/01/22. doi:10.1038/nrm3047

Sui, H., Zhou, M., Imamichi, H., Jiao, X., Sherman, B. T., Lane, H. C., et al. (2017). STING Is an Essential Mediator of the Ku70-Mediated Production of IFN-Λ1 in Response to Exogenous DNA. *Sci. Signal.* 10, eaah5054. doi:10.1126/scisignal.aah5054

Sui, H., Chen, Q., and Imamichi, T. (2021a). Cytoplasmic-translocated Ku70 Senses Intracellular DNA and Mediates Interferon-lambda1 Induction. *Immunology* 163, 323–337. doi:10.1111/imm.13318

Sui, H., Hao, M., Chang, W., and Imamichi, T. (2021b). The Role of Ku70 as a Cytosolic DNA Sensor in Innate Immunity and beyond. *Front. Cel. Infect. Microbiol.* 11, 761983. doi:10.3389/fcimb.2021.761983

Sun, L., Wu, J., Du, F., Chen, X., and Chen, Z. J. (2013). Cyclic GMP-AMP Synthase Is a Cytosolic DNA Sensor that Activates the Type I Interferon Pathway. *Science* 339, 786–791. doi:10.1126/science.1232458

Taffoni, C., Steer, A., Marines, J., Chamma, H., Vila, I. K., and Laguette, N. (2021). Nucleic Acid Immunity and DNA Damage Response: New Friends and Old Foes. *Front. Immunol.* 12, 660560. Epub 2021/05/14. doi:10.3389/fimmu.2021.660560

Takeuchi, O., and Akira, S. (2010). Pattern Recognition Receptors and Inflammation. *Cell.* 140, 805–820. Epub 2010/03/23. doi:10.1016/j.cell.2010.01.022

Tatematsu, M., Nishikawa, F., Seya, T., and Matsumoto, M. (2013). Toll-like Receptor 3 Recognizes Incomplete Stem Structures in Single-Stranded Viral RNA. *Nat. Commun.* 4, 1833. Epub 2013/05/16. doi:10.1038/ncomms2857

Tigano, M., Vargas, D. C., Tremblay-Belzile, S., Fu, Y., and Sfeir, A. (2021). Nuclear Sensing of Breaks in Mitochondrial DNA Enhances Immune Surveillance. *Nature* 591, 477–481. Epub 2021/02/26. doi:10.1038/s41586-021-03269-w

Timme, C. R., Rath, B. H., O'Neill, J. W., Camphausen, K., and Tofilon, P. J. (2018). The DNA-PK Inhibitor VX-984 Enhances the Radiosensitivity of Glioblastoma Cells Grown *In Vitro* and as Orthotopic Xenografts. *Mol. Cancer Ther.* 17, 1207–1216. doi:10.1158/1535-7163.mct-17-1267

Tisi, R., Vertemara, J., Zampella, G., and Longhese, M. P. (2020). Functional and Structural Insights into the MRX/MRN Complex, a Key Player in Recognition and Repair of DNA Double-Strand Breaks. *Comput. Struct. Biotechnol. J.* 18, 1137–1152. doi:10.1016/j.csbj.2020.05.013

Trinchieri, G., and Sher, A. (2007). Cooperation of Toll-like Receptor Signals in Innate Immune Defence. *Nat. Rev. Immunol.* 7, 179–190. Epub 2007/02/24. doi:10.1038/nri2038

Uematsu, N., Weterings, E., Yano, K.-i., Morotomi-Yano, K., Jakob, B., Taucher-Scholz, G., et al. (2007). Autophosphorylation of DNA-PKCS Regulates its Dynamics at DNA Double-Strand Breaks. *J. Cel. Biol.* 177, 219–229. doi:10.1083/jcb.200608077

Uziel, T., Lerenthal, Y., Moyal, L., Andegeko, Y., Mittelman, L., and Shiloh, Y. (2003). Requirement of the MRN Complex for ATM Activation by DNA Damage. *EMBO J.* 22, 5612–5621. Epub 2003/10/09. doi:10.1093/emboj/cdg541

Volkman, H. E., Cambier, S., Gray, E. E., and Stetson, D. B. (2019). Tight Nuclear Tethering of cGAS Is Essential for Preventing Autoreactivity. *Elife* 8, e47491. doi:10.7554/eLife.47491

Vyncke, L., Bovijn, C., Pauwels, E., Van Acker, T., Ruyssinck, E., Burg, E., et al. (2016). Reconstructing the TIR Side of the Myddosome: a Paradigm for TIR-TIR Interactions. *Structure* 24, 437–447. Epub 2016/02/16. doi:10.1016/j.str.2015.12.018

Wang, B., and Yin, Q. (2017). AIM2 Inflammasome Activation and Regulation: A Structural Perspective. *J. Struct. Biol.* 200, 279–282. Epub 2017/08/17. doi:10.1016/j.jsb.2017.08.001

Wang, Q., Wang, Y., Ding, J., Wang, C., Zhou, X., Gao, W., et al. (2020). A Bioorthogonal System Reveals Antitumour Immune Function of Pyroptosis. *Nature* 579, 421–426. Epub 2020/03/20. doi:10.1038/s41586-020-2079-1

Wang, Y., Fu, Z., Li, X., Liang, Y., Pei, S., Hao, S., et al. (2021a). Cytoplasmic DNA Sensing by KU Complex in Aged CD4+ T Cell Potentiates T Cell Activation and Aging-Related Autoimmune Inflammation. *Immunity* 54, 632–647. Apr 13e639Epub 2021/03/06. doi:10.1016/j.immuni.2021.02.003

Wang, Y., Wang, M., Djekidel, M. N., Chen, H., Liu, D., Alt, F. W., et al. (2021b). eccDNAs Are Apoptotic Products with High Innate Immunostimulatory Activity. *Nature* 599, 308–314. Epub 2021/10/22. doi:10.1038/s41586-021-04009-w

Watson, R. O., Manzanillo, P. S., and Cox, J. S. (2012). Extracellular *M. tuberculosis* DNA Targets Bacteria for Autophagy by Activating the Host DNA-Sensing Pathway. *Cell* 150, 803–815. Epub 2012/08/21. doi:10.1016/j.cell.2012.06.040

West, A. P., Khoury-Hanold, W., Staron, M., Tal, M. C., Pineda, C. M., Lang, S. M., et al. (2015). Mitochondrial DNA Stress Primes the Antiviral Innate Immune Response. *Nature* 520, 553–557. Epub 2015/02/03. doi:10.1038/nature14156

Wilson, D. R., Sen, R., Sunshine, J. C., Pardoll, D. M., Green, J. J., and Kim, Y. J. (2018). Biodegradable STING Agonist Nanoparticles for Enhanced Cancer

Immunotherapy. *Nanomedicine: Nanotechnology, Biol. Med.* 14, 237–246. Epub 2017/11/12. doi:10.1016/j.nano.2017.10.013

Woo, S.-R., Fuertes, M. B., Corrales, L., Spranger, S., Furdyna, M. J., Leung, M. Y. K., et al. (2014). STING-dependent Cytosolic DNA Sensing Mediates Innate Immune Recognition of Immunogenic Tumors. *Immunity* 41, 830–842. Nov 20Epub 2014/12/18. doi:10.1016/j.immuni.2014.10.017

Woodrick, J., Gupta, S., Camacho, S., Parvathaneni, S., Choudhury, S., Cheema, A., et al. (2017). A New Sub-pathway of Long-patch Base Excision Repair Involving 5′ gap Formation. *Embo J.* 36, 1605–1622. doi:10.15252/embj.201694920

Woods, D., and Turchi, J. J. (2013). Chemotherapy Induced DNA Damage Response. *Cancer Biol. Ther.* 14, 379–389. Epub 2013/02/06. doi:10.4161/cbt.23761

Wu, J., Sun, L., Chen, X., Du, F., Shi, H., Chen, C., et al. (2013). Cyclic GMP-AMP Is an Endogenous Second Messenger in Innate Immune Signaling by Cytosolic DNA. *Science* 339, 826–830. doi:10.1126/science.1229963

Xiao, W., Singh, K. K., Chen, B., and Samson, L. (1993). A Common Element Involved in Transcriptional Regulation of Two DNA Alkylation Repair Genes (MAG and MGT1) of *Saccharomyces cerevisiae. Mol. Cell Biol* 13, 7213–7221. Epub 1993/12/01. doi:10.1128/mcb.13.12.7213-7221.1993

Xie, B., Liang, X., Yue, W., Ma, J., Li, X., Zhang, N., et al. (2021). Targeting Cytokinesis Bridge Proteins to Kill High-CIN Type Tumors. *Fundam. Res.* 1, 752–766. doi:10.1016/j.fmre.2021.08.015

Xie, H., Wang, W., Xia, B., Jin, W., and Lou, G. (2020). Therapeutic Applications of PARP Inhibitors in Ovarian Cancer. *Biomed. Pharmacother.* 127, 110204. Epub 2020/05/19. doi:10.1016/j.biopha.2020.110204

Xu, S., Wang, L., and Liu, Z. (2021). Molecularly Imprinted Polymer Nanoparticles: An Emerging Versatile Platform for Cancer Therapy. *Angew. Chem. Int. Ed. Engl.* 19 (60), 3858–3869. Epub 2020/08/14. doi:10.1002/anie.202005309

Yamamoto, M., Sato, S., Hemmi, H., Hoshino, K., Kaisho, T., Sanjo, H., et al. (2003). Role of Adaptor TRIF in the MyD88-independent Toll-like Receptor Signaling Pathway. *Science* 301, 640–643. Epub 2003/07/12. doi:10.1126/science.1087262

Yilmaz, D., Furst, A., Meaburn, K., Lezaja, A., Wen, Y., Altmeyer, M., et al. (2021). Activation of Homologous Recombination in G1 Preserves Centromeric Integrity. *Nature* 600, 748–753. Epub 2021/12/03. doi:10.1038/s41586-021-04200-z

Yoneyama, M., Kikuchi, M., Matsumoto, K., Imaizumi, T., Miyagishi, M., Taira, K., et al. (2005). Shared and Unique Functions of the DExD/H-Box Helicases RIG-I, MDA5, and LGP2 in Antiviral Innate Immunity. *J. Immunol.* 175, 2851–2858. Epub 2005/08/24. doi:10.4049/jimmunol.175.5.2851

Yoneyama, M., Kikuchi, M., Natsukawa, T., Shinobu, N., Imaizumi, T., Miyagishi, M., et al. (2004). The RNA Helicase RIG-I Has an Essential Function in Double-Stranded RNA-Induced Innate Antiviral Responses. *Nat. Immunol.* 5, 730–737. doi:10.1038/ni1087

Zandarashvili, L., Langelier, M. F., Velagapudi, U. K., Hancock, M. A., Steffen, J. D., Billur, R., et al. (2020). Structural Basis for Allosteric PARP-1 Retention on DNA Breaks. *Science* 368, eaax6367. Apr 3Epub 2020/04/04. doi:10.1126/science.aax6367

Zhang, C., Shang, G., Gui, X., Zhang, X., Bai, X.-c., and Chen, Z. J. (2019). Structural Basis of STING Binding with and Phosphorylation by TBK1. *Nature* 567, 394–398. Epub 2019/03/08. doi:10.1038/s41586-019-1000-2

Zhang, J.-Z., Liu, Z., Liu, J., Ren, J.-X., and Sun, T.-S. (2014a). Mitochondrial DNA Induces Inflammation and Increases TLR9/NF-Kb Expression in Lung Tissue. *Int. J. Mol. Med.* 33, 817–824. doi:10.3892/ijmm.2014.1650

Zhang, X., Shi, H., Wu, J., Zhang, X., Sun, L., Chen, C., et al. (2013). Cyclic GMP-AMP Containing Mixed Phosphodiester Linkages Is an Endogenous High-Affinity Ligand for STING. *Mol. Cel.* 51, 226–235. doi:10.1016/j.molcel.2013.05.022

Zhang, X., Wu, J., Du, F., Xu, H., Sun, L., Chen, Z., et al. (2014b). The Cytosolic DNA Sensor cGAS Forms an Oligomeric Complex with DNA and Undergoes Switch-like Conformational Changes in the Activation Loop. *Cell Rep.* 6, 421–430. Epub 2014/01/28. doi:10.1016/j.celrep.2014.01.003

Zhao, B., Du, F., Xu, P., Shu, C., Sankaran, B., Bell, S. L., et al. (2019). A Conserved PLPLRT/SD Motif of STING Mediates the Recruitment and Activation of TBK1. *Nature* 569, 718–722. Epub 2019/05/24. doi:10.1038/s41586-019-1228-x

Zheng, L., Asprodites, N., Keene, A. H., Rodriguez, P., Brown, K. D., and Davila, E. (2008). TLR9 Engagement on CD4 T Lymphocytes Represses γ-radiation-induced Apoptosis through Activation of Checkpoint Kinase Response Elements. *Blood* 111, 2704–2713. doi:10.1182/blood-2007-07-104141

Zhong, X., Thornton, K., and Reed, E. (2000). Computer Based Analyses of the 5'-flanking Regions of Selected Genes Involved in the Nucleotide Excision Repair Complex. *Int. J. Oncol.* 17, 375–380. Epub 2000/07/13. doi:10.3892/ijo.17.2.375

Zhu, M., Zhao, H., Limbo, O., and Russell, P. (2018). Mre11 Complex Links Sister Chromatids to Promote Repair of a Collapsed Replication fork. *Proc. Natl. Acad. Sci. U S A.* 115 (115), 8793–8798. Epub 2018/08/15. doi:10.1073/pnas.1808189115

Zierhut, C., Yamaguchi, N., Paredes, M., Luo, J.-D., Carroll, T., and Funabiki, H. (2019). The Cytoplasmic DNA Sensor cGAS Promotes Mitotic Cell Death. *Cell.* 178, 302–315. e323Epub 2019/07/13. doi:10.1016/j.cell.2019.05.035

Zimmer, A. S., Gillard, M., Lipkowitz, S., and Lee, J.-M. (2018). Update on PARP Inhibitors in Breast Cancer. *Curr. Treat. Options. Oncol.* 19, 21. Apr 11Epub 2018/04/13. doi:10.1007/s11864-018-0540-2

11

RRM2 Mediates the Anti-Tumor Effect of the Natural Product Pectolinarigenin on Glioblastoma Through Promoting CDK1 Protein Degradation by Increasing Autophagic Flux

Haiping Jiang[1,2,3], *Dongzhi Zhang*[1,2,3,4], *Karpov Denis Aleksandrovich*[1,2,3,5], *Junyi Ye*[1,2,3], *Lixiang Wang*[1,2,3], *Xiaofeng Chen*[1,2,3], *Ming Gao*[1,2,3], *Xinzhuang Wang*[1,2,3], *Tao Yan*[1,2,3], *He Yang*[1,2,3], *Enzhou Lu*[1,2,3], *Wenwu Liu*[1,2,3], *Cheng Zhang*[6], *Jianing Wu*[7], *Penglei Yao*[7], *Zhenying Sun*[7], *Xuan Rong*[7], *Sokhatskii Andrei Timofeevich*[1,2,3,5], *Safin Shamil Mahmutovich*[5], *Zhixing Zheng*[1,2,3], *Xin Chen*[1,2,3]* and *Shiguang Zhao*[1,2,3,7]*

[1] Department of Neurosurgery, The First Affiliated Hospital of Harbin Medical University, Harbin, China, [2] Department of Neurosurgery, Key Colleges and Universities Laboratory of Neurosurgery in Heilongjiang Province, Harbin, China, [3] Institute of Neuroscience, Sino-Russian Medical Research Center, Harbin Medical University, Harbin, China, [4] Department of Neurosurgery, The Affiliated Cancer Hospital of Harbin Medical University, Harbin, China, [5] Department of Neurosurgery and Medical Rehabilitation, Bashkir State Medical University, Ufa, Russia, [6] Department of Undergraduate, Suffolk University, Boston, MA, United States, [7] Department of Neurosurgery, Shenzhen University General Hospital, Shenzhen, China

***Correspondence:**
Shiguang Zhao
guangsz@hotmail.com
Xin Chen
chenxin_tracy@yeah.net

The natural product pectolinarigenin exerts anti-inflammatory activity and anti-tumor effects, and exhibits different biological functions, particularly in autophagy and cell cycle regulation. However, the antineoplastic effect of pectolinarigenin on glioblastoma (GBM) remains unclear. In the present study, we found that pectolinarigenin inhibits glioblastoma proliferation, increases autophagic flux, and induces cell cycle arrest by inhibiting ribonucleotide reductase subunit M2 (RRM2), which can be reversed by RRM2 overexpression plasmid. Additionally, pectolinarigenin promoted RRM2 protein degradation *via* autolysosome-dependent pathway by increasing autophagic flow. RRM2 knockdown promoted the degradation of CDK1 protein through autolysosome-dependent pathway by increasing autophagic flow, thereby inhibiting the proliferation of glioblastoma by inducing G2/M phase cell cycle arrest. Clinical data analysis revealed that RRM2 expression in glioma patients was inversely correlated with the overall survival. Collectively, pectolinarigenin promoted the degradation of CDK1 protein dependent on autolysosomal pathway through increasing autophagic flux by inhibiting RRM2, thereby inhibiting the proliferation of glioblastoma cells by inducing G2/M phase cell cycle arrest, and RRM2 may be a potential therapeutic target and a prognosis and predictive biomarker in GBM patients.

Keywords: pectolinarigenin, glioblastoma, RRM2, CDK1, autophagic flux

INTRODUCTION

Glioblastoma (World Health Organization grade IV), the most malignant form of intracranial tumor found in adults, accounting for 54% of all gliomas, is incurable due to its high proliferation ability, high invasiveness, resistance to various therapies, and high rate of postoperative recurrence (1). Despite improvements in patients outcomes with the combined radiotherapy and temozolomide regimen since 2005, the median survival duration after the initial diagnosis remains at 15 months with a 5-year survival rate of 7.2% (2). Thus, effective therapeutic approaches for patients with GBM are urgently needed.

Pectolinarigenin (PECT), a dual inhibitor of cyclooxygenase-2/5-lipoxygenase, which is abundantly present in and can be extracted from the Chinese herbal plant *Chromolaena odorata*, has been proven to have numerous pharmacological characteristics, including, anti-inflammatory, anticancer, and anti-allergy activities (3). A previous study also reported that the cancer-specific cytotoxic activity of PECT was mainly attributable to the suppression of proliferative cell cycle, the induction of apoptosis, and the regulation of autophagy (4). However, the benefits of PECT in GBM treatment is not known.

Ribonucleotide reductase subunit M2 (RRM2) encodes the catalytic subunit of ribonucleotide reductase (RNR), which is a hetero-tetramer consisting of two RRM1 and two RRM2 subunits and is involved in regulating DNA synthesis and modifying proteins (5), and is a rate-limiting molecule during the conversion of ribonucleoside triphosphates into dNTPs in the G2 phase of cell cycle (6) and shows elevated levels in some cancers (7, 8). Recent studies demonstrated that overexpression of RRM2 is essential for the cellular response to abnormal dNTP levels, which leads to malignant biological phenotypes such as angiogenesis, epithelial to mesenchymal transition, relapse and drug- or radio-resistance (5, 8). In precision medicine for tumors, targeting of RRM2 has emerged as a therapeutic method for some cancers as it inhibits proliferative cell cycle and regulates autophagy pathways to suppress tumor progress (9). Autophagy is a cellular catabolic process that maintains normal cellular physiological functions by degrading and/or recycling intracellular macromolecules and dysfunctional organelles (10). Moreover, autophagy activation is essential for promoting tumor cell survival and malignant transformation. However, excessive activation or inhibition of autophagy can suppress tumor proliferation and induce cell cycle arrest, and some autophagy genes are involved in cell cycle regulation (11, 12). For example, p62 depletion has been shown to induce cell cycle arrest by promoting cyclin-dependent kinase 1 (CDK1) degradation in human breast cancer (13). In contrast, autophagy related 7 (Atg7) -deficient cells fail to induce p21 expression, thereby impairing p53-mediated cell cycle arrest (14). Although RRM2 is involved in regulating autophagy pathway and cell cycle arrest, it is unclear whether the two biological phenomena are played a role in the anti-tumor effect of PECT on GBM. In this study, we investigate how RRM2 mediates the anti-tumor effect of PECT on GBM *via* reducing CDK1 protein expression and examined the functional significance of autophagy and cell cycle in GBM treatment.

MATERIALS AND METHODS

Patients and Specimens

Normal human brain specimens (n = 6) and fresh glioma specimens (n = 19) were obtained from the Department of Neurosurgery, First Affiliated Hospital of Harbin Medical University. The study protocol was approved by the Clinical Research Ethics Committee of Harbin Medical University. All patients provided written informed consent, and the study was conducted in accordance with the Declaration of Helsinki.

Cell Lines and Chemical Reagents

The U251, U87, and HUVEC cell lines were provided by the China Infrastructure of Cell Line Resource (National Science and Technology Infrastructure) and cultured in Dulbecco's Modified Eagle medium (RNBK0465, Sigma-Aldrich, St. Louis, MO, USA) supplemented with 10% fetal bovine serum (AllBio Science, Taichung, Taiwan). MG132, chloroquine (CQ), and PECT were from MedChemExpress (Monmouth Junction, NJ, USA).

MTT Assay and Clone Formation Assay

The cells were added to a 96-well plate at a density of 5,000 cells/well. At different time points, 10 μL of 3-(4,5-dimethylthiazol-2-yl)-2,5-diphenyl-2H-tetrazolium bromide (MTT; cat# HY-15924, MedChemExpress) dye was added to each well and incubated for 4 h. Finally, we replaced the medium with 150 μL of dimethyl sulfoxide and measured the cell viability (Infinite M200 PRO; Tecan Trading AG, Männedorf, Switzerland). The GBM cells were centrifuged and evenly inoculated into a six-well plate at a density of 800 cells/well. After 14 days of culture at distinct concentrations of PECT, the colonies were measured using the ChemiDoc™ MP imaging software (Bio-Rad Laboratories, Inc., CA, USA).

Immunofluorescence Analysis

After fixation, permeabilization, and sealing, the treated cells and paraffin-embedded glioma tissue sections were incubated with primary antibody and fluorescent secondary antibody, and images were observed with a fluorescence microscope (Lionheart FX; BioTek, Beijing, China). The following primary antibodies were used: CDK1 (BF0091, 1:500, Affinity, USA), p62 (A19700, 1:100, Abclonal, Wuhan, China), LAMP2 (66301-1-lg, 1:100, Proteintech, Hubei, China), Ki67 (A2094, 1:100, Abclonal, Wuhan, China).

Cell Transfection

GBM cells were interfered with siRNA, plasmid, and lentiviruses. The siRNA-NC/RRM2 and RRM2 overexpression plasmid pEnter-NC/RRM2 were from Miaolingbio (Wuhan, China) and lentiviruses were from GeneChem (Shanghai, China). The sequences of siRNA-NC/RRM2 and LV-shNC/LV-shRRM2 are shown in **Table 1**.

Transmission Electron Microscopy

U251 cells were first fixed with 2.5% glutaraldehyde at 4°C, and post-fixed with 1% osmium tetroxide. The immobilized cells were then dehydrated in increasing concentrations of ethanol and acetone. Finally, Transmission Electron Microscopy (TEM) was used to observe autophagic vesicles.

Western Blot Analysis

For Western Blot (WB) analysis, the tissues and treated cells were first extracted and lysed. After separating the proteins using 12.5% sodium dodecyl sulfate-polyacrylamide gel electrophoresis, they were transferred to a polyvinylidene fluoride membrane, which was blocked and then incubated with primary antibodies and fluorescent-dye conjugated secondary antibodies. Protein bands were imaged using a ChemiDoc™ MP Imaging System (Bio-Rad, Hercules, CA, USA). The following primary antibodies were used: RRM2 (BS7520, 1:1,000, BioWorld, Nanjing, China); LAMP2 (66301-1-lg, 1:1,000, Proteintech, Hubei, China); LC3B (83506S, 1:1,000, Cell Signaling Technology, USA); CCNA2 (A7632, 1:1,000), CCNB1 (A2056, 1:1,000), CDK1 (A0220, 1:1,000) and p62 (A19700, 1:1,000) were purchased from Abclonal (Wuhan, China).

Flow Cytometric Analysis

The treated cells were first digested with 0.25% trysin, centrifuged, and then fixed with 70% ethyl alcohol at 4°C. The next day, the digested cells were stained using a cell cycle analysis kit (P0010, Beyotime, Shanghai, China). Finally, a flow cytometer (Agilent NovoCyte, China) was used to measure the cell cycle distribution.

RFP-GFP-LC3 Lentivirus Transfection and Fluorescence Imaging

After treatment under different conditions, U251 cells transfected with RFP-GFP-LC3 lentivirus were fixed and used to measure autophagy flux. The fluorescence intensity was analyzed using a FluoView FV300 confocal microscope (Olympus Corporation, Tokyo, Japan).

Quantitative Real-Time Polymerase Chain Reaction Assay

Total RNA was extracted from the clinical samples or treated cells using TRIzol (Sigma-Aldrich), and then one microgram of total RNA was reverse-transcribed into cDNA using a ReverTra Ace qPCR RT Kit (Toyobo, Osaka, Japan). Quantitative Real-Time Polymerase Chain Reaction (qRT-PCR) was performed on triplicate samples in a reaction mixture of SYBR Green (Roche, Basel, Switzerland) with a Gene Amp PCR System 9700 (Thermo Fisher Scientific, Waltham, MA, USA). The data were normalized to glyceraldehyde 3-phosphate dehydrogenase (GAPDH) using the ΔΔCt method. The primer sequences for GAPDH, RRM2 and CDK1 are shown in **Table 1**.

Co-Immunoprecipitation

First, the primary antibody was added to Protein A/G Plus-Agarose and incubated at 4°C for 2 h, and then the cell protein lysates were added and incubated at 4°C overnight. We next separated the magnetic beads, collected the supernatant, and performed WB.

Liquid Chromatography-Mass Spectrometry

Each tumor bearing mice brain tissue sample was mixed with methanol (containing 5 μg/mL 2-chloro-L-phenylalanine as an internal standard) and mixed with a vortex mixer for homogenization. The samples were centrifuged and transferred to sampler vial. An in-house quality control (QC) sample was prepared by mixing equal amounts of each sample. We performed Liquid Chromatography-Mass Spectrometry (LC-MS) analysis of the QC samples. The raw data was converted to a common format, and the degree of aggregation of QC samples was assessed using the principal component analysis modeling method and PCA modeling method was used to check the aggregation degree of QC simples.

In Vivo Studies

BALB/c nude mice were purchased from Beijing Vital River Laboratory Animal Technology Co., Ltd. (Beijing, China). For each mouse, 5×10^6 U251 cells were subcutaneously implanted into the right flank, or 1×10^6 U251 cells were implanted into the brain. The mice were randomly divided into control and PECT groups (six mices per group). PECT (25mg/kg every other day, prepared as a 150 mM stock solution in DMSO and stored at -20°C) diluted with 100 μL PBS was administered intraperitoneally for 3 weeks, whereas the control group treated with the same amount of DMSO diluted with 100 μL PBS. Additionally, 1×10^6 U251 cells transfected with LV-shNC or LV-shRRM2 per mice were implanted into the brain. All animal study protocols were approved by the Animal Experiments Ethics Committee of Harbin Medical University and the study was conducted in accordance with the Declaration of Helsinki.

TABLE 1 | Sequences of siRNA, primers, and lentiviruses.

siRNA sequences	
si-NC	5′UUCUCCGAACGUGUCACGUTT3′
RRM2-si RNA1	5′GGCUCAGCUUGGUCGACAA3′, 5′UUGUCGACCAAGCUGAGCC3′
RRM2-si RNA2	5′GGAGAGAGUAAGAGAAAUATT3′
RRM2-si RNA3	5′GAAGAGAGUAGGCGAGUAUTT3′
Primer sequences	
GAPDH	F-5′CACCCACTCCTCCACCTTTGA3′, R-5′ACCACCCTGTTGCTGTAGCCA3′
CDK1	F-5′AAACTACAGGTCAAGTGGTAGCC3′, R-5′TCCTGCATAAGCACATCCTGA3′
RRM2	F-5′TGCCATTGAAACGATGCCTT 3′, R-5′ACTGCAGCAAAGGCTACAAC 3′
Lentivirus sequences	
LV-shNC	5′ TTCTCCGAACGTGTCACGT 3′
LV-shRRM2 1	5′ccCATTTGACTTTATGGAGAA3′
LV-shRRM2 2	5′ gcTCAAGAAACGAGGACTGA3′
LV-shRRM2 3	5′ gcAGATGTATAAGAAGGCAGA3′

Hematoxylin and Eosin Staining and Immunohistochemical Staining

After dehydration and paraffin embedding, the mice brain tumor and organ sections were stained with Hematoxylin and Eosin (H&E). For Immunohistochemical (IHC) assay, tumors were first formalin-fixed, paraffin-embedded, and sliced, and then the sample sections were immunostained with primary antibodies and an anti-mouse/rabbit secondary antibody.

RNA-Sequencing and Bioinformatics Analyses

We used DESeq2 or edgeR to analyze differences in expression and identify enriched functional terms and pathways (*via* Gene Ontology [GO] and Kyoto Encyclopedia of Genes and Genomes [KEGG]). The clinical information and mRNA sequencing data of the 1,038 patients with glioma were obtained from the Chinese Glioma Genome Atlas (CGGA) database http://www.cgga.org.cn/index.jsp, which included data from 625 low-grade glioma (LGG), 388 GBM, and 20 non-glioma patients. OS was determined among 592 LGG and 374 GBM cases, and the median was used as the demarcation point.

Statistical Analysis

Differences between two groups and multiple groups were estimated using Student *t*-test and one-way analysis of variance, respectively. The statistical significance of OS between different groups was evaluated by log-rank test. All statistical analyses were carried using GraphPad Prism version 7.0 software (GraphPad, Inc., San Diego, CA, USA), and a value of $p < 0.05$ was considered to indicate statistically significant results.

RESULTS

PECT Suppresses GBM Cells Proliferation *In Vitro* and *In Vivo*

The 2D structure of PECT is presented in **Figure 1A**. Firstly, human GBM cells U87 and U251, and human normal cell HUVEC were used to verify the anti-proliferation effect of PECT. MTT results showed that PECT inhibited GBM cells proliferation in dose- and time-dependent manners, but not that of HUVECs. The half-maximal inhibitory concentration (IC_{50}) values of PECT for 48 h among U87 and U251 cells were 21.17 and 21.00 μM, respectively (**Figure 1B**). Therefore, the drug concentration closest to IC_{50} of 20 μM was selected for follow-up experiments. Subsequently, we used clonogenic assays to verify the sensitivity of GBM cells to PECT and founded that PECT can prevent the tumor sphere formation in a dose-dependent manner (**Figure 1C**). Additionally, PECT inhibited GBM cells proliferation as shown using ki67 staining (**Figure 1D**). Therefore, PECT inhibited GBM cells proliferation and can be administered safely *in vitro*.

The mice accepted the treatment of PECT showed a much smaller brain tumor size than another (**Figure 1E**) and had a significantly prolonged lifespan (**Figure 1F**). In addition, we performed LC-MS assays to detect the concentration of PECT in gliomas and found that PECT can penetrate the blood-brain barrier (BBB) (**Figures 1G, H, Figure S1**), which was consistent with the outcomes described in the traditional Chinese medicine systems pharmacology database and analysis platform (TCMSP) (http://lsp.nwu.edu.cn/tcmsp.php) (**Table S1**) (15). These data indicate that PECT had an anti-tumor effect on GBM *in vivo*.

PECT Downregulates RRM2 Expression and Increased Autophagy Flux *In Vitro*

To determine the mechanism of the anti-tumor effect of PECT on GBM, we screened differentially expressed genes (DEGs) using RNA-Sequencing (RNA-Seq) analysis after PECT treatment, and detected 1,279 DEGs (662 upregulated genes and 617 downregulated genes, $|\log2 \text{ fold-change}|>1.0$, $p<0.05$), the top 50 of which are shown in **Figure 1I**. The functional annotation analysis of the DEGs using GO. DNA replication and cell cycle regulation were the mainly GO terms (p.adjust <0.05) (**Figure 1J**). In addition, KEGG enrichment pathway (*p*.adjust <0.05) analysis revealed that the DNA replication, cell cycle, lysosomal, and proteasome pathways were the major signs pathways influenced by PECT (**Figure 1K**). Among the top 50 of DEGs, RRM2 was closely correlated with DNA replication, cell cycle, lysosomal and proteasome pathways, so we hypothesized that RRM2 may be a key target gene for the anti-tumor effect of PECT on GBM. To verify the changes of RRM2 expression, we exposed GBM cells to PECT for 48 h and founded that RRM2 mRNA and protein expression gradually decreased with increasing PECT concentrations (**Figures 2A, B**).

Next, we investigated whether PECT regulates autophagy in GBM cells. TEM results revealed that autophagic vacuoles gradually increased after adding PECT to U251 cells from 0 h to 48 h (**Figure 2C**); simultaneously, LC3B-II and LAMP2 protein expression increased and p62 protein expression decreased (**Figure 2E**), indicating that PECT increased autophagic vacuoles in GBM cells by increasing autophagic flux. Further, we performed a RFP-GFP-LC3 transfection assay on U251 cells to re-confirm the above results, and found that both free red puncta (autolysosomes) and yellow puncta (autophagosomes) increased in the merged sections of U251 cells treated with PECT in a time-dependent manner, and the red puncta increased more (**Figure 2D**), validating the increase of autophagic flux.

Subsequently, we investigated whether the autolysosome was involved in RRM2 degradation. chloroquine (CQ), a late-stage autophagy inhibitor, of which low dose that can partially inhibit pH value increase and block protein degradation in the autolysosome, but has no effect on cell activity (16), was used. The results showed that 2 μM CQ did not affect the cell viability of GBM (**Figure S2**), but increased p62 and LC3B-II protein expression, indicating inhibition of autophagic flux (**Figure 2F**). Therefore, 2 μM CQ was selected. An increased number of yellow puncta but a decreased number of free red puncta was observed in the merged sections of the PECT+CQ-treated groups compared to the PECT-treated groups (**Figure 2G**); simultaneously, the reduction of the p62 and RRM2 protein expression was partially recovered, but the LC3B-II protein expression further increased (**Figure 2F**), indicating that CQ

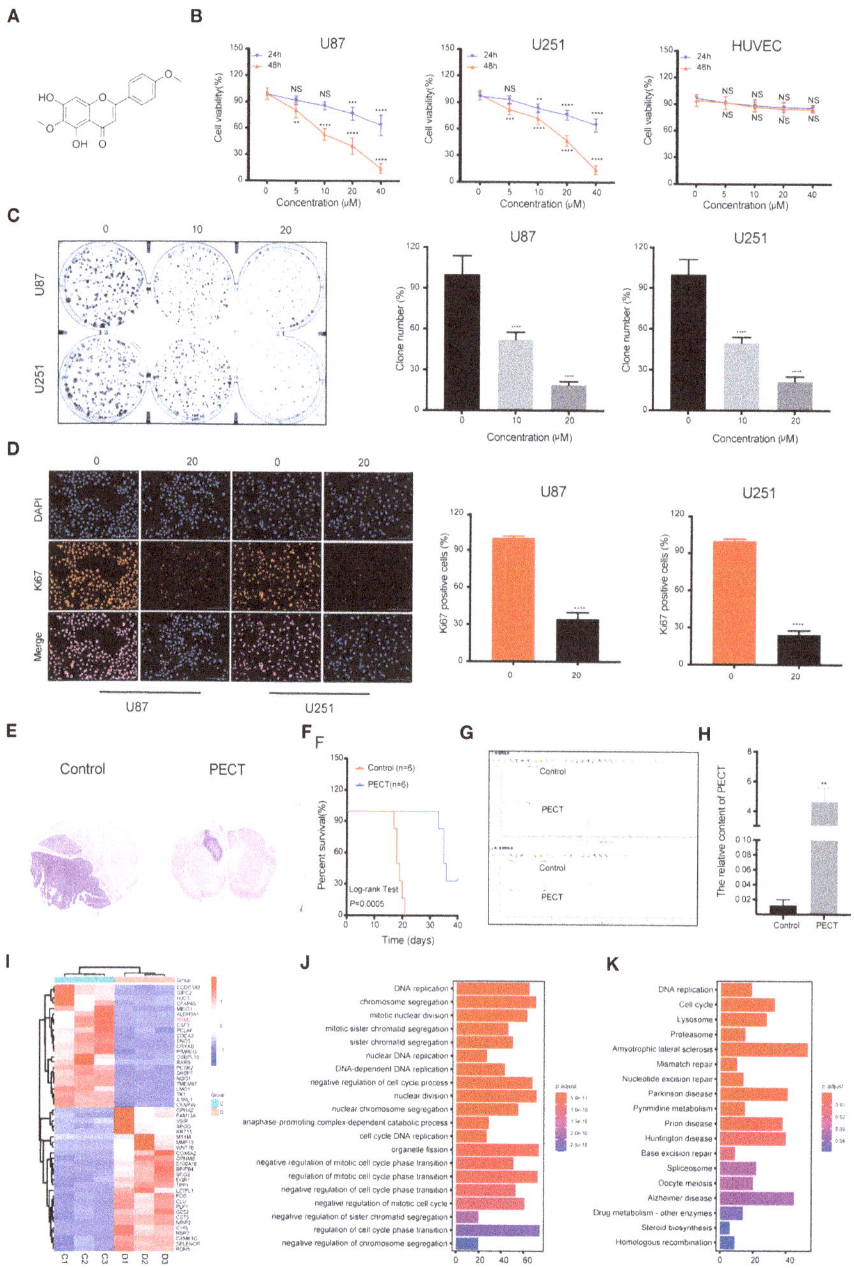

FIGURE 1 | PECT inhibits GBM cells proliferation both *in vitro* and *in vivo*, and RNA-sequencing analysis. **(A)** Structure of PECT. **(B)** After exposuring to different concentrations of PECT for 24 or 48 h, cell viability of U87, U251 and HUVECs cells was assessed using MTT. **(C)** Representative images of colony formation on U87 and 251 cells treated with PECT for different concentrations. **(D)** After U87 and U251 cells were cultured with or without PECT (20 μM, 48 h), Ki67 staining was observed by fluorescence microscopy. Scale bar: 200 μm. **(E)** H&E images of brain sections of mice orthotopically xenografted tumor with U251 cells treated with PECT. Scale bar: 1000 μm. **(F)** Kaplan-Meier survival curve of mice orthotopically xenografted tumor with U251 cells treated with PECT. **(G, H)** LC-MS analysis of PECT content in the tumor bearing mice brain homogenate samples. **(I)** Heatmap of top 50 up- or down-regulated DEGs after PECT treatment. C1-3: control group, D1-3: PECT-treated group. **(J)** GO and **(K)** KEGG analysis of DEGs. The data are presented as the mean ± SD (n=3). NS, non-significant. $^{**}P < 0.01$, $^{***}P < 0.001$, $^{****}P < 0.0001$.

blocked the autophagic flux induced by PECT and inhibited RRM2 protein degradation. As expected, immunofluorescence assay of LAMP2 [a lysosomal membrane marker that is involved in autophagy and critical for some proteins degradation in lysosomes (17)] and RRM2 showed that PECT treatment resulted in more LAMP2 protein expression but less RRM2 protein expression in U251 cells, and increased the cytoplasmic co-localization of LAMP2 and RRM2 (**Figure 2H**), further indicating that RRM2 depends on autolysosome pathway degradation.

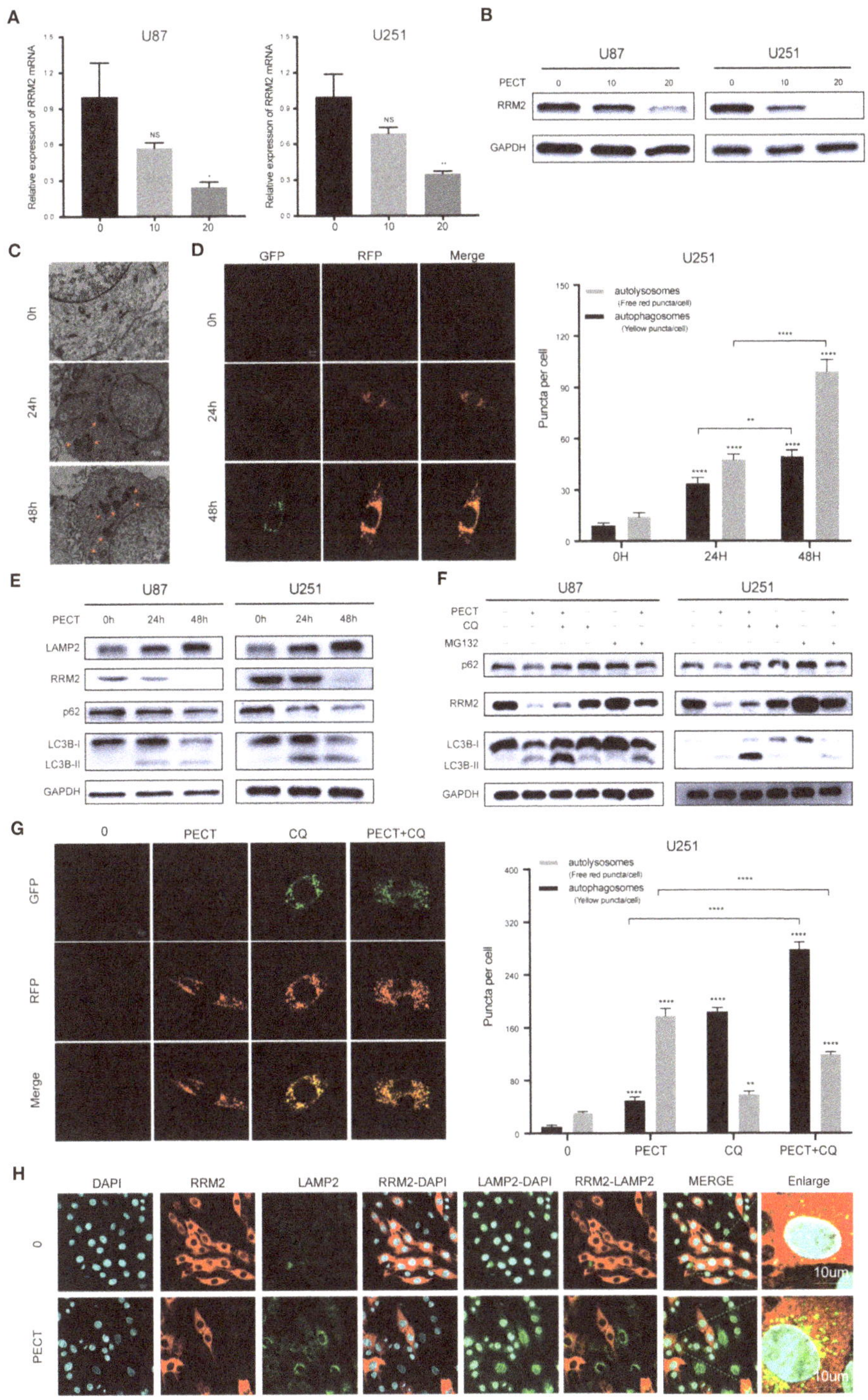

FIGURE 2 | PECT downregulates RRM2 expression and increases autophagy flux *in vitro*. **(A, B)** After culturing U87 and U251 cells with different concentrations of PECT for 48h, RRM2 mRNA and protein expression were examined by qRT-PCR and western blot assay, respectively. **(C)** TEM images of U251 cells exposed to PECT (20 μM) for 0h, 24h, and 48 h. Autophagic vacuole (red arrows). Scale bar: 10 μm. **(D)** After U251 cells cultured with PECT (20 μM) for 0h, 24h, and 48 h, autophagic flux was analyzed using the RFP-GFP-LC3 construct. Scale bar: 20 μm. **(E)** Western blot analysis of RRM2, p62, LC3B and LAMP2 protein expression in U87 and U251 cells cultured with PECT (20 μM) for 0h, 24h, and 48 h. **(F)** Western blot analysis of RRM2, p62 and LC3B protein expression in U87 and U251 cells cultured with PECT (20 μM, 48 h) or CQ (2 μM, 2 h) or MG132 (2 μM, 3 h). **(G)** After U251 cells cultured with PECT (20 μM, 48h) or CQ (2 μM, 2h), autophagic flux was analyzed using the RFP-GFP-LC3 construct. Scale bar: 20 μm. **(H)** Immunofluorescence analysis of RRM2 (red) and LAMP2 (green) in U251 cells treated with or without PECT(20 μM, 48 h). The nuclei were stained with DAPI. Scale bar: 10 μm. The data are presented as the mean ± SD (n=3). NS, non-significant. $^{*}P < 0.05$, $^{**}P < 0.01$, $^{****}P < 0.0001$.

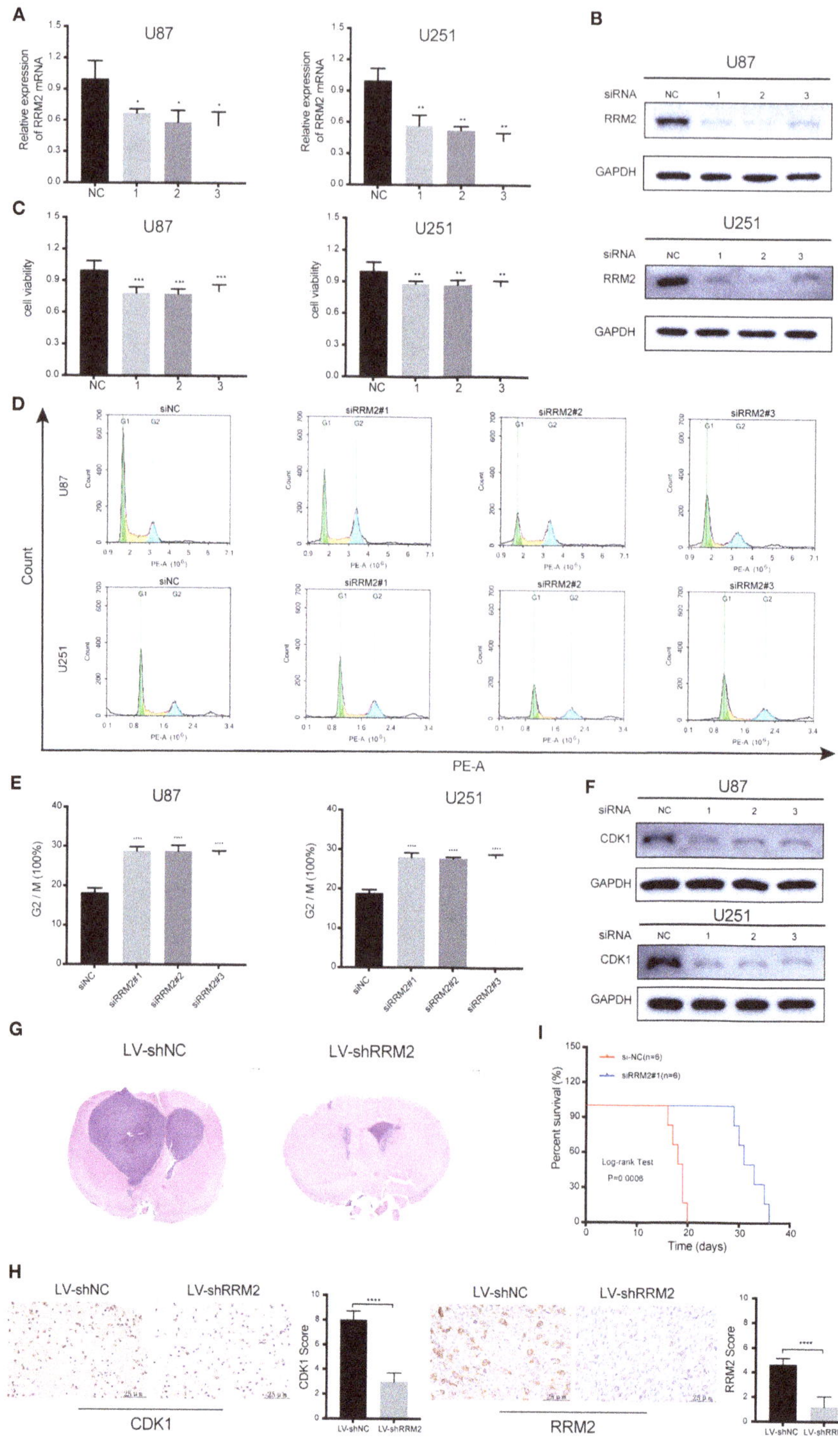

FIGURE 3 | RRM2 knockdown inhibits GBM proliferation and induces cell cycle arrest both *in vitro* and *in vivo*. After transfecting U87 and U251 cells with RRM2 siRNA for 48h, **(A)** RRM2 mRNA expression was examined by qRT-PCR, **(B)** RRM2 protein expression was analyzed by western blot assay, **(C)** cells viability were assessed using MTT, **(D, E)** cells cycle distribution were analyzed using flow cytometry. (green: G0-G1, yellow: S, and blue: G2-M). **(F)** CDK1 protein expression was analyzed by western blot assay. **(G)** H&E images of brain sections of mice orthotopically xenografted with U251 cells transfected with LV-shNC and LV-shRRM2. Scale bar: 1000 μm. **(H)** IHC staining of CDK1 and RRM2 in consecutive brain sections of mice orthotopically xenografted with U251 cells transfected with LV-shNC and LV-shRRM2. Scale bar: 25 μm. **(I)** The survival time of nude mice orthotopically xenografted with U251 cells transfected with LV-shNC and LV-shRRM2. The data are presented as the mean ± SD (n=3). $^*P < 0.05$, $^{**}P < 0.01$, $^{***}P < 0.001$, $^{****}P < 0.0001$.

Additionally, we verified that the proteasome is also involed in RRM2 protein degradation, which can be partly reversed by the proteasome inhibitor MG132 (**Figure 2F**).

Overall, our *in vitro* data confirmed that PECT treatment can increase autophagy flux in GBM cells, and RRM2 protein reduction after PECT treatment is not only dependent on transcriptional inhibition but also proteasomal and autolysosomal degradation.

RRM2 Knockdown Inhibits GBM Proliferation and Induces Cell Cycle Arrest *In Vitro* and *In Vivo*

To assess the effect of RRM2 on GBM, we used siRNA to interfere with RRM2 expression in GBM cells. The siRNA efficiency was shown in **Figure 3A**; similarly, RRM2 knockdown not only decreased RRM2 protein expression (**Figure 3B**) but also suppressed GBM cells viability (**Figure 3C**). Moreover, we founded that the proportion of G2/M phase cells increased (**Figures 3D, E**) and CDK1 protein expression was decrease with RRM2 knockdown (**Figure 3F**), but CCNA2 and CCNB1 protein expression no change (**Figure S3**). In addition, we founded that the expression of CDK1 mRNA was also not change (**Figure S4**). These results demonstrated that G2/M cell cycle arrest is caused by the decrease of CDK1 protein, which is consistent with previous reports (18, 19).

Subsequently, RRM2 knockdown was induced by RRM2 lentivirus in U251 cells. After testing the transfection efficiency (**Figure S5**), lentivirus-treated cells were implanted into the brains of 5-week-old nude mice. Mice treated with RRM2 lentivirus showed much smaller tumor volumes compared to controls (**Figure 3G**) and exhibited significantly prolonged survival time (**Figure 3I**). IHC analysis showed that compared with the LV-shNC group, the protein expression of CDK1 and RRM2 decreased in LV-shRRM2 group (**Figure 3H**).

Taken together, our results revealed that RRM2 knockdown could induce G2/M phase cell cycle arrest by reducing the level of CDK1 protein and inhibit GBM cells proliferation *in vitro* and *in vivo*.

RRM2 Knockdown Induces Cell Cycle Arrest in GBM *via* Promoting CDK1 Protein Degradation by Increasing Autophagic Flux *In Vitro*

Firstly, we founded that RRM2 knockdown can promote the autophagic vacuoles accumulated in U251 cells (**Figure 4A**). Simultaneously, a RFP-GFP-LC3 transfection assay revealed that both free red puncta and yellow puncta increased in the merged sections of si-RRM2#1 U251 cells compared with that in si-NC U251 cells, but the free red puncta increased more (**Figure 4B**), indicating the autophagic flux increased.

Subsequently, we sought to determine whether autophagy is required for RRM2-mediated cell cycle progression. The data showed that RRM2 knockdown promoted G2/M phase cell cycle arrest, while this effect was reversed by CQ, an inhibitor of autophagic flux that prevents autophagosome-lysosome fusion and lysosomal protein degradation (**Figures 4C, D**). Interestingly, the change in CDK1 protein level was consistent with the cell cycle distribution (**Figure 4E**). These data indicate that the blockage of G2/M phase cell cycle induced by RRM2 knockdown is dependent on the function of RRM2 in autophagy.

To further investigate the mechanism regarding whether the degradation of CDK1 protein depends on the autolysosomal pathway during RRM2 knockdown, we performed Co-Immunoprecipitation (Co-IP) assays to analyze the interaction between CDK1 and p62, an adapter protein, is required for some protein degradation through the autolysosome pathway (20). As shown in **Figure 4F**, p62 was able to interact with CDK1. Additionally, immunofluorescence analysis showed that CDK1 could co-localize with p62 in U251 cell, but the co-localization of p62 with CDK1 decreased after RRM2 knockdown (**Figure 4G**). Thus, our results demonstrated that RRM2 knockdown induced cell cycle arrest in GBM *via* promoting CDK1 protein degradation by increasing autophagic flux *in vitro*.

PECT Inhibits GBM Proliferation, Promotes Cell Cycle Arrest, and Increases Autophagic Flux by Decreasing RRM2 Expression *In Vitro*

To verify whether RRM2 mediates the anti-tumor effect of PECT on GBM, we overexpressed RRM2 and exposed them to PECT, and founded that GBM cells viability (**Figure 5A**) were partially rescued with RRM2 expression upregulation (**Figures 5B, C**). Similarly, the increased proportion of G2/M phase GBM cells (**Figures 5D, E**) and the downregulation of p62 and CDK1 protein and upregulation of LAMP2 and LC3B-II protein caused by PECT were partially recovered with RRM2 expression upregulation (**Figure 5F**). Overall, our results showd that PECT can inhibit GBM proliferation and promote G2/M phase cell cycle arrest as well as increase autophagic flux by decreasing RRM2 expression *in vitro*.

PECT Inhibits GBM Proliferation *In Vivo*

In vivo, our results showed that PECT suppressed tumor proliferation, accompanied by reducing tumor weight (**Figures 6A, B**) and tumor weight/mouse weight (**Figure 6C**), and downregulating RRM2 mRNA (**Figure 6D**) and protein (**Figure 6E**) expression compared to that in controls. However, the body weight of mice in each group did not differ significantly (**Figure 6F**). Moreover, we founded that PECT itself did not induce additional toxicities by evaluating morphological changes in tissues in all groups (**Figure 6G**). IHC results showed that compared with the control group, the protein expression of LC3B and LAMP2 increased while that of Ki67, RRM2, p62, and CDK1 decreased in xenograft tumors administered with PECT (**Figure 6H**). Taken together, PECT exerts an anti-tumor effect in GBM and can be safely administered *in vivo*.

RRM2 Is Increased in GBM Tissues and Inversely Correlated With the Prognosis of Glioma Patients

To verify the clinical significance of RRM2 in glioma patients, firstly, we performed IHC staining analysis, and founded that

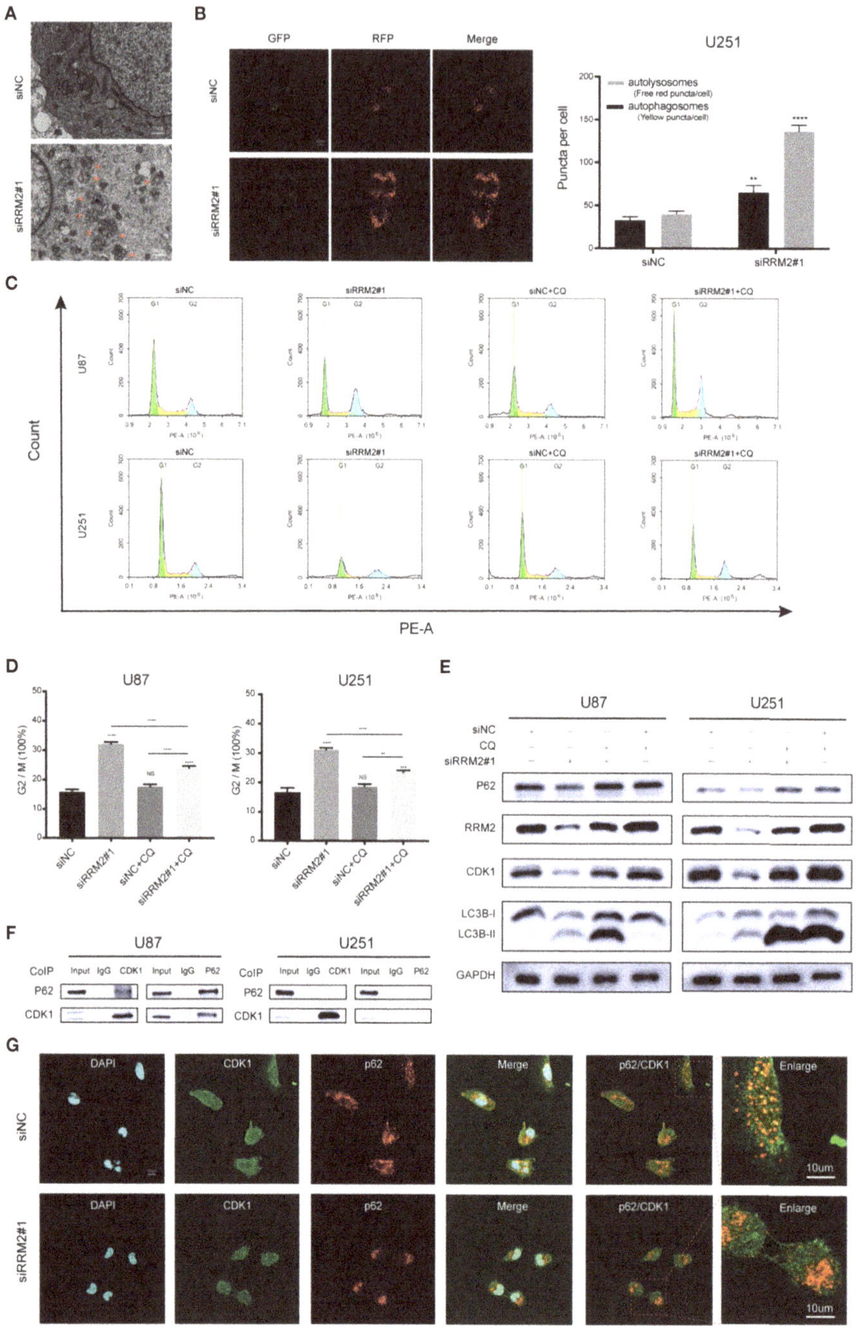

FIGURE 4 | RRM2 knockdown induces cell cycle arrest in GBM *via* promoting CDK1 protein degradation by increasing autophagic flux *in vitro*. **(A)** TEM images of U251 cells transfected with RRM2 siRNA for 48h. Autophagic vacuole (red arrows). Scale bar: 10 μm. **(B)** U251 cells transfected with RRM2 siRNA for 48h, autophagic flux was analyzed using the RFP-GFP-LC3 construct. Scale bar: 20 μm. **(C, D)** After U87 and U251 cells transfected with RRM2 siRNA for 48 h or cultured with CQ (2 μM, 2 h), cells cycle distribution were analyzed using flow cytometry. (green: G0-G1, yellow: S, and blue: G2-M). **(E)** After U87 and U251 cells transfected with RRM2 siRNA for 48 h or cultured with CQ (2 μM, 2 h), CDK1, RRM2, p62 and LC3B proteins expression were analyzed by western blot assay. **(F)** Total protein lysates of U87 or U251 cells were prepared for Co-IP using CDK1 or p62 antibody. **(G)** Immunofluorescence assay of the co-localization of p62 (red) and CDK1 (green) in U251 cells after transfection with RRM2 siRNA for 48 h. Scale bar: 10 μm. The data are presented as the mean ± SD (n=3). NS, non-significant. $^{**}P < 0.01$, $^{***}P < 0.001$, $^{****}P < 0.0001$.

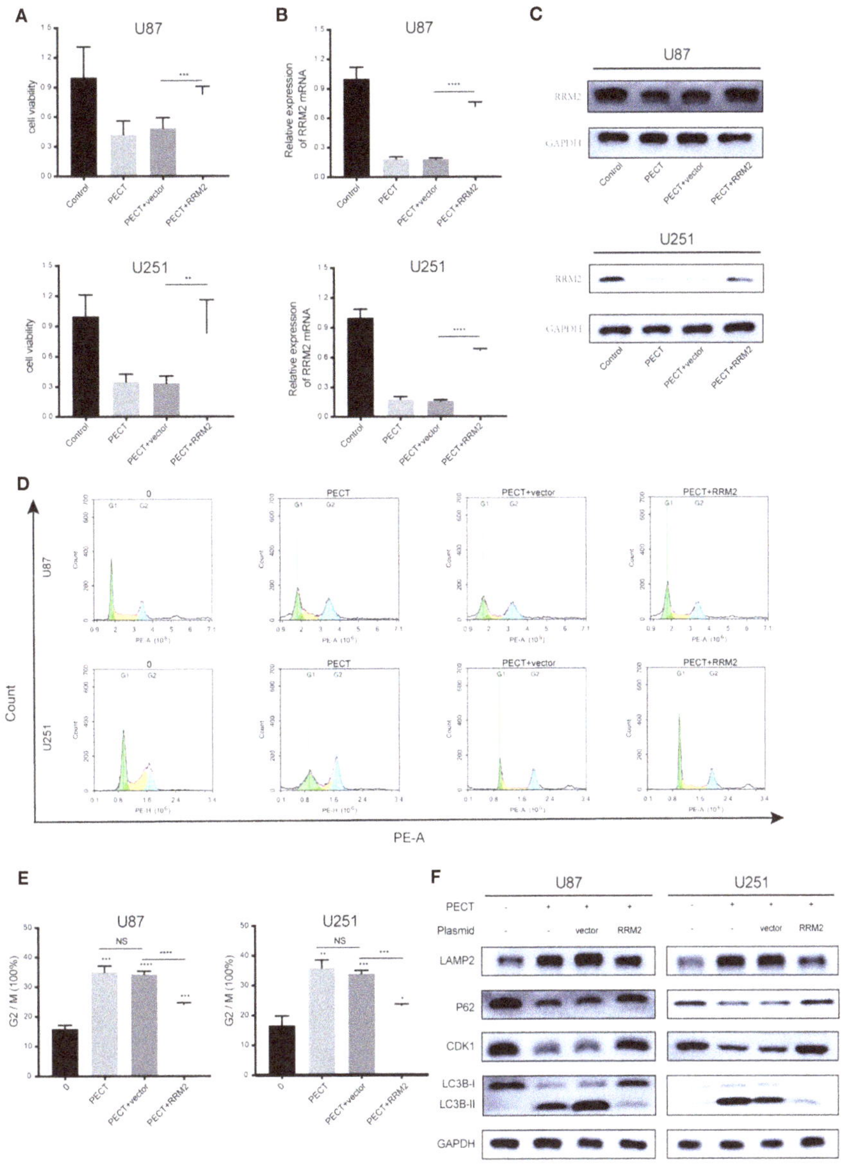

FIGURE 5 | PECT inhibits GBM proliferation, promotes cell cycle arrest, and increases autophagic flux by decreasing RRM2 expression *in vitro*. After U87 and U251 cells transfected with RRM2 overexpression plasmid or cultured with PECT (20 μM, 48 h), **(A)** cells viability were assessed using MTT, **(B)** RRM2 mRNA expression was examined by qRT-PCR, **(C)** RRM2 protein expression was analyzed by western blot assay, **(D, E)** cells cycle distribution were analyzed using flow cytometry. (green: G0-G1, yellow: S, and blue: G2-M). **(F)** CDK1, p62, LAMP2 and LC3B protein expression were analyzed by western blot assay. Vector and RRM2 represent negative control plasmid and RRM2 overexpression plasmid, respectively. The data are presented as the mean ± SD (n=3). NS: non-significant. *$P < 0.05$, **$P < 0.01$, ***$P < 0.001$, ****$P < 0.0001$.

compared with normal human brain tissues, RRM2, CDK1, and p62 protein expression had increase in distinct grades of glioma, especially in GBM tissues (**Figure 7A**). Additionally, according to the CGGA data and qRT-PCR results, compared with non-tumor brain tissues, RRM2 mRNA expressions gradually increased with increasing the degree of glioma malignancy (**Figure 7B**). WB analysis revealed that RRM2 and CDK1 protein expression in human GBM tissue was higher than that in LGG and normal human brain tissues, but no significant difference between LGG and normal human brain tissues, indicating that RRM2 may be a predictive marker of GBM (**Figures 7C, D**).

We confirmed that p62 can directly interact with CDK1 and is an adapter for the degradation of CDK1 protein in autolysosome *in vitro*. Therefore, we performed immunofluorescence staining, and founded that p62 and CDK1 protein are co-located in the lesional cells from human GBM cases, which indicated that p62 and CDK1 protein could interact directly *in vivo* (**Figure 7E**). More importantly, we examined the clinical data of patients with glioma in the CGGA database and revealed that RRM2

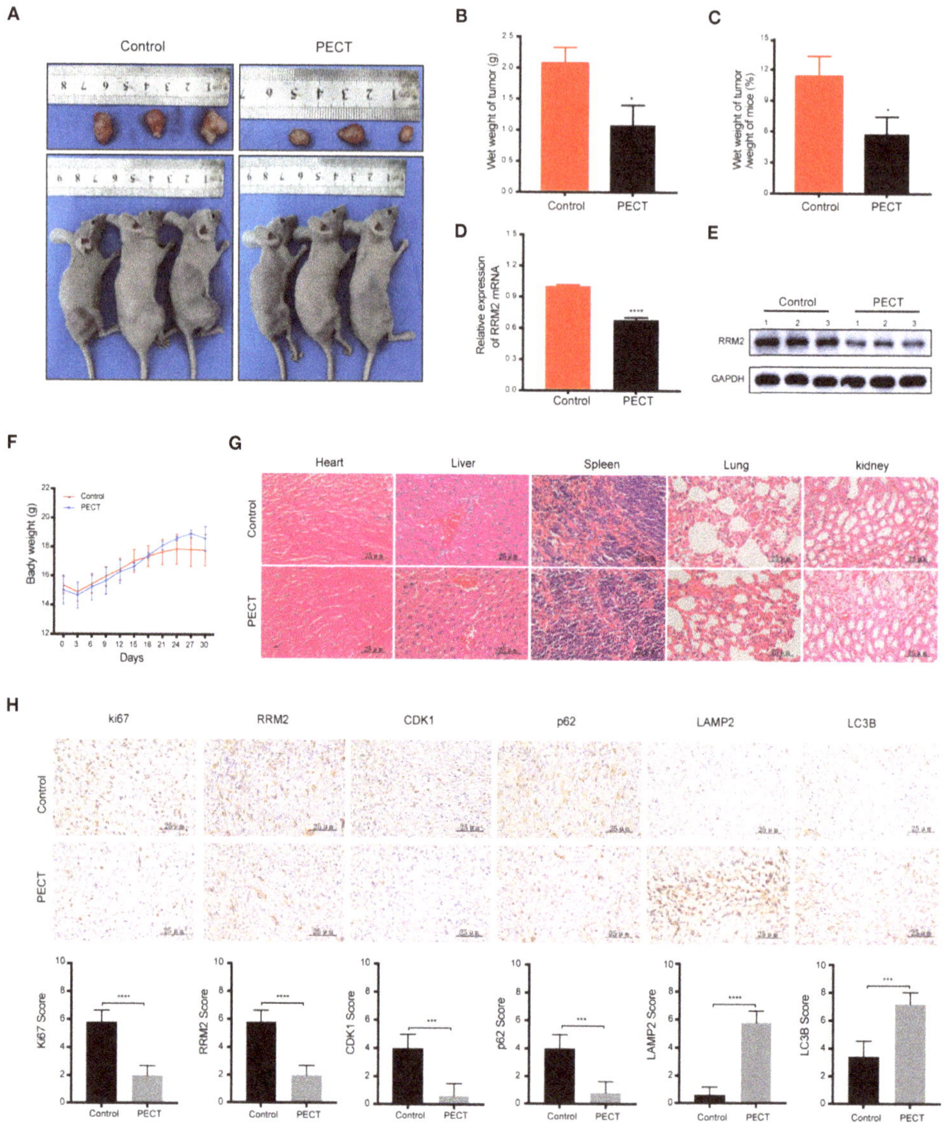

FIGURE 6 | PECT inhibits GBM proliferation *in vivo*. **(A)** Dissected images of mices and tumors, **(B)** tumor wet weight and **(C)** wet weight of tumor/weight of mice between the control and PECT groups. **(D, E)** RRM2 mRNA and protein expressions in mouse tumors with or without PECT treatment. **(F)** Body weight changes in the mouse models. **(G)** Representative images of H&E staining of the organs from mice with or without PECT treatment. Scale bar: 25 μm. **(H)** IHC staining for Ki67, RRM2, CDK1, p62, LAMP2, and LC3B in xenograft tumors between the control and PECT groups. Scale bar: 25 μm. The data are presented as the mean ± SD (n=3). **P* < 0.05, ****P* < 0.001, *****P* < 0.0001.

expression was inversely correlated with the OS time, indicating that RRM2 may be a prognosis marker of GBM (**Figure 7F**).

DISCUSSION

Chemotherapy is one of the conventional treatments for GBM. However, the existing chemotherapeutic drugs are insufficient to provide a survival period of more than 15 months to GBM patients (21, 22). Nearly a third of the drugs used in clinical care, currently, to treat cancer, come from natural products or its derivatives (23), indicating an attractive prospect for the development of natural products as a novel GBM therapy. PECT, a natural flavonoid, has demonstrated several anticancer activities, including autophagy and G2/M phase cell cycle arrest induction, cell proliferation, and migration inhibition (3, 24, 25). In the present study, we demonstrated for the first time that PECT can suppress GBM proliferation both *in vitro* and *in vivo*. More importantly, PECT significantly suppressed GBM cells, but not HUVECs, proliferation and did not caused morphological changes in organ tissues, indicating that PECT can inhibit tumor growth and can be safely administered *in vitro* and *in vivo*. Effective drugs for treating GBM are currently limited; one of the major limitations to drug development is that therapeutic agents

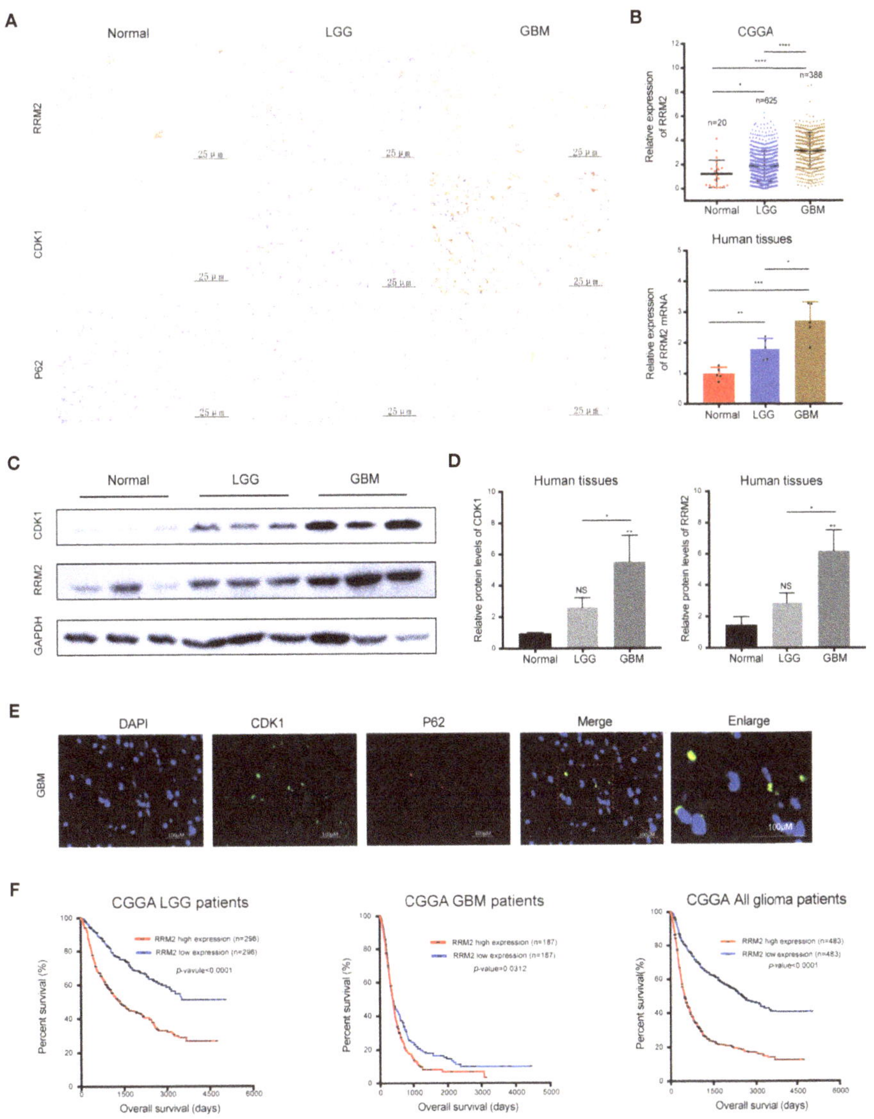

FIGURE 7 | RRM2 is increased in GBM tissues and inversely correlated with the prognosis of glioma patients. **(A)** IHC analysis of RRM2, CDK1, and p62 in sections obtained from primary glioma sample tissues and normal human brain sample tissues. **(B)** Analysis of RRM2 mRNA expression in GBM samples compared to normal human brain samples and LGG samples according to the CGGA data and qRT-PCR results. **(C, D)** WB analysis of RRM2 and CDK1 in GBM sample tissues compared to normal human brain sample tissues and LGG sample tissues. **(E)** Immunofluorescence double-staining analysis showing co-localization of p62 and CDK1 in the same lesional cells in human GBM cases. **(F)** OS curves of patients with glioma according to the median of RRM2. The data are presented as the mean ± SD (n=3). NS, non-significant. *$P < 0.05$, **$P < 0.01$, ***$P < 0.001$, ****$P < 0.0001$.

must possess the ability to cross BBB (26). Our results revealed that PECT can not only cross BBB, but also suppress the growth of intracranial GBM in nude mice and prolonged their effective survival time. However, the underlying molecular mechanism of the antineoplastic effect of PECT on GBM remains unclear.

We performed RNA-Seq analysis and found PECT treatment could inhibit the expression of RRM2 in U251 cells and affect the signal pathways such as DNA replication, cell cycle, lysosomal, and proteasome. In addition, qRT-PCR and western blotting assays further verified that PECT could reduce the expression of RRM2 mRNA and protein in GBM cells. RRM2 is the catalytic subunit of heterodimeric tetramer RNR and catalyzes *de novo* formation of dNTPs (27). The level of RRM2 changes continuously during the cell cycle to maintain the balance between dNTP production and DNA synthesis. Multiple cancers, such as melanoma, colorectal cancer, prostate cancer, liver cancer, breast cancer, glioma, and ovarian cancer, benefit from therapy targetting RRM2 (5, 28, 29). Sun and coworkers have shown that silencing RRM2 can induce G2/M phase cell cycle arrest of U87 cells (30). Chen et al. reported that RRM2 knockdown can reverse the resistance of human lung squamous carcinoma cells to gemcitabine by inducing autophagy (31). Our

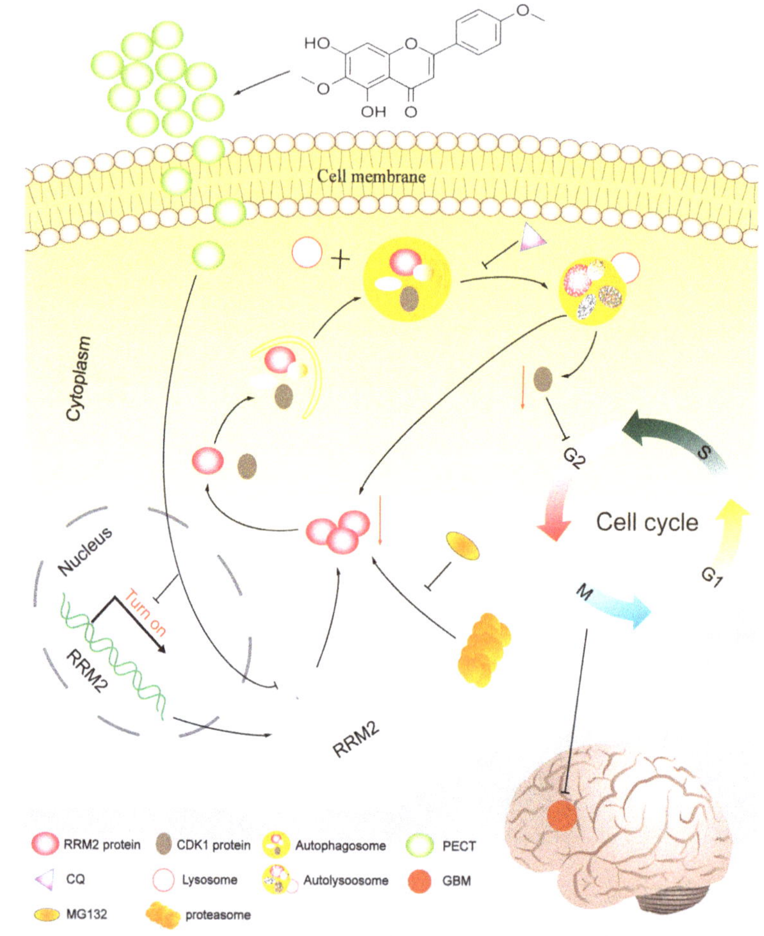

FIGURE 8 | The schematic diagram of RRM2 mediates the anti-tumor effect of PECT on GBM.

results showed that PECT can induce G2/M phase cell cycle arrest and increase autophagic flux of glioblastoma cells by inhibting RRM2 expression, which can be reversed by RRM2 overexpression plasmid.

Additionally, we found that PECT could inhibit RRM2 transcription and promote RRM2 protein degradation through a proteasome-dependent pathway, consistent with previous report. Such as RRM2 is ubiquitinated by APC/CCDH1 or cyclin F, and then degraded through the proteasome-dependent pathway (32, 33). Transcription factors, including Sp1, AP-2, BRCA, E2F1 and MYBL2, bind to the DNA sequence in the promoter region of *RRM2* and regulate their expression in response to DNA damage in cancer cells (34, 35). We did not thoroughly explore the effect of PECT on RRM2 transcription suppression and proteasome degradation, which will be verified in furture studies. However, we found that in addition to transcriptional suppression and proteasome-dependent degradation, RRM2 protein also depend on autophagy-lysosome pathway degradation. It was reported that excessive activation of autophagy could result in type II programmed cell death, which differs from necrosis and apoptosis (36). Additionally, the dual role of autophagy in response to anticancer therapy is well-known. Although there was some controversy regarding whether autophagy should be turned on or off to treat cancer (12), at least in this context, our data confirmed that RRM2 downregulation mediates the anti-proliferation effect of PECT on GBM, which depended on the increase of autophagic flux. Because PECT inhibited RRM2 expression, which can be inhibited by autophagy inhibitor CQ. In addition, immunofluorescence assay showed that RRM2 can co-localize with LAMP2 in U251 cells, while PECT treatment can increase the intracellular co-localization of LAMP2 and RRM2, and decrease the RRM2 protein expression. Thus, these further demonstrated that PECT could promote RRM2 protein degradation by autolysosome-dependent pathway in GBM.

In proliferating cells, RRM2 overexpression is regulated in a G2/M phase cell cycle-dependent manner (37, 38). Additionally, RRM2 downregulation has been demonstrated to promote autophagy-dependent cell death by decreasing intracellular dNTP levels (31). Reduction in RNR activity could suppress DNA replication and damage repair, resulting in cell cycle arrest (9, 39), and Autophagy has played a role in various cellular processes like DNA damage repair and cell cycle regulation (11, 40, 41). However, the effect of autophagy as a multifunctional regulator on cell cycle progression in GBM remains unclear. In the present study, we confirmed that RRM2 knockdown can induce G2/M phase cell cycle arreste by decreasing CDK1 protein expression, which can be reversed by the inhibition of autophagy. CDK1, an essential kinase regulating cell cycle progression, is upregulated in multiple cancers. CDK1 depletion promote cell-cycle arrest and ultimately inhibit tumor cell proliferation (42–44). Additionally, p62 is an adapter that is widely involved in protein interactions. Our results demonstrated that CDK1 can interact with p62, which provided a basis for autophagy to degrade CDK1. Simultaneously, immunofluorescence assay showed that CDK1 can co-localize with p62 in U251 cells, and RRM2 knockdown can decrease the intracellular co-localization of CDK1 and p62, and decrease the CDK1 protein expression. These data indicated that autophagy is required for RRM2 to inhibit GBM cell proliferation through inducing G2/M phase cell cycle arrest by promoting CDK1 protein degradation, which supported by previous studies that p62-HDAC6 promoted CDK1 degradation through an autophagy-lysosome pathway in breast cancer (13). However, the exact binding site at which CDK1 binds p62 was not identified.

Clinical data revealed that RRM2 is increased in GBM tissues and inversely correlated with glioma sufferers OS time, which suggests RRM2 as a potential therapeutic target, as well as a prognosis and predictive biomarker. Additionally, we found that p62 and CDK1 protein were co-located in the lesional cells from human GBM cases, indicating that autophagy and cell cycle may be related to the occurrence and development of GBM, which may play a certain role for GBM clinical research. We also demonstrated that PECT or RRM2 knockdown was involved in regulating GBM cells migration, and PECT could directly bind to RRM2, and promote CDK1 protein degradation through proteasomal pathway, although the corresponding molecular mechanisms remain to be determined.

CONCLUSIONS

In summary, Our study provides a novel insight into the mechanisms by which PECT promoted the degradation of CDK1 protein dependent on autolysosomal pathway through increasing autophagic flow by inhibiting RRM2 (**Figure 8**). Additionally, RRM2 may be a potential therapeutic target and a prognosis and predictive biomarker in GBM patients, and manipulation of RRM2-mediated autophagy offers promising clinical therapeutic directions for GBM. However, the precise molecular mechanism of RRM2 to regulate autophagy in GBM should be further addressed in the future.

ETHICS STATEMENT

The study protocol was approved by the Clinical Research Ethics Committee of Harbin Medical University. All patients provided written informed consent, and the study was conducted in accordance with the Declaration of Helsinki. The patients/participants provided their written informed consent to participate in this study. All animal study protocols were approved by the Animal Experiments Ethics Committee of Harbin Medical University and the study was conducted in accordance with the Declaration of Helsinki.

AUTHOR CONTRIBUTIONS

HJ designed, conceived, planned, implemented the experiment, and wrote the original draft. LW, HY and EL assisted in collecting clinical samples. TY assisted in imaging. JY, XW and MG provided experimental guidance, and DZ assisted in completing experiments. KD, WL, CZ, JW, PY, ZS, XR, SA and SS participated in the investigation. XiaoC and ZZ provided financial sponsorship. XinC and SZ supervised and funded the research. All authors contributed to the article and approved the submitted version.

ACKNOWLEDGMENTS

We would like to thank Editage (www.editage.cn) for English language editing.

SUPPLEMENTARY MATERIAL

Supplementary Figure 1 | LC-MS of PECT content using Principal component analysis (PCA).

Supplementary Figure 2 | The cytotoxicity effect of chloroquine on U87 and U251 cells analyzed using MTT assays

Supplementary Figure 3 | CCNA2 and CCNB1 protein expression no change after RRM2 was silenced.

Supplementary Figure 4 | CDK1 mRNA expression no change after RRM2 was silenced.

Supplementary Figure 5 | The transfection efficiency of RRM2 lentivirus in U251 cells.

REFERENCES

Li Y, Zhang ZX, Huang GH, Xiang Y, Yang L, Pei YC, et al. A Systematic Review of Multifocal and Multicentric Glioblastoma. *J Clin Neurosci* (2021) 83:71–6. doi: 10.1016/j.jocn.2020.11.025

De Waele J, Verhezen T, van der Heijden S, Berneman ZN, Peeters M, Lardon F, et al. A Systematic Review on Poly(I:C) and Poly-ICLC in Glioblastoma: Adjuvants Coordinating the Unlocking of Immunotherapy. *J Exp Clin Cancer Res* (2021) 40:213. doi: 10.1186/s13046-021-02017-2

Liu S, Zhang J, Yang H, Zhang Q, Chen M. Pectolinarigenin Flavonoid Exhibits Selective Anti-Proliferative Activity in Cisplatin-Resistant Hepatocellular Carcinoma, Autophagy Activation, Inhibiting Cell Migration and Invasion, G2/M Phase Cell Cycle Arrest and Targeting ERK1/2 MAP Kinases. *J BUON* (2020) 25:415–20.

Lee HJ, Saralamma VVG, Kim SM, Ha SE, Raha S, Lee WS, et al. Pectolinarigenin Induced Cell Cycle Arrest, Autophagy, and Apoptosis in Gastric Cancer Cell *via* PI3K/AKT/mTOR Signaling Pathway. *Nutrients* (2018) 10(8):1043. doi: 10.3390/nu10081043

Zhan Y, Jiang L, Jin X, Ying S, Wu Z, Wang L, et al. Inhibiting RRM2 to Enhance the Anticancer Activity of Chemotherapy. *BioMed Pharmacother* (2021) 133:110996. doi: 10.1016/j.biopha.2020.110996

Engstrom Y, Eriksson S, Jildevik I, Skog S, Thelander L, Tribukait B. Cell Cycle-Dependent Expression of Mammalian Ribonucleotide Reductase. Differential Regulation of the Two Subunits. *J Biol Chem* (1985) 260:9114– 6. doi: 10.1016/S0021-9258(17)39337-7

Liu Q, Guo L, Qi H, Lou M, Wang R, Hai B, et al. A MYBL2 Complex for RRM2 Transactivation and the Synthetic Effect of MYBL2 Knockdown With WEE1 Inhibition Against Colorectal Cancer. *Cell Death Dis* (2021) 12:683. doi: 10.1038/s41419-021-03969-1

Li S, Mai H, Zhu Y, Li G, Sun J, Li G, et al. MicroRNA-4500 Inhibits Migration, Invasion, and Angiogenesis of Breast Cancer Cells *via* RRM2- Dependent MAPK Signaling Pathway. *Mol Ther Nucleic Acids* (2020) 21:278– 89. doi: 10.1016/j.omtn.2020.04.018

Li ZN, Shu Y, Chen CG, Li XQ, Li MY, Zhao XH, et al. Acquired Tamoxifen Resistance is Surmounted by GW8510 Through Ribonucleotide Reductase M2 Downregulation-Mediated Autophagy Induction. *Biochem Biophys Res Commun* (2020) 528:554–60. doi: 10.1016/j.bbrc.2020.05.149

Li X, He S, Ma B. Autophagy and Autophagy-Related Proteins in Cancer. *Mol Cancer* (2020) 19:12. doi: 10.1186/s12943-020-1138-4

Li H, Peng X, Wang Y, Cao S, Xiong L, Fan J, et al. Atg5-Mediated Autophagy Deficiency in Proximal Tubules Promotes Cell Cycle G2/M Arrest and Renal Fibrosis. *Autophagy* (2016) 12:1472–86. doi: 10.1080/15548627.2016.1190071

Lim SM, Mohamad Hanif EA, Chin SF. Is Targeting Autophagy Mechanism in Cancer a Good Approach? The Possible Double-Edge Sword Effect. *Cell Biosci* (2021) 11:56. doi: 10.1186/s13578-021-00570-z

Galindo-Moreno M, Giraldez S, Saez C, Japon MA, Tortolero M, Romero F. Both P62/SQSTM1-HDAC6-Dependent Autophagy and the Aggresome Pathway Mediate CDK1 Degradation in Human Breast Cancer. *Sci Rep* (2017) 7:10078. doi: 10.1038/s41598-017-10506-8

Lee IH, Kawai Y, Fergusson MM, Rovira II, Bishop AJ, Motoyama N, et al. Atg7 Modulates P53 Activity to Regulate Cell Cycle and Survival During Metabolic Stress. *Science* (2012) 336:225–8. doi: 10.1126/science.1218395

Ru J, Li P, Wang J, Zhou W, Li B, Huang C, et al. TCMSP: A Database of Systems Pharmacology for Drug Discovery From Herbal Medicines. *J Cheminform* (2014) 6:13. doi: 10.1186/1758-2946-6-13

Bi Y, Shen C, Li C, Liu Y, Gao D, Shi C, et al. Inhibition of Autophagy Induced by Quercetin at a Late Stage Enhances Cytotoxic Effects on Glioma Cells. *Tumour Biol* (2016) 37:3549–60. doi: 10.1007/s13277-015-4125-4

Yamamoto K, Venida A, Yano J, Biancur DE, Kakiuchi M, Gupta S, et al. Autophagy Promotes Immune Evasion of Pancreatic Cancer by Degrading MHC-I. *Nature* (2020) 581:100–5. doi: 10.1038/s41586-020-2229-5

Sunada S, Saito H, Zhang D, Xu Z, Miki Y. CDK1 Inhibitor Controls G2/M Phase Transition and Reverses DNA Damage Sensitivity. *Biochem Biophys Res Commun* (2021) 550:56–61. doi: 10.1016/j.bbrc.2021.02.117

Xu G, Yan X, Hu Z, Zheng L, Ding K, Zhang Y, et al. Glucocappasalin Induces G2/M-Phase Arrest, Apoptosis, and Autophagy Pathways by Targeting CDK1 and PLK1 in Cervical Carcinoma Cells. *Front Pharmacol* (2021) 12:671138. doi: 10.3389/fphar.2021.671138

Zhou C, Liang Y, Zhou L, Yan Y, Liu N, Zhang R, et al. TSPAN1 Promotes Autophagy Flux and Mediates Cooperation Between WNT-CTNNB1 Signaling and Autophagy *via* the MIR454-FAM83A-TSPAN1 Axis in Pancreatic Cancer. *Autophagy* (2021) 17:3175–95. doi: 10.1080/ 15548627.2020.1826689

Qazi MA, Vora P, Venugopal C, Sidhu SS, Moffat J, Swanton C, et al. Intratumoral Heterogeneity: Pathways to Treatment Resistance and Relapse in Human Glioblastoma. *Ann Oncol* (2017) 28:1448–56. doi: 10.1093/annonc/mdx169

Lim M, Xia Y, Bettegowda C, Weller M. Current State of Immunotherapy for Glioblastoma. *Nat Rev Clin Oncol* (2018) 15:422–42. doi: 10.1038/s41571-018-0003-5

Mann J. Natural Products in Cancer Chemotherapy: Past, Present and Future. *Nat Rev Cancer* (2002) 2:143–8. doi: 10.1038/nrc723

Bonesi M, Tundis R, Deguin B, Loizzo MR, Menichini F, Tillequin F, et al. *In Vitro* Biological Evaluation of Novel 7-O-Dialkylaminoalkyl Cytotoxic Pectolinarigenin Derivatives Against a Panel of Human Cancer Cell Lines. *Bioorg Med Chem Lett* (2008) 18:5431 –4. doi: 10 .1016/ j.bmcl.2008.09.037

Wu T, Dong X, Yu D, Shen Z, Yu J, Yan S. Natural Product Pectolinarigenin Inhibits Proliferation, Induces Apoptosis, and Causes G2/M Phase Arrest of HCC *via* PI3K/AKT/mTOR/ERK Signaling Pathway. *Onco Targets Ther* (2018) 11:8633–42. doi: 10.2147/OTT.S186186

Arvanitis CD, Ferraro GB, Jain RK. The Blood-Brain Barrier and Blood- Tumour Barrier in Brain Tumours and Metastases. *Nat Rev Cancer* (2020) 20:26–41. doi: 10.1038/s41568-019-0205-x

Rahman MA, Amin AR, Wang D, Koenig L, Nannapaneni S, Chen Z, et al. RRM2 Regulates Bcl-2 in Head and Neck and Lung Cancers: A Potential Target for Cancer Therapy. *Clin Cancer Res* (2013) 19:3416–28. doi: 10.1158/ 1078-0432.CCR-13-0073

Lee Y, Vassilakos A, Feng N, Lam V, Xie H, Wang M, et al. GTI-2040, an Antisense Agent Targeting the Small Subunit Component (R2) of Human Ribonucleotide Reductase, Shows Potent Antitumor Activity Against a Variety of Tumors. *Cancer Res* (2003) 63:2802–11.

Shao J, Liu X, Zhu L, Yen Y. Targeting Ribonucleotide Reductase for Cancer Therapy. *Expert Opin Ther Targets* (2013) 17:1423–37. doi: 10.1517/14728222.2013.840293

Sun H, Yang B, Zhang H, Song J, Zhang Y, Xing J, et al. RRM2 is a Potential Prognostic Biomarker With Functional Significance in Glioma. *Int J Biol Sci* (2019) 15:533–43. doi: 10.7150/ijbs.30114

Chen P, Wu JN, Shu Y, Jiang HG, Zhao XH, Qian H, et al. Gemcitabine Resistance Mediated by Ribonucleotide Reductase M2 in Lung Squamous Cell Carcinoma is Reversed by GW8510 Through Autophagy Induction. *Clin Sci (Lond)* (2018) 132:1417–33. doi: 10.1042/CS20180010

Chabes AL, Pfleger CM, Kirschner MW, Thelander L. Mouse Ribonucleotide Reductase R2 Protein: A New Target for Anaphase-Promoting Complex- Cdh1-Mediated Proteolysis. *Proc Natl Acad Sci USA* (2003) 100:3925–9. doi: 10.1073/pnas.0330774100

D'Angiolella V, Donato V, Forrester FM, Jeong YT, Pellacani C, Kudo Y, et al. Cyclin F-Mediated Degradation of Ribonucleotide Reductase M2 Controls Genome Integrity and DNA Repair. *Cell* (2012) 149:1023–34. doi: 10.1016/j.cell.2012.03.043

Fang Z, Gong C, Liu H, Zhang X, Mei L, Song M, et al. E2F1 Promote the Aggressiveness of Human Colorectal Cancer by Activating the Ribonucleotide Reductase Small Subunit M2. *Biochem Biophys Res Commun* (2015) 464:407–15. doi: 10.1016/j.bbrc.2015.06.103

Gong C, Liu H, Song R, Zhong T, Lou M, Wang T, et al. ATR-CHK1-E2F3 Signaling Transactivates Human Ribonucleotide Reductase Small Subunit M2 for DNA Repair Induced by the Chemical Carcinogen MNNG. *Biochim Biophys Acta* (2016) 1859:612 – 2 6 . d oi: 10.1016/ j.bbagrm.2016.02.012

Talukdar S, Pradhan AK, Bhoopathi P, Shen XN, August LA, Windle JJ, et al. MDA-9/Syntenin Regulates Protective Autophagy in Anoikis-Resistant Glioma Stem Cells. *Proc Natl Acad Sci USA* (2018) 115:5768–73. doi: 10.1073/pnas.1721650115

Chen CW, Li Y, Hu S, Zhou W, Meng Y, Li Z, et al. DHS (Trans-4,4'-Dihydroxystilbene) Suppresses DNA Replication and Tumor Growth by Inhibiting RRM2 (Ribonucleotide Reductase Regulatory Subunit M2). *Oncogene* (2019) 38:2364–79. doi: 10.1038/s41388-018-0584-6

Shu Z, Li Z, Huang H, Chen Y, Fan J, Yu L, et al. Cell-Cycle-Dependent Phosphorylation of RRM1 Ensures Efficient DNA Replication and Regulates Cancer Vulnerability to ATR Inhibition. *Oncogene* (2020) 39:5721–33. doi: 10.1038/s41388-020-01403-y

Gandhi M, Gross M, Holler JM, Coggins SA, Patil N, Leupold JH, et al. The lncRNA lincNMR Regulates Nucleotide Metabolism *via* a YBX1 - RRM2 Axis in Cancer. *Nat Commun* (2020) 11:3214. doi: 10.1038/s41467-020- 17007-9

Pathania AS, Guru SK, Kumar S, Kumar A, Ahmad M, Bhushan S, et al. Interplay Between Cell Cycle and Autophagy Induced by Boswellic Acid Analog. *Sci Rep* (2016) 6:33146. doi: 10.1038/srep33146

Lin TY, Chan HH, Chen SH, Sarvagalla S, Chen PS, Coumar MS, et al. BIRC5/ Survivin is a Novel ATG12-ATG5 Conjugate Interactor and an Autophagy- Induced DNA Damage Suppressor in Human Cancer and Mouse Embryonic Fibroblast Cells. *Autophagy* (2020) 16:1296–313. doi: 10.1080/15548627.2019.1671643

Gan H, Qi M, Chan C, Leung P, Ye G, Lei Y, et al. Digitoxin Inhibits HeLa Cell Growth Through the Induction of G2/M Cell Cycle Arrest and Apoptosis *In Vitro* and *In Vivo*. *Int J Oncol* (2020) 57:562–73. doi: 10.3892/ijo.2020.5070

Pack LR, Daigh LH, Meyer T. Putting the Brakes on the Cell Cycle: Mechanisms of Cellular Growth Arrest. *Curr Opin Cell Biol* (2019) 60:106– 13. doi: 10.1016/j.ceb.2019.05.005

Roskoski R Jr. Cyclin-Dependent Protein Serine/Threonine Kinase Inhibitors as Anticancer Drugs. *Pharmacol Res* (2019) 139:471–88. doi: 10.1016/j.phrs.2018.11.035

12

CD44-Targeted Nanocarrier for Cancer Therapy

Prashant Kesharwani[1*†], *Rahul Chadar*[1†], *Afsana Sheikh*[1†], *Waleed Y. Rizg*[2] *and Awaji Y Safhi*[3]

[1]Department of Pharmaceutics, School of Pharmaceutical Education and Research, Jamia Hamdard, New Delhi, India, [2]Department of Pharmaceutics, Faculty of Pharmacy, King Abdulaziz University, Jeddah, Saudi Arabia, [3]Department of Pharmaceutics, Faculty of Pharmacy, Jazan University, Jazan, Saudi Arabia

***Correspondence:**
Prashant Kesharwani
prashantdops@gmail.com

†These authors have contributed equally to this work

Cluster of differentiation 44 (CD44) is a cell surface glycoprotein overexpressed in varieties of solid tumors including pancreatic, breast, ovary, brain, and lung cancers. It is a multi-structural glycoprotein of the cell surface which is majorly involved in cell proliferation, cell-to-cell interaction, cellular migration, inflammation, and generation of immune responses. Numerous studies focus on the development of nanocarriers for active targeting of the CD44 receptor to improve efficacy of targeting chemotherapy and achieve precise chemotherapy by defining the release, uptake, and accumulation of therapeutic agents. The CD44 receptor has a selective binding affinity towards hyaluronic and chondroitin sulfate (CS). Taking this into consideration, this review focused on the role of CD44 in cancer and its therapy using several nanocarriers such as polymeric/non-polymeric nanoparticles, dendrimer, micelles, carbon nanotubes, nanogels, nanoemulsions etc., for targeted delivery of several chemotherapeutic molecules and nucleic acid. This review also illuminates the role of hyaluronic acid (HA) in cancer therapy, interaction of HA with CD44, and various approaches to target CD44-overexpressed neoplastic cells.

Keywords: CD44, targeted drug delivery, gene delivery, hyaluronic acid, anticancer therapy, nanocarrier

INTRODUCTION

Among the recent statistics of most life-threatening diseases, cancer poses a major issue by being the most dangerous and fatal disease causing the death of millions of people worldwide every year; the number of deaths due to cancer is gradually rising. Cancer is the major challenge of the 21st century, that does not have any limit, it can occur in any organ of the body and can migrate to nearby tissue (Bharali and Mousa, 2010). Cancer can originate in any part of the human body, comprising of trillions of cells. In general, cells grow, multiply, become old/damaged, die, and new cells replace the old cells, but in the case of cancer, this orderly process breaks down, causing tumors or lumps of tissue (Kateb et al., 2011; Singh S. et al., 2021). The process of cancer treatment is very complex because of its molecular complexity at genetic and phenotypic levels. Due to molecular complexity, cancer cells exhibit clinical diversity and therapeutic resistance. There are numerous strategies, such as surgical removal, radiation therapy, chemotherapy, and hormonal therapy, that have been developed for cancer treatment but each of them possesses drawbacks and side effects. Chemotherapy is the most commonly used anticancer therapy for cancer management (Kamal et al., 2012; Zhao and Rodriguez, 2012; Sheikh and Kesharwani, 2021). In most cases, due to non-specific delivery, chemotherapeutic agents fail to deliver desired therapeutic effects along with generating multiple side effects (Chadar et al., 2021; Kaur and Kesharwani, 2021; Singh and

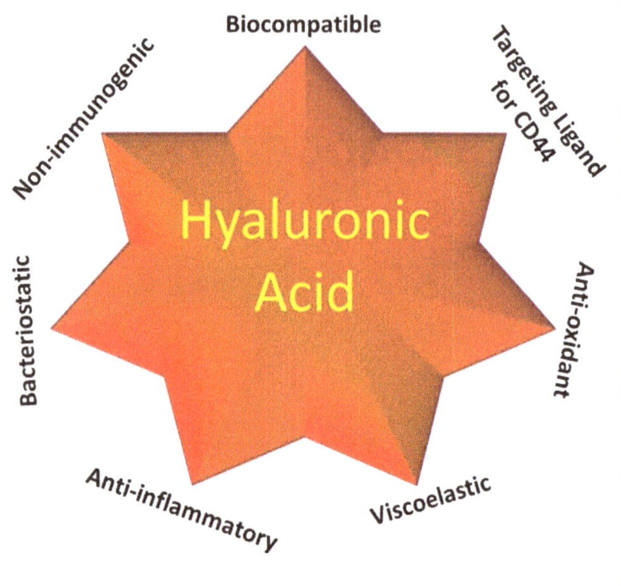

FIGURE 1 | Potential of hyaluronic acid in pharmaceutical drug delivery.

Kesharwani, 2021). Development of cancer therapy is a very complex, challenging, and expensive process, thus, the future of cancer therapy is associated with cutting edge research in polymer chemistry and electronic engineering. Differentiation between cancerous and normal cells poses another challenge for physicians and oncology scientists. Therefore, engineering of drugs in such a framework can recognize tumor cells to inhibit cell growth and proliferation. Conventional chemotherapy (CC) interacts with normal tissues causing numerous undesired effects including organ failure/damage (Mousa and Bharali, 2011).

To overcome the challenges associated with conventional chemotherapy, currently various evolving nanotechnology-based nanocarriers have been developed. Several nanocarriers such as dendrimers, liposomes, micelles, nanogels, emulsions, carbon nanotubes, polymeric/non-polymeric nanoparticles, and quantum dots displayed great potential to deliver chemotherapeutic agents at the target of interest. The potential of nanocarriers includes improvement in physicochemical properties of chemotherapeutic molecules, reduced side effects, targetability, reduced doses of drugs, enhanced blood circulation time, and many others. Nanoparticles (NPs) can be used for both passive targeting and active targeting, but passive targeting is associated with some limitations, so that development of actively targeting NPs or "intelligent" NPs is of utmost importance as they can deliver their cargo to cancerous cells by binding with overexpressed biomarkers present on the surface of cancer cells. As mentioned earlier, the molecular structure of cancer is different from the normal cell. Several receptors such as integrin, folate receptors (FR), transferrin, EGFR, sigma, GPCR, and CD44 are overexpressed in tumor cells. Thus, development of a system to target such cells could provide a way for efficient and active delivery of chemotherapeutic agents.

Cluster of differentiation 44 (CD44) is overexpressed in several types of cancer including breast, lungs, ovary, brain, and hepatic carcinoma which are responsible for many metabolic activities of cancer cells such as cellular differentiation, migration, proliferation hematopoiesis, angiogenesis, and cell and tumor metastasis (Kesharwani et al., 2015a; Kesharwani et al., 2015b). The CD44 receptor after binding with hyaluronic acid (HA), is activated and potentiates cancer cell growth. Utilizing such a process of tumor cell growth, researchers concluded that the CD44 receptor could be a promising target for anticancer therapy (Goodison et al., 1999; Luo et al., 2019). The CD44 receptor has a remarkable affinity towards glycosaminoglycan polymers like HA and chondroitin sulfate (CS). HA, a biocompatible, biodegradable, low immunogenic hydrophilic polymer is mainly located in the epithelial, neural, and connective tissue (Salari et al., 2021) (**Figure 1**). Most importantly, HA could bind to the CD44 receptor *via* H-bond or van der Waals forces, depending on the variant and expression level of the CD44 receptor (Banerji et al., 2007; Dosio et al., 2016; Kim et al., 2019; Spadea et al., 2019; Li et al., 2021). The HA molecule contains several functional groups such as -COOH, -OH and N-acetyl groups through which it could easily be conjugated with different types of nanomaterials and with different chemotherapeutics drugs like doxorubicin (DOX), paclitaxel (PTX), docetaxel (DTX), and camptothecin (CPT) (Cai et al., 2019; Luo et al., 2019). CS is another ligand for targeting the CD44 receptor with a similar chemical structure to HA, thereby drawing interest of formulation scientists towards such targeting ligands. Likewise, CS also possesses many functional groups through which it can conjugate with different nanomaterials and drugs. In a study, Onishi et al. reported that DOX and PTX conjugate with CS particles (Lee et al., 2016a; Jin et al., 2017; Onishi et al., 2019). It is important to understand the binding ability of HA with its receptor. Low molecular weight HA binds to monomeric CD44 receptors and activates TLR 2/4 receptors showing a pro-inflammatory characteristic, while the high molecular weight HA inhibits TLR activation and induces an anti-inflammatory characteristic (Lesley et al., 2000). Moreover, the receptor binding of HA depends on the following factors: HA is required to bind at multiple sites as a single interaction could be weak, for binding with more than one receptor, more than 20 residues of oligosaccharide are required and the molecular weight of HA should be more than 31 kDa as one below 31 kDa can attach with a single receptor while those above 132 kDa could interact with five to eight receptors (Oommen et al., 2014).

Structure of the Target CD44

The type I transmembrane receptor protein known as CD44 bears a common structure consisting of four major domains: the stem region, the cytoplasmic region, extracellular domain, and the transmembrane region (Dzwonek and Wilczyński, 2015). The cytoplasmic domain of CD44 constitutes both a short and long tail that demonstrate its ability in the transcription process and nuclear localization (Naor et al., 2008). The extracellular domain interacts and senses the stimuli with/in the external microenvironment (Hill et al., 2006). The transmembrane domain provides a platform for interaction of the adaptor protein with co-factors. It also helps in directing the homing of lymphocytes (Williams et al., 2013).

The target protein of CD44 is encoded by single genes comprising of 20 exons. The endothelial cells, fibroblast, neurons, and leukocytes along with many vertebrate cells show high expression of exons 1–5, 16–18, and 20 (Naor et al., 2008). The exons between 6–15 present in the middle of the CD44 gene are spliced alternatively to form a variant of CD44 (CD44V) to develop its isoform showing variable function in the stem region (Naor et al., 1997). The amino group present on the periphery of exons basically contains two binding sites; the linking site comprising of 32–132 amino acids and exterior binding motif to the linking site that comprises 150–158 amino acid groups. In between the N-terminal globular domain and the transmembrane site, there lies 46 amino acids in a stretch forming a star-shaped structure. This shape contains numerous cleavable sites which are extra-glycosylated. The stretch could further be modified by inserting various exons (Kalniņa et al., 2005). The cytoplasmic tail and *O*-glycosylation demonstrates its localization on the cell membrane and thus enables the crosstalk between HA and CD44 (Neame and Isacke, 1993). The CD44 isoforms can be modified through fabrication with O-glycans, N-glycans, and glycosaminoglycans, such as chondroitin sulfate and heparan sulfate (Greenfield et al., 1999; Gomari et al., 2021). The binding of CD44 with its agonist and antagonist is dependent on the activation state of the CD44 receptor. Apart from binding with HA, CD44 also interact with the extracellular proteins such as matrix metalloproteinases (MMPs), growth factors, fibronectin, cytokines, collagens, and chemokines (Ma et al., 2019).

NANOTECHNOLOGY IN CANCER TARGETING

Nanotechnology is an umbrella term defined as the scientific principles, process, methodologies, techniques, and other scientific activity dealing in the size range from a few nanometers to several hundred nm, depending upon their intended use (Peer et al., 2007; Dubey et al., 2021; Srivastava et al., 2021; Kumar et al., 2021). Nanotechnology has become the focused area of interest over the last few decades for emerging drug delivery systems because it offers several unique advantages over the conventional drug delivery system (Malam et al., 2009; Zeeshan et al., 2021). It is also a promising and intelligent approach for the theranosis of many dangerous diseases like cancer, as it is able to deliver its cargo directly to its target. Nanotechnology is actively implemented in several cancer therapies mainly for detection, diagnosis, imaging, and treatment of different types of cancers. A significant amount of research and advancement is being carried out to find the most precise cancer treatment with minimal side effects encountered by conventional therapy. Multiple nanocarriers have been designed to modify therapeutic drugs in such a way that could overcome limitations such as biological barrier, unintended intermolecular interactions, and distribution to many intact or normal tissues. Nanoparticles' unique characteristics such as being modifiable could be utilized for optical, magnetic, electronic, and biological observation offering several advantages over macro nanoparticles (Park, 2007; Praetorius and Mandal, 2008; Patnaik et al., 2021; Surekha et al., 2021).

Nanotechnology has revolutionized the field of biomedicine, especially in cancer therapy for selective targeting of tumor cells. Characteristics of several nanocarriers can be modified such as size, shape, and texture by chemical or physical modification, making them important candidates for desired delivery action at specific sites. Nanoparticles could be programmed towards selective tumor cells either *via* active targeting or passive targeting (Singh V. et al., 2021; Gupta et al., 2021; Zafar et al., 2021; Zhang et al., 2021) (**Figure 2**).

Nanotechnology-Based Active Drug Targeting

Active targeting is the delivery of drugs and other therapeutic molecules directly to the tumor cells. For active targeting, chemotherapeutic-loaded nanocarriers have been framed in a such way that they can directly interact with or recognize tumor cells. Several pathophysiological changes of cancers cells form the basis of active targeting by recognizing overexpressed biomarkers and genes. Basically, nanoparticle surfaces can be decorated with ligands which can easily be recognized by tumor cells, that act either by ligand receptor binding or antigen-antibody binding (Guo and Szoka, 2003; Cho et al., 2008; Jin et al., 2020). A targeting drug delivery system based on nanotechnology mainly consist of three parts, first, cell death-causing agents (chemotherapeutic drugs), second, targeting ligand/penetration enhancers, and third, a nanocarrier. Today, numerous materials are used to construct nanocarriers but most commonly used materials include polymers (Kavand et al., 2020), lipids (Shankar et al., 2018), ceramics (Cisterna et al., 2016), and metals (Yezhelyev et al., 2006; Cho et al., 2008; Hitchcock et al., 2020). Usually, natural and synthetic polymers and lipids are most commonly used as vectors for drug delivery (Duncan, 2006; Schroeder et al., 2012). Early clearance of nanoparticles from circulation *via* an RES system is a major limitation of nanocarriers, which can be solved by polymeric modification. NPs modified by hydrophilic polymers allows them to remain in the circulation system for a long period of time or for the duration of NPs' interaction with cancerous cells. Due to surface modification, hydrophilic nanoparticles avoid cellular opsonization by repelling plasma proteins (Jeon et al., 1991; Brigger et al., 2002; Francis et al., 2004). There are innumerable hydrophilic polymers available that are used for the targeted delivery of chemotherapeutics, a few examples of such polymers include poly ethylene glycol (PEG), poloxamines, poloxamers, polysaccharides (hyaluronic acid), etc. (Storm et al., 1995; Torchilin and Trubetskoy, 1995). As mentioned earlier, the molecular structure of cancer cells is different from healthy cells, that show overexpression of some receptors on their surface making them selectively targetable for drug delivery. When a ligand-modified nanocarrier is administered, it is easily recognized by the overexpressed receptor on tumor cells that

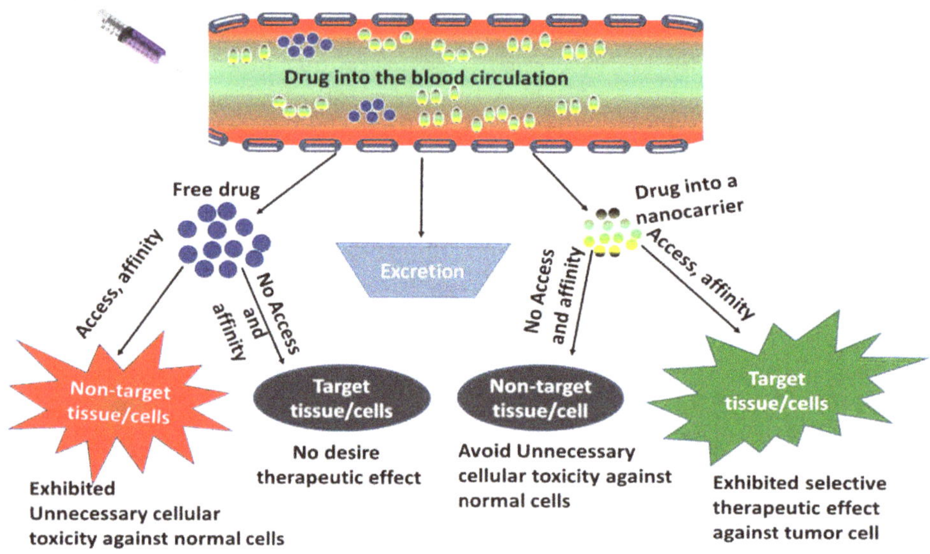

FIGURE 2 | Basic principle of drug targeting.

can be identified, bound, and rapidly internalized by receptor-mediated endocytosis or phagocytosis of tumor cells. Once well-decorated NPs are internalized into the tumor cell, the NPs release their cargo intracellularly, which leads to apoptosis (Peer et al., 2007). Receptors such as the folate receptor, CD44 receptor, transferrin receptor, luteinizing hormone-releasing hormone receptor, and asialo glycol protein (ASGP), are some examples of receptors which are most often discussed for cancer targeting therapy.

Nanotechnology-Based Passive Targeting

As reported in several studies, the metabolic activities of tumor cells rise to fulfil the energy demand required by rapidly growing tumor cells. The blood vessels linked with tumor cells form leaky vasculature due to basement membrane irregularity, which enhances the penetration of molecules to pass through the blood vessel. The size of this leaky vasculature ranges from 100–780 nm, so the NPs below this size can easily pass across the leaky vasculature of tumor cells. Due to lack of a well-defined lymphatic network, the retention time of the entered drug into the tumor interstitium increases, facilitating the EPR effect, that could enhance drug accumulation. It is well reported that NPs deliver their therapeutic effect *via* both active and passive targeting approaches (Maeda et al., 2000; Maeda, 2001; Alavi and Hamidi, 2019).

ROLE OF CD44 IN CANCER TARGETING

CD44 is a kind of glycoprotein overly expressed in a variety of mammalian tumor cells including prostate, breast, colon, gastric, head, and squamous cell carcinoma. It is also majorly involved in a number of non-cancerous diseases such as arthritis, bacterial and viral infections, lung disease, wound healing, and cardiovascular issues (Sherman et al., 1994). CD44 cells are associated with a wide variety of vital cellular functions like lymphocyte activation, recirculation, hematopoiesis, cell division, migration, adhesion, and signaling, etc. CD44 cells are comprised of nine variable axons 1–5 and 16–20, resulting in the formation of a variety of CD44 splice variants (Cao H. et al., 2016). Inflammatory response and cellular damage alter the cellular expression and functions of the CD44 cells. Oxley and Sackstein established a relation between CD44 cell antigens with cell-cell interactions, downstream signaling, cell adhesion, and proliferation (Oxley and Sackstein, 1994). The non-sulfated glycosaminoglycan hyaluronic acid (HA) is the most common or principle substrate of CD44 cells; other than HA, osteopontin, collagens, and matrix metalloproteinase (MMP) also interact with CD44 receptors (Senbanjo and Chellaiah, 2017). Such a substrate plays an important role in the regulation of cell signaling in accordance with several other factors such as post-translational modification, varied expression of isoform, along with spatial distribution of the CD44 receptor on the cell surface that contributes to control CD44 functions (Misra et al., 2015). The thrust areas that determine the role of CD44 in cancer metastasis and growth are divided into two main categories, one is HA-dependent, and another is HA-independent. HA-independent cancer signaling of CD44 cells depends on the interactions of the intracellular domain of CD44 cells and cytoskeletal proteins or kinases. HA-dependent signaling relies on the interaction of its native ligand HA with CD44 cells, almost all isoform of CD44 cells show affinity for its most specific and robust ligand, HA. The stem cell niches mainly comprise of HA, which is a chief constituent of the cancer matrix. CD44 is strongly associated with matrix assembly, thus the association of CD44 and HA could not only aid in arresting cancerous cells but also

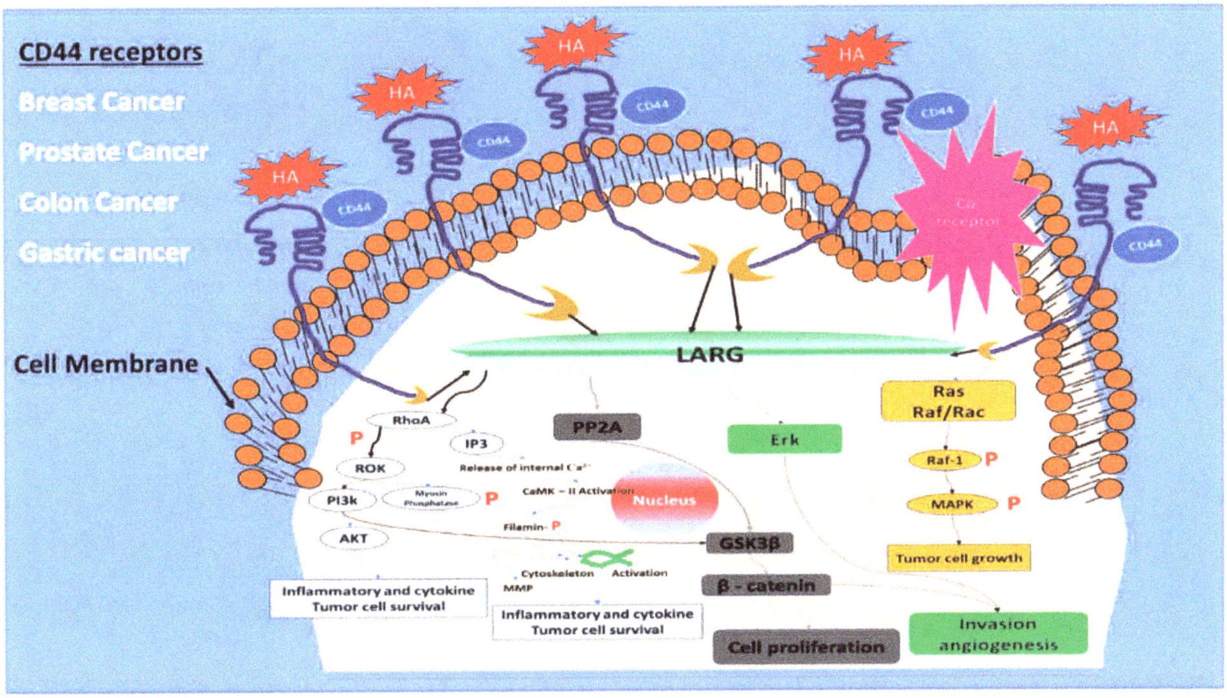

FIGURE 3 | Cell signaling pathways associated with the CD44 receptor.

facilitate modification of tissue matrix to maintain colonization (Hill et al., 2006; Kuhn and Tuan, 2010). Matrix component perturbation could alter the cell shape and intracellular tension, exhibiting shifting of signaling events that modify gene expression (Wang et al., 2009). CD44 isoforms such as CD44v3, CD44v5, and CD44v6 are also involved in matrix assembly whereas CD44v5, CD44v6, and CD44v7-8 play key roles in lymph node metastasis (Jung et al., 2009). The isoform of CD44 encodes for various peptides inside the juxta membrane domain causing conformational changes along with providing binding sites for growth factors and cytokines. Such binding mediates tumor growth and associated activities such as prognosis and metastasis. Many studies identified tumor cells with stem-like characteristics [cancer stem cells (CSCs)] that have self-renewal, tumor metastatic, and recurrent characteristics. In many cancers such as colon and breast cancer, CD44 acts as a significant marker on CSCs, however in many situations the specific isoforms are still unknown (Zeilstra et al., 2008). CD44v6 isoforms have been investigated as colon cancer stem cell markers with metastatic propensity suggesting CD44v6 targeting in colon tumors could potentially provide significant results. However, CD44 isoforms are also present in tumor cells that respond to drugs as well. However, to improve the tumor homing effect, a ligand is required (Alves and Konstantopoulos, 2012). Several metabolic pathways like PI3K/Akt, PPA2, Erk, and Ras/Raf are also associated with CD44 cell signaling (**Figure 3**). Such pathways regulate inflammation/cytokines through the NF-κB pathway, proliferation through B-catenin, invasion/angiogenesis, and cytoskeleton rearrangement, respectively (Chen et al., 2018). Isoforms CD44/CD44-V6 are also reported as important anti-apoptotic genes. Expression of CD44-V9 and CD44-V6 are mainly controlled by cytokines like TNFα and IFN3. CD44 plays key roles in tumor development through the above metabolic pathways and other physiological events. Under normal conditions, CD44 regulates normal function and maintains cellular homeostasis. But in the case of a tumor, it fails to maintain such cellular function. As described earlier, CD44 cells have high affinity for several ligands, HA is considered as one of the best ligands for CD44. Interaction of HA with CD44 activates the FAK-linked PI3K/Akt and ERK signaling pathways (Misra et al., 2011). Various studies reported a high chance of CD44 isoform transition in tumor cells, thereby developing different types of cancers by the activation of HA. Overexpression of CD44-V6 and CD44-V10 isoforms are also associated with colorectal carcinoma. The CD44-V6 isoform is the strongest and most active variant among all other variants that are involved in cell migration and metastasis activated by the Wnt/B-catenin pathway (Thapa and Wilson, 2016). The upregulated CD44-V6 shows high viability in comparison to its other variants after treatment with standard chemotherapy. In breast cancer, the role of CD44 depends upon many factors, like CD44 expression, ligand binding ability, cell variants, methylation/splicing events, etc. (Afify et al., 2009). Bourguignon et al. studied the interaction of HA with CD44 causing expression of Pgp (MDR) along with the anti-apoptotic Bcl gene in breast cancer, thereby mediating proliferation and survival of breast tumor cells (Chen and Bourguignon, 2014). Treatment strategies based on targeting CD44 decreases the glucose consumption and ATP by the cancerous cells. The expression of CD44 might be associated with B-catenin and

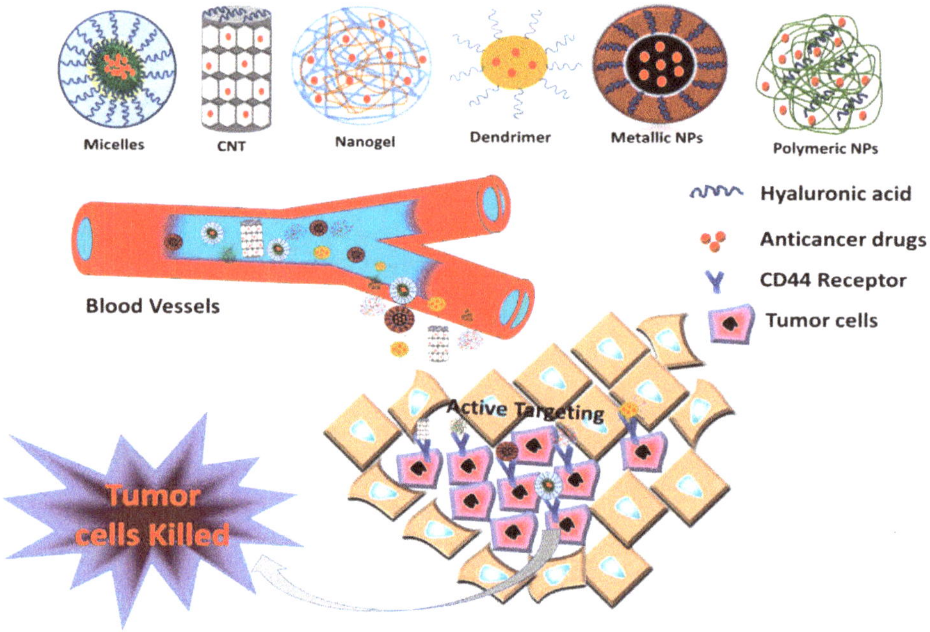

FIGURE 4 | Schematic illustration of CD44-targeted delivery of anticancer drugs.

AKT pathways, so CD44 expression could be regulated by inhibiting either pathway or both. CD44 cells also play a major role in metastatic cascade in various carcinomas. Metastatic cascade is regulated by epidermal growth factor receptor (EGFR)/ErbB1 and ErbB2/Her 2 receptors whose overexpression form the most aggressive kind of breast cancer. Ras/SOS is activated by the interactions of HA/other ligands with CD44, and regulates the growth and invasion cascade (Nam et al., 2016). In a study, the CD44 role in Smad-dependent invasion was reported along with its effect on TGFb receptor 1 and 2 triggering CD44 binding. The activation of Rho ATPase by CD44 enhances the cytoskeletal transformation and invasion, while other pathways like PI3K-AKT and MAPK-Ras enhances tumor cell growth, survival, and invasion (Bourguignon, 2019).

CD44 ENGINEERED NANOCARRIERS FOR CANCER THERAPY

Owing to good biodegradability and biocompatibility, NPs targeting the CD44 receptor could deliver the therapeutic agent directly to the cell in a controlled manner, sparing its effect on normal cells (Lai et al., 2021). Such a nano-drug delivery system also offers modification with attachment on the surface that could elevate its uptake and prompt apoptosis. Nanocarriers also offer multiple advantages, for instance, ease of production, high drug loading capacity, improved solubility and bioavailability, improved distribution of drug inside the body, enhanced permeability to physiological barriers, and decreased drug toxicity (Khurana et al., 2017) (**Figure 4**).

CD44 Engineered Liposomes for Cancer Therapy

Liposomes are spherical vesicles composed of phospholipid bilayers with an enclosed aqueous core. The lipid bilayer may be natural or synthetic, single bilayer vesicles are known as unilamellar vesicles; multiple bilayer vesicles are termed as multilamellar vesicles. Liposomes can encapsulate both hydrophilic and hydrophobic drug molecules into their bilayers. They may vary in size, surface, composition, and methods of preparations. Nowadays, the liposome is the most commonly used model nanocarrier for the delivery of numerous bioactive molecules such as drugs, vaccines, cosmetics, genes, nutraceuticals, and various combination therapies (Deshpande et al., 2013; Torchilin, 2005). It is also a preferred carrier for targeting delivery, especially for anticancer drugs, that shows various advantages over the conventional system of which targeting delivery is among the most considered (**Figure 5**). It helps in reduction of side effects of many chemotherapeutics agents by preventing them from distribution to non-targeted sites. Liposomes can alter the pharmacokinetics of drug carriers by their surface functionalization (Sharma et al., 2006). They can easily be functionalized with the various targeting moieties, such as polysaccharides [folate (FA), hyaluronic acid (HA), chitosan (CH), etc.], peptides, genes, and antibodies (Accardo and Morelli, 2015; Ruttala et al., 2017; Sofou and Sgouros, 2008; Zylberberg et al., 2017) for delivering chemotherapeutics to specific tumor cells. Here, we have discussed liposome-based nanocarriers targeting CD44 tumor cells by using the most potent ligand hyaluronic acid (HA) to bind with target CD44 cells (**Table 1**). Song et al. had designed hyaluronic acid (HA)-modified

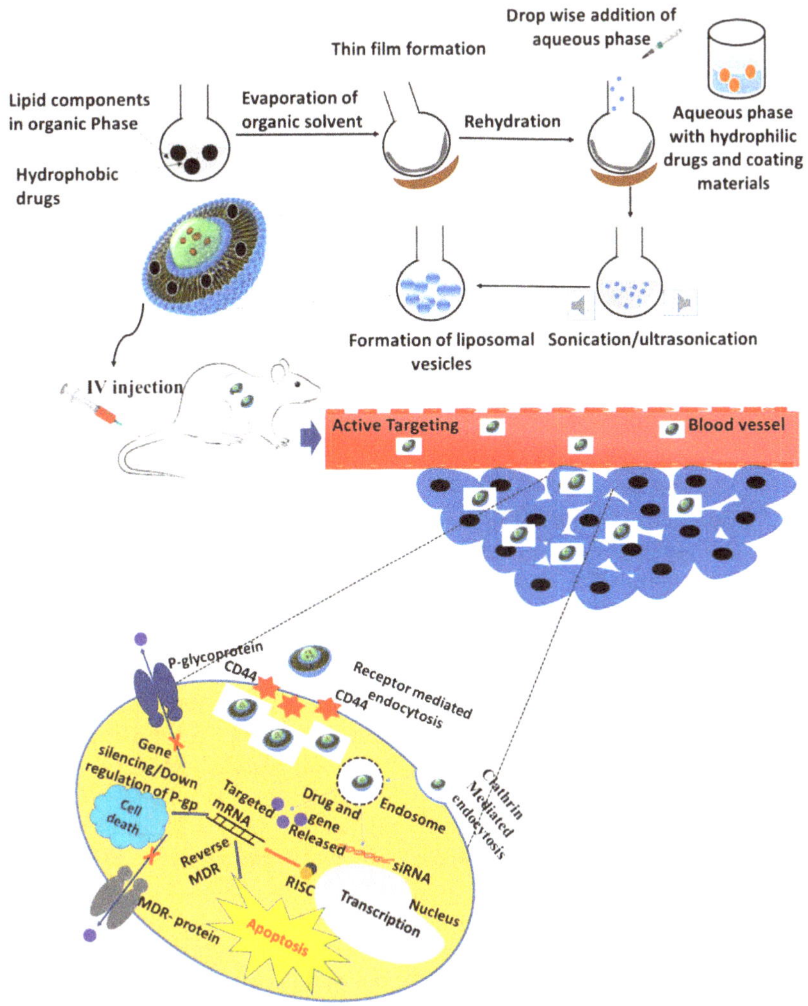

FIGURE 5 | Schematic illustration of liposome-based CD44-targeted delivery of anticancer drugs/genes.

TABLE 1 | Summary of liposome-targeted CD44 cells for cancer therapy.

Types of liposomes	Therapeutic agents	Types of cancer	X′ cell lines	Animal model	References
HA-modified liposomes	DOX and PTX	Breast cancer	MCF-7 and HepG2	–	Song et al. (2019)
Cationic liposomes	Cabazitaxel and silibinin	Prostate cancer	PC-3 and DU-145	–	Mahira et al. (2019)
Cationic liposomes	Gemcitabine and docetaxel	TNBC	MCF-7 and MDA-MB-231	Mice	Fan et al. (2017)
PEGylated liposomes	Anti-CD44 2′-F pyrimidine RNA aptamer	Lung and breast	A549 and MDA-MB-231	–	Alshaer et al. (2015)
HNPs	Paclitaxel	Metastatic breast cancer	4T1, MCF-7, A549, and NIH/3T3 cells	Mice	Lv et al. (2018)
PEGylated liposomes	Stigmasterol and DOX	Breast cancer	MCF-7 and MDA-MB-231	Mice	Gautam et al. (2020)
Polymersomes (PEG-PCL)	DOX	Breast cancer	MCF-7 and 4T1	Mice	Shahriari et al. (2019)

liposomes for targeting CD44 cells expressed on breast cancer and codelivery of paclitaxel (PTX) and doxorubicin (DOX). Firstly, paclitaxel, hydrogenated lecithin, and cholesterol in a particular ratio was dissolved into a solution of methanol: chloroform at a ratio of 1:3. The organic solvent was then evaporated by a rotary evaporator to form a thin film, the overnight-dried film was hydrated with ammonium solution at 47°C for 1 h, and subsequently sonicated to achieve the desired vesicle size. DOX was also loaded into the liposomes by the thin film hydration method with minor changes. Both DOX and paclitaxel was loaded into the HA-modified liposomes using the post-insertion method with small variation Briefly, a small amount of cholesterol-conjugated HA was incubated with the above solutions containing DOX and paclitaxel-loaded liposomes for half an hour at the temperature of 50°C. The prepared formulation showed a particle size range between 90 and 130 nm and PDI <0.25. HA conjugation with liposome increased the particle size of the liposome, and also changed its surface charge. The negative charge of unmodified liposomes changed to a positive charge due to the carboxy group of HA. HA conjugation of liposomes acts as a PEG molecule in circulation, which increases the blood retention time by escaping clearance *via* the RES system. Encapsulation efficiency (EE) of HA-decorated liposomes (HA-D-P-liposome) was 93.6 % and 70.4% for DOX and paclitaxel, respectively. TEM images exhibited spherical shape and uniform size distribution particles of HA-D-P-liposome. The amount of cholesterol-HA into the HA-modified lipid was determined by the carbazole method, that was found to be 9.5% mol of the total lipids. *In vitro* comparative cellular uptake of HA-DOX-liposome, DOX-liposome, and free DOX was also evaluated using MCF-7 ($CD44^+$ receptors) and HepG2 ($CD44^-$ receptor) cell lines through confocal microscopic imaging. Fluorescent intensity of HA-DOX-liposome was higher than the free DOX and DOX-liposome treated in MCF-7 cells, whereas HepG2 cells showed comparatively less fluorescence intensity. This is due to overexpression of CD44 receptor on MCF-7 cells, which enhanced the receptor ligand (HA)-mediated transport of HA-DOX-liposome (active targeting) whereas in HepG2 cells due to low expression of CD44 cells, the ligand (HA)-mediated transport of HA-DOX-liposome was hampered, however, free DOX and DOX-liposome traversed by passive diffusion. Scientists also demonstrated the high uptake of HA-DOX-liposome on MCF-7 cell lines which were majorly due to caveolae, clathrin-mediated endocytosis, and the ligand housing effect. MCF-7 cell lines pre-treated with the free HA significantly decreased the HA-DOX-liposome cellular uptake. This demonstrated the ligand binding capability of HA towards CD44. A cytotoxicity study revealed that both HA-DOX-liposome and HA-PTX-liposome showed higher cytotoxicity than free and unmodified drug-loaded liposomes. The IC50 value for drug-loaded HA-modified liposomes was lower than free or drug-loaded unmodified liposomes, the reason for such an effect may be due to high cellular uptake, control release, and drug resistance. As compared to individual drug treatment, co-loaded treatment had superior cytotoxicity. The IC50 value for DOX/PTX-liposome and HA-D/P-liposome was 0.51 and 0.14, respectively, HA-D/P-liposome showed the overall lowest IC50 value among the formulations, illustrating that the HA-modified codelivery system had a synergistic cytotoxic effect (Song et al., 2019). In another similar study, Mahira et al. targeted the CD44 receptor overexpressed on prostate cancer stem cells (CSCs) using anionic polysaccharide-coated cationic liposomes. In this study, researchers had co-loaded cabazitaxel (CBX) and silibinin (SIL) in liposomes to evaluate the anticancer effect against CSCs. Liposomes were prepared by dissolving cationic phospholipid N-[1-(2,3-Dioleoyloxy) propyl] N, N, N-trimethyl ammonium chloride (DOTAP), cholesterol, CBX, and SIL in common solvent (ethanol). The mixture was added dropwise into the aqueous solution of TPGS under continuous stirring followed by solvent evaporation. For the preparation of HA-coated liposomes, HA was dissolved into the aqueous solution with TPGS followed by dropwise addition to the organic phase. Researchers selected HA-wrapped liposomes with 10% w/w drug loading, a 1/5 phase volume ratio, and 0.1% HA concentration from the diverse batches due to their small size and PDI. Anionic polysaccharide with a concentration of 0.1 mg/ml showed optimum results which masked the cationic surface charge of liposomes, resulting in reduced toxicity of liposomes due to cationic surface charge and finally helped to target tumor cells. Comparative cellular reduced CD44 cells were studied for active HA receptor targeting on PC-3 and DU-145 prostate cancer cells. HA-coated liposomes showed 4.03 times more CD44 population suppression as compared to other formulations. Obtained results proved the concept of active targeting of CD44 cells, which enhanced the therapeutic benefits and reduced non-specific distribution leading to reduced toxicity. Cytotoxicity results showed IC50 values of 78 ng/ml, 46 μg/ml, and 23 ng/ml, respectively for CS-Sol, CS-liposome and HA-CS-LP (C and S-loaded HA-modified liposomes) in PC-3 cells, whereas, 17.6 ng/ml, 160 ng/ml, 29 ng/ml, respectively in DU-145 cells for HCS-LP, CS-LP, and CS-sol. HCS-LP comparatively exhibited efficient cell growth inhibition with the lowest IC50 value in both cell lines. These outcomes again denoted that HA coating encouraged efficiency of combined drug treatments. Cell cycle inhibition results revealed that CS-loaded HA-liposome showed strong knockdown of PC cells by arresting the cell cycle at the G2/M phase due to the increment in the intracellular concentration of both drugs. The synergistic therapeutic effect of C and S by HA-coated liposomes targeting the CD44 receptor against CSCs was also concluded from this study (Mahira et al., 2019). Fan and co-workers reported a new combination of nanocomplex for co-delivery of gemcitabine (GEM) and docetaxel (DTX) against triple negative breast cancer. GEM was linked with HA by esterification. This HA-modified nanocarrier had great potency for active targeting of overexpressed CD44 receptors on MDA-MB-231 cell lines. DTX-loaded liposome (DTX-LP) was prepared by usual thin film hydration methods. Finally, the GEM/DTX coloaded nanocomplex was obtained by dropwise addition of DTX-LP into the HA-GEM solution under continuous stirring at 4°C. Prepared NCs exhibited suitable characteristics with a size range <200 nm, PDI <0.2, zetapotential −31.1 mV, sufficient drug loading (GEM 9.3% and DTX 3.1%), and stimuli-responsive release characteristics. The prepared formulation showed higher *in vitro* cellular uptake in MDA-MB-231 cell lines than MCF-7 cell lines. A HA receptor block assay was also performed to confirm receptor-meditated endocytosis, that revealed that the fluorescence intensity for HA/C6-CL NCs decreased drastically in MDA-MB-231 cell lines while there was no change in fluorescence intensity in MCF-7 cell lines. Thus, it was concluded that the CD44 receptor-mediated endocytosis is strongly receptor-dependent. Moreover, higher cellular uptake in the MDA-MB-231 cells than MCF-7 cells was due to its overexpression of CD44 receptors. An *in vitro* cytotoxicity study revealed that among the different formulations, cells treated with a nanocomplex exhibited increased cytotoxicity compared to free drugs showing an IC50 value of 0.67 ng/ml, which was 0.14-fold more than the free drug. This further confirms the successful uptake of the nanocomplex mediated by the CD44 tumor homing effect with successful endosomal and lysosomal escape. Moreover, the minimum inhibitory concentration and cell apoptosis confirms that both drugs could induce synergistic cytotoxic effect in combination with better targeting potential. The nanocomplex also elevated the S phase/cell cycle inhibition capability and modification of CDA and dCK balance *via* decreasing mRNA expression of CDA (Fan et al., 2017). In another study, Alshaer et al. evaluated the targeting effect of aptamer-mediated PEGylated liposomes against CD44 receptor positive cells (A549 and MDA-MB-231 cell). The PEGylated liposomes were prepared by the thin film evaporation method *via* a thiol-maleimide click reaction. Here, cholesterol, and DSPE-PEG (2000)- Mal were dissolved in common solvent (chloroform). The thin film was obtained after evaporation of chloroform followed by hydration with PBS solution. Rhodamine-linked liposomes were used as the blank control. PEG-Mal-liposomes was conjugated with an anti-CD44 2′-F-pyrimidineRNA aptamer by the thiol-maleimide click chemistry reaction. The aptamer selectively binds to CD44-expressing tumor cells. Conjugation of the aptamer with the liposome was confirmed by change in size, zeta potential, and gel electrophoresis. The hydrodynamic size of Mal-Lip increased from 129 ± 5 nm to 140 ± 6 nm after conjugation with the aptamer. Similarly, zetapotential shifted from −17.5 ± 0.9 mV for Mal-Lip to −31.0 ± 2.3 mV. An increase in size and zeta potential confirmed successful binding of the aptamer to liposomes. The binding affinity of the aptamer-liposome complex (Kd = 6.2 ± 1.6 nM) was comparatively better than the free aptamer (Kd = 21.5 ± 3.3 nM). Moreover, the free aptamer exhibited higher binding saturation than the aptamer-liposome complex which blanketed a large portion of beads causing steric hindrance of the residual free binding sites. This was further confirmed by *in vitro* flow cytometry and a confocal microscopy assay, showing higher uptake of the aptamer-liposome complex than rhodamine-loaded liposomes. However, in CD44 negative cells (NIH/3T3), there were no significant change in fluorescent intensity after treatment with targeted and non-targeted liposomes confirming the affinity of aptamer to target specific cells without affecting the normal human cellular structure (Alshaer et al., 2015). With the surge in oncology-based research, experts are studying the tumor microenvironment (TME) to get familiar with the reason of tumor progression, metastasis, and drug resistance. The TME is composed of immune cells, fibroblasts, and majorly the extracellular matrix (ECM). Any alteration in the ECM affects cell progression and metastasis by regulating the TME. Matrix metalloproteinases degrades the ECM, for instance fibronectins, gelatin, and collagen causing a surge in tumor progression. To overcome such a hurdle, Lv et al. designed self-assembled hybrid nanoparticles (H_Np) using the PTX-HA prodrug and Matt-loaded lysolipid-based thermosensitive liposomes for targeting TME and CD44 positive metastatic breast carcinoma. Matt is an enzyme inhibitor that suppresses the progression of tumors by affecting their metastasis. The formed (H_Np) exhibited a particle size, PDI, and surface potential of 95.60 ± 1.10 nm, 0.24 ± 0.01, and −1.62 ± 1.25 mV, respectively. H_Np released its payload into the extracellular environments triggered by hyperthermia. The thermosensitive dual targeted H_Np was rapidly up taken by 4T1 tumor cells due to its high binding affinity of CD44 towards HA with 1.6-fold tumor accumulation, 10-fold tumor growth inhibition activity, and 10-fold angiogenesis as compared to non-targeted preparation.

Notably, H_Np inhibited >5-fold expression and activity of MMP, and also blocked activation of fibroblasts *via* the suppressing expression of TGF-β and downregulated extracellular matrix degradation. Finally, PTX-HA active compound and H_Np were easily self-assembled into a multifunctional nanocarrier for simultaneously targeting TME and CD44 cells (Lv et al., 2018). Thus, this study offered a proof of concept that self-assemble nanoparticles dual targeting TME and CD44 cancer cells using PTX-HA and Matt with H_Np was efficient for the treatment of metastatic breast cancer. Gautam et al. had fabricated HA-modified PEGylated phyto-liposome for the targeted delivery of stigmasterol (STS) and DOX for breast cancer treatment. Optimized formulation exhibited acceptable particle size and surface characteristics. After coating with HA, surface charge changed from +17.1 ± 0.8 mV to −9.5 ± 0.2, while the particle size and PDI were found to be 173.9 ± 2.4 nm and 0.26 ± 0.01, respectively. These parameters confirmed that the drug-loaded liposomes (HA-STS-DOX-Lip) were coated with HA. The targeted liposomes exhibited a sustained release profile over a period of 48 h. *In vitro* confocal microscopy displayed a significantly higher uptake of HA-STS-DOX-Lip in CD44-overexpressed MDA-MB-231 cells than MCF-7, this might be due to CD44 receptor-mediated endocytosis, where HA interacted with membrane-bound CD44 protein. At the same condition, uptake of HA-STS-DOX-Lip into MDA-MB-231 cells declined in the presence of free HA, which means free HA competes with HA-STS-DOX-Lip for CD44 binding. HA-STS-DOX-Lip also exhibited deep penetration into the nucleus showing higher apoptosis in MDA-MB-231 cells as compared to free DOX and STS. Accumulation of HA-STS-DOX-Lip was observed into the tumor site only which might be due to CD44 homing and ERP effect. The *in vivo* anticancer study revealed significant higher efficacy of targeted preparation than free DOX, STS, and STS-DOX-lip showing much less toxicity than the free drug (Gautam et al., 2020). In another study, Shahriari et al. had designed a novel polymer-based formulation for CD44-targeted delivery of DOX. In this study, HA was used as a ligand to target CD44 cells of breast cancer. Initially carboxylated polycaprolactone (PCL-COOH) was obtained by dissolving and treating 1, 4 dioxane with succinic anhydride, DMAP, and triethylamine. The PCL was activated with the treatment of EDC or NHS. NHS-activated PCL was coupled with aminated HA by dissolving in DMF and DIPEA under gentle stirring. HA-PCL was formed by amide linkage between HA and PCL functional groups. The nanoprecipitation method was used to prepare blank PCL-HA polymersome and DOX-loaded HA-PCL polymersome. Moreover, DOX was loaded into the PEG-PCL NPs by the double emulsification method. *In vitro* comparative cellular uptake along with cancer targeting results of formulations such as PCL-HA-DOX, PEGylated-PCL-DOX along with free DOX in the MCF-7 and 4T1 cells revealed that PCL-HA-DOX NPs exhibited higher cellular uptake than PEGylated-PCL-DOX and free DOX in both cells. A decrease in uptake of PCL-HA-DOX NPs was observed when cells were pre-treated with HA. HA bound and occupied the CD44 receptors overexpressed in cancer cells causing decreased cellular uptake of PCL-HA-DOX. Due to surface modification of nanoparticles by HA, *in vivo* antitumor efficacy, bio-distribution parameters, and tumor tissue necrosis ability were elevated (Shahriari et al., 2019).

CD44-Engineered Nanoparticles for Cancer Therapy

Nanoparticles may be defined as a small particle ranging between 1–100 nm in size. They show notably physical as well as chemical properties different from their parents' larger materials. For example, reduction in size of any materials to nano size range increases the surface area, enabling a higher chance of interaction with the surrounding materials affecting their reactivity. Such an alteration in physicochemical properties of NPs also influences the alteration/change in electric, magnetic, electric, chemical, and optical properties (Jeevanandam et al., 2018).

Application of nanoparticles in the field of medicine is increasing day by day. NP-based drug delivery systems are a focused research area in cancer therapy and other prominent and emerging diseases. NPs can influence the pharmacokinetics, distribution, and accumulation of therapeutic moiety into the specific site which reduces toxicity. In comparison to conventional drug delivery for cancer theragnostics, nanoparticle-based therapy provided better results. Nanoparticles improved several physicochemical properties of many therapeutic drug molecules, increased aqueous solubility, and modified the release pattern providing significant accumulation of the drug at the site of the tumor (Rizvi and Saleh, 2018).

Numerous methods are available for the manufacturing of NPs. However, most NPs are prepared by two methods namely 1) the top-down method (chemical etching, mechanical milling, sputtering, electro explosion, and laser ablation) and 2) bottom-up method (solvent evaporation, solvent precipitation, laser photolysis, atomic and molecular condensation, and biological synthesis by bacteria, virus, yeast, or fungi). Due to their nanometric size, NPs possess several unique advantages such as passive tumor targeting of incorporated therapeutic molecules, which accumulate passively into the leaky vasculature of tumor cells through the ERP effect. Their small size of <20 nm can pass through blood vessel walls, and it allows for IV, IM, and SC administration, these injections reduce irritation reactions at injection sites due to their small size. To deliver efficient cargos at specific sites in a controlled way, NPs are manufactured in a defined way using specific materials. There are many types of NPs based on material construct which are mainly carbon-based NPs (CNT), metallic NPs (Au, Fe2O3), ceramic NPs, polymeric NPs, and lipid-based NPs. Tailoring nanocarriers suitable for combination therapy is challenging and requires multiple refinement processes. NPs can be decorated as per need (Wolfbeis, 2015; Khan et al., 2019) (**Table 2**).

Polymeric Nanoparticles

There are lots of synthetic or natural polymers that can be used as NP constructs for the therapeutic delivery of anticancer molecules; most used polymers are biodegradable. Most of these polymers can easily conjugate with hyaluronic acid and other targeting ligands to achieve targeted drug delivery against different types of cancer (Begines et al., 2020).

Muntimadugu et al. designed and developed a poly (lactic-co-glycolic acid) (PLGA) nanoparticle for the CD44-targeted delivery of anticancer drug molecules, salinomycin (SLM) to kill cancer stem cells (CSCs) and paclitaxel to weaken cancerous cells. The PLGA nanoparticle was prepared by the emulsion solvent diffusion method. To carry out the cellular uptake study, FITC-loaded NPs were also prepared. The prepared targeted and non-targeted nanoparticles were characterized using DLS to measure the size and PDI. The wrapped SLM-NPs with HA showed concentration-dependent charge inversion. The entrapment efficiency increased from 63.5 ± 1.2% to 71.2 ± 3.4% after coating with HA, which is due to more surface availability due to the coating of nanoparticles. *In vitro* cytotoxicity into the non-sorted, non-isolated MCF-7 cells showed concentration-dependent cytotoxicity. A 100 μM concentration of SLM-HA-NP-treated cells exhibited poor cell viability of 6.9 due to CD44 receptor-mediated cellular uptake. The IC50 value also confirmed the idea of receptor-mediated cellular uptake by showing a 4.1-fold lower IC50 value of SLM-FA-NPs than SLM. FITC-HA-NPs exhibited 1.5 times higher uptake than non-targeted FITC-NPs. The % cell inhibition was obtained in the following order PTX < SLM < SLM/PTX, additionally a significant decrease in CD44 + cell count was observed in SLM-HA-NPs, confirming active targeting ability of HA-coated NPs (Muntimadugu et al., 2016). Saneja et al. used PEGylated PLGA-HA for the targeted delivery of a thio-tetrazoly analogue of a clinical candidate IC87114 (TTQ). HA-modified PEGylated PLGA nanoparticles exhibited significant greater cellular internalization and cell cytotoxicity as compared to HA-non-modified PEGylated PLGA nanoparticles. Cellular uptake and cytotoxicity results of PLGA-PEG-HA NPs were found in the following order MCF-7 >MDA-MB-231 >MiaPaca-2 cells, these differences in the cellular internalization in different cell lines depended on the level of CD44 receptor expression. The level of expression of CD44 receptors in the following cell lines MCF-7, MDA-MB-231, and MiaPaca-2 were low, medium, and large. The therapeutic benefit of the prepared targeted delivery system was based on binding of the HA ligand on to the CD44 overexpressed receptor on the tumor cells (Saneja et al., 2017).

TABLE 2 | Outline of nanoparticle-targeted CD44 cells against cancer.

Polymers used to prepare NPs	Therapeutic agents	Types of study (*in vitro*/*in vivo*)	Cancer types	Cell lines	Animal model	References
PLGA	SLM and PTX	Both	Mammary gland	MCF-7	SD rats	Muntimadugu et al. (2016)
PLGA	TTQ	*In vitro*	Multiple	MCF-7, MDA-MB-231, and MiaPaca-2	——	Saneja et al. (2017)
Chitosan, chondroitin SO4, and PLGA	HCPT	Both	Colon cancer	C-26	Mice	Liu D et al. (2019)
HA	DOX and cisplatin	Both	Mammary carcinoma	4T1 and NIH-3T3	Female BALB/c mice	Yu et al. (2020)
PLL	PTX and GEM	Both	Biliary	HuCCT1 and SCK	BALB/c nude mice	Noh et al. (2015)
LbL lipid NPs	Berberine and rapamycin	Both	Lung	A549	Male Albino mice	Kabary et al. (2018)
PLGA	Bromelain	Both	Mammary gland	HEK293, MCF-7, A549	Swiss albino mice	Bhatnagar et al. (2016)
BSA	ATRA	Both	Lung cancer	B16F10 cells	Mouse	Li et al. (2018)
SLN	DTX	Both	Skin	B16F10 CD44+/αvβ3+	C57BL/6 mice	Shi et al. (2016)
PAMAM	DTX and alendronate	Both	Lung	RAW264.7	Nude mice	Bai et al. (2019)
HA	MTX and alendronate	*In vitro*	Cervical Carcinoma	HeLa, A549, and HUVEC cells	-	Gao et al. (2021)
PEI and PEG	Daunorubicin	Both	AML	HL60 cells	BALB/c mice	Bai et al. (2021)
MSNs	MTX	*In vitro* and in silico	Mammary gland	MDA-MB-231 and MCF-7	-	Sargazi et al. (2018)
MSNs	Au	Both	Cervical cancer	HeLa and U87MG cells	Mice	Li et al. (2015)
MSNs	FI	Both	Cervical cancer	HeLa and U87MG cells	Mice	Li et al. (2014)
MSNs and PEI	OXL	Both	Colon cancer	HT-29	BALB/c nude mice	Yang et al. (2019)
MSNs	-	*In vitro*	Cervical	HeLa cells	—	Nairi et al. (2018)
MSNs	-	*In vitro*	Breast	MDA-MB-231 and A2780	—	Ricci et al. (2018)
MAL and PEG	DTX	Both	Breast	MCF-7	BALB/c nude mice	Lee H et al. (2020)
HA ceramide FA	Dox	Both	Ovarian	SKOV-3	BALB/c nude mice	Lee et al. (2016b)
PEG-gelatin	Epigallocatechin-3-gallate	Both	Prostate	PC3	Nude mice	Huang et al. (2016)
Adipic dihydrazide	Curcumin	Both	Mammary gland	4T1 and MCF-7	Mice	Lai et al. (2021)

In another study, Liu et al. prepared chitosan (CN) and chondroitin sulfate (CS)-modified PLGA NPs for the targeted delivery of an anticancer drug (10-hydroxy camptothecin) (HCPT). Tirella et al. reported CS had a hyaluronic acid-like structure, so can be identified by the HA receptor (CD44) (Wang et al., 2016; Tirella et al., 2019). Prepared NPs were denoted as HCPT-CN-PLGA NP and HCPT-CS-CN-PLGA NP. *In vitro* cellular uptake results into the Colon-26 cells exhibited around a 40% higher uptake of Cy5-CS-CN-PLGA NP than Cy5-CN-PLGA NP, due to the overexpression of the CD44 receptor on C26 cells, which is due to the affinity towards the CS ligand. Numbers of tumor nodules after treatment of tumor-induced mice reduced by both HCPT-CS-CN-PLGA NP and HCPT-CN-PLGA NP formulations, the model group exhibited 23.6 tumor modules. HCPT-CS-CN-PLGA NP dramatically reduced TNF-α and IL-1β levels in tumor tissues than HCPT-CN-PLGA NP. Such results are attributed to surface modifications by CS which helped the ingestion of the formulation into tumor cells resulting in cell death (Liu D. et al., 2019). Lee et al. designed a chondroitin sulfate A and MAL-based nanostructure which enhanced tumor targeting and penetration due to selective CD44 receptor binding and selective binding of MAL to the thiol group of blood components and cellular membrane (Lee H. et al., 2020). Huang et al. had successfully delivered a polyphenol extract of green tea epigallocatechin-3-gallate (EGCG) by HA-PEG-gelatin NPs to inhibit MMP associated with tumor metastasis and invasion against prostate cancer. In this study, EGCG-loaded HA-PEG-gelatin-based NPs showed inhibition of tumor metastasis, cell cycle arrest at the G2/M phase, and inhibited the growth of prostate cancer. The *in vivo* results also showed CD44 receptor-based anticancer activity against prostate cancer (Huang et al., 2016).

Yu and co-workers evaluated CD44-targeted antitumor activity of HA-modified DOX-CDDP (cis-diamminedichloroplatinum, cisplatin) NPs. *In vitro* cellular uptake was evaluated by flow cytometry and CLSM against 3T3 and 4T1 cells incubated with free drug and HA-coated DOX-CDDP for 6 h cells. HA-coated DOX-CDDP-treated 4T1 (CD44 +) cells displayed significantly higher internalization than the group treated with free drugs and pre-treated with HA, while in 3T3 (CD44 low expression) cells, internalization of free drug was higher than other formulations. These results prove the uptake of nanoparticles is mediated by the presence of CD44 in cells. *In vitro* cytotoxicity of the HA-coated DOX-CDDP-treated group showed significant higher cytotoxicity against 4T1 cells than other groups. An *in vivo* biodistribution study showed 2.1 times higher fluorescence intensity in the tumor cell treated with HA-coated DOX-CDDP than the free drug group 12 h after injection. Histopathological analysis revealed a 56.3% ± 5.8% tissue necrosis area for the HA-coated DOX-CDDP-treated group which was higher than the free drugs (35.65 ± 6.5%) and non-treated groups (1.5% ± 0.8%). Conclusively, for reducing side effects, targeting drugs specifically to receptor overexpressed cells can potentiate therapeutic advantage (Yu et al., 2020). In another study, *Noh and co-workers* co-delivered two anticancer drugs namely PTX and GEM *via* a HA-modified poly (L-lysine) carboxylate nanocarrier. The study revealed, *in vitro* and *in vivo*, that the prepared PTX/GEM-loaded HA-conjugated treatment exhibited significantly higher anticancer effect in HuCCT1 (high level of CD44 receptor expression) cells than that of SCK (high level of CD44 receptor expression). Both drugs synergistically induced apoptosis against HuCCT1 cells. These results suggested HA-dependent CD44 receptor-mediated endocytosis playing a crucial role in cancer apoptosis (Noh et al., 2015). Kabarya et al. co-delivered berberine (BER) and rapamycin (RAP) by designing layer by layer NPs functionalized using tumor targeting polymers lactoferrin (LF) and HA. *In vitro* cytotoxicity results showed that LBL NPs coated with polymers had significantly increased cytotoxicity against A549 cell lines than non-coated LBL, *via* increased cellular uptake by specific binding with overexpressed CD44 receptors. HA-based CD44 receptor-mediated endocytosis was also verified *in vivo*, both drugs loaded with LBL-HA exhibited an 88.09% average number of microscopic tumor foci reduction which was remarkably higher than free drugs, moreover BER-RAP-loaded LBL-HA reduced VEGF (tumor growth factor) 3.1 times compared to positive control (Kabary et al., 2018).

Bhatnagar et al. used a HA-grafted PLGA copolymer for the targeted delivery of anticancer phytoconstituents bromelain (BL). The BL-loaded copolymer (BL-HA-PLGA NPs) showed a size ranging between 140 nm and 281 nm. BL-HA-PLGA NPs exhibited significant higher cell cytotoxicity than free BL or BL-PLGA NPs. BL-HA-PLGA NPs also showed significant reduction in IC50 value than free BL and BL-PLGA NPs, which clearly indicates enhanced capability of BL-HA-PLGA NPs to kill tumor cells more effectively. Remarkably, cytotoxic results are mediated by active and passive targeting by BL-HA-PLGA. Fluorescence (F)-labeled BL-HA-PLGA NPs showed 3.5 times higher cellular uptake than PLGA-NPs and free drugs with higher accumulation in MCF-7 cell than A549 cells. This prominent difference was contributed *via* the expression level of CD44 receptor on tumor cells. HA receptor-mediated cellular internalization was also confirmed in the presence/absence of free FA. *In vivo* cell anticancer activity of free BL, BL-PLGA-NPs, BL-HA-PLGA NPs, and control group showed 90–95% cell viability. Non-targeted BL-PLGA NPs reduced viability to 40 ± 3.75%, whereas BL-HA-PLGA NPs reduced cancer viability to 11 ± 2.18% which was significantly better than free BL and BL-PLGA NPs. Targeted nanoparticles showed better anti-cancer activity with improved survival rate in mice than non-targeted preparations (Bhatnagar et al., 2016).

Similarly, Li et al. used the naturally occurring derivative of retinoic acid called all trans retinoic acid (ATRA) and successfully loaded it into the HA-modified albumin nanoparticles. The prepared cationic albumin nanoparticle showed 93% encapsulation efficiency and 8.37% drug loading for ATRA, with spherical shape, and uniform size and with a highly stable nanoparticle. HA-coated nanoparticles exhibited significantly higher uptake into the CD44 $^{+}$ B16F10 cells than non-targeted NPs which is due to higher affinity of the HA CD44 + receptor. The targeted nanoparticles showed a decrease in tumor size compared to the non-targeted preparation explaining the effect of ligand-mediated endocytosis (Li et al., 2018).

Shi et al. designed and developed a novel dual targeting system to enhance the targeting efficiency of chemotherapeutic therapy. A dual targeting system conjugated HA (ligand for CD44 receptor) and tertaiodo-thyroacetic acid (tetrac) (ligand for αvβ3) to a solid lipid nanoparticle for synergistic active targeted delivery of DTX. Prepared NPs were denoted as SLN/DTX, Te-SLNs/DTX, HA-SLNs/DTX, and TeHA-SLN/DTX. TeHA-SLN/DTX exhibited DTX >91.6% encapsulation efficiency showing toroid morphology. Results of *in vivo* imaging and vessel distribution tests showed significantly higher synergistic active targeting efficiency for TeHA-SLNs toward αvβ3 and CD44 receptors than that for ERP-mediated passive targeting. These obtained results strongly recommended that an enhancement in the efficacy TeHA-SLNs/DTX against tumor cells was strongly reliant on the specific interactions between TeHA ligands and CD44/αvβ3 receptors, both ligands did not inhibit the interactions with their particular target but exhibited a synergistic dual active targeting effect (Shi et al., 2016). In another study, by Bai et al., the CD44 receptor of osteoclasts and bone metastatic tumor cells was effectively targeted and inhibited osteoclast and bone metastasis of lung cancer by using a DTX-loaded alendronate (ALN)-HA-PAMAM (AHP) nanocarrier. Scientists investigated therapeutic effectiveness of this formulation both *in vitro* and *in vivo*, and reported its effectiveness in both studies, in which CD44 receptor-mediated endocytosis played a significant role (Bai et al., 2019). Recently, in another study, Gao and co-worker investigated the *in vitro*/*in vivo* antitumor activity of dual receptor-targeted HA-modified alendronate-methotrexate (HA-ALN-MTX-NPs) and they found that HA-ALN-MTX-NPs had a significantly higher cytotoxic effect against A549 (overexpressed CD44 receptor cells) than that of HUVECs (normal tissue) cells. This is due to selective uptake by tumor cells through specific binding of HA with the CD44 receptor on tumor cells (Gao et al., 2021).

Most recently, Bai et al. reported a pH-responsive, dual targeting nano system for the treatment of acute myeloid leukemia (AML). They targeted CXCR4 and CD44 overexpressed receptor on AML. Here, PEG-grafted PEI *via* benzoic imine bond decorated with Prussian blue NPs (PBNPs) were prepared, which was further functionalized with CXCR4 targeting peptide E5 and HA. Daunorubicin (DNR)-

loaded dual-targeted PBNPs efficiently escaped endosomal uptake and increased circulation time in the physiological condition. Dual-targeted PBNPs also showed significantly enhanced cellular uptake and anti-HL60 cell effect leading to reduced tumor migration than mono-targeted PBNPs. *In vivo* results of DNR-loaded dual-targeted PBNPs exhibited significantly improved anticancer and anti-metastatic results against AML treatment (Bai et al., 2021). Lee et al. synthesized unique types of dual-targeting nanocarriers consisting of hyaluronic acid and ceramide folic acid (HACE-FA) in which the -COOH group of FA was reacted with the -OH group of HA to bind *via* the ester bond. DOX was loaded into the HACE-FA and was successfully delivered against SKOV-3 cells (CD44 and FR positive cells). Accumulation of HACE-FA NPs was significantly higher than HACE NPs, while conjugation of FA to HACE NPs enhanced uptake efficiency around 67%. *In vivo* NIRF imaging also confirmed the dual targetability of DOX-loaded HACE-FA NPs by showing 3.81-fold higher fluorescence intensity in the tumor group than that of DOX-loaded HACE NPs. HACE-FA NPs were primarily accumulated in the tumor site and exhibited around a 4.82-fold higher fluorescent signal than HACE-FA NPs. Finally, the researcher suggested that DOX-loaded HACE-FA NPs were synergistic in *in vitro* and *in vivo* therapeutic results by active targeted CD44 receptor and FR receptor internalization (Lee et al., 2016b). Lai and co-workers recently prepared self-assembled amphiphilic HA-modified adipic dihydrazide (ADH) conjugates loaded with hydrophobic drug curcumin for CD44 targeted delivery. Prepared HA-modified CUR NPs internalized very efficiently into 4T1 and MCF-7 cells which might be due to CD44-mediated endocytosis releasing its cargo intracellularly into lysosomes. Due to HA modification, this nanocarrier showed a significantly higher accumulation into the tumor cells as compared to free CUR and showed prominent tumor growth inhibition *in vivo*. These results were attributed to the EPR effect and CD44-mediated endocytosis (Lai et al., 2021).

Metallic Nanoparticles

The various inorganic and organic NPs in the biomedical field have gained significant attention due to their unique structural characteristics and functionality over the past years. Particularly, magnetic iron oxide (Fe3O4) NPs and AuNPs are used in the field of disease diagnosis and treatment therapy. Several properties like magnetic resonance, thermal, X-ray attenuation, and CT imaging makes them very useful in the biomedical field. Due to variability of cancer conditions, it becomes important to design a theranostic platform that would be able to provide both diagnosis and chemotherapy simultaneously. By using these particles, a multifunctional nanoplatform could be possible, that is able to solve complex problems related to cancer *in vitro* and *in vivo* (Li C. et al., 2014; Tian et al., 2014).

Sargazi et al. reported HA-conjugated PEGylated MNPs for the targeted delivery of mitoxantrone (MTX). The MNPs were prepared using Fe3O4 and the surface of MNPs were modified by dopamine hydro bromide (DPA -polyethylene glycol to form DPA-PEG-MNPs. DPA was used to prevent NP agglomeration. DPA-PEG-Fe3O4 NPs were conjugated with HA, followed by MTX loading to form MTX-FA-MNPs. *In vitro* cytotoxicity results against MDA-MBA-231 and MCF-7 cell lines revealed that about 32% MDA-MB-231 cell viability was reduced by MTX-FA-MNPs treatment whereas the cytotoxic effect of MTX-FA-MNPs against the MCF-7 cell line was not much higher as that for the MDA-MB-231 cell line. The reason behind this difference was the expression of the CD44 receptor, the MCF-7 cell line expressed a significantly smaller amount of CD44 receptor on its surface as compared to MDA-MB-231 cells. Flow cytometry results of MTX-FA-MNPs exhibited approximately 70.3% apoptosis against MDA-MB-231 cell lines whereas apoptosis against MCF-7 cell lines showed only 5%. These results were attributed to the high affinity of HA-conjugated MNPs towards the CD44 receptor. The significant high affinity of MTX-HA-MNPs compared to HA towards CD44 receptor was also confirmed by molecular docking simulation. Conclusively, HA-mediated MNPs could be a good choice for CD44-targeted delivery of MTX (Sargazi et al., 2018).

Li and co-workers designed a novel multifunctional theranostic approach for diagnosis and photothermal anticancer therapy against different types of cancer. In this study, Fe3O4@Ag NPs were used as the seed to prepare an Fe3O4@Ag nano star (Fe3O4@Ag NSs). The prepared Fe3O4@Ag NSs were used as triple-response NPs such as magnetic resonance (MR), computer tomography (CT), thermal imaging, and photothermal therapy against cancer cells. Fe3O4@Ag NSs were again decorated with polyethyleneimine (PEI) and HA to form Fe3O4@Ag- HA-NSs, in this formulation Fe3O4 was a core of NPs while the star-shaped Au was the shell. The *in vitro* and *in vivo* xenograft tumor model revealed that this multifunctional nanocarrier can be used as a nano probe for effective magnetic resonance and CT imaging. Moreover thermal absorption characteristics allowed it to be used as a nano probe for thermal imaging of a tumor *in vitro* and *in vivo*. HA-mediated cellular uptake of Fe3O4@Au-HA NSs was evaluated in HeLa cells and U87MG cells, both cells were incubated with the same concentration of Au but uptake of Au from Fe3O4@Au-HA NSs in HeLa cells was significantly higher than that of U87MG cells. This difference in cellular uptake was contributed by the expression of the CD44 receptor on the cell lines, HeLa cells were CD44-enriched cells while U87MG cells do not express CD44 receptor. Thus, the role of HA in CD44 receptor-mediated specific cellular internalization of NPs was justified (Li et al., 2015). In another study, Li et al. also evaluated CD44 targeting ability and tumor magnetic resonance imaging of HA-modified MNPs *in vitro* and *in vivo*. The *in vitro* cell cytotoxicity and hemolysis results illustrated that formulation was biocompatible. This study also showed CD44 receptor-dependent therapeutic efficacy *in vitro* and *in vivo* against HeLa and U87MG cells (Li J. et al., 2014).

Ceramic Nanoparticles

Ceramic NPs are non-metallic solids, mainly consisting of oxide, carbides, phosphates and carbonates of metals, and metalloids such as calcium, titanium, silicon, etc., generally prepared by heating followed by cooling. These particles have a wide range of use due to a number of favorable properties such as high heat resistance, amorphous, polycrystalline, dense, porous/hollow, and chemical inertness attributes (Sigmund et al., 2006). They can also be used as catalysis, photocatalysis, photodegradation, and imaging agents (Thomas et al., 2015). MSNs could be easily decorated with polymeric moieties on the external surface, which make them more controllable in the field of drug delivery. Recently Yang et al. prepared MSNs for targeted delivery of oxaliplatin (OXL) and miRNA-204-5p. OX-mi-HSMN showed significantly higher uptake efficiency and higher cell cytotoxicity than all other formulations in CD44 overexpressed receptors present on HT-29 cells demonstrating internalization *via* HA receptor-mediated endocytosis, which leads to increased anticancer activity of OX-mi-HSMN. OX-mi-HSMN also showed 43.9% pre-apoptosis which had significantly higher anticancer efficacy in terms of apoptosis potentials. Remarkably, OX-mi-HSMN exhibited significantly higher noticeable downregulation of tumor growth than free OXL and OXL-MSNs. Conclusively, delivery of OXL and miRNA by HA-targeted MSNs showed synergistic anticancer effect against colon cancer (Yang et al., 2019). In another study by Nairi et al., biocompatible MSN-based nanoparticles were prepared. This researcher took three HA samples of different molecular weights, HAS (8–15 kDa), HAM (30–50 kDa), and HAL (90–130 kDa). The formed NPs were denoted as MSN-HAS, MSN-HAM, and MSN-HAL. Zeta potential results showed an increase in negative value with the length of the HA chain. Cellular uptake results for different formulations on HeLa cells at 37°C were investigated by optical and electron microscopy. These results showed that cellular uptake of MSN-NH2/MSN-HAS was higher as compared to MSN-HAM and MSN-HAL, the reason behind the lower internalization of the high molecular weight polymer might be the large size of the sample. A similar study at 4°C exhibited the internalization of MSN-HA samples but not for MSN-NH2, these results suggest that the internalization of samples was mediated *via* two different mechanisms. MSN-NH2 internalization primarily occurred due to electrostatic interactions between cellular phospholipids and MSN-NH2, whereas MSN-HA uptake was mainly driven by CD44 receptor-mediated endocytosis (Nairi et al., 2018). In another study, researchers evaluated the effect of molecular weight of the polymer and methods of preparation on the physicochemical and biological performance of MSNs. In this study, two different MW Has namely HA200 and HA 6.4 kDa were conjugated with MSNs *via* two different methods, in the first method "A," both MW HAs were preactivated followed by addition of NPs and in the second method "B," both MW HAs were activated in the presence of NPs; formed NPs were denoted as HA200A, HA6.4A and HA200B, HA6.4B, respectively for methods A and B. All four samples exhibited the same solubility but variation in the loading of HA, texture, surface charge, and stability. Method A could not perform well in these parameters showing low HA loading and stability in biological conditions. In contrast to this, method B performed well with high molecular weight HA, this high MW of HA loading onto the MSNs reflected the biological results of NPs. *In vitro* cellular uptake of different formulations against MDA-MB-231 ($CD44^+$) and A2780 ($CD44^-$) cell lines showed significantly higher uptake of HA200B, HA6.4B into the MDA-MB-231 ($CD44^+$) than A2780 ($CD44^-$) cells. More precise uptake of HA6.4B into MDA-MB-231 ($CD44^+$) was due to HA-dependent CD44 receptor-mediated endocytosis of formulation (Ricci et al., 2018).

CD44-Engineered Dendrimer for Cancer Therapy

Between 1970–1990, Buhleier et al. and Tomalia et al. synthesized dendrimers for the first time. Dendrimers have a precise controlled structure, suitable for surface functionalization with different ligands (Kokare et al., 2021). The word dendrimer is derived from a Greek term dendron which means tree, that is because of their distinctive architecture with a number of branching units. Dendrimers may be defined as synthetic polymer macromolecules, with high branching points, 3D globular shape, monodispersity, and a nanometric (1–100 nm) size range. Due to nanoscopic size and monodispersity, the dendrimer is also popularly known as cascade molecules, arborols, dendritic molecules, and nano-metric architectures (Kesharwani et al., 2012, Kesharwani et al., 2014a, Kesharwani et al., 2014b; Kesharwani et al., 2015b; Gawande et al., 2021). The dendrimer architecture is primarily composed of three different domains, i.e., a "core" center consisting of an atom/molecule with at least two identical chemical functional groups, "branches" originating from the core, a repeat unit with at least one branch junction, this repetition is organized in a geometrical progression that results in a series of radially concentric layers known as "generation," and a "terminal functional group" which determines the properties of the dendritic macromolecules (Fréchet, 1994). The dendrimer is an ideal nanocarrier to achieve passive targeting due to permeability and retention effects in tumor sites. Due to its surface functional group, the dendrimer also offers active targeting of different sites of dendrimers. The use of a plain PAMAM dendrimer was limited to achieve targeted delivery of anticancer molecules due to its intrinsic surface cationic charge, which caused high cytotoxicity because of non-specific interactions with both normal and cancer cells. To solve this problem, there are a number of approach available such as PEGylation, coating with different polymers, and conjugation of targeting ligands. Among these approaches, ligand conjugation is one of the best approaches. Conjugation of ligands with dendrimers not only reduces inherent cytotoxicity of PAMAM but provides some other benefits such as enhancement in solubility, increase in drug loading, sustained/controlled drug release, and improvement in stability, biodistribution, and pharmacokinetics (Duncan and Izzo, 2005; Jain et al., 2010; Kesharwani et al., 2015c; Kesharwani and Iyer, 2015). Kesharwani et al. designed a CD44-targeted 3, 4-difluorobenzylidene curcumin (CDF)-loaded G4 PAMAM dendrimer functionalized with HA and evaluated its therapeutic activity against MiaPaCa-2 and AsPC-1 cells. Initially, HA was conjugated with the NH2 group of dendrimers *via* the EDC coupling reaction. The COOH- group of HA was easily conjugated with the amine functional group of dendrimers by amide bond formation in the presence of EDC, conjugation was confirmed by TEM images, which exhibited 7.6 ± 1.7 and 9.3 ± 1.5 nm sizes for the PAMAM dendrimer and HA-PAMAM dendrimer, respectively. HA-PAMAM-CDF showed 1.42-fold higher entrapment efficiency than PAMAM-CDF, which might be due to HA on the surface of the PAMAM periphery having more space to load a higher amount of CDF. Due to steric hindrance, HA-PAMAM-CDF showed sustained and delayed release of CDF at pH 7.4. HA-PAMAM-CDF comparatively showed better cytotoxicity, due to the CD44 receptor-mediated uptake of the formulation. Moreover, HA-PAMAM-CDF exhibited higher anticancer activity in MiaPaCa-2 cells than AsPC-1 cells because the expression of CD44 receptor was comparatively higher on MiaPaCa-2 cells than AsPC-1 cells. Targeting efficiency of HA-PAMAM-CDF was reconfirmed by the receptor blocked study, here firstly the CD44 receptor was blocked by the presence of an excess of free HA. The IC50 value was found to be 405 ± 6.32 nM for HA-PAMAM-CDF, without a HA-blocked receptor, whereas with the HA-blocked receptor, the formulation exhibited an IC50 value of 694 ± 8.36 nM for HA-PAMAM-CDF. A significant difference was observed in the cytotoxicity curve of HA-PAMAM-CDF as compared to free CDF and PAMAM-CDF, which clearly indicated that the CD44 receptor is a major pathway for HA-PAMAM-CDF uptake. Higher HA-PAMAM-CDF uptake through the CD44 receptor due to the presence of HA on the periphery of the PAMAM was also confirmed by the fluorescence microscopic studies (Kesharwani et al., 2015d). In another similar study, Qi et al. fabricated a dual functional HA-conjugated PAMAM dendrimer for long systemic circulation and active targeting of CD44 receptor and delivery of topotecan HCl (TPT). HA was conjugated with PAMAM in the presence of NHS/EDC to form HA-PAMAM, additionally HA-PAMAM was linked with fluorescence isothiocyanate (FITC) to form FITC-conjugated FA-PAMAM. A hemolytic study revealed that HA conjugation with the PAMAM significantly reduced the hemolytic toxicity of PAMAM at low as well as higher concentrations. HA-PAMAM showed 2.67-fold higher drug encapsulation than PAMAM, due to the presence of HA on the PAMAM surface. Due to HA conjugation, TPT-loaded HA-PAMAM exhibited sustained release of TPT. *In vitro* cytotoxicity study was evaluated in the HCT-116 cell lines, these cell lines are reported to be CD44 + receptor cell lines. After 48 h of incubation, the IC50 value found to be 38.029 nM and 4.966 nM for HA-PAMAM and PAMAM, respectively, clearly indicating that the HA conjugation significantly decreased the cytotoxicity of the PAMAM dendrimer. Cell cytotoxicity for free TPT and TPT-loaded HA-PAMAM were also evaluated in HCT-116 cell lines, the IC50 values were 0.262 and 0.086 nM for the free TPT and TPT-loaded HA-PAMAM, respectively. These results revealed that TPT-loaded HA-PAMAM had relatively higher cytotoxicity at lower concentrations. To evaluate CD44 receptor-mediated uptake of the formulation, the HCT-116 cell line was incubated with FITC-labeled HA-PAMAM with or without HA treatment. Fluorescence microscopy showed competitive binding for the CD44 receptor, meaning a significant reduction in fluorescence intensity of HA-PAMAM-FITC in the pre-incubated HA HCT-116 cell lines. This result was reconfirmed by flow cytometric analysis. Pharmacokinetics of preparation were also evaluated for free TPT, TPT-PAMAM, and TPT-HA-PAMAM in normal rates. MRT was found to be 0.56, 2.53, and 7.09 h for free TPT given in PBS, TPT in PAMAM, and TPT in HA-PAMAM, respectively. TPT-loaded HA-PAMAM exhibited higher MRT as compared to other preparation, as HA may shield all the surface charge of PAMAM and prevent opsonization, thus due to this effect, HA increased the MRT of HA-PAMAM. Tissue distribution results showed 3.6-fold higher TPT distribution in the kidney and 1.7-fold higher distribution in the liver due the HA modification. *In vivo* antitumor results in S-180 mice were also examined for all groups namely, free TPT, PAMAM/TPT, and HA-PAMAM-TPT, here also HA-conjugated PAMAM/TPT was found to have comparatively higher anticancer activity (Qi et al., 2015). Zhanga et al. developed mixed dendrimer micelles (MDM) based on dendrimers for the co-delivery of MDM-1-siRNA and DOX, for the inhibition of genes which are involved in the development of MDR. Additionally, a dendriplex was prepared by mixing MDM-1-siRNA with PAMAM *via* electrostatic interactions, HA had no effect on the complexation between PAMAM and siRNA. HA-DOPE/MDM/siRNA and HA/MDM/siRNA dendriplexes were evaluated for stability. Gel electrophoresis results revealed that approximately 85% of siRNA was intact after 30 min. In the presence of RNAse, indicated formulations were able to protect the dendriplexes from RNAse-mediated degradation. Cytotoxicity of free MDM and HA-modified formulations were evaluated in the A2780ADR, MDA-MB-231, and HCT-116 cell lines. Due to the anionic charge of HA, the cationic charge of PAMAM was masked, hence both HA/HA-DOPE functionalizations increased the cytotoxicity of formulations in all cell lines. HA/MDM exhibited comparatively lower cytotoxicity than HA-DOPE/MDM in MDA-MB-231 cell lines, this is because the HA covered the complete surface of MDM. The DOPE moiety promotes strong binding of HA with an MDM structure. Cytotoxicity of combinations, namely MDM loaded with DOX (MDM-D), HA-DOPE-MDM-DOX, and HA-DOPE-MDM-DOX-siMDR-1, was evaluated on all three cell lines; results were DOX concentration and quantity of CD44 receptor expression-dependent. HA-DOPE-MDM-DOX with 10 μM DOX exhibited higher cytotoxicity than MDM-DOX in both HCT116 and MDA-MB-231 cell lines. In A2780 ADR cell lines, HA-mediated cytotoxicity was not observed because of lower CD44 receptor expression in A2780 ADR compared to HCT116 and MDA-MB-231 cell lines. Membrane-bound P-gp was overexpressed in both HCT116 and MDA-MB-231 cell lines; co-delivery of DOX and siRNA in HA-DOPE-MDM can further increase the specificity and cytotoxicity in CD44 and P-gp overexpressed tumor cells (Zhang et al., 2020).

Tang et al. designed and developed a synergistic anticancer system to achieve chemotherapy and phototherapy simultaneously. HA-PAMAM-COOH-TMZ (HPCT) and HA-PAMAM-COOH-ICG (HPCI) were prepared which showed spherical, monodispersed, uniform, and better distributed particles than non-modified PAMAM. HPCT exhibited 44.91

and 16.64% EE and LC, respectively for TMZ while HPCI showed 99.87% and 28.55% EE and LC, respectively for ICG. Release of TMZ was significantly increased at pH 5.0, because at this pH hyaluronidase caused enzymatic hydrolysis of HA. For the photothermal therapy, HPCI was better than free ICG because in HPCI, ICG was present in the PAMAM cavity, which made it stable in the solution and in increased laser irradiation. Additionally, HPCI generated higher singlet-oxygen than the free ICG. In cell viability results, HPCT + HPCI + NIR combinedly exhibited the highest anticancer activity and exhibited 17.1% cell viability, which is better than the HPCT + NIR, HPCI + NIR (36.3% cell viability), and ICG + NIR (48.9%) groups. These results established synergistic anticancer activity of HPCT + HPCI under laser irradiation. *In vivo* biological distribution of NPs was studied in nude mice after IV injection in the tail vein that exhibited strong fluorescence in tumor cells 72 h after injection. These results indicated that HPCI and HPCT mainly accumulated in cancer cells which was further proved by NIR irradiation effective 24 h after injection. *In vivo* anticancer results of HPCT + HPCI + NIR groups showed complete disappearance of the tumor. Biodistributions of NPs to the normal tissues were evaluated, showing no damage to normal tissue by treatment of combined therapy. There was no significant change into the level of alanine aminotransferase, aspartate aminotransferase, total bilirubin, creatinine, urea N2, uric acid, and creatine phosphate in tumor-bearing mice and normal mice groups (Tang et al., 2018). Therapeutic benefits of many anticancer molecules were compromised due to MDR, this MDR was mostly due to the Pgp-mediated efflux of drugs. It is considered that nanocarriers escaped from Pgp efflux by endocytosis and internalized drugs into the cytoplasm, but in some cases another protein called major vault protein may be involved in the development of drug resistance, which transport drugs like DOX out from the target site (nucleus) to the cytoplasm (Van Zon et al., 2006; Abbasi et al., 2013). To overcome this problem, Han et al. has designed a HA-functionalized PAMAM dendrimer for the codelivery of DOX and MVP-siRNA against MCF-7/ADR cells. Firstly, HA–PAMAM were prepared then DOX was loaded into HA-PAMAM to form DOX-HA-PAMAM. The DOX-HA-PAMAM/siRNA dendriplex was prepared by adding 20 μM of siRNA into the specified amount of DOX-HA-PAMAM solution (1:100 w/w, siRNA: polymer) and incubated for 20 min at RT. Negatively charged siRNA bind electrostatically with positively charged polymers. Gel electrophoresis confirmed the binding ability and stability of siRNA with HA-PAMAM. DOX-HA-PAMAM exhibited higher *in vivo* bioavailability and MRT (AUC, 4.79 h μg/ml and MRT, 21.8 h) compared to the free DOX solution group (AUC, 0.98 h μg/ml and MRT, 3.1 h), which indicated sustained DOX release from HA-coated PAMAM. HA decoration on PAMAM played an important role in these results, due to HA, the nanocarrier was internalized into the tumor cell by overexpressed CD44 receptor-mediated endocytosis. In MCF-7/ADR cells, accumulation of DOX was much less than MCF-7 cells because MCF-7/ADR overexpressed Pgp which caused Pgp-mediated efflux of DOX. DOX loaded into HA-PAMAM avoided/bypassed Pgp and significantly increased the accumulation of DOX into both MCF-7 and MCF-7/ADR cell lines. Pre-treatment with HA or chloropromazine (CPZ) significantly decreased the accumulation of DOX into cell lines, which indicated HA-PAMAM uptake was CD44 receptor-mediated through clathrin-dependent endocytosis. DOX–HA–PAMAM exhibited comparatively higher cytotoxicity (IC50, 11.3 μM) compared to the free DOX solution (IC50, 48.5 μM) in MCF-7/ADR cell lines. Western blot assay revealed that the MVP-siRNA solution and MVP-siRNA lipofectamine 2000 were not effective in downregulating the MVP expression in MCF-7/ADR cells, while PAMAM-HA was able to downregulate MVP protein expression as compared to untreated cells. Intracellular localization of DOX in MCF-7/ADR cells was evaluated by confocal microscopy with or without MVP-siRNA treatment. Initially no significant difference in intracellular DOX fluorescence intensity between free DOX solution and DOX-HA-PAMAM was observed but after 24 h, DOX was observed outside the nucleus, whereas the MVP downregulated cell still exhibited significant strong fluorescent in the nucleus. Conclusive co-delivery of DOX and MVP-siRNA by PAMAM-HA could enter into the nucleus without MVP-siRNA pre-treatment and induce gene silencing and cytotoxicity (Han et al., 2012). A summary of dendrimers used against cancer therapy has been illustrated in **Table 3**.

CD44-Engineered Carbon Nanotube for Cancer Therapy

In 1991, Iijima first observed a tubular carbon structure by TEM, called a carbon nanotube (CNT). CNTs can be defined as graphite sheets, wrapped up into cylindrical shapes (Iijima, 1991). It is composed of derivatives of both carbon fibers and fullerene with molecules of 60 carbon atoms arranged in specific tubes. Based on layers, there are two types of carbon nanotubes namely single-walled carbon nanotubes (SWCNTs) and multi-walled carbon nanotubes (MWCNTs). SWCNTs are composed of a single layer of graphene of between 0.4 and 2.0 nm in diameter whereas MWCNTs consist of two or more graphene cylinders with a diameter of 1–3 nm (He et al., 2013). Currently CNTs are under the scrutiny for use as a new tool for biomedical applications. A CNT has many characteristics such as ordered structure with high aspect ratio, low weight, high mechanical strength, high electrical and thermal conductivity, and the length of the CNT is in the form of micrometers with a diameter of about 100 nm (Polizu et al., 2006). Due to these unique characteristics, CNTs have the potential for diverse applications including biomedicals (Lacerda et al., 2006). A CNT can easily cross the plasma membrane and reach directly into the targeted cells because of its needle-shaped structure, and be internalized into the cell by the endocytosis mechanism without causing cell lysis (Cai et al., 2005). The prominent properties, mainly controlled and targeted drug delivery, makes them potential carriers for therapeutic benefit. The multifunctional surface group of a CNT allows them to conjugate different targeting ligands for targeted delivery of many anticancer therapeutic agents. A number of HA-functionalized CNTs were reported for targeting overexpressed CD44 receptor

TABLE 3 | Analysis of dendrimers used against tumor cells overexpressing CD44.

Types and generation of dendrimers	Therapeutic agents	Types of cancer	Cell lines	Animal model	References
G4 PAMAM	CDF	Pancreatic cancer	MiaPaCa-2 and AsPC-1 cells	–	Kesharwani et al. (2015c)
G4 PAMAM	Topotecan	Colorectal cancer	HCT-116 cells	Normal rate/S-180 mice	Qi et al. (2015)
G4 PAMAM	DOX and siMDR-1	–	HCT116, A2780 ADR and MDA-MB-231	–	Zhang et al. (2020)
G5 PAMAM	TMZ and ICG	Melanoma	A375 cells	Mice	Tang et al. (2018)
G5 PAMAM	DOX and MVP - siRNA	Breast cancer	MCF-7/ADR and MCF-7	Mice	Han et al. (2012)

TABLE 4 | Summary of CNT-targeted CD44 cells.

Types of CNTs	Therapeutic agents	Types of cancer	Types of study (*in vitro*/*in vivo*)	Cell lines	Animal model	References
MWCNTs	DOX	Breast Cancer	*In vitro*	MDA-MB-231	–	Singhai et al. (2020)
MWCNTs	GEM	Colon cancer	Both	HT-29	Sprague-Dawley rat	Prajapati et al. (2019)
SWCNTs	DOX	TNBC	*In vitro*	MDA-MB-231	–	Liu Z et al. (2019)
MWCNTs	DOX	Cervical cancer	*In vitro*	HeLa and L929	–	Cao et al. (2015)
SWCNTS	SAL and PTX	Breast cancer	Both	MDA-MB-231 and CSC-/CSC $^+$	Mice	Al Faraj et al. (2016)

on various tumor cells (Klumpp et al., 2006) (**Table 4**). Singhai et al. used an MWCNT functionalized with HA and α-Tocopheryl succinate (α-TOS) for the targeted delivery of DOX against TNBC cells. Prepared different formulations namely aminated MWCNTs/DOX, α-TOS-MWCNTs/DOX, HA-MWCNTs/DOX, and α-TOS-HA-MWCNTs/DOX exhibited drug loading of 56.25 ± 1.77, 65.54 ± 2.13, 67.76 ± 2.98, and 76.23 ± 1.76, respectively. α-TOS-HA-MWCNTs/DOX exhibited comparatively higher drug loading compared to other formulations which might be due to conjugation of two different polymers with CNTs, providing a large space to load a large amount of the drug. A cellular uptake study against MDA-MB-231 cell lines revealed that α-TOS-HA-MWCNTs/DOX exhibited significant higher cellular internalization than aminated MWCNTs/DOX, α-TOS-MWCNTs/DOX, HA-MWCNTs/DOX, and free DOX. Plain or free DOX rarely entered into the tumor cell while aminated MWCNTs/DOX exhibited better uptake than plain DOX. Cellular internalization was improved with α-TOS-MWCNTs/DOX but HA-MWCNTs/DOX showed even better cellular internalization than α-TOS-MWCNTs/DOX. Results confirmed the role of HA in cellular uptake by CD44 receptor-mediated endocytosis. *In vitro* cytotoxicity results showed comparatively significant higher cytotoxicity and the lowest IC50 value for α-TOS-HA-MWCNTs/DOX (IC50, 0.810 ± 0.017; $p < 0$ 0.001). Combination of both polymers in α-TOS-HA-MWCNTs/DOX (IC50, 0.810 ± 0.017) exhibited lower IC50 than the individual polymer. Dual ligands conjugated on MWCNT surfaces enhanced cellular uptake of α-TOS-HA-MWCNTs/DOX through which more DOX was available to exhibit its therapeutic effect on the tumor cell. This was attributed to CD44 receptor-mediated cell internalization which led to a decrease in IC50 values (Singhai et al., 2020). Prajapati et al. designed gemcitabine-loaded HA-PEG-MWCNTs for colon cancer targeting and evaluated them *in vitro* and *in vivo*. GEM/HA-PEG-MWCNTs exhibited maximum entrapment efficiency 90.2 ± 1.9% which was higher than GEM-MWCNTs, GEM/HA-MWCNTs, and GEM/PEGMWCNTs. An intracellular uptake study of FITC-labeled GEM/HA-MWCNTs exhibited significant higher cellular uptake among all other formulations, this was attributed to uptake of the formulation through HA receptor-mediated endocytosis. GEM/HA-PEG-MWCNTs showed lower cellular uptake than GEM/HA-MWCNTs, which might be due to the hydrophilic chain of PEG on the CNT inhibiting interactions between the formulation and cell membrane. *In vitro* cytotoxicity against HT-29 cells showed that HA-coated CNTs exhibited comparatively higher cytotoxicity than non-HA-coated CNTs. GEM/HA-PEG-MWCNTs were relatively more compatible in the blood (less hemolytic) than other preparations. Pharmacokinetic parameters of GEM such as C_{max}, $t_{1/2}$, MRT, and AUC were comparatively improved by GEM/HA-PEG-MWCNTs. *In vivo* antitumor activity was investigated in tumor-bearing female rats (Sprague-Dawley strain) by measuring tumor growth. GEM/HA-MWCNTs and GEM/HAPEG-MWCNTs both decreased tumor volume significantly compared to free GEM. GEM/HA-MWCNTs exhibited higher antitumor activity than GEM/HAPEG-MWCNTs because of receptor-mediated accumulation and intracellular internalization (Prajapati et al., 2019). Leu et al. prepared a targeted delivery system for DOX against TNBC cell lines. They used HA-conjugated aminated single-walled carbon nanotubes (NH2 SWCNTs), where HA was non-covalently coated on to the CNT surface. Surface morphology and size of CNTs was significantly changed after HA coating, the size of nano-NH2-SWCNTs and SWCNTs-DOX was around 2000 nm which was reduced to around 262.5 ± 0.9 nm after HA coating. As reported in many studies, adsorption and desorption are the main characteristics of CNTs. Hence in this study, SWCNTs-DOX-HA showed 81.5 ± 1.0% DOX adsorption. *In vitro* drug release and desorption of DOX from SWCNTs-DOX-HA was pH-triggered. At pH 7.4, desorption of DOX from SWCNTs-DOX and SWCNTs-DOX-HA was slow which was around 11% and 8% in 24 h, respectively, whereas in pH 5.5, the PBS desorption rate of DOX from SWCNTs-DOX-HA increased to 34.5% in 24 h. *In vitro* cellular uptake of SWCNTs-DOX and SWCNTs-DOX-HA into the MDA-MB-231 cell lines were also evaluated, flow cytometry results revealed that SWCNTs-DOX-HA had 2.1-fold higher uptake of DOX than the SWCNTs-DOX. Cellular uptake results were reconfirmed by confocal microscopy, which was also consistent with cellular uptake results of flow cytometry. Higher cellular uptake of SWCNTs-DOX-HA than SWCNTs-DOX was possibly due to HA receptor-mediated endocytosis. The SRB assay revealed that SWCNTs-DOX-HA and SWCNTs-DOX showed dose-dependent anticancer activity, additionally SWCNTs-DOX-HA exhibited significant higher anticancer activity as well as MDA-MB-231 cell migration inhibition than SWCNTs-DOX, which was maximum at 1.0 μg/ml. The *in vitro* apoptosis rate by flow cytometry was 2.33 ± 0.56%, 9.25 ± 1.62%, 37.72 ± 1.03%, and 73.45 ± 1.54% respectively for control, SWCNTs-DOX, SWCNTs-DOX-HA, and free DOX groups. SWCNTs-DOX-HA was better than SWCNTs-DOX, the difference in the results was mainly attributed to HA modification (Liu Z. et al., 2019). Cao and co-worker also evaluated the targeted ability of DOX-loaded PEI-modified MWCNTs covalently attached with FI and FA, the final prepared product was denoted as MWCNT/PEI-FI-HA/DOX. As mentioned earlier, loading and unloading of drugs onto the CNTs was pH-dependent, here the MWCNT/PEI-FI-HA/DOX complex showed DOX loading was 72.0% at basic pH which was significantly higher than at an acidic pH. In an acidic condition, DOX was protonated showing increased hydrophilicity which prohibited hydrophobic π-π interactions with CNTs, while at basic pH DOX was deprotonated and quite hydrophobic, which facilitated hydrophobic π-π interaction with CNTs leading to higher drug loading. Due to effect of the pH on loading/unloading, the DOX release rate was higher at acidic pH (5.8) at 54.6% whereas at physiological pH it was 40.8% after 48 h pH-triggered release of DOX from prepared complexes was beneficial for tumor targeting. The CD44 receptor targeted efficiency of HA-conjugated complex was investigated in HeLa cells and normal L929 cells. Flow cytometry results of prepared complexes showed seven times higher uptake into HeLa cells than L929 cells. Obtained results confirmed the idea of CD44 receptor-mediated endocytosis of prepared complexes into the HeLa cells, enhancing its uptake. Confocal microscopy results were also consistent with flow cytometry results. An MTT assay was also performed to determine % viability in both HeLa and L929 cells treated with prepared complexes. After 2 h of incubation, HeLa cells showed 50% viability while almost all L929 cells were alive. All these results indicated HA mediated targeted inhibition of tumor cells *via* CD44-mediated endocytosis and intracellular uptake (Cao et al., 2015). Faraj et al. reported a novel approach of combination therapy against breast cancer cells and cancer stem cells (CSCs). In this study, they loaded paclitaxel and salinomycin (SAL) onto SWCNTs, and biocompatible CD44 antibody was conjugated on SWCNT surfaces by a hydrazone linker. Here, prepared conjugates were denoted as SWCNT-PEG-Hyd-5HP-SAL-CD44 and SWCNT-PEG-Hyd-LEV-PTX-CD44 for the salinomycin and PTX-loaded CNTs, respectively. The *in vitro* cytotoxicity study was evaluated using CSC−, CSC^+, and MDA-MB-231 cell lines. These cell lines were incubated with different formulation samples for 24, 48, and 72 h. The MTT assay revealed that the SAL and PTX-loaded SWCNT-treated cells exhibited a prominent effect on cell viability compared to free drugs, moreover, co-delivery of both formulations showed maximum cytotoxic activity as compared to individual delivery. Combined treatment with SWCNT-SAL and SWCNT-PTX showed cell viability of 20.3 ± 1.2%, 26.1 ± 1.3%, and 22.9 ± 0.9% respectively against MDA-MB-231, CSC^-, and CSC^+ after 72 h of incubation. To confirm these results, bioluminescence signal (BLI) measurement was performed on all three cell lines. Combined delivery of both drugs by nanocarriers showed a significant reduction in bioluminescence. Like the above results, BLI also confirmed a higher antitumor capability of SWCNT-SAL and SWCNT-PTX than free drugs. In this study, *in vivo* anticancer activity of the drug-loaded SWCNT conjugate was also evaluated by MRI and BLI imaging. The tumor volume of MDA-MB-231 cell-bearing mice was 200 ± 20 mm^3 observed by non-invasive MRI and radiance efficiency of $47.5 \pm 2.1 \times 10^6$ ρ/s/cm^2/sr by non-invasive BLI. The radiance efficiency in the control mice group (non-treated) gradually increased with time, which reached up to $139.6 \pm 8.4 \times 10^6$ in 5 weeks. The signal of BLI was reduced after the 3rd dose of salinomycin injection, it was reduced in a significantly higher amount after paclitaxel injection and injection of combined drugs. Radiance efficiency reduction reached $75.8 \pm 7.5 \times 10^6$ in the SAL + PTX-injected mice group up to the last investigation. An equivalent dose of both drugs reached a radiance efficiency of $35.6 \pm 7.1 \times 10^6$ (salinomycin formulations) and $23.7 \pm 8.9 \times 10^6$ (paclitaxel formulations) at 5 weeks of investigation. Combined drug conjugates significantly reduced the radiance efficiency to $2.4 \pm 2.1 \times 10^6$ ρ/s/cm^2/sr. MRI results were also consistent with BRI results; the tumor volume of the non-treated group was 615 ± 50 mm^3 at the last MRI measurement, whereas the combined drug-conjugated treatment group exhibited a tumor volume of 15.5 ± 13.0 mm^3 up to the last measurement which was significant less than all other formulations. Here CD44 antibody-conjugated SWCNTs had a very significant role in selective active targeting of CSCs, which improved the therapeutic efficiency of this tumor therapy (Al Faraj et al., 2016). Another study reported a CD44 targeting novel nanotube which is known as a halloysite nanotube and modified with HA for acquiring targeted therapy. As evidenced by confocal microscopy, the cellular uptake was enhanced due to the tumor homing effect. Moreover, the preparation showed improved therapeutic effect due to internalization of DOX inside the cell (Mo et al., 2021).

CD44-Engineered Nanoemulsion for Cancer Therapy

The term "nanoemulsion" (NE) or mini-emulsion means fine oil/water or water/oil dispersion stabilized by an interfacial film of a surfactant molecule with a droplet size range of 20–600 nm (Jaiswal et al., 2015). Due to their small size, nanoemulsions are transparent in appearance. Many other unique properties of NEs include amorphous surface, solid sphere, high drug loading, and negatively charged particles. Nanoemulsions are mainly composed of oil, surfactant, and co-surfactant. They are extensively used as a carrier for poorly soluble chemotherapeutic drugs to enhance their solubility *via* their solubilizing capacity (Tadros et al., 2004). As a parenteral drug carrier, NEs have numerous advantages over other nanocarriers such as simple manufacturing process, high BA and solubilizing capacity, and long shelf-life, etc. Attachment of targeting moieties to NEs is quite challenging because of the weak bond with targeting moieties. Therefore, a highly advanced approach and thorough study is needed before preparing a tumor-targeted drug delivery system (Gupta et al., 2015; Hörmann and Zimmer, 2016). Kim et al. used hyaluronan-modified nanoemulsions (HNEs) for the targeted delivery of poorly soluble drug paclitaxel. The stability results revealed that HNEs were stable for 96 h which was significantly higher than Taxol®, which was stable only for 72 h. HNEs showed significantly higher uptake into the SK-OV-3 compared to the OVCAR cell lines, uptake efficiency of HNEs into the SK-OV-3 cell lines was directly related to the quantity of HA attached to the HNE surface. SK-OV-3 and OVCAR-3 cell lines displayed around 10 times higher targeting affinity for HNEs than the NEs. These results were further confirmed by confocal microscopy; confocal images showed that in SK-OV-3 cells, a remarkably higher binding affinity and cellular uptake was observed. Finally, researchers concluded that HA-modified NEs were stable, were able to solubilize poorly soluble drugs, were highly stable, and had high drug loading with efficient active targeting ability (Kim and Park, 2017a). In another study by the same research group, PTX-loaded HA-modified solid NEs (PTX-HSNs) were evaluated. In this study, the nanoemulsion was prepared by the high pressure homogenization method, the concentration of PTX loading was reduced to 3 mg/ml with approximately 100% entrapment efficiency. The HA-modified PTX-NEs exhibited 100-fold *in vitro* binding affinity in SK-OV-3 and OVCAR-3 cells as compared to non-HA-modified PTX nanoemulsions. The targeted preparation showed efficient tumor reduction with enhanced pharmacokinetic profile (Kim and Park, 2017b). Wang et al. developed a CD44-targeted microemulsion loaded with shikonin (SKN) and docetaxel (DTX) for the treatment of glioma. Targeted delivery of chemotherapeutic agents to the brain is a very challenging task due to the blood-brain barrier (BBB). The SKN and DTX-loaded microemulsion was bifunctionalized with A1411 aptamer and HA that exhibited targeted delivery *via* specifically binding with CD44/nucleolin-overexpressed glioma. The *in vitro* cytotoxicity study against U87 cells treated with HA loaded with both SKN and DTX showed an IC50 value of 3.4 ± 0.3 mg/ml which was reduced to 2.0 ± 0.3 mg/ml when U87 cells were treated with the HA-modified microemulsion, the IC50 value further declined after the conjugation of aptamer AS1411. The dual targeted preparation enhanced the apoptosis of U87 cells by 71.3 ± 4.2%. Cancer stem cell-enriched U87 cell spheroids were efficiently inhibited by the bifunctional system leading to downregulation of CD133 expression.

The apparent permeability coefficient of the prepared microemulsion was increased as assessed by an artificial BBB model. Additionally, targeted formulations significantly inhibited the growth of brain tumors and showed higher survival period than non-targeted groups. Conclusively, the HA/A1411-modified microemulsion exhibited its superior activity due to effective targeted delivery of the formulation at the targeted site and receptor-mediated endocytosis (Wang et al., 2019). The abovementioned studies proved that emulsions can be used as nanocarriers for the CD44-mediated targeted delivery of many chemotherapeutics (**Table 5**).

CD44-Engineered Micelles for Cancer Therapy

Micelles are lipidic nanocarriers that assemble themselves in a spherical form in aqueous solutions. They have an amphiphilic architecture which contains both a hydrophobic region (a long hydrophobic chain "core") and hydrophilic regions (a polar head group "shell") (Oh et al., 2004). The hydrophobic core of micelles enables them to load hydrophobic drugs while the hydrophilic shell allows binding of water-soluble drugs (Adams et al., 2003). Micelles are biocompatible, stable at biological conditions, and can be used to solubilize highly insoluble pharmaceutical agents/drugs. These properties led to development of many drug-loaded micelles, some of which are in the preclinical and clinical stages currently (Sahoo and Labhasetwar, 2003; Kateb et al., 2011). Micelles possess important characteristics such as nanometric size (diameter <50 nm) and hydrophilicity providing protection for polymeric micelles from elimination by the RES, leading to enhanced retention time and direct delivery to tumor cells. Targeted delivery of anticancer molecules by micelles may be achieved by the ERP effect, or employing several block copolymers, or by conjugating specific targeting ligands to the special surface functional groups of micelles (Dabholkar et al., 2006). Micelles can be easily conjugated with hyaluronic acid (HA) for active tumor targeting, and can efficiently deliver drugs intracellularly by binding with its specific CD44 receptor which has been illustrated in **Table 6**. It was reported in several studies that CD44 receptors overexpressed in several cancer cells causes MDR. Kesharwani et al. has designed a HA-linked co-poly (styrene maleic acid) (HA-SMA) nano-micellar system for targeted delivery of anticancer molecules (CDF) for the treatment of MDR pancreatic cancer. Nano-micelles (HA-SMA-CDF) were characterized by DLS, and TEMDLS exhibited 96.5 ± 3.1 nm particle size and 0.228 ± 0.14 PDI for SMA-CDF, while 114.1 ± 2.7 nm particle size and 0.236 ± 0.11 PDI was obtained for the HA-SMA-CDF. TEM images showed a particle size range of 70.3 ± 1.8 and 89.5 ± 2.8 nm respectively for SMA-CDF and HA-SMA-CDF with smooth surface and spherical geometry. HA conjugation significantly improved the

TABLE 5 | Examples of nanoemulsion-targeted CD44 cells.

Oils, surfactants, and other materials	Therapeutic agents	Types of study (*in vitro*/*in vivo*)	Cancer types	Cell lines	Animal model	References
Soyabean oil, polysorbate 80, dl-a-tocopheryl acetate and Fecl3	PTX	*In vitro*	Ovarian	SK-OV-3 and OVCAR-3	–	Kim and Park, (2017a)
Soyabean oil, polysorbate 80, dl-a-tocopheryl acetate, and Fecl3	PTX	Both	Ovarian	SK-OV-3 and OVCAR-3	BALB/cAnNCrjBgi-nu/nu nude mice	Kim and Park, (2017b)
Mal-DSPE-PEG	Shikonin and DTX	Both	Brain	U87 cell	BALB/C (nu/nu) nude mice	Wang et al. (2019)

TABLE 6 | Examples of micelle-targeted CD44 cells.

Main characteristics of micelles	Therapeutic agents	Types of study (*in vitro*/*in vivo*)	Types of cancer	Cell lines	Animal model	References
Nano micelles	CDF	*In vitro*	Pancreatic	MiaPaCa-2 and AsPC-1	–	Kesharwani et al. (2015b)
Nano micelles	CDF	Both	TNBC	MDAMB- 231 and MDAMB- 268	Mice	Wang et al. (2018)
Hybrid micelles	Dox	Both	TNBC	4T1, CT26, MDA-MB-231, and NIH 3T3	Female mice	Yang et al. (2020)
pH-sensitive micelles	DTX	Both	Breast cancer	MCF-7	Mice	Du et al. (2018)
pH-sensitive micelles	PTX	Both	Breast cancer	MCF-7	Mice	Zhong et al. (2016)
pH-sensitive micelles	PTX	Both	Breast cancer	MCF-7	Mice	Liu et al. (2018)
Mixed micelles	Curcumin	*In vitro*	TNBC	MDA-MB-231	–	Soleymani et al. (2021)

entrapment efficiency of CDF due to HA that enhanced the CDF interaction with the nano-micelles. HA-SMA-CDF was found to be sufficiently stable at RT in the dark than at 0°C/60°C. The percentage of cell viability was found to be 28.47 ± 2.29%, 15.62 ± 5.74%, and 8.51 ± 1.99% for CDF, CDF-SMA, and HA-SMA-CDF, respectively at a 1,000 nM equivalent concentration in MiaPaCa-2 cells. Similar results were observed in AsPC-1 cells, where HA conjugates showed significantly higher anticancer activity. HA-SMA-CDF also exhibited comparatively lower IC50 values in both MiaPaCa- 2 and AsPC-1 cell lines. To confirm CD44 receptor-mediated cellular internalization, a receptor blocked study was performed. For HA-SMA-CDF, the IC50 value obtained was 182 ± 6.68 nM before blocking by excess HA, whereas the value changed to 234 ± 8.24 nM after pre-treatment of cells with HA. These results clearly established that pre-treated cell lines with free HA significantly enhanced the IC50 values which means pre-treated free HA molecules occupied CD44 receptors and availability of the CD44 receptor for HA-SMA-CDF binding was limited and competitive. Western blot results revealed a significant reduction in CD44 expression level in HA-SMA-CDF-treated cells compared to free CDF and SMA-CDF-treated cells (Kesharwani et al., 2015b). Similarly, Wang et al. has designed CDF-loaded HA-SMA-TPGS nano-micelles for CD44-targeted delivery, specially functionalized for NIR imaging. Targeted (HA-SMA-TPGS-CDF) preparation exhibited strong red fluorescence intensity compared to the non-targeted preparation that indicates targeted formulations accumulated faster than non-targeted preparations. This higher accumulation of HA-SMA-TPGS-CDF is possibly due to the high affinity of the HA ligand towards the CD44 receptor. Anticancer activity was also found to be highest for HA-SMA-TPGS-CDF as compared to free CDF and SMA-TPGS-CDF against both cell lines. The high cell killing activity of HA-SMA-TPGS-CDF was possibly due to active tumor targeting due to CD44 receptor-mediated endocytosis. The targeted formulation induced significantly higher apoptosis than free CDF and non-targeted formulations. In this study, researchers have also described the mechanistic pathway behind the apoptosis of TNBC cells, as apoptosis was induced due to the downregulation of NF-κB and upregulation of PTEN in the TNBC cell lines (Kesharwani et al., 2015b). A western blot study displayed significant upregulation of PTEN and downregulation of PTEN and NF-κB protein expression in the HA-SMA-TPGS-CDF-treated cells as compared to free CDF and SMA-TPGS-CDF, and HA-targeted ability of HA-SMA-TPGS was evaluated *in vivo* for the early diagnosis of TNBC by NIR imaging. HA-SMA-TPGS or SMA-TPGS was conjugated with S0456 high contrast dye, which revealed significantly higher fluorescence intensity in the tumor tissue than other normal tissues also indicating the tumor homing effect by the ligand (Wang et al., 2018). Recently, Yang and co-workers developed stable hybrid micelles for targeted delivery of chemotherapeutic agents DOX against TNBC. Here stable hybrid micelles (HT-LT) were prepared by mixing hyaluronic acid-D-α-tocopheryl succinate (HA-TOS, HT) and low molecular weight heparin-TOS (LT). Prepared HT-LT NPs had better stability, prolonged release at pH 5.5 which might be due to breaking of the ester bond. The western blot technique was utilized to investigate the expression of CD44 receptor on different cell lines. It was estimated that CD44 was expressed on 4T1, CT26, and MDA-MB-231 cells but much less in NIH 3T3 cells. CLSM results showed a stronger uptake signal for HT-LT than LT and HT in 4T1 cells. Lysosomal release was also evaluated by lysotracker, which exhibited a strong signal for HT-LT into the lysosome which was due to breaking of the ester bond due to presence of esterases that enabled prolonged release of DOX. Here HT-LT showed 2.2 times higher (highest) uptake efficiency of DOX in 4T1 cells whereas LT showed 1.5 times uptake than that with the lowest efficiency. *In vitro* cellular migration was effectively inhibited by HT-LT NPs more than other formulations. *In vivo* tumor targeting was investigated by loading HT, LT, and HT-LT NPs with fluorescence probe DiD in place of DOX and observed under CLSM. DiD-loaded HT-LT NPs exhibited comparatively stronger fluorescence in the tumor site that commenced after 1 h of administration and persisted for 24 h. Additionally, *ex vivo* tumor images also showed increased tumor accumulation and decreased liver distribution of HT-LT/DiD NPs than others. *In vivo* antitumor activity was investigated in 4T1-bearing Balb/c female mice, the tumor growth inhibition rate was calculated as 20.96%, 32.60%, 46.89%, and 77.39%, respectively for free DOX, HT/DOX NPs, LT/DOX NPs, and HT-LT/DOX NPs. Ki -67 is a marker for cell growth, here researchers found high expression of Ki -67 in the PBS group whereas lower expression in the HT-LT/DOX NP group. These results confirmed the superiority of HT-LT/DOX NP over other formulations (Yang et al., 2020). In another study, Du et al. has developed biocompatible, pH-sensitive, and charge-conversion micelles bearing a half-generation PAMAM dendrimer (G4.5 sPA) decorated with HA-conjugated poly (lactide) (PLA) and loaded with docetaxel. Formed micelles were uniformly distributed, spherical in shape, and had a smooth surface. As reported previously, HA could improve biocompatibility of polymers of carriers with drugs. Here the cationic surface charge of PALA was masked by HA to improve the biocompatibility of micelles. Drug release results revealed that the drug release from the formulation was dependent on HA degradation, which was HAase-mediated and pH-dependent, hence HA-conjugated micelles reached the tumor site through CD44 receptor-mediated tumor targeting, HA was degraded in the tumor site due to the effect of pH and HAase. Formulations such as free docetaxel (DTX), Taxotere®, PALA-DTX, and HA-PALA-DTX were compared for their cytotoxicity against MCF-7 cell lines, in this, HA-PALA-DTX exhibited significantly higher cytotoxicity than free DTX and Taxotere®. The IC50 value for HA-PALA-DTX was found to be 5.92 ng/ml which was notably lower than that of free DTX (264.91 ng/ml) and Taxotere® (76.56 ng/ml). Cellular uptake of different coumarin-6 (C6)-conjugated formulations were analyzed by CLSM, C6-HA-PALA showed significantly higher intracellular fluorescence intensity than other preparations in the MCF-7 cell lines. *In vivo* biodistribution results by *in vivo* imaging and results of DiR-loaded micelles groups (DiR-HA-PALA) showed the majority of fluorescence at the tumor site and this fluorescence persisted for 12 h, whereas free DiR was not found at the tumor site. The HA modification formulation was internalized by CD44-mediated endocytosis. *In vivo* antitumor activity in the S180 tumor-bearing mice HA-PALA-DTX-treated group showed approximately 72.32% tumor cell inhibition which was highest amongst all other groups. This highest anticancer activity was attributed to the HA modification of micelles. HA-modified formulations also performed well in preliminary *in vivo* safety evaluation. Hence the prepared carrier was viable and efficient to use for targeted delivery of chemotherapeutic agents (Du et al., 2018). Zhong et al. designed and developed similar types of preparation consisting of paclitaxel-loaded HA-modified -b- dendritic oligoglycerol (HA-dOG-PTX) polymeric micelles (PM). Prepared PM exhibited a diameter of 155 nm, low CMC (6.8 mg/L), and 0.12 PDI. Release of PTX from the HA-modified formulation was pH-dependent which showed 20%, 48%, and 81% release at pH- 7.4, pH 6.0, and pH 5.0, respectively. At acidic pH, maximum released PTX was obtained which might be due to degradation of HA at low pH. *In vivo* pharmacokinetic parameters evaluated in the distribution phase at $t_{1/2}$ were equal to 1.63 and 0.12 h, whereas the elimination phase half-lives were 4.32 and 0.23 h, respectively for HA-dOG-PTX-PM and Taxol. HA-dOG-PTX-PM had an AUC of 158.4 mg x h/L, that was 68 times higher than free PTX (2.3 mg x h/L). *In vivo* tumor targeting activity was similar to the above study, where DiR-HA-dOG-PTX-PM exhibited significantly higher fluorescence activity 4 h after injection that reached maximum after 12 h and persisted for 48 h post injection. This indicates that DiR-HA-dOG-PTX-PM was up taken very efficiently by MCF-7 cell lines. Thus, HA modification improved the pharmacokinetics, biodistribution, and *in vivo* antitumor activity due to CD44 receptor targeting (Zhong et al., 2016). In another study, Liu et al. designed p -sensitive dual-functionalized HA–deoxycholic acid histidine (HA-DOCA-His) micelles for CD44-targeted delivery of PTX and to overcome MDR. PTX-loaded HA-DOCA-His showed significantly improved cytotoxicity having greater MDR overcoming activity against MCF-7/ADR cell lines, this was due to the maximum intracellular accumulation of PTX *via* the CD44 receptor-mediated pathway and endosomal pH-triggered release of PTX. Pharmacokinetic parameters such as long blood circulation time, larger AUC, and less V_d and CL were achieved by PTX-loaded HA-DOCA-His which was comparatively better than PTX. PTX-loaded HA-DOCA-His exhibited significantly higher antitumor activity in MCF-7/Adr tumor-bearing mice compared to PTX/HA-DOCA micelles and free PTX. Conclusively, PTX-loaded HA-DOCA-His showed better antitumor activity as well as established outstanding MDR reversal ability (Liu et al., 2018). Similarly, Soleymani et al. has designed mixed nano-micelles for targeted delivery of curcumin. In this study, hydrophobic curcumin was encapsulated into the hydrophobic cavity of pluronic F127/dodecyl dimethyl ammonium bromide (PD) *via* the film hydration method, after curcumin encapsulation, the positively charged surface of micelles was interacted with negatively charged HA through electrostatic interaction. HA-coated micelles showed a change in average hydrodynamic size from 19.8 to 35.8 nm and also increased *in vitro* cytotoxicity against MDA-MB-231 cell lines compared to non-coated micelles and free micelles. The IC50 value for HA-coated PD was found to be 2.83 μg/ml which was less than free curcumin and non-HA coated micelles. On the basis of these

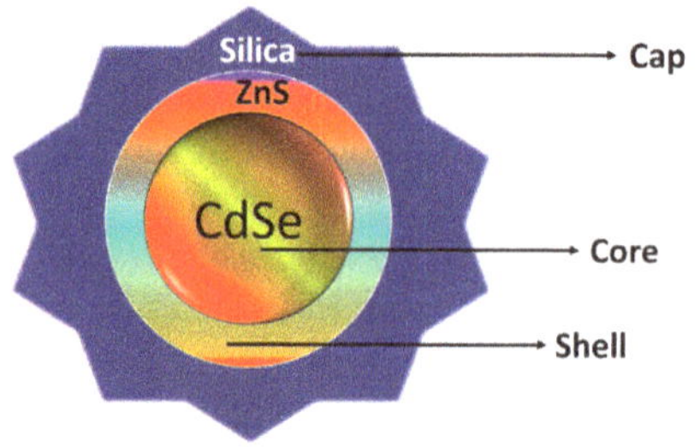

FIGURE 6 | Schematic illustration of quantum dots.

results, the author suggested that curcumin-loaded HA-PD micelles would be a potential system for targeted delivery of hydrophobic drugs to breast cancer as well as other cancers in which the CD44 receptor was overexpressed (Soleymani et al., 2021). Finally, we can conclude that the variety of micelles modified by HA are able to deliver drug molecules to overexpressed CD44 receptors on various cancer cells.

CD44-Engineered Quantum Dots for Cancer Therapy

In 1980, Russian physicist Alexei Ekimov first discovered quantum dots (QDs) in solids (glass crystals), later in 1982, a chemist from the US, Louis E. Brus discovered QDs in colloidal solutions (Tokihiro and Hanamura, 1984; Zhu et al., 2013). In 1990, Canham reported optical properties of QDs for first time in silicon (Canham, 1990). QDs are most commonly used for drug delivery and targeting as well as diagnosis and imaging purposes, along with this, QDs are also used for sensing DNA and oligonucleotides (Jaiswal et al., 2004; Mitchell et al., 1999). Quantum dots are semiconductor nanosized crystals having optical and electronic properties which are different from the larger particles because of quantum mechanics. Generally, QDs are mainly composed of three parts, i.e., first, the "core" made up of semiconductor materials, second, the "shell," a coating that surrounds the semiconductor core, which improves the optical feature of QDs, and third, the "cap" outer layer of QDs encapsulating both the core and shell, mainly consisting of materials like silica, that improve solubility (**Figure 6**) (Aqel et al., 2012; Chen et al., 2006). There are four basic steps of QD preparation such as core synthesis, shell growth, aqueous solubility, and biomolecular attachment which are involved in the design of QDs for biological applications (Mishra et al., 2017). Steps of QDs like shell growth and surface functionalization enhance stability and photoluminescence of the QD core. QDs are gaining the significant attention of researchers as a part of the technological future, demonstrating various unique physicochemical properties which are required for imaging and targeting purposes into the living cell and whole animals. There are many unique features of QDs like optical properties, aqueous solubility, lower cytotoxicity, biocompatibility, and reduced cost which make them preferred nanocarriers for drug delivery and targeting delivery in the cancer patient (Gerion, 2007; Liu et al., 2012). Recently, Karakoçak et al. used HA-modified nitrogen carbon quantum dots (CQDs) for bioimaging of tumor cells. Firstly, HA-modified nitrogen CQDs were prepared by the coupling reaction of the NH2 group of nCQDs and the COOH group of HA. An *in vitro* comparative biocompatibility study evaluated the dots in both ARPE-19 and CHO cells lines, and revealed that the HA-modified nitrogen CQDs exhibited enhanced biocompatibility in both cell lines and significantly decreased the intracellular ROS concentration in both cell lines. HA-mediated cellular internalization was confirmed by *in vitro* investigation of HA-modified nitrogen CQDs and nitrogen CQDs treated with both ARPE-19 and CHO cells lines, CLSM imaging of these cell lines revealed that HA-modified nitrogen CQDs were efficiently internalized into both cell lines. When the same study was performed on additional cells pre-treated with HA, which remarkably resulted in cellular internalization of HA-modified nitrogen CQDs into both cells, there was not much change in internalizations of nitrogen CQDs. The selective cellular uptake of HA-modified nitrogen CQD and nCQD conjugates was reconfirmed by treating NIH 3T3, ARPE-19, and CHO cell lines with HA-modified nitrogen CQDs. *In vitro* results showed that uptake of HA-modified nitrogen CQDs into the NIH 3T3 cell was comparatively less than that of ARPE-19 cells and CHO cells, this difference in uptake of HA-modified nitrogen CQDs was related to the expression of CD44 receptor in the cell lines. The NIH 3T3 cell lines had much lower expression of CD44 receptor than ARPE-19 cells and CHO cells, so that NIH3T3 cells exhibited less cellular uptake. These results suggested that the HA-modified nitrogen CQDs were facilitated *via* CD44 receptor-mediated internalization by selective HA and CD44 binding. *In vivo* results also revealed that HA-modified nitrogen CQDs accumulated in the tumor site 15 min after injection and the fluorescence signal for HA-modified nitrogen CQDs was detected at the tumor site whereas no fluorescence signal was found for non-HA-conjugated nCQDs. A similar pattern of fluorescence signal was observed in another experiment, in which HA-modified nitrogen CQDs and non-HA-conjugated nCQDs were given *via* IV to mice bearing WHIM4 tumors, 150 min after injection a fluorescence signal at the tumor site was observed for HA-modified nitrogen CQDs, but there was no signal for non-HA-conjugated nCQDs at the tumor site. These results further confirmed the ability of HA-modified nitrogen CQDs to target CD44 receptor (Karakoçak et al., 2021). In another study, Zhang et al. reported HA-functionalized CQDs, prepared by the hydrothermal carbonization method. Formed HA-CQDs were stable, biocompatible, highly hydrophilic, and had uniform size distribution with a heterogeneous multi-layered solid structure. A CCK8 assay showed that the prepared HA-CQDs were biocompatible with Hela and MCF-7 cells. Due to excellent fluorescence properties of HA-functionalized CQDs, labelled MCF-7 and Hela cells could be examined and noticed by using CLSM and flow cytometry. In HA-CQD-treated HeLa and U251 cells, CLSM images exhibited that the HA-CQDs were localized to the cytoplasmic regions, mainly around the nucleus, it seemed that a major amount of HA-CQDs was internalized by tumor cells which could be controlled by receptor-mediated endocytosis. CD44 receptor-mediated

TABLE 7 | Illustration of quantum dot-targeted CD44 cells.

QDs	Therapeutic agents	Types of study (*in vitro*/*in vivo*)	Cancer types	Cell lines	Animal model	References
Nitrogen CQDs	–	Both	Breast cancer	ARPE-19 and CHO	NSG mice	Karakoçak et al. (2021)
CQDs	–	*In vitro*	Human gland	HeLa and MCF-7	–	Zhang et al. (2016)
HA-cysteamine polymer-wrapped QDs	–	*In vitro*	Breast cancer	MDA-MB-231, and MCF-7	–	Wang et al. (2014)
S-S- PEG-diethylenetriamine QDs	Histamine	*In vitro*	Breast	MCF-7 and A549 cells	–	Fu et al. (2019)

cellular internalization was also confirmed by the quantitative analysis *via* flow cytometry, these results revealed that the HeLa cells efficiently took up HA-CQDs while MCF-7 took up a very small amount of HA-CQDs. Notably, internalization of HA-CQDs in HeLa cells decreased when HeLa cells were pre-treated with free HA, but there was not much change in uptake of HA-CQDs in the MCF-7 cells. This is due to the expression of CD44 receptor on HeLa cells which was significantly higher than that in MCF-7 cell lines, so more CD44 receptors were able to selectively bind with HA and get internalized very efficiently. These outcomes were attributed to HA receptor-mediated endocytosis (Zhang et al., 2016). Wang et al. synthesized a HA-modified cysteamine polymer, encapsulating (CdSe) CdZnS QDs to form a final HA polymer-wrapped QD *via* the reverse micelle method. The HA polymer-wrapped QD showed enough stability in PBS and BSA mixed culture medium and in the entire pH range. To assess biocompatibility, MDA-MB-231 cell lines were treated with the HA polymer-wrapped QD, and 83% viability was found even 24 h after incubation. This result revealed that the HA polymer-wrapped QD was biocompatible. CD44-targeted imaging was investigated in MCF-7 and MD-MB-231 cell lines, the NIH/3T3 cell line was used as negative control. All these cell lines were treated with different concentrations of HA polymer-wrapped QDs, and strong fluorescence was observed on MCF-7 and MD-MB-231 cell lines but not on NIH/3T3 ($CD44^-$) cell lines. These results showed the targeted ability of the HA polymer-wrapped QDs. The receptor blocked assay also confirmed the CD44 receptor imaging of HA polymer-wrapped QD-treated MCF-7 cell lines (Wang et al., 2014). In another recent study, similar results were obtained for multifunctional redox-sensitive HA-modified S-S-PEGylated histamine-loaded diethylenetriamine QDs. The prepared completely decorated QDs exhibited high mono-dispersibility, high stability, high drug loading efficiency, and biocompatibility. Most importantly, the formed multifunctional HA-modified nanocarriers exhibited CD44 receptor-mediated endocytosis, which facilitated targeted bioimaging and other therapeutic benefits of the nanocarrier (**Table 7**) (Fu et al., 2019).

CD44-Engineered Nanogel for Cancer Therapy

Nanogels (NGs) are nanocarriers prepared by combining a hydrogel and a cross-linked hydrophilic polymer. NGs have

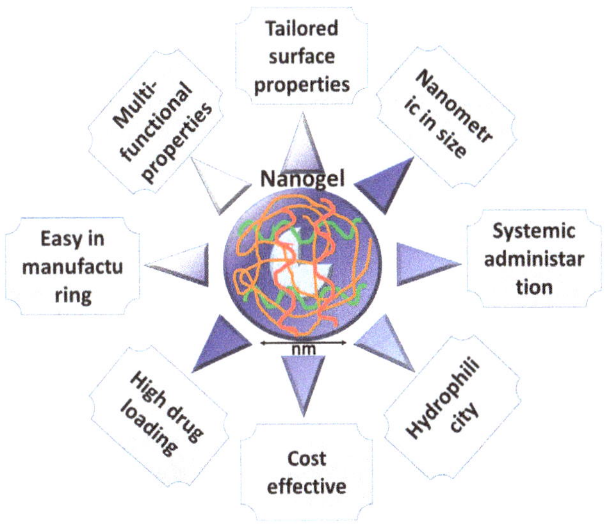

FIGURE 7 | Schematic illustration of the different characteristics of nanogels.

attracted significant attention as promising drug-carrying agents for targeting cancer cells because they can exert unique properties such as greater functionality, easy formation, and improved targetability compared to traditional drug delivery systems. NGs are also known for some other features like high drug loading, better release capability, and easy tailoring (Cao Z et al., 2016; Nita et al., 2016; Qiao et al., 2016) (**Figure 7**). Wei and co-worker have designed and developed HA-based NG drug conjugates for the targeted delivery of etoposide (ETO), salinomycin (SAL), and curcumin (CUR). Here, the cholesteryl-hyaluronic acid (CHA) and non-HA nanogel was conjugated with ETO, SAL, and CUR by binding covalently through the degradable ester bond. Prepared CHA-drug conjugates exhibited particle sizes of 32.17 ± 5.66, 36.48 ± 6.23, and 29.15 ± 5.37 nm, respectively for CHA-ETO, CHA-SAL, and CHA-CUR. All preparations passively accumulated in the tumor cells *via* an enhanced permeability retention effect. *In vitro* cytotoxicity of CHA-drug conjugates was investigated in MDA-MB-231/F and MIA PaCa-2 cells, the IC50 value for CHA-ETO, CHA-SAL, and CHA-CUR was found to be 3.0, 0.9, and 9.0, respectively, which was comparatively better compared to free drugs. Notably, HA-modified drug nanogels exhibited about 2-7-

fold greater cell cytotoxicity against MDA-MB-231/F and MIA PaCa-2 cells than that of free drugs and unmodified HA-drug conjugates. This difference in cytotoxicity results was attributed to the efficient cellular internalization of the HA-modified nanogel through CD44-mediated endocytosis. Also, after conjugation with cholesterol moieties, tumor accumulation of formulations was improved. The HA-modified drug nanogel was efficiently up taken into the multicellular spheroids and exhibited significantly higher anticancer activity in the modeling tumor environment as compared to free drugs and only HA drug conjugates, which means cholesterol played an important role into the activity of CHA-drug conjugates. Finally, it was concluded that the HA-modified drug nanogels prominently enhanced drug BA, tumor targeting, and therapeutic efficacy against resistant cancer cells (Wei et al., 2013). In similar study, Ma et al. used HA-based self-targeted nanogels for intracellular delivery of DOX and cisplatin to avoid MDR breast cancer. In this study, HA-based nanogels (HANGs) were coloaded with two anticancer molecules namely DOX and cisplatin. The formed nanogels exhibited intertumoral accumulation of drugs, synchronized pharmacokinetics, and prolonged blood distribution time. HA-modified nanogels loaded with both drugs exhibited efficient drug delivery into the multi-drug-resistant MCF-7/ADR breast cancer cells and exerted its anticancer activity intracellularly. By thoroughly understanding the mechanisms behind the internalization of HA-modified NGs into the MDR MCF-7/ADR tumor cells, researchers found that MCF-7/ADR and MCF-7 tumor cells overexpressed CD44 receptors, so that drug-loaded HA-modified NGs were efficiently internalized by tumor cells because of strong affinity of HA towards CD44 receptors which facilitated selective internalization of their cargo into CD44 + tumor cells. The nanogel avoided drug resistance *via* the following pathways, 1) the intracellular environment of tumor cells enriched with NGs due to specific internalization *via* CD44-mediated endocytosis leads to reduced P-gp efflux of NGs, 2) combination of DOX and cisplatin tackled clinical MDR, and 3) drugs were released at tumor pH because of disintegration of the compacted structure at acidic pH. This mechanism was confirmed by using the immunofluorescence staining and western blot technique. Finally, the researcher concluded that the HANGs had CD44 tumor targeting, reversing of MDR, and pH-responsive release effect for both drugs intracellularly (Ma et al., 2021). Seok et al. used a biodegradable, renewal, and cost-effective cross polymer called “Zein” for the preparation of a HA-modified nanogel for targeted delivery of anticancer drug curcumin (CRC). Here, the HA-coated Zein nanogel was prepared by the modified precipitation method. The formed HA-coated Zein NGs showed drug loading efficiency of 9.41% and drug encapsulation efficiency of 94.15%. *In vitro* selective cellular uptake was evaluated by a HA competitive assay, results of this assay revealed that the HA-coated Zein NGs were up taken *via* HA receptor-mediated endocytosis. *In vitro* anticancer efficacy of HA-coated Zein-CRC NGs was comparatively higher against CT26 cells than that of NIH3T3 cells. The IC50 value was 37 µg/ml and 94 µg/ml respectively, against CT26 and NIH3T3 cells. This anticancer efficacy difference of HA-coated Zein-CRC NGs between the CT26 and NIH3T3 cells was attributed to glutathione S-transferases (GST) level in the CT26 cells and also due to the level of CD44 receptors in the cells. *In vitro* stability and biocompatibility studies suggested that the HA-coated Zein-CRC NGs have sufficient stability in serum and compatibility of blood components. *In vivo* biodistribution of the conjugated HA-coated Zein-CRC NGs was investigated in a CT26 tumor model *via* conjugations with IR-780 dye. Higher tumor accumulation of HA-coated Zein-CRC NGs than Zein-CRC NGs led to improved therapeutic efficiency of CRC. These results were reconfirmed by histopathological analysis, which exhibited a higher apoptotic area in the HA-coated Zein-CRC NG-treated group than the untreated or free drug-treated groups. Finally, it was concluded that the CD44-targeted delivery of CRC by HA-coated Zein-CRC NGs could be a potential approach for anticancer therapy (Seok et al., 2018). Ma and co-worker designed and developed multifunctional HA-based NGs (HNPs). Here, all-trans retinoid acid (ATRA)/aggregation-induced emission luminogen (AIEgen) fluorophores were conjugated with HA *via* the disulphide bond. The developed NG was used for targeted delivery of DOX. The formed HA-modified NGs showed better drug loading efficiency with a sufficient stability profile at normal biological environments, DOX was rapidly released from the formulation in tumor microenvironments. *In vitro* cellular localization results revealed that the DOX was successfully transported into the cytoplasm of tumor cells through HNPs. This selective tumor accumulation of DOX-loaded HNPs was mainly attributed to targeted specific binding of HA to the CD44 receptor or LYCE-1 receptor. Higher intracellular accumulation of DOX-loaded HNPs caused significantly higher tumor cell suppression than the control and free drug. An *in vitro* real-time imaging biodistribution and uptake study of DOX-loaded HNPs exhibited CD44-mediated tumor accumulation and uptake in the tumor cells (Ma et al., 2018). In all the above studies, HA-decorated nanogels exhibited outstanding results which was due to binding of HA specifically to the CD44 receptor which promoted cellular internalization of nanocarriers, leading to release of their cargo into the tumor microenvironment because generally at low pH bonding between HA and its cargo could be broken. Importantly CD44-mediated internalization is the best way to bypass the Pgp reflux system and reverse MDR. Illustration of nanogel targeting CD44 cells is highlighted in **Table 8**.

SIRNA-BASED CD44-MEDIATED NANOCARRIER FOR TREATMENT OF VARIOUS CANCERS

In the current scenario, due to potent, effective, and specific gene silencing effects, siRNAs have gained great recognition as therapeutic molecules for the treatment of many dangerous diseases like cancers, neurological diseases, etc. (Elbashir et al., 2001; Kim et al., 2008). However, translation of siRNA in clinical use poses a major challenge because naked siRNA possesses

TABLE 8 | Outline of CD44-targeted therapy using nanogels.

Material	Therapeutic agents	Types of study (*in vitro*/*in vivo*)	Cancer types	Cell lines	Animal model	References
Cholesteryl chloroformate and HA	ETO, SAL, and CUR	*In vitro*	Breast	MDA-MB-231 and MIA PaCa-2	–	Wei et al. (2013)
FA	DOX and cisplatin	Both	Breast	MCF-7/ADR	BALB/c mice	Ma et al. (2021)
Zein	Curcumin	Both	Colon	CT26 and NIH3T3 normal cells	Mice	Seok et al. (2018)
HA-ATRA	Dox	*In vitro*	Hepatic	HepG-2 and 293 T cells	–	Ma et al. (2018)

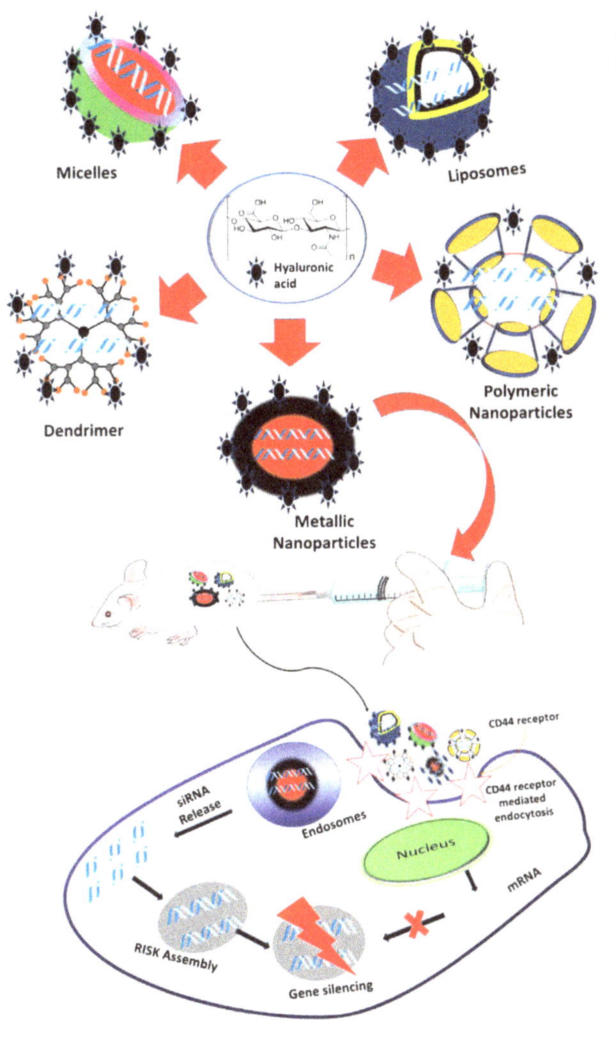

FIGURE 8 | CD44-mediated siRNA delivery.

several intrinsic problems like poor cellular membrane penetration, inadequate stability in biological fluids, and most importantly a lack of targetability. To overcome this problem, numerous nanocarriers have been designed depending on the viral and non-viral vectors (Oishi et al., 2005). Use of a viral vector for the siRNA delivery is limited due to potential immune response of viral vectors, thus, researchers now focus more on non-viral vectors namely cationic liposomes, several polymers, and dendrimers, that could easily bind with the siRNA and deliver it to the targeted site (**Figure 8**) (Chen et al., 2009; Park et al., 2006). Moreover, by realizing the great potential of siRNA, it could be complexed with different nanocarriers that could impart the following properties, such as high targetability, high intracellular uptake, and site-specific release of siRNA (mostly into cytosol). In the following section, we discuss a few studies in which siRNA was delivered by a CD44-engineered nanocarrier, mostly by incorporating HA as a targeting ligand (**Table 9**) (Matsumoto et al., 2009; Kesharwani et al., 2015b). Yoon et al. has designed and developed a biodegradable, biocompatible HA cross-linked poly (dimethyl amino ethyl methacrylate) HPD conjugate which can easily form a complex with siRNA *via* the formation of the cross-linked disulfide bond. Gel electrophoresis results revealed among uncross-linked siRNA-HPD and cross-linked siRNA-HPD, crosslinked HPD efficiently formed a stable complex with the siRNA. An *in vitro* cell cytotoxicity study evaluated the conjugates in B16F10 and normal cells (NIH3T3 and CV-1 cell) and it was found that cross-linked siRNA-HPD caused a significance decrease in B16F10 cell viability at the maximum concentration >10 µg/ml while no observable viability changes were observed in CV-1 and NIH3T3 cells. Obtained results showed that the cytotoxicity of the complexes was regulated by expression of the CD44 receptor on cell lines. *In vitro* cellular uptake and gene silencing exhibited the best fluorescent signal for both cross-linked siRNA-HPD and uncross-linked siRNA-HPD in the B16F10 cells but an insignificant fluorescence signal was obtained in the NIH3T3 cells, similar types of results were also observed in an *in vivo* study. The *in vivo* fluorescence signal for both cross-linked siRNA-HPD and uncross-linked siRNA-HPD was reported in the initial 3 h due to the complex in the circulation, but after 3 h, the intensity of the fluorescence signal in the tumor site increased gradually, this may be due to HA-mediated selective uptake *via* the CD44 receptor at the tumor site. Importantly cross-linked siRNA-HPD always exerted a stronger signal than uncross-linked siRNA-HPD. A real-time NIRF technique revealed better *in vivo* gene silencing efficacy of both complexes in RFP-B16F10 tumor-bearing mice. The cross-linked siRNA-HPD complex showed around 6.6-fold less fluorescence intensity than that of control in the excised tumor. Finally, it was concluded that the cross-linked siRNA-HPD complex exhibited the best therapeutic results mainly *via* HA receptor-mediated endocytosis (Yoon et al.,

TABLE 9 | Examples of siRNA-based CD44-mediated nanocarriers.

Material	Therapeutic agents	Types of study (*in vitro/in vivo*)	Cancer types	Cell lines	Animal model	References
HPD	siRNA	Both	Melanoma	B16F10 and NIH3T3	RFP-B16F10 tumor-bearing mice	Yoon et al. (2013)
LHRH–PPI	siRNA	Both	Ovarian	Ascitic cells	Female athymic nu/nu mice	Shah et al. (2013)
PEI with GAG and HSA	siRNA	*In vitro*	—	hMSCs	—	Herrera and Shastri, (2019)
Β-cyclodextrin- PLL	DOX and oligo RNA	Both	Hepatic cancer	MHCC-97H and HepG2	HCC xenograft mouse	Xiong et al. (2017)

2013). Shah et al. has designed a CD44-targeted nanocarrier for the delivery of siRNA and anticancer drug PTX for the purpose of CD44 cell suppression and cancer cell death initiation in ovarian cancer. The anticancer drug PTX was first linked to the PPI dendrimer *via* succinic acid as a spacer, additionally, luteinizing hormone–releasing hormone (LHRH) peptide as the targeting ligand was conjugated to the PEG polymer which surrounds the DTBP-caged dendrimer. Then, the PPI dendrimer was complexed with siRNA (PPI-siRNA). The LHRH–PPI–siRNA and LHRH–PPI–paclitaxel complexes showed decreased viability in ascitic cells around 10-fold that of control cells, > 5-fold that of the free PTX and >2 fold when compared to the non-targeted PPI–paclitaxel–siRNA complex. These results suggested the important role of LHRH peptide in mediating cellular cytotoxicity. Cellular uptake and distribution results showed significant higher fluorescence for PPI siRNA conjugated in cellular cytoplasm while very low fluorescence intensity was observed for naked siRNA in the tumor cell, which revealed that conjugated siRNA can easily penetrate and distribute intracellularly into the tumor cell, but naked siRNA cannot. In support of *in vitro* results, *in vivo* investigation of different formulations was carried out in nude mouse xenografts. The PPI-siRNA complex with HA suppressed the CD44 protein of the tumor cell while the other formulation did not show a significant change in expression of CD44 protein. Moreover, the PPI-siRNA conjugate exhibited extensive accumulation of dendrimer in the tumor cells, whereas the other formulation showed distribution in other tissues like liver, kidney, lungs, spleen, and heart. All the above results were attributed to the specific binding of LHRH peptide to the overexpressed CD44 receptor on tumor cells (Shah et al., 2013). Herrera et al. used ternary and quaternary polyplexes made up of siRNA-bPEI, modified with three different glycosaminoglycan (GAGs) polysaccharides, like HA, CS, and HA, alone or along with HSA for silencing of human mesenchymal stem cells (hMSCs) expressing green fluorescent protein. MSC or mesenchymal stem cells or multipotent stromal cells are employed in tissue repair sites and are also involved in immunomodulation, anti-inflammatory processes, and paracrine signaling. These cells are exceptional targets for genetic engineering. As reported in several studies, the N/P ratio plays an important role in stability and therapeutic efficiency of polyplexes, so here a balance between the polymer and siRNA was achieved at N/P 40 and above this. At an N/P ratio between 40–50, significant gene silencing of polyplex and stability in the cell cytosol condition was effectively obtained. As reported, there are several markers expressed on the hMSC surface and CD44 receptor. Thus, caveolae-mediated uptake of the whole polyplex is most probably driven by HA interactions with specifically overexpressed CD44 receptors on hMSC. Most importantly, increased cellular caveolae-mediated uptake of the HA-modified polyplex showed more than 97% GFP gene expression on hMSC cells (Herrera and Shastri, 2019). In another study, Xiong et al. designed and developed a codelivery system for anticancer drug DOX and a gene decorated with HA against hepatocellular carcinoma. The targeted nanoparticle showed enhanced uptake compared to the non-targeted nanoparticle. Similar to *in vitro* anticancer results, HA-modified NPs significantly showed higher accumulation of HA-modified NPs at the tumor site with maximum fluorescent intensity 24 h after injection. According to many previous studies, it was concluded that HA-modified NPs showed its better therapeutic effect due to selective binding of HA with CD44 receptor which was overexpressed on HCC cells (Xiong et al., 2017).

CHONDROITIN SULFATE AND CHONDROITIN SULFATE-BASED NANOCARRIER

Among the types of glycosaminoglycans, CS is found in the extracellular matrix and plays a crucial role in cellular functions by modifying them. The structure of CS depends on the position of sulfation which is distinctively divided into four structures such as 1) chondroitin-4,6-sulfate, 2) chondroitin2,6-sulfate, 3) chondroitin-6-sulfate, and 4) chondroitin-4-sulfate. As a naturally occurring mucopolysaccharide, CS is extensively found in skin, cartilage, and bone. CS has high specificity towards CD44 receptors present on cancer cells. Due to such an effect, CS-modified nanocarriers have been formulated and have shown extraordinary benefit towards cancer therapy. A very recent study reported a docetaxel-loaded Zein nanoparticle modified with CS for effective treatment against prostate cancer. It is worth noting that the targeted preparation displayed improved pharmacokinetics with approximately a 9-fold half-life than free docetaxel. Moreover, a higher accumulation was observed in PC-3 tumor cell-bearing mice that indicated enhanced accumulation at the tumor site. Hence, a CS-based nanoparticle imparts the hope of effective therapy (Lee et al., n.d.). Another study reported a temozolomide-loaded albumin nanoparticle fabricated with CS for brain-targeted delivery. The preparation was characterized for surface charge, particle size, DSC, XRD, FTIR, and TEM, and revealed suitable results. Moreover, the biodistribution results exhibited a higher accumulation of drugs in the brain by the targeted preparation as compared with the pure drug that significantly confirmed the brain targeting ability of nanoparticles (Kudarha and Sawant, 2021). Oommen et al. confirmed the anti-cancer effect against breast and colon cancer cells by using CS and HA nanoparticles loaded with doxorubicin (Oommen et al., 2016). Luo et al. explored the targeting effect of a CS-modified DOX and retinoic acid-loaded lipid nanoparticle against liver cancer. The resulting preparation was found to be accumulated in Golgi bodies and also inhibited the ECM production proving its targeting potential against the most dangerous cancer (Luo et al., 2020). Hence, to obtain a profound therapeutic effect with low toxicity and off-site effect, a targeting therapy based on CS and HA is highly effective.

CONCLUSION AND FUTURE PERSPECTIVE

Active targeting holds promise regarding target identification, efficient tumor cell death, and reduced off-target effect and toxicities of chemotherapeutic agents. Nowadays, interest has been increasing towards targeted delivery of chemotherapeutics to design effective and efficient formulations. The CD44 receptor is the most expressed receptor on several tumor cells and it has a great affinity towards two polymers HA and CS which are natural targets for formulations. A nanocarrier modified by HA/CS coating or used as a targeting ligand/moiety could be the backbone of a nanocarrier against CD44. In the current review, many nanocarriers such as dendrimers, nanoparticles, micelles, nanoemulsions, CNTs, quantum dots, nanogels, and other polymeric carriers coated with HA/CS can effectively/efficiently binding with the CD44 receptor facilitating cellular internalization of nanocarriers loaded with cargo into the tumor cells. In some reports, CD44-mediated endocytosis could enable the bypass of MDR or the Pgp system. In several cases, the CD44 receptor had a significant role in intracellular and safe delivery of several genes against the most dangerous and fatal cancers. The CD44 receptor can be targeted by various agents such as antibodies, single chain variable fragments, peptides, and macromolecules such as hyaluronic acid and chondroitin which show a tumor homing effect, sparing the normal cells. Thus, the toxicity of treatment could be reduced. However, the major limitation is the heterogeneity of the tumor cells that show different isoforms of CD44. Thus, a thorough study of proteomics is required to overcome such pitfalls. Thus, it could be established that the CD44 receptor has great potential as a therapeutic target against several cancers.

AUTHOR CONTRIBUTIONS

All authors listed have made a substantial, direct, and intellectual contribution to the work and approved it for publication.

REFERENCES

Abbasi, M., Lavasanifar, A., and Uludag, H. (2013). Recent Attempts at RNAi-Mediated P-Glycoprotein Downregulation for Reversal of Multidrug Resistance in Cancer. *Med. Res. Rev.* 33, 33–53. doi:10.1002/med.20244

Accardo, A., and Morelli, G. (2015). Review Peptide-Targeted Liposomes for Selective Drug Delivery: Advantages and Problematic Issues. *Biopolymers.* 104, 462–479. doi:10.1002/bip.22678

Adams, M. L., Lavasanifar, A., and Kwon, G. S. (2003). Amphiphilic Block Copolymers for Drug Delivery. *J. Pharm. Sci.* 92, 1343–1355. doi:10.1002/jps.10397

Afify, A., Purnell, P., and Nguyen, L. (2009). Role of CD44s and CD44v6 on Human Breast Cancer Cell Adhesion, Migration, and Invasion. *Exp. Mol. Pathol.* 86, 95–100. doi:10.1016/j.yexmp.2008.12.003

Al Faraj, A., Shaik, A. S., Ratemi, E., and Halwani, R. (2016). Combination of Drug-Conjugated SWCNT Nanocarriers for Efficient Therapy of Cancer Stem Cells in a Breast Cancer Animal Model. *J. Control Release.* 225, 240–251. doi:10.1016/j.jconrel.2016.01.053

Alavi, M., and Hamidi, M. (2019). Passive and Active Targeting in Cancer Therapy by Liposomes and Lipid Nanoparticles. *Drug Metab. Pers. Ther.* 34. doi:10.1515/dmpt-2018-0032

Alshaer, W., Hillaireau, H., Vergnaud, J., Ismail, S., and Fattal, E. (2015). Functionalizing Liposomes with Anti-CD44 Aptamer for Selective Targeting of Cancer Cells. *Bioconjug. Chem.* 26, 1307–1313. doi:10.1021/bc5004313

Alves, C. S., and Konstantopoulos, K. (2012). PDGF Suppresses the Sulfation of CD44v and Potentiates CD44v-Mediated Binding of Colon Carcinoma Cells to Fibrin under Flow. *PLoS One.* 7, e41472. doi:10.1371/JOURNAL.PONE.0041472

Aqel, A., El-Nour, K. M. M. A., Ammar, R. A. A., and Al-Warthan, A. (2012). Carbon Nanotubes, Science and Technology Part (I) Structure, Synthesis and Characterisation. *Arabian J. Chem.* 5, 1–23. doi:10.1016/j.arabjc.2010.08.022

Bai, H., Wang, T., Kong, F., Zhang, M., Li, Z., Zhuang, L., et al. (2021). CXCR4 and CD44 Dual-Targeted Prussian Blue Nanosystem with Daunorubicin Loaded for Acute Myeloid Leukemia Therapy. *Chem. Eng. J.* 405, 126891. doi:10.1016/j.cej.2020.126891

Bai, S. B., Liu, D. Z., Cheng, Y., Cui, H., Cui, M. X., Zhang, B. L., et al. (2019). Osteoclasts and Tumor Cells Dual Targeting Nanoparticle to Treat Bone Metastases of Lung Cancer. *Nanomedicine.* 21, 102054. doi:10.1016/j.nano.2019.102054

Banerji, S., Wright, A. J., Noble, M., Mahoney, D. J., Campbell, I. D., Day, A. J., et al. (2007). Structures of the Cd44-Hyaluronan Complex Provide Insight into a Fundamental Carbohydrate-Protein Interaction. *Nat. Struct. Mol. Biol.* 14, 234–239. doi:10.1038/nsmb1201

Begines, B., Ortiz, T., Pérez-Aranda, M., Martínez, G., Merinero, M., Argüelles-Arias, F., et al. (2020). Polymeric Nanoparticles for Drug Delivery: Recent Developments and Future Prospects. *Nanomaterials.* 10, 1403. doi:10.3390/nano10071403

Bharali, D. J., and Mousa, S. A. (2010). Emerging Nanomedicines for Early Cancer Detection and Improved Treatment: Current Perspective and Future Promise. *Pharmacol. Ther.* 128, 324–335. doi:10.1016/j.pharmthera.2010.07.007

Bhatnagar, P., Pant, A. B., Shukla, Y., Panda, A., and Gupta, K. C. (2016). Hyaluronic Acid Grafted PLGA Copolymer Nanoparticles Enhance the Targeted Delivery of Bromelain in Ehrlich's Ascites Carcinoma. *Eur. J. Pharm. Biopharm.* 105, 176–192. doi:10.1016/j.ejpb.2016.06.002

Bourguignon, L. Y. W. (2019). Matrix Hyaluronan-CD44 Interaction Activates MicroRNA and LncRNA Signaling Associated With Chemoresistance, Invasion, and Tumor Progression. *Front. Oncol.* 9, 492. doi:10.3389/fonc.2019.00492

Brigger, I., Dubernet, C., and Couvreur, P. (2002). Nanoparticles in Cancer Therapy and Diagnosis. *Adv. Drug Deliv. Rev.* 54 (5), 631–51. doi:10.1016/S0169-409X(02)00044-3

Cai, D., Mataraza, J. M., Qin, Z. H., Huang, Z., Huang, J., Chiles, T. C., et al. (2005). Highly Efficient Molecular Delivery into Mammalian Cells Using Carbon Nanotube Spearing. *Nat. Methods.* 2, 449–454. doi:10.1038/nmeth761

Cai, J., Fu, J., Li, R., Zhang, F., Ling, G., and Zhang, P. (2019). A Potential Carrier for Anti-tumor Targeted Delivery-Hyaluronic Acid Nanoparticles. *Carbohydr. Polym.* 208, 356–364. doi:10.1016/j.carbpol.2018.12.074

Canham, L. T. (1990). Silicon Quantum Wire Array Fabrication by Electrochemical and Chemical Dissolution of Wafers. *Appl. Phys. Lett.* 57, 1046–1048. doi:10.1063/1.103561

Cao, H., Heazlewood, S. Y., Williams, B., Cardozo, D., Nigro, J., Oteiza, A., et al. (2016). The Role of CD44 in Fetal and Adult Hematopoietic Stem Cell Regulation. *Haematologica.* 101, 26–37. doi:10.3324/haematol.2015.135921

Cao, Z., Zhou, X., and Wang, G. (2016). Selective Release of Hydrophobic and Hydrophilic Cargos from Multi-Stimuli-Responsive Nanogels. *ACS Appl. Mater. Inter.* 8, 28888–28896. doi:10.1021/acsami.6b10360

Cao, X., Tao, L., Wen, S., Hou, W., and Shi, X. (2015). Hyaluronic Acid-Modified Multiwalled Carbon Nanotubes for Targeted Delivery of Doxorubicin into Cancer Cells. *Carbohydr. Res.* 405, 70–77. doi:10.1016/j.carres.2014.06.030

Chadar, R., Afzal, O., Alqahtani, S. M., and Kesharwani, P. (2021). Carbon Nanotubes as an Emerging Nanocarrier for the Delivery of Doxorubicin for Improved Chemotherapy. *Colloids Surf. B.* 208, 112044. doi:10.1016/J.COLSURFB.2021.112044

Chen, C., Zhao, S., Karnad, A., and Freeman, J. W. (2018). The Biology and Role of CD44 in Cancer Progression: Therapeutic Implications. *J. Hematol. Oncol.* 11, 64. doi:10.1186/s13045-018-0605-5

Chen, L., and Bourguignon, L. Y. (2014). Hyaluronan-CD44 Interaction Promotes C-Jun Signaling and miRNA21 Expression Leading to Bcl-2 Expression and Chemoresistance in Breast Cancer Cells. *Mol. Cancer.* 13, 52. doi:10.1186/1476-4598-13-52

Chen, L. D., Li, Y., Yuan, H. Y., and Pang, D. W. (2006). *Quantum Dots and Their Applications in Cancer Research.* Ai Zheng.

Chen, Y., Sen, J., Bathula, S. R., Yang, Q., Fittipaldi, R., and Huang, L. (2009). Novel Cationic Lipid that Delivers siRNA and Enhances Therapeutic Effect in Lung Cancer Cells. *Mol. Pharm.* 6, 696–705. doi:10.1021/mp800136v

Cho, K., Wang, X., Nie, S., Chen, Z., and Shin, D. M. (2008). Therapeutic Nanoparticles for Drug Delivery in Cancer. *Clin. Cancer Res.* 14, 1310–1316. doi:10.1158/1078-0432.CCR-07-1441

Cisterna, B. A., Kamaly, N., Choi, W. I., Tavakkoli, A., Farokhzad, O. C., and Vilos, C. (2016). Targeted Nanoparticles for Colorectal Cancer. *Nanomedicine.* 11, 2443–2456. doi:10.2217/nnm-2016-0194

Dabholkar, R. D., Sawant, R. M., Mongayt, D. A., Devarajan, P. V., and Torchilin, V. P. (2006). Polyethylene Glycol-Phosphatidylethanolamine Conjugate (PEG-PE)-based Mixed Micelles: Some Properties, Loading with Paclitaxel, and Modulation of P-Glycoprotein-Mediated Efflux. *Int. J. Pharm.* 315, 148–157. doi:10.1016/j.ijpharm.2006.02.018

Deshpande, P. P., Biswas, S., and Torchilin, V. P. (2013). Current Trends in the Use of Liposomes for Tumor Targeting. *Nanomedicine.* 8, 1509–1528. doi:10.2217/nnm.13.118

Dosio, F., Arpicco, S., Stella, B., and Fattal, E. (2016). Hyaluronic Acid for Anticancer Drug and Nucleic Acid Delivery. *Adv. Drug Deliv. Rev.* 97, 204–236. doi:10.1016/j.addr.2015.11.011

Du, X., Yin, S., Wang, Y., Gu, X., Wang, G., and Li, J. (2018). Hyaluronic Acid-Functionalized Half-Generation of Sectorial Dendrimers for Anticancer Drug Delivery and Enhanced Biocompatibility. *Carbohydr. Polym.* 202, 513–522. doi:10.1016/j.carbpol.2018.09.015

Dubey, S. K., Kali, M., Hejmady, S., Saha, R. N., Alexander, A., and Kesharwani, P. (2021). Recent Advances of Dendrimers as Multifunctional Nano-Carriers to Combat Breast Cancer. *Eur. J. Pharm. Sci.* 164, 105890. doi:10.1016/j.ejps.2021.105890

Duncan, R., and Izzo, L. (2005). Dendrimer Biocompatibility and Toxicity. *Adv. Drug Deliv. Rev.* 57, 2215–2237. doi:10.1016/j.addr.2005.09.019

Duncan, R. (2006). Polymer Conjugates as Anticancer Nanomedicines. *Nat. Rev. Cancer.* 6, 688–701. doi:10.1038/nrc1958

Dzwonek, J., and Wilczynski, G. M. (2015). CD44: Molecular Interactions, Signaling and Functions in the Nervous System. *Front. Cell. Neurosci.* 9, 175. doi:10.3389/FNCEL.2015.00175

Elbashir, S. M., Harborth, J., Lendeckel, W., Yalcin, A., Weber, K., and Tuschl, T. (2001). Duplexes of 21-nucleotide RNAs Mediate RNA Interference in Cultured Mammalian Cells. *Nature.* 411, 494–498. doi:10.1038/35078107

Fan, Y., Wang, Q., Lin, G., Shi, Y., Gu, Z., and Ding, T. (2017). Combination of Using Prodrug-Modified Cationic Liposome Nanocomplexes and a Potentiating Strategy via Targeted Co-delivery of Gemcitabine and Docetaxel for CD44-Overexpressed Triple Negative Breast Cancer Therapy. *Acta Biomater.* 62, 257–272. doi:10.1016/j.actbio.2017.08.034

Francis, M. F., Cristea, M., and Winnik, F. M., 2004. Polymeric Micelles for Oral Drug Delivery: Why and How. *Pure Appl. Chem.* 76, 1321–1335. doi:10.1351/pac200476071321

Fréchet, J. M. J. (1994). Functional Polymers and Dendrimers: Reactivity, Molecular Architecture, and Interfacial Energy. *Science.* 263, 1710–1715. doi:10.1126/science.8134834

Fu, Y., Jang, M. S., Wu, T., Lee, J. H., Li, Y., Lee, D. S., et al. (2019). Multifunctional Hyaluronic Acid-Mediated Quantum Dots for Targeted Intracellular Protein Delivery and Real-Time Fluorescence Imaging. *Carbohydr. Polym.* 224, 115174. doi:10.1016/j.carbpol.2019.115174

Gao, C., Wang, M., Zhu, P., and Yan, C. (2021). Preparation, Characterization and *In Vitro* Antitumor Activity Evaluation of Hyaluronic Acid-Alendronate-Methotrexate Nanoparticles. *Int. J. Biol. Macromol.* 166, 71–79. doi:10.1016/j.ijbiomac.2020.10.088

Gautam, M., Thapa, R. K., Gupta, B., Soe, Z. C., Ou, W., Poudel, K., et al. (2020). Phytosterol-loaded CD44 Receptor-Targeted PEGylated Nano-Hybrid Phyto-Liposomes for Synergistic Chemotherapy. *Expert Opin. Drug Deliv.* 17, 423–434. doi:10.1080/17425247.2020.1727442

Gawande, V., Choudhury, H., and Kesharwani, P. (2021). Dendrimer Nomenclature and Synthesis Methods. *Dendrimer-Based Nanotherapeutics.*, 75–94. doi:10.1016/B978-0-12-821250-9.00009-3

Gerion, D. (2007). "Fluorescence Imaging in Biology Using Nanoprobes," in *Nanotechnologies for the Life Sciences* (Wiley-VCH Verlag GmbH & Co. KGaA). doi:10.1002/9783527610419.ntls0024

Gomari, M. M., Farsimadan, M., Rostami, N., mahmoudi, Z., Fadaie, M., Farhani, I., et al. (2021). CD44 Polymorphisms and its Variants, as an Inconsistent Marker in Cancer Investigations. *Mutat. Research/Reviews Mutat. Res.* 787, 108374. doi:10.1016/J.MRREV.2021.108374

Goodison, S., Urquidi, V., and Tarin, D. (1999). CD44 Cell Adhesion Molecules. *Mol. Pathol.* 52, 189–196. doi:10.1136/mp.52.4.189

Greenfield, B., Wang, W. C., Marquardt, H., Piepkorn, M., Wolff, E. A., Aruffo, A., et al. (1999). Characterization of the Heparan Sulfate and Chondroitin Sulfate Assembly Sites in CD44. *J. Biol. Chem.* 274, 2511–2517. doi:10.1074/JBC.274.4.2511

Guo, X., and Szoka, F. C. (2003). Chemical Approaches to Triggerable Lipid Vesicles for Drug and Gene Delivery. *Acc. Chem. Res.* 36, 335–341. doi:10.1021/ar9703241

Gupta, A., Mathur, R., Singh, S., Bag, N., Khan, U. A., Ahmad, F. J., et al. (2021). 99mTc-Methionine Gold Nanoparticles as a Promising Biomaterial for Enhanced Tumor Imaging. *J. Pharm. Sci.* 110, 888–897. doi:10.1016/j.xphs.2020.11.008

Gupta, R., Shea, J., Scafe, C., Shurlygina, A., and Rapoport, N. (2015). Polymeric Micelles and Nanoemulsions as Drug Carriers: Therapeutic Efficacy, Toxicity, and Drug Resistance. *J. Control Release.* 212, 70–77. doi:10.1016/j.jconrel.2015.06.019

Han, M., Lv, Q., Tang, X. J., Hu, Y. L., Xu, D. H., Li, F. Z., et al. (2012). Overcoming Drug Resistance of MCF-7/ADR Cells by Altering Intracellular Distribution of Doxorubicin via MVP Knockdown with a Novel siRNA Polyamidoamine-Hyaluronic Acid Complex. *J. Control Release.* 163, 136–144. doi:10.1016/j.jconrel.2012.08.020

He, H., Pham-Huy, L. A., Dramou, P., Xiao, D., Zuo, P., and Pham-Huy, C. (2013). Carbon Nanotubes: Applications in Pharmacy and Medicine. *Biomed. Res. Int.* 2013, 1–12. doi:10.1155/2013/578290

Herrera, L. C., and Shastri, V. P. (2019). Silencing of GFP Expression in Human Mesenchymal Stem Cells Using Quaternary Polyplexes of siRNA-PEI with Glycosaminoglycans and Albumin. *Acta Biomater.* 99, 397–411. doi:10.1016/j.actbio.2019.09.006

Hill, A., McFarlane, S., Johnston, P. G., and Waugh, D. J. (2006). The Emerging Role of CD44 in Regulating Skeletal Micrometastasis. *Cancer Lett.* 237, 1–9. doi:10.1016/J.CANLET.2005.05.006

Hitchcock, J., White, A. L., Hondow, N., Hughes, T. A., Dupont, H., Biggs, S., et al. (2020). Metal-shell Nanocapsules for the Delivery of Cancer Drugs. *J. Colloid Interf. Sci.* 567, 171–180. doi:10.1016/j.jcis.2019.12.018

Hörmann, K., and Zimmer, A. (2016). Drug Delivery and Drug Targeting with Parenteral Lipid Nanoemulsions - A Review. *J. Controlled Release.* 223, 85–98. doi:10.1016/j.jconrel.2015.12.016

Huang, W. Y., Lin, J. N., Hsieh, J. T., Chou, S. C., Lai, C. H., Yun, E. J., et al. (2016). Nanoparticle Targeting CD44-Positive Cancer Cells for Site-Specific Drug Delivery in Prostate Cancer Therapy. *ACS Appl. Mater. Inter.* 8, 30722–30734. doi:10.1021/acsami.6b10029

Iijima, S. (1991). Helical Microtubules of Graphitic Carbon. *Nature.* 354, 56–58. doi:10.1038/354056a0

Jain, K., Kesharwani, P., Gupta, U., and Jain, N. K. (2010). Dendrimer Toxicity: Let's Meet the challenge. *Int. J. Pharm.* 394, 122–142. doi:10.1016/J.IJPHARM.2010.04.027

Jaiswal, J. K., Goldman, E. R., Mattoussi, H., and Simon, S. M. (2004). Use of Quantum Dots for Live Cell Imaging. *Nat. Methods.* 1, 73–78. doi:10.1038/nmeth1004-73

Jaiswal, M., Dudhe, R., and Sharma, P. K. (2015). Nanoemulsion: an Advanced Mode of Drug Delivery System. *Biotech.* 5, 123–127. doi:10.1007/s13205-014-0214-0

Jeevanandam, J., Barhoum, A., Chan, Y. S., Dufresne, A., and Danquah, M. K. (2018). Review on Nanoparticles and Nanostructured Materials: History, Sources, Toxicity and Regulations. *Beilstein J. Nanotechnol.* 9, 1050–1074. doi:10.3762/bjnano.9.98

Jeon, S. I., Lee, J. H., Andrade, J. D., and De Gennes, P. G. (1991). Protein-surface Interactions in the Presence of Polyethylene Oxide. *J. Colloid Interf. Sci.* 142, 149–158. doi:10.1016/0021-9797(91)90043-8

Jin, C., Wang, K., Oppong-Gyebi, A., and Hu, J. (2020). Application of Nanotechnology in Cancer Diagnosis and Therapy - A Mini-Review. *Int. J. Med. Sci.* 17, 2964–2973. doi:10.7150/ijms.49801

Jin, Y., Ma, X., Zhang, S., Meng, H., Xu, M., Yang, X., et al. (2017). A Tantalum Oxide-Based Core/shell Nanoparticle for Triple-Modality Image-Guided Chemo-thermal Synergetic Therapy of Esophageal Carcinoma. *Cancer Lett.* 397, 61–71. doi:10.1016/j.canlet.2017.03.030

Jung, T., Castellana, D., Klingbeil, P., Cuesta Hernández, I., Vitacolonna, M., Orlicky, D. J., et al. (2009). CD44v6 Dependence of Premetastatic Niche Preparation by Exosomes. *Neoplasia.* 11, 1093–1105. doi:10.1593/NEO.09822

Kabary, D. M., Helmy, M. W., Elkhodairy, K. A., Fang, J. Y., and Elzoghby, A. O. (2018). Hyaluronate/lactoferrin Layer-By-Layer-Coated Lipid Nanocarriers for Targeted Co-delivery of Rapamycin and Berberine to Lung Carcinoma. *Colloids Surf. B Biointerfaces.* 169, 183–194. doi:10.1016/j.colsurfb.2018.05.008

Kalniņa, Z., Zayakin, P., Siliņa, K. n., and Line, A. (2005). Alterations of Pre-mRNA Splicing in Cancer. *Genes Chromosom. Cancer.* 42, 342–357. doi:10.1002/GCC.20156

Kamal, M. A., Jabir, N., Tabrez, G. M., Ashraf, S., Shakil, G. A., and Damanhouri, M. A. (2012). Nanotechnology-based Approaches in Anticancer Research. *Int. J. Nanomedicine.* 7, 4391. doi:10.2147/IJN.S33838

Karakoçak, B. B., Laradji, A., Primeau, T., Berezin, M. Y., Li, S., and Ravi, N. (2021). Hyaluronan-Conjugated Carbon Quantum Dots for Bioimaging Use. *ACS Appl. Mater. Inter.* 13, 277–286. doi:10.1021/acsami.0c20088

Kateb, B., Chiu, K., Black, K. L., Yamamoto, V., Khalsa, B., Ljubimova, J. Y., et al. (2011). Nanoplatforms for Constructing New Approaches to Cancer Treatment, Imaging, and Drug Delivery: What Should Be the Policy? *Neuroimage.* 54, S106–S124. doi:10.1016/j.neuroimage.2010.01.105

Kaur, H., and Kesharwani, P. (2021). Advanced Nanomedicine Approaches Applied for Treatment of Skin Carcinoma. *J. Control Release.* 337, 589–611. doi:10.1016/J.JCONREL.2021.08.003

Kavand, A., Anton, N., Vandamme, T., Serra, C. A., and Chan-Seng, D. (2020). Synthesis and Functionalization of Hyperbranched Polymers for Targeted Drug Delivery. *J. Controlled Release.* 321, 285–311. doi:10.1016/j.jconrel.2020.02.019

Kesharwani, P., Gajbhiye, V., and Jain, N. K. (2012). A Review of Nanocarriers for the Delivery of Small Interfering RNA. *Biomaterials.* 33, 7138–7150. doi:10.1016/J.BIOMATERIALS.2012.06.068

Kesharwani, P., and Iyer, A. K. (2015). Recent Advances in Dendrimer-Based Nanovectors for Tumor-Targeted Drug and Gene Delivery. *Drug Discov. TodayToday.* 20, 536–547. doi:10.1016/j.drudis.2014.12.012

Kesharwani, P., Jain, K., and Jain, N. K. (2014a). Dendrimer as Nanocarrier for Drug Delivery. *Prog. Polym. Sci.* 39, 268–307. doi:10.1016/j.progpolymsci.2013.07.005

Kesharwani, P., Tekade, R. K., and Jain, N. K. (2014b). Generation Dependent Cancer Targeting Potential of Poly(propyleneimine) Dendrimer. *Biomaterials.* 35, 5539–5548. doi:10.1016/j.biomaterials.2014.03.064

Kesharwani, P., Banerjee, S., Gupta, U., Mohd Amin, M. C. I., Padhye, S., Sarkar, F. H., et al. (2015a). PAMAM Dendrimers as Promising Nanocarriers for RNAi Therapeutics. *Mater. Today.* 18, 565–572. doi:10.1016/j.mattod.2015.06.003

Kesharwani, P., Banerjee, S., Padhye, S., Sarkar, F. H., and Iyer, A. K. (2015b). Hyaluronic Acid Engineered Nanomicelles Loaded with 3,4-Difluorobenzylidene Curcumin for Targeted Killing of CD44+ Stem-like Pancreatic Cancer Cells. *Biomacromolecules.* 16, 3042–3053. doi:10.1021/acs.biomac.5b00941

Kesharwani, P., Mishra, V., and Jain, N. K. (2015c). Generation Dependent Hemolytic Profile of Folate Engineered Poly(propyleneimine) Dendrimer. *J. Drug Deliv. Sci. Technology.* 28, 1–6. doi:10.1016/j.jddst.2015.04.006

Kesharwani, P., Xie, L., Banerjee, S., Mao, G., Padhye, S., Sarkar, F. H., et al. (2015d). Hyaluronic Acid-Conjugated Polyamidoamine Dendrimers for Targeted Delivery of 3,4-difluorobenzylidene Curcumin to CD44 Overexpressing Pancreatic Cancer Cells. *Colloids Surf. B. Biointerfaces.* 136, 413–423. doi:10.1016/j.colsurfb.2015.09.043

Khan, I., Saeed, K., and Khan, I. (2019). Nanoparticles: Properties, Applications and Toxicities. *Arabian J. Chem.* 12, 908–931. doi:10.1016/j.arabjc.2017.05.011

Khurana, R. K., Beg, S., Burrow, A. J., Vashishta, R. K., Katare, O. P., Kaur, S., et al. (2017). Enhancing Biopharmaceutical Performance of an Anticancer Drug by Long Chain PUFA Based Self-Nanoemulsifying Lipidic Nanomicellar Systems. *Eur. J. Pharm. Biopharm.* 121, 42–60. doi:10.1016/j.ejpb.2017.09.001

Kim, J. E., and Park, Y. J. (2017a). High Paclitaxel-Loaded and Tumor Cell-Targeting Hyaluronan-Coated Nanoemulsions. *Colloids Surf. B Biointerfaces.* 150, 362–372. doi:10.1016/j.colsurfb.2016.10.050

Kim, J. E., and Park, Y. J. (2017b). Paclitaxel-loaded Hyaluronan Solid Nanoemulsions for Enhanced Treatment Efficacy in Ovarian Cancer. *Int. J. Nanomedicine.* 12, 645–658. doi:10.2147/IJN.S124158

Kim, K., Choi, H., Choi, E. S., Park, M. H., and Ryu, J. H. (2019). Hyaluronic Acid-Coated Nanomedicine for Targeted Cancer Therapy. *Pharmaceutics.* 11, 301. doi:10.3390/pharmaceutics11070301

Kim, S. H., Jeong, J. H., Lee, S. H., Kim, S. W., and Park, T. G. (2008). Local and Systemic Delivery of VEGF siRNA Using Polyelectrolyte Complex Micelles for Effective Treatment of Cancer. *J. Control Release.* 129, 107–116. doi:10.1016/j.jconrel.2008.03.008

Klumpp, C., Kostarelos, K., Prato, M., and Bianco, A. (2006). Functionalized Carbon Nanotubes as Emerging Nanovectors for the Delivery of Therapeutics. *Biochim. Biophys. Acta (Bba) - Biomembranes.* 1758, 404–412. doi:10.1016/j.bbamem.2005.10.008

Kokare, C. R., Khot, S. V., Gorain, B., and Kesharwani, P. (2021). "Characterization of Dendrimers," in *Dendrimer-Based Nanotherapeutics* (Elsevier), 125–141. doi:10.1016/B978-0-12-821250-9.00006-8

Kudarha, R. R., and Sawant, K. K. (2021). Chondroitin Sulfate Conjugation Facilitates Tumor Cell Internalization of Albumin Nanoparticles for Brain-Targeted Delivery of Temozolomide via CD44 Receptor-Mediated Targeting. *Drug Deliv. Transl. Res.* 11, 1994–2008. doi:10.1007/s13346-020-00861-x

Kuhn, N. Z., and Tuan, R. S. (2010). Regulation of Stemness and Stem Cell Niche of Mesenchymal Stem Cells: Implications in Tumorigenesis and Metastasis. *J. Cell. Physiol.* 222, 268–277. doi:10.1002/JCP.21940

Kumar, A. V. P., Dubey, S. K., Tiwari, S., Puri, A., Hejmady, S., Gorain, B., et al. (2021). Recent Advances in Nanoparticles Mediated Photothermal Therapy Induced Tumor Regression. *Int. J. Pharmaceutics.* 606, 120848. doi:10.1016/J.IJPHARM.2021.120848

Lacerda, L., Bianco, A., Prato, M., and Kostarelos, K. (2006). Carbon Nanotubes as Nanomedicines: From Toxicology to Pharmacology. *Adv. Drug Deliv. Rev.* 58, 1460–1470. doi:10.1016/j.addr.2006.09.015

Lai, H., Ding, X., Ye, J., Deng, J., and Cui, S. (2021). pH-Responsive Hyaluronic Acid-Based Nanoparticles for Targeted Curcumin Delivery and Enhanced Cancer Therapy. *Colloids Surf. B Biointerfaces.* 198, 111455. doi:10.1016/j.colsurfb.2020.111455

Lee, H., Kang, N.-W., Kim, H., Kim, D. H., Chae, J.-w., Lee, W., et al. (2020). Chondroitin Sulfate-Hybridized Zein Nanoparticles for Tumor-Targeted Delivery of Docetaxel. *Carbohydr. Polym.* 253, 117187. doi:10.1016/j.carbpol.2020.117187

Lee, J., Lee, H. S., Kang, N. W., Lee, S. Y., Kim, D. H., Kim, S., et al. (2020). Blood Component Ridable and CD44 Receptor Targetable Nanoparticles Based on a

Maleimide-Functionalized Chondroitin Sulfate Derivative. *Carbohydr. Polym.* 230, 115568. doi:10.1016/j.carbpol.2019.115568

Lee, J. Y., Park, J. H., Lee, J. J., Lee, S. Y., Chung, S. J., Cho, H. J., et al. (2016a). Polyethylene Glycol-Conjugated Chondroitin Sulfate A Derivative Nanoparticles for Tumor-Targeted Delivery of Anticancer Drugs. *Carbohydr. Polym.* 151, 68–77. doi:10.1016/j.carbpol.2016.05.043

Lee, J. Y., Termsarasab, U., Park, J. H., Lee, S. Y., Ko, S. H., Shim, J. S., et al. (2016b). Dual CD44 and Folate Receptor-Targeted Nanoparticles for Cancer Diagnosis and Anticancer Drug Delivery. *J. Control Release.* 236, 38–46. doi:10.1016/j.jconrel.2016.06.021

Lesley, J., Hascall, V. C., Tammi, M., and Hyman, R. (2000). Hyaluronan Binding by Cell Surface CD44. *J. Biol. Chem.* 275, 26967–26975. doi:10.1074/JBC.M002527200

Li, C., Chen, T., Ocsoy, I., Zhu, G., Yasun, E., You, M., et al. (2014). Gold-Coated Fe3O4 Nanoroses with Five Unique Functions for Cancer Cell Targeting, Imaging and Therapy. *Adv. Funct. Mater.* 24, 1772–1780. doi:10.1002/adfm.201301659

Li, J., He, Y., Sun, W., Luo, Y., Cai, H., Pan, Y., et al. (2014). Hyaluronic Acid-Modified Hydrothermally Synthesized Iron Oxide Nanoparticles for Targeted Tumor MR Imaging. *Biomaterials.* 35, 3666–3677. doi:10.1016/j.biomaterials.2014.01.011

Li, J., Hu, Y., Yang, J., Wei, P., Sun, W., Shen, M., et al. (2015). Hyaluronic Acid-Modified Fe3O4@Au Core/shell Nanostars for Multimodal Imaging and Photothermal Therapy of Tumors. *Biomaterials.* 38, 10–21. doi:10.1016/j.biomaterials.2014.10.065

Li, M., Sun, J., Zhang, W., Zhao, Y., Zhang, S., and Zhang, S. (2021). Drug Delivery Systems Based on CD44-Targeted Glycosaminoglycans for Cancer Therapy. *Carbohydr. Polym.* 251, 117103. doi:10.1016/j.carbpol.2020.117103

Li, Y., Shi, S., Ming, Y., Wang, L., Li, C., Luo, M., et al. (2018). Specific Cancer Stem Cell-Therapy by Albumin Nanoparticles Functionalized with CD44-Mediated Targeting. *J. Nanobiotechnology.* 16, 99–15. doi:10.1186/s12951-018-0424-4

Liu, C., Zhang, P., Zhai, X., Tian, F., Li, W., Yang, J., et al. (2012). Nano-carrier for Gene Delivery and Bioimaging Based on Carbon Dots with PEI-Passivation Enhanced Fluorescence. *Biomaterials.* 33, 3604–3613. doi:10.1016/j.biomaterials.2012.01.052

Liu, D., Zhang, Q., Wang, J., Fan, L., Zhu, W., and Cai, D. (2019). Hyaluronic Acid-Coated Single-Walled Carbon Nanotubes Loaded with Doxorubicin for the Treatment of Breast Cancer. *Pharmazie.* 74, 83–90. doi:10.1691/ph.2019.8152

Liu, Z., Li, L.-F., Xia, S.-S., Tian, H.-P., Yan, Z.-H., Zhang, G.-J., et al. (2019). Chondroitin Sulfate Modification Enhances the Targeting and Therapeutic Effect of Nanomedicine on AOM/DSS-induced Mouse colon Cancer. *J. Drug Deliv. Sci. Technology.* 52, 1–7. doi:10.1016/j.jddst.2019.04.010

Liu, Y., Zhou, C., Wei, S., Yang, T., Lan, Y., Cao, A., et al. (2018). Paclitaxel Delivered by CD44 Receptor-Targeting and Endosomal pH Sensitive Dual Functionalized Hyaluronic Acid Micelles for Multidrug Resistance Reversion. *Colloids Surf. B Biointerfaces.* 170, 330–340. doi:10.1016/j.colsurfb.2018.06.024

Luo, J., Gong, T., and Ma, L. (2020). Chondroitin-modified Lipid Nanoparticles Target the Golgi to Degrade Extracellular Matrix for Liver Cancer Management. *Carbohydr. Polym.* 249, 116887. doi:10.1016/j.carbpol.2020.116887

Luo, Z., Dai, Y., and Gao, H. (2019). Development and Application of Hyaluronic Acid in Tumor Targeting Drug Delivery. *Acta Pharmaceutica Sinica B.* 9, 1099–1112. doi:10.1016/j.apsb.2019.06.004

Lv, Y., Xu, C., Zhao, X., Lin, C., Yang, X., Xin, X., et al. (2018). Nanoplatform Assembled from a CD44-Targeted Prodrug and Smart Liposomes for Dual Targeting of Tumor Microenvironment and Cancer Cells. *ACS Nano.* 12, 1519–1536. doi:10.1021/acsnano.7b08051

Ma, L., Dong, L., and Chang, P. (2019). CD44v6 Engages in Colorectal Cancer Progression. *Cell Death Dis.* 10, 30. doi:10.1038/S41419-018-1265-7

Ma, W., Chen, Q., Xu, W., Yu, M., Yang, Y., Zou, B., et al. (2021). Self-targeting Visualizable Hyaluronate Nanogel for Synchronized Intracellular Release of Doxorubicin and Cisplatin in Combating Multidrug-Resistant Breast Cancer. *Nano Res.* 14, 846–857. doi:10.1007/s12274-020-3124-y

Ma, Y., Zhou, H., Hu, F., Pei, Z., Xu, Y., and Shuai, Q. (2018). Multifunctional Nanogel Engineering with Redox-Responsive and AIEgen Features for the Targeted Delivery of Doxorubicin Hydrochloride with Enhanced Antitumor Efficiency and Real-Time Intracellular Imaging. *Artif. Cell Nanomed Biotechnol.* 46, S900. doi:10.1080/21691401.2018.1518910

Maeda, H. (2001). The Enhanced Permeability and Retention (EPR) Effect in Tumor Vasculature: The Key Role of Tumor-Selective Macromolecular Drug Targeting. *Adv. Enzyme Regul.* 41, 189–207. doi:10.1016/S0065-2571(00)00013-3

Maeda, H., Wu, J., Sawa, T., Matsumura, Y., and Hori, K. (2000). Tumor Vascular Permeability and the EPR Effect in Macromolecular Therapeutics: A Review. *J. Control Release.* 65, 271–284. doi:10.1016/S0168-3659(99)00248-5

Mahira, S., Kommineni, N., Husain, G. M., and Khan, W. (2019). Cabazitaxel and Silibinin Co-encapsulated Cationic Liposomes for CD44 Targeted Delivery: A New Insight into Nanomedicine Based Combinational Chemotherapy for Prostate Cancer. *Biomed. Pharmacother.* 110, 803–817. doi:10.1016/j.biopha.2018.11.145

Malam, Y., Loizidou, M., and Seifalian, A. M. (2009). Liposomes and Nanoparticles: Nanosized Vehicles for Drug Delivery in Cancer. *Trends Pharmacol. Sci.* 30, 592–599. doi:10.1016/j.tips.2009.08.004

Matsumoto, S., Christie, R. J., Nishiyama, N., Miyata, K., Ishii, A., Oba, M., et al. (2009). Environment-responsive Block Copolymer Micelles with a Disulfide Cross-Linked Core for Enhanced siRNA Delivery. *Biomacromolecules.* 10, 119–127. doi:10.1021/bm800985e

Mishra, V., Gurnany, E., and Mansoori, M. H. (2017). "Quantum Dots in Targeted Delivery of Bioactives and Imaging," in *Nanotechnology-Based Approaches for Targeting and Delivery of Drugs and Genes* (Elsevier), 427–450. doi:10.1016/B978-0-12-809717-5.00015-4

Misra, S., Heldin, P., and Hascall, V. C. (2011). HA/CD44 Interactions as Potential Targets for Cancer Therapy[WWW Document]. *FEBS J.* 278, 1429. doi:10.1111/j.1742-4658.2011.08071.x

Misra, S., Hascall, V. C., Markwald, R. R., and Ghatak, S. (2015). Interactions between Hyaluronan and its Receptors (CD44, RHAMM) Regulate the Activities of Inflammation and Cancer. *Front. Immunol.* 6, 201. doi:10.3389/fimmu.2015.00201

Mitchell, G. P., Mirkin, C. A., and Letsinger, R. L. (1999). Programmed Assembly of DNA Functionalized Quantum Dots. *J. Am. Chem. Soc.* 121, 8122–8123. doi:10.1021/ja991662v

Mo, X., Wu, F., Li, Y., and Cai, X. (2021). Hyaluronic Acid-Functionalized Halloysite Nanotubes for Targeted Drug Delivery to CD44-Overexpressing Cancer Cells. *Mater. Today Commun.* 28, 102682. doi:10.1016/J.MTCOMM.2021.102682

Mousa, S. A., and Bharali, D. J. (2011). Nanotechnology-Based Detection and Targeted Therapy in Cancer: Nano-Bio Paradigms and Applications. *Cancers.* 3, 2888–2903. doi:10.3390/cancers3032888

Muntimadugu, E., Kumar, R., Saladi, S., Rafeeqi, T. A., and Khan, W. (2016). CD44 Targeted Chemotherapy for Co-eradication of Breast Cancer Stem Cells and Cancer Cells Using Polymeric Nanoparticles of Salinomycin and Paclitaxel. *Colloids Surf. B Biointerfaces.* 143, 532–546. doi:10.1016/j.colsurfb.2016.03.075

Nairi, V., Magnolia, S., Piludu, M., Nieddu, M., Caria, C. A., Sogos, V., et al. (2018). Mesoporous Silica Nanoparticles Functionalized with Hyaluronic Acid. Effect of the Biopolymer Chain Length on Cell Internalization. *Colloids Surf. B Biointerfaces.* 168, 50–59. doi:10.1016/j.colsurfb.2018.02.019

Nam, K., Oh, S., and Shin, I. (2016). Ablation of CD44 Induces Glycolysis-To-Oxidative Phosphorylation Transition via Modulation of the C-Src-Akt-LKB1-Ampkα Pathway. *Biochem. J.* 473, 3013–3030. doi:10.1042/BCJ20160613

Naor, D., Sionov, R. V., and Ish-Shalom, D. (1997). CD44: Structure, Function, and Association with the Malignant Process. *Adv. Cancer Res.* 71, 241–319. doi:10.1016/S0065-230X(08)60101-3

Naor, D., Wallach-Dayan, S. B., Zahalka, M. A., and Sionov, R. V. (2008). Involvement of CD44, a Molecule with a Thousand Faces, in Cancer Dissemination. *Semin. Cancer Biol.* 18, 260–267. doi:10.1016/J.SEMCANCER.2008.03.015

Neame, S. J., and Isacke, C. M. (1993). The Cytoplasmic Tail of CD44 Is Required for Basolateral Localization in Epithelial MDCK Cells but Does Not Mediate Association with the Detergent-Insoluble Cytoskeleton of Fibroblasts. *J. Cell Biol.* 121, 1299–1310. doi:10.1083/JCB.121.6.1299

Nita, L. E., Chiriac, A. P., Diaconu, A., Tudorachi, N., and Mititelu-Tartau, L. (2016). Multifunctional Nanogels with Dual Temperature and pH Responsiveness. *Int. J. Pharm.* 515, 165–175. doi:10.1016/j.ijpharm.2016.10.017

Noh, I., Kim, H. O., Choi, J., Choi, Y., Lee, D. K., Huh, Y. M., et al. (2015). Co-delivery of Paclitaxel and Gemcitabine via CD44-Targeting Nanocarriers as a Prodrug with Synergistic Antitumor Activity against Human Biliary Cancer. *Biomaterials.* 53, 763–774. doi:10.1016/j.biomaterials.2015.03.006

Oh, K. T., Bronich, T. K., and Kabanov, A. V. (2004). Micellar Formulations for Drug Delivery Based on Mixtures of Hydrophobic and Hydrophilic Pluronic Block Copolymers. *J. Control Release.* 94, 411–422. doi:10.1016/j.jconrel.2003.10.018

Oishi, M., Nagasaki, Y., Itaka, K., Nishiyama, N., and Kataoka, K. (2005). Lactosylated Poly(ethylene Glycol)-siRNA Conjugate through Acid-Labile Beta-Thiopropionate Linkage to Construct pH-Sensitive Polyion Complex Micelles Achieving Enhanced Gene Silencing in Hepatoma Cells. *J. Am. Chem. Soc.* 127, 1624–1625. doi:10.1021/ja044941d

Onishi, H., Ikeuchi-Takahashi, Y., Kawano, K., and Hattori, Y. (2019). Preparation of Chondroitin Sulfate-Glycyl-Prednisolone Conjugate Nanogel and its Efficacy in Rats with Ulcerative Colitis. *Biol. Pharm. Bull.* 42, 1155–1163. doi:10.1248/bpb.b19-00020

Oommen, O. P., Duehrkop, C., Nilsson, B., Hilborn, J., and Varghese, O. P. (2016). Multifunctional Hyaluronic Acid and Chondroitin Sulfate Nanoparticles: Impact of Glycosaminoglycan Presentation on Receptor Mediated Cellular Uptake and Immune Activation. *ACS Appl. Mater. Inter.* 8, 20614–20624. doi:10.1021/acsami.6b06823

Oommen, O. P., Garousi, J., Sloff, M., and Varghese, O. P. (2014). Tailored Doxorubicin-Hyaluronan Conjugate as a Potent Anticancer Glyco-Drug: an Alternative to Prodrug Approach. *Macromol. Biosci.* 14, 327–333. doi:10.1002/MABI.201300383

Oxley, S. M., and Sackstein, R. (1994). Detection of an L-Selectin Ligand on a Hematopoietic Progenitor Cell Line. *Blood.* 84, 3299–3306. doi:10.1182/blood.v84.10.3299.bloodjournal84103299

Park, K. (2007). Nanotechnology: What it Can Do for Drug Delivery. *J. Controlled Release.* 120, 1–3. doi:10.1016/j.jconrel.2007.05.003

Park, T., Jeong, J., and Kim, S. (2006). Current Status of Polymeric Gene Delivery Systems☆. *Adv. Drug Deliv. Rev.* 58, 467–486. doi:10.1016/j.addr.2006.03.007

Patnaik, S., Gorain, B., Padhi, S., Choudhury, H., Gabr, G. A., Md, S., et al. (2021). Recent Update of Toxicity Aspects of Nanoparticulate Systems for Drug Delivery. *Eur. J. Pharm. Biopharm.* 161, 100–119. doi:10.1016/j.ejpb.2021.02.010

Peer, D., Karp, J. M., Hong, S., Farokhzad, O. C., Margalit, R., and Langer, R. (2007). Nanocarriers as an Emerging Platform for Cancer Therapy. *Nat. Nanotech.* 2, 751–760. doi:10.1038/nnano.2007.387

Polizu, S., Savadogo, O., Poulin, P., and Yahia, L. (2006). Applications of Carbon Nanotubes-Based Biomaterials in Biomedical Nanotechnology. *J. Nanosci. Nanotechnol.* 6, 1883–1904. doi:10.1166/jnn.2006.197

Praetorius, N. P., and Mandal, T. K. (2008). Engineered Nanoparticles in Cancer Therapy. *Recent Pat. Drug Deliv. Formul.* 1, 37–51. doi:10.2174/187221107779814104

Prajapati, S. K., Jain, A., Shrivastava, C., and Jain, A. K. (2019). Hyaluronic Acid Conjugated Multi-Walled Carbon Nanotubes for colon Cancer Targeting. *Int. J. Biol. Macromol.* 123, 691–703. doi:10.1016/j.ijbiomac.2018.11.116

Qi, X., Fan, Y., He, H., and Wu, Z. (2015). Hyaluronic Acid-Grafted Polyamidoamine Dendrimers Enable Long Circulation and Active Tumor Targeting Simultaneously. *Carbohydr. Polym.* 126, 231–239. doi:10.1016/j.carbpol.2015.03.019

Qiao, L., Wang, X., Gao, Y., Wei, Q., Hu, W., Wu, L., et al. (2016). Laccase-mediated Formation of Mesoporous Silica Nanoparticle Based Redox Stimuli-Responsive Hybrid Nanogels as a Multifunctional Nanotheranostic Agent. *Nanoscale.* 8, 17241–17249. doi:10.1039/c6nr05943k

Ricci, V., Zonari, D., Cannito, S., Marengo, A., Scupoli, M. T., Malatesta, M., et al. (2018). Hyaluronated Mesoporous Silica Nanoparticles for Active Targeting: Influence of Conjugation Method and Hyaluronic Acid Molecular Weight on the Nanovector Properties. *J. Colloid Interf. Sci.* 516, 484–497. doi:10.1016/j.jcis.2018.01.072

Rizvi, S. A. A., and Saleh, A. M. (2018). Applications of Nanoparticle Systems in Drug Delivery Technology. *Saudi Pharm. J.* 26, 64–70. doi:10.1016/j.jsps.2017.10.012

Ruttala, H. B., Ramasamy, T., Gupta, B., Choi, H. G., Yong, C. S., and Kim, J. O. (2017). Multiple Polysaccharide-Drug Complex-Loaded Liposomes: A Unique Strategy in Drug Loading and Cancer Targeting. *Carbohydr. Polym.* 173, 57–66. doi:10.1016/j.carbpol.2017.05.062

Sahoo, S. K., and Labhasetwar, V. (2003). Nanotech Approaches to Drug Delivery and Imaging. *Drug Discov. Today.* 8 (24), 1112–20. doi:10.1016/S1359-6446(03)02903-9

Salari, N., Mansouri, K., Valipour, E., Abam, F., Jaymand, M., Rasoulpoor, S., et al. (2021). Hyaluronic Acid-Based Drug Nanocarriers as a Novel Drug Delivery System for Cancer Chemotherapy: A Systematic Review. *DARU J. Pharm. Sci.* 29, 439–447. doi:10.1007/S40199-021-00416-6

Saneja, A., Nayak, D., Srinivas, M., Kumar, A., Khare, V., Katoch, A., et al. (2017). Development and Mechanistic Insight into Enhanced Cytotoxic Potential of Hyaluronic Acid Conjugated Nanoparticles in CD44 Overexpressing Cancer Cells. *Eur. J. Pharm. Sci.* 97, 79–91. doi:10.1016/j.ejps.2016.10.028

Sargazi, A., Shiri, F., Keikha, S., and Majd, M. H. (2018). Hyaluronan Magnetic Nanoparticle for Mitoxantrone Delivery toward CD44-Positive Cancer Cells. *Colloids Surf. B Biointerfaces.* 171, 150–158. doi:10.1016/j.colsurfb.2018.07.025

Schroeder, A., Heller, D. A., Winslow, M. M., Dahlman, J. E., Pratt, G. W., Langer, R., et al. (2012). Treating Metastatic Cancer with Nanotechnology. *Nat. Rev. Cancer.* 12, 39–50. doi:10.1038/nrc3180

Senbanjo, L. T., and Chellaiah, M. A. (2017). CD44: A Multifunctional Cell Surface Adhesion Receptor Is a Regulator of Progression and Metastasis of Cancer Cells. *Front. Cell Dev. Biol.* 5, 18. doi:10.3389/fcell.2017.00018

Seok, H. Y., Sanoj Rejinold, N., Lekshmi, K. M., Cherukula, K., Park, I. K., and Kim, Y. C. (2018). CD44 Targeting Biocompatible and Biodegradable Hyaluronic Acid Cross-Linked Zein Nanogels for Curcumin Delivery to Cancer Cells: *In Vitro* and *In Vivo* Evaluation. *J. Control Release.* 280, 20–30. doi:10.1016/j.jconrel.2018.04.050

Shah, V., Taratula, O., Garbuzenko, O. B., Taratula, O. R., Rodriguez-Rodriguez, L., and Minko, T. (2013). Targeted Nanomedicine for Suppression of CD44 and Simultaneous Cell Death Induction in Ovarian Cancer: An Optimal Delivery of siRNA and Anticancer Drug. *Clin. Cancer Res.* 19, 6193–6204. doi:10.1158/1078-0432.CCR-13-1536

Shahriari, M., Taghdisi, S. M., Abnous, K., Ramezani, M., and Alibolandi, M. (2019). Synthesis of Hyaluronic Acid-Based Polymersomes for Doxorubicin Delivery to Metastatic Breast Cancer. *Int. J. Pharm.* 572, 118835. doi:10.1016/j.ijpharm.2019.118835

Shankar, R., Joshi, M., and Pathak, K. (2018). Lipid Nanoparticles: A Novel Approach for Brain Targeting. *Pharm. Nanotechnol.* 6, 81–93. doi:10.2174/2211738506666180611100416

Sharma, G., Anabousi, S., Ehrhardt, C., and Ravi Kumar, M. N. V. (2006). Liposomes as Targeted Drug Delivery Systems in the Treatment of Breast Cancer. *J. Drug Target.* 14, 301–310. doi:10.1080/10611860600809112

Sheikh, A., and Kesharwani, P. (2021). An Insight into Aptamer Engineered Dendrimer for Cancer Therapy. *Eur. Polym. J.* 159, 110746. doi:10.1016/J.EURPOLYMJ.2021.110746

Sherman, L., Sleeman, J., Herrlich, P., and Ponta, H. (1994). Hyaluronate Receptors: Key Players in Growth, Differentiation, Migration and Tumor Progression. *Curr. Opin. Cell Biol.* 6, 726–733. doi:10.1016/0955-0674(94)90100-7

Shi, S., Zhou, M., Li, X., Hu, M., Li, C., Li, M., et al. (2016). Synergistic Active Targeting of Dually Integrin αvβ3/CD44-targeted Nanoparticles to B16F10 Tumors Located at Different Sites of Mouse Bodies. *J. Control Release.* 235, 1–13. doi:10.1016/j.jconrel.2016.05.050

Sigmund, W., Yuh, J., Park, H., Maneeratana, V., Pyrgiotakis, G., Daga, A., et al. (2006). Processing and Structure Relationships in Electrospinning of Ceramic Fiber Systems. *J. Am. Ceram. Soc.* 89, 395–407. doi:10.1111/j.1551-2916.2005.00807.x

Singh, S., Numan, A., Maddiboyina, B., Arora, S., Riadi, Y., Md, S., et al. (2021). The Emerging Role of Immune Checkpoint Inhibitors in the Treatment of Triple-Negative Breast Cancer. *Drug Discov. Today.* 26, 1721–1727. doi:10.1016/j.drudis.2021.03.011

Singh, V., Sahebkar, A., and Kesharwani, P. (2021). Poly (Propylene Imine) Dendrimer as an Emerging Polymeric Nanocarrier for Anticancer Drug and Gene Delivery. *Eur. Polym. J.* 158, 110683. doi:10.1016/j.eurpolymj.2021.110683

Singh, V., and Kesharwani, P. (2021). Recent Advances in Microneedles-Based Drug Delivery Device in the Diagnosis and Treatment of Cancer. *J. Control Release.* 338, 394–409. doi:10.1016/J.JCONREL.2021.08.054

Singhai, N. J., Maheshwari, R., and Ramteke, S. (2020). CD44 Receptor Targeted 'smart' Multi-Walled Carbon Nanotubes for Synergistic Therapy of Triple-

Negative Breast Cancer. *Colloid Interf. Sci. Commun.* 35, 100235. doi:10.1016/j.colcom.2020.100235

Sofou, S., and Sgouros, G. (2008). Antibody-targeted Liposomes in Cancer Therapy and Imaging. *Expert Opin. Drug Deliv.* 5, 189–204. doi:10.1517/17425247.5.2.189

Soleymani, M., Velashjerdi, M., and Asgari, M. (2021). Preparation of Hyaluronic Acid-Decorated Mixed Nanomicelles for Targeted Delivery of Hydrophobic Drugs to CD44-Overexpressing Cancer Cells. *Int. J. Pharm.* 592, 120052. doi:10.1016/j.ijpharm.2020.120052

Song, M., Liang, Y., Li, K., Zhang, J., Zhang, N., Tian, B., et al. (2019). Hyaluronic Acid Modified Liposomes for Targeted Delivery of Doxorubicin and Paclitaxel to CD44 Overexpressing Tumor Cells with Improved Dual-Drugs Synergistic Effect. *J. Drug Deliv. Sci. Technology.* 53, 101179. doi:10.1016/j.jddst.2019.101179

Spadea, A., Rios De La Rosa, J. M., Tirella, A., Ashford, M. B., Williams, K. J., Stratford, I. J., et al. (2019). Evaluating the Efficiency of Hyaluronic Acid for Tumor Targeting via CD44. *Mol. Pharm.* 16, 2481–2493. doi:10.1021/acs.molpharmaceut.9b00083

Srivastava, S., Mahor, A., Singh, G., Bansal, K., Singh, P. P., Gupta, R., et al. (2021). Formulation Development, *In Vitro* and *In Vivo* Evaluation of Topical Hydrogel Formulation of Econazole Nitrate-Loaded β-Cyclodextrin Nanosponges. *J. Pharm. Sci.* 110, 3702–3714. doi:10.1016/J.XPHS.2021.07.008

Storm, G., Belliot, S. O., Daemen, T., and Lasic, D. D. (1995). Surface Modification of Nanoparticles to Oppose Uptake by the Mononuclear Phagocyte System. *Adv. Drug Deliv. Rev.* 17 (1), 31–48. doi:10.1016/0169-409X(95)00039-A

Surekha, B., Kommana, N. S., Dubey, S. K., Kumar, A. V. P., Shukla, R., and Kesharwani, P. (2021). PAMAM Dendrimer as a Talented Multifunctional Biomimetic Nanocarrier for Cancer Diagnosis and Therapy. *Colloids Surf. B Biointerfaces.* 204, 111837. doi:10.1016/j.colsurfb.2021.111837

Tadros, T., Izquierdo, P., Esquena, J., and Solans, C. (2004). Formation and Stability of Nano-Emulsions. *Adv. Colloid Interf. Sci.* 108-109, 303–318. doi:10.1016/j.cis.2003.10.023

Tang, J., Zhou, H., Hou, X., Wang, L., Li, Y., Pang, Y., et al. (2018). Enhanced Anti-tumor Efficacy of Temozolomide-Loaded Carboxylated Poly(amido-Amine) Combined with Photothermal/photodynamic Therapy for Melanoma Treatment. *Cancer Lett.* 423, 16–26. doi:10.1016/j.canlet.2018.03.002

Thapa, R., and Wilson, G. D. (2016). The Importance of CD44 as a Stem Cell Biomarker and Therapeutic Target in Cancer. *Stem Cell Int.* 2016, 1–15. doi:10.1155/2016/2087204

Thomas, S. C., Harshita, B. S. P., Mishra, P. K., and Talegaonkar, S. (2015). Ceramic Nanoparticles: Fabrication Methods and Applications in Drug Delivery. *Curr. Pharm. Des.* 21, 6165–6188. doi:10.2174/1381612821666151027153246

Tian, Q., Wang, Q., Yao, K. X., Teng, B., Zhang, J., Yang, S., et al. (2014). Multifunctional polypyrrole@Fe(3)O(4) Nanoparticles for Dual-Modal Imaging and *In Vivo* Photothermal Cancer Therapy. *Small.* 10, 1063–1068. doi:10.1002/smll.201302042

Tirella, A., Kloc-Muniak, K., Good, L., Ridden, J., Ashford, M., Puri, S., et al. (2019). CD44 Targeted Delivery of siRNA by Using HA-Decorated Nanotechnologies for KRAS Silencing in Cancer Treatment. *Int. J. Pharm.* 561, 114–123. doi:10.1016/j.ijpharm.2019.02.032

Tokihiro, T., and Hanamura, E. (1984). Multi-polariton Scattering via Excitonic Molecules. *Solid State. Commun.* 52, 771–774. doi:10.1016/0038-1098(84)90002-4

Torchilin, V. P. (2005). Recent Advances with Liposomes as Pharmaceutical Carriers. *Nat. Rev. Drug Discov.* 4, 145–160. doi:10.1038/nrd1632

Torchilin, V. P., and Trubetskoy, V. S. (1995). Which Polymers Can Make Nanoparticulate Drug Carriers Long-Circulating? *Adv. Drug Deliv. Rev.* 16 (2–3), 141–155. doi:10.1016/0169-409X(95)00022-Y

Van Zon, A., Mossink, M. H., Houtsmuller, A. B., Schoester, M., Scheffer, G. L., Scheper, R. J., et al. (2006). Vault Mobility Depends in Part on Microtubules and Vaults Can Be Recruited to the Nuclear Envelope. *Exp. Cell Res.* 312, 245–255. doi:10.1016/j.yexcr.2005.10.016

Wang, H., Zhu, Z., Zhang, G., Lin, F., Liu, Y., Zhang, Y., et al. (2019). AS1411 Aptamer/Hyaluronic Acid-Bifunctionalized Microemulsion Co-loading Shikonin and Docetaxel for Enhanced Antiglioma Therapy. *J. Pharm. Sci.* 108, 3684–3694. doi:10.1016/j.xphs.2019.08.017

Wang, H., Sun, H., Wei, H., Xi, P., Nie, S., and Ren, Q. (2014). Biocompatible Hyaluronic Acid Polymer-Coated Quantum Dots for CD44+ Cancer Cell-Targeted Imaging. *J. Nanopart Res.* 16, 1–13. doi:10.1007/s11051-014-2621-x

Wang, N., Tytell, J. D., and Ingber, D. E. (2009). Mechanotransduction at a Distance: Mechanically Coupling the Extracellular Matrix with the Nucleus. *Nat. Rev. Mol. Cell Biol.* 10, 75–82. doi:10.1038/nrm2594

Wang, S., Sugahara, K., and Li, F. (2016). Chondroitin Sulfate/dermatan Sulfate Sulfatases from Mammals and Bacteria. *Glycoconj. J.* 33, 841–851. doi:10.1007/s10719-016-9720-0

Wang, Z., Sau, S., Alsaab, H. O., and Iyer, A. K. (2018). CD44 Directed Nanomicellar Payload Delivery Platform for Selective Anticancer Effect and Tumor Specific Imaging of Triple Negative Breast Cancer. *Nanomedicine.* 14, 1441–1454. doi:10.1016/j.nano.2018.04.004

Wei, X., Senanayake, T. H., Warren, G., and Vinogradov, S. V. (2013). Hyaluronic Acid-Based Nanogel-Drug Conjugates with Enhanced Anticancer Activity Designed for the Targeting of Cd44-Positive and Drug-Resistant Tumors. *Bioconjug. Chem.* 24, 658–668. doi:10.1021/bc300632w

Williams, K., Motiani, K., Giridhar, P. V., and Kasper, S. (2013). CD44 Integrates Signaling in normal Stem Cell, Cancer Stem Cell and (Pre) metastatic Niches. *Exp. Biol. Med. (Maywood).* 238, 324–338. doi:10.1177/1535370213480714

Wolfbeis, O. S. (2015). An Overview of Nanoparticles Commonly Used in Fluorescent Bioimaging. *Chem. Soc. Rev.* 44, 4743–4768. doi:10.1039/c4cs00392f

Xiong, Q., Cui, M., Bai, Y., Liu, Y., Liu, D., and Song, T. (2017). A Supramolecular Nanoparticle System Based on β-cyclodextrin-conjugated Poly-L-Lysine and Hyaluronic Acid for Co-delivery of Gene and Chemotherapy Agent Targeting Hepatocellular Carcinoma. *Colloids Surf. B Biointerfaces.* 155, 93–103. doi:10.1016/j.colsurfb.2017.04.008

Yang, H., Liu, Y., Qiu, Y., Ding, M., and Zhang, Y. (2019). MiRNA-204-5p and Oxaliplatin-Loaded Silica Nanoparticles for Enhanced Tumor Suppression Effect in CD44-Overexpressed colon Adenocarcinoma. *Int. J. Pharm.* 566, 585–593. doi:10.1016/j.ijpharm.2019.06.020

Yang, Y., Long, Y., Wang, Y., Ren, K., Li, M., Zhang, Z., et al. (2020). Enhanced Anti-tumor and Anti-metastasis Therapy for Triple Negative Breast Cancer by CD44 Receptor-Targeted Hybrid Self-Delivery Micelles. *Int. J. Pharm.* 577, 119085. doi:10.1016/j.ijpharm.2020.119085

Yezhelyev, M. V., Gao, X., Xing, Y., Al-Hajj, A., Nie, S., and O'Regan, R. M. (2006). Emerging Use of Nanoparticles in Diagnosis and Treatment of Breast Cancer. *Lancet Oncol.* 7 (8), 657–67. doi:10.1016/S1470-2045(06)70793-8

Yoon, H. Y., Kim, H. R., Saravanakumar, G., Heo, R., Chae, S. Y., Um, W., et al. (2013). Bioreducible Hyaluronic Acid Conjugates as siRNA Carrier for Tumor Targeting. *J. Control Release.* 172, 653–661. doi:10.1016/j.jconrel.2013.09.008

Yu, T., Li, Y., Gu, X., and Li, Q. (2020). Development of a Hyaluronic Acid-Based Nanocarrier Incorporating Doxorubicin and Cisplatin as a pH-Sensitive and CD44-Targeted Anti-Breast Cancer Drug Delivery System. *Front. Pharmacol.* 11, 532457. doi:10.3389/fphar.2020.532457

Zafar, A., Alruwaili, N. K., Imam, S. S., Alharbi, K. S., Afzal, M., Alotaibi, N. H., et al. (2021). Novel Nanotechnology Approaches for Diagnosis and Therapy of Breast, Ovarian and Cervical Cancer in Female: A Review. *J. Drug Deliv. Sci. Technology.* 61, 102198. doi:10.1016/j.jddst.2020.102198

Zeeshan, F., Madheswaran, T., Panneerselvam, J., Taliyan, R., and Kesharwani, P. (2021). Human Serum Albumin as Multifunctional Nanocarrier for Cancer Therapy. *J. Pharm. Sci.* 110, 3111–3117. doi:10.1016/j.xphs.2021.05.001

Zeilstra, J., Joosten, S. P., Dokter, M., Verwiel, E., Spaargaren, M., and Pals, S. T. (2008). Deletion of the WNT Target and Cancer Stem Cell Marker CD44 in Apc(Min/+) Mice Attenuates Intestinal Tumorigenesis. *Cancer Res.* 68, 3655–3661. doi:10.1158/0008-5472.CAN-07-2940

Zhang, M., Dai, Z., Theivendran, S., Gu, Z., Zhao, L., Song, H., et al. (2021). Nanotechnology Enabled Reactive Species Regulation in Biosystems for Boosting Cancer Immunotherapy. *Nano Today.* 36, 101035. doi:10.1016/j.nantod.2020.101035

Zhang, M., Fang, Z., Zhao, X., Niu, Y., Lou, J., Zhao, L., et al. (2016). Hyaluronic Acid Functionalized Nitrogen-Doped Carbon Quantum Dots for Targeted Specific Bioimaging. *RSC Adv.* 6, 104979–104984. doi:10.1039/c6ra22210b

Zhang, X., Pan, J., Yao, M., Palmerston Mendes, L., Sarisozen, C., Mao, S., et al. (2020). Charge Reversible Hyaluronic Acid-Modified Dendrimer-Based Nanoparticles for siMDR-1 and Doxorubicin Co-delivery. *Eur. J. Pharm. Biopharm.* 154, 43–49. doi:10.1016/j.ejpb.2020.06.019

Zhao, G., and Rodriguez, L. B. (2012). Molecular Targeting of Liposomal Nanoparticles to Tumor Microenvironment. *Int. J. Nanomedicine.* 8, 61. doi:10.2147/IJN.S37859

13

PI3K/Akt/mTOR Pathway and its Role in Cancer Therapeutics: Are we Making Headway?

Yan Peng[1], Yuanyuan Wang[2], Cheng Zhou[3], Wuxuan Mei[2] and Changchun Zeng[3]*

[1] Department of Obstetrics, Longhua District Central Hospital, Shenzhen, China, [2] Xianning Medical College, Hubei University of Science and Technology, Xianning, China, [3] Department of Medical Laboratory, Shenzhen Longhua District Central Hospital, Guangdong Medical University, Shenzhen, China

***Correspondence:**
Changchun Zeng
zengchch@glmc.edu.cn

Cancer is a severe public health issue that is a leading cause of mortality globally. It is also an impediment to improving life expectancy worldwide. Furthermore, the global burden of cancer incidence and death is continuously growing. Current therapeutic options are insufficient for patients, and tumor complexity and heterogeneity necessitate customized medicine or targeted therapy. It is critical to identify potential cancer therapeutic targets. Aberrant activation of the PI3K/AKT/mTOR pathway has a significant role in carcinogenesis. This review summarized oncogenic PI3K/Akt/mTOR pathway alterations in cancer and various cancer hallmarks associated with the PI3K/AKT/mTOR pathway, such as cell proliferation, autophagy, apoptosis, angiogenesis, epithelial-to-mesenchymal transition (EMT), and chemoresistance. Importantly, this review provided recent advances in PI3K/AKT/mTOR inhibitor research. Overall, an in-depth understanding of the association between the PI3K/AKT/mTOR pathway and tumorigenesis and the development of therapies targeting the PI3K/AKT/mTOR pathway will help make clinical decisions.

Keywords: PI3K/Akt/mTOR pathway, targeted therapy, precision medicine, cancer, oncogenic alterations

INTRODUCTION

The mammalian target of rapamycin complex 1 (mTORC1) and the mammalian target of rapamycin complex 2 (mTORC2) are two distinct complexes formed by the mTOR. Growth factors, rapamycin, insulin, phosphatidic acid, certain amino acids, and oxidative stress affect the activity of mTOCR1, which is comprised of mTOR, Raptor, MLST8, PRAS40, and DEPTOR. The most classical targets downstream of mTOCR1 are S6K and 4EBP1, which play critical roles in protein synthesis, nutritional response, and tumor development. mTORC2 is composed of mTOR, RICTOR, mLST8, PROTOR1/2, DEPTOR, and mSIN1. mTORC2 interacts with PDK1 to activate AKT *via* phosphorylating it. Moreover, mTORC2 plays a critical role in the actin cytoskeleton, cell cycle, and survival (1–5). Receptor tyrosine kinases (RTKs), alterations in PIK3CA and its effectors, reduced PTEN expression, and other events contribute to oncogenic stimulation of the PI3K/Akt/mTOR pathway (6–8). In this review, we mainly described the genetic alterations of the PI3K/Akt/mTOR pathway. The mutations and amplification of PIK3CA are the most occurring events in cancer, and abnormal PI3K activity is a transforming event in the disease process (9). Alteration in AKT can cause an abnormal increase in the phosphorylated level of Akt in cancer cells (10). PTEN is another component of the PI3K/Akt signaling pathway, and its dysregulation can enhance cell growth, proliferation, and survival. Loss of heterozygosity (LOH), mutations, promoter methylation, and post-translational inhibition of PTEN are events in tumors and are involved in the pathogenesis of tumors (11, 12).

In this era of precision medicine, there are some advances in tailored, targeted therapies that inhibit specific pathways, potentially halting the evolution and spread of cancer. Understanding the abnormal expression of cancer pathway genes that play a vital role in cancer genesis and progression will contribute to cancer therapies. Based on current cancer genomic investigations, several critical cancer pathways are abnormally regulated (13). The PI3K/AKT/mTOR signaling pathway has been described as one of the most commonly disrupted pathways in cancer, making it an attractive candidate for therapeutic intervention. The PI3K/AKT/mTOR pathway is crucial for cell motility, growth, survival, and metabolism in cancer (14, 15). The current commercially accessible targeted inhibitors for cancer patients with abnormal activation of the PI3K/AKT/mTOR pathway include everolimus (mTOR inhibitor), sirolimus (mTOR inhibitor), temsirolimus (mTOR inhibitor), alpelisib (PI3K inhibitor), duvelisib (PI3K inhibitor), copanlisib (PI3K inhibitor), idelalisib (PI3K inhibitor), umbralisib (PI3K inhibitor). Phase III clinical trials of AKT inhibitors, such as capivasertib and ipatasertib, have been proceeded in cancer (**Figure 1** and **Table 1**) (6, 16, 17). Preclinical and clinical trials have shown encouraging outcomes for these targeted medicines. However, resistance to these medications is a drawback to their clinical usage. The rising prevalence of cancer necessitates the development of increasingly effective targeted medicines. Additionally, drugs targeting the PI3K/AKT/mTOR pathway in combination with chemotherapy drugs or other targeted drugs can inhibit tumor development (18). This review highlights the importance of the PI3K/AKT/mTOR pathway in

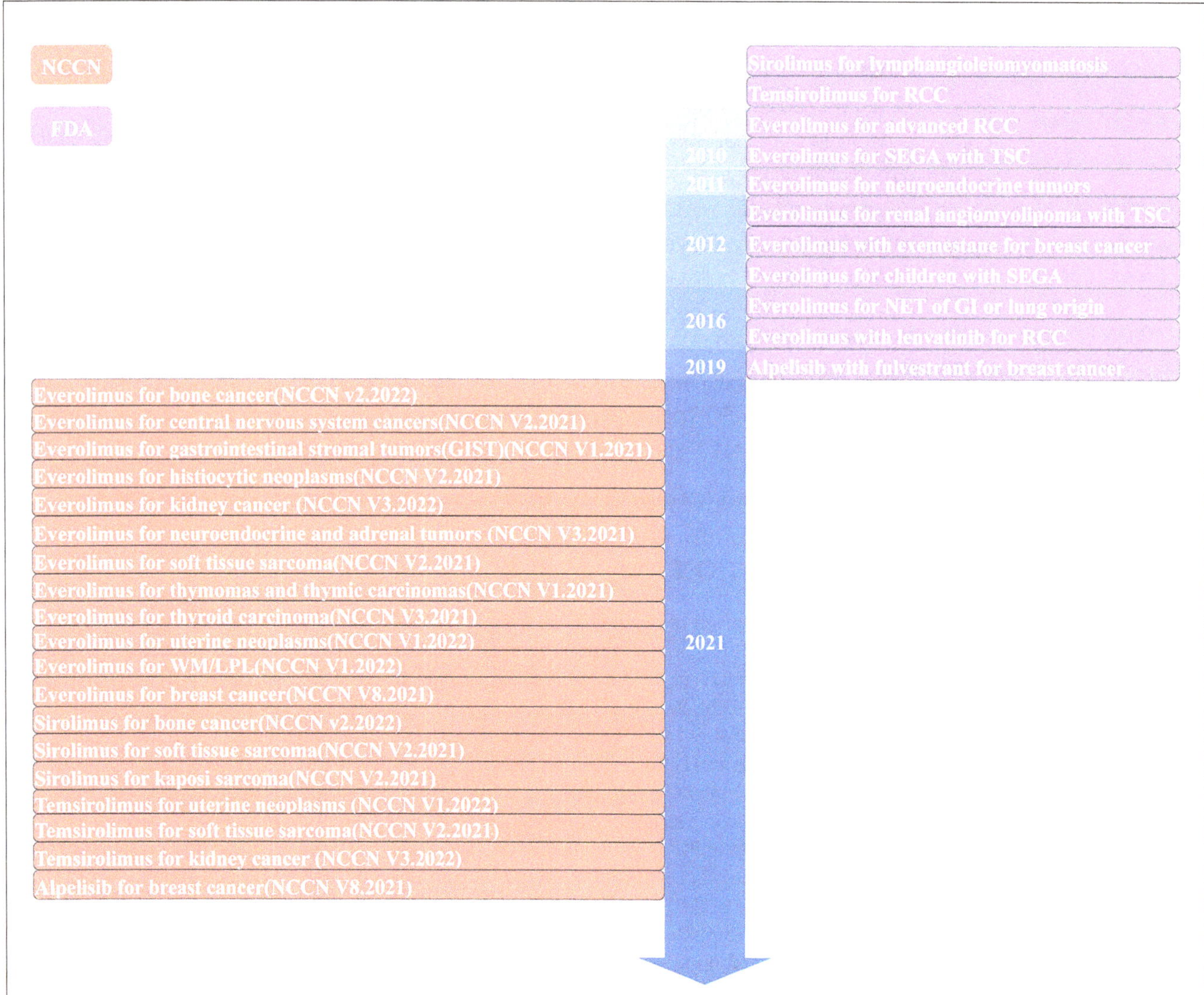

FIGURE 1 | Timeline of The Food and Drug Administration (FDA)-approved or the National Comprehensive Cancer Network (NCCN) recommended inhibitors targeting the PI3K/AKT/mTOR pathway in solid tumors. WM, Waldenstrom macroglobulinemia; LPL, lymphoplasmacytic lymphoma; RCC, renal cell carcinoma; SEGA, subependymal giant cell astrocytoma; TSC, tuberous sclerosis complex; NET, neuroendocrine tumor; GI, gastrointestinal.

TABLE 1 | PI3K/AKT/mTOR pathway inhibitors.

Inhibitors	Targets	FDA-approved status	Clinical trial	Condition
Piqray (alpelisib) 2019 year	PI3Kα	Yes	NCT02437318(Phase III)	In combination with fulvestrant for postmenopausal women, and men, with HR-positive, HER2-negative, PIK3CA-mutated, advanced or metastatic breast cancer.
Copiktra (duvelisib) 2018 year	PI3Kδ, PI3Kγ	Yes	NCT02004522(Phase III);NCT02204982 (Phase III)	Adult patients with relapsed or refractory CLL or SLL or FL after at least two prior therapies.
Aliqopa (copanlisib) 2017 year	PI3Kδ, PI3Kα	Yes	NCT01660451(Phase II)	Copanlisib for the treatment of adult patients with relapsed FL.
Zydelig (idelalisib) 2014 year	PI3Kδ	Yes	NCT01539512(Phase III)	Chronic lymphocytic leukemia, relapsed follicular B-cell non-Hodgkin lymphoma, and relapsed small lymphocytic lymphoma.
Ukoniq (umbralisib) 2021year	PI3Kδ, CK1ε	Yes	NCT02793583 (Phase II/III)	MZL and FL.
Sonolisib (PX-866) 2015 year	PI3Kα, PI3Kγ, PI3Kδ	No	NCT01259869(Phase II)	Glioblastoma multiforme at the time of first relapse or progression.
Buparlisib (NVP-BKM120) 2018 year	PI3Kα, PI3Kβ, PI3Kγ, PI3Kδ	No	NCT01633060(Phase III)	In combination fulvestrant, in postmenopausal women with HR-positive HER2-negative aromatase inhibitor-treated, locally advanced or metastatic breast cancer who progressed on or after mTOR inhibitor-based treatment.
Afinitor (everolimus) 2009 year	mTORC1, mTORC2	Yes	NCT00863655(Phase III); NCT00510068 (Phase III); NCT01524783(Phase III); NCT00412061(Phase III); NCT00410124 (Phase III)	Advanced HR+, HER2- breast cancer; PNET; progressive NET of gastrointestinal or lung origin; advanced renal cell carcinoma; SEGA and renal angiomyolipomas associated with tuberous sclerosis.
Rapamune (Sirolimus) 1999 year	mTORC1, mTORC2	Yes	NCT00414648(Phase III)	The prophylaxis of organ rejection in patients aged 13 years or older receiving renal transplants, and LAM.
Torisel (temsirolimus) 2007year	mTORC1, mTORC2	Yes	NCT00065468(Phase III)	Advanced renal cell carcinoma.
Capivasertib (AZD5363) 2020 year	AKT1, AKT2, AKT3	No	NCT03997123(Phase III)	Locally advanced or metastatic triple-negative breast cancer
Ipatasertib (GDC-0068) 2021 year	AKT1, AKT2, AKT3	No	NCT03072238(Phase III)	Ipatasertib plus abiraterone and prednisolone in metastatic castration-resistant prostate cancer
MK-2206 2020 year	AKT1, AKT2, AKT3	No	NCT01042379(Phase II)	HER2-positive and/or HR-negative breast cancer

HR: hormone receptor; HER2: epidermal growth factor receptor 2; CLL: chronic lymphocytic leukemia; SLL: small lymphocytic lymphoma; FL: follicular lymphoma; MZL: marginal zone lymphoma; PNET: progressive neuroendocrine tumors of pancreatic origin; NET: neuroendocrine tumors; SEGA: subependymal giant cell astrocytoma; LAM: lymphangioleiomyomatosis.

cancer genesis and progression and summarizes inhibitors of this axis for cancer prevention and treatment.

ONCOGENIC PI3K/AKT/MTOR PATHWAY ALTERATIONS IN CANCER

Genetic Alterations in the PIK3CA Gene

The p110 α (p110α) subunit encoded by the PIK3CA gene is the most prevalent altered catalytic subunit of the phosphatidylinositol 3-kinase (PI3K) isoform in cancer. PI3K, comprised of a catalytic subunit (p110α) and a regulatory subunit (p85α), is a class of lipid kinases that participates in cellular functions, including cell proliferation, growth, differentiation, migration, and survival (**Figure 2A**). Numerous receptor tyrosine kinases, such as ERBB2, EGFR, MET, RET, and VEGFR, transform extracellular stimuli into intracellular signals and bind PI3K to the plasma membrane through scaffold proteins like IRS1 or by activation of RAS. After being stimulated, PI3K-110α transforms its lipid substrate phosphatidylinositol-4,5-bisphosphate (PIP2) to phosphatidylinositol- 3,4,5-bisphosphate (PIP3), triggering the AKT/mTOR pathway (19).

According to various studies, the mutation frequency of the PIK3CA gene ranges from 11% to 14% in cancer. PIK3CA activation mutations are identified in multiple tumor types, such as breast cancer, uterine corpus endometrial carcinoma, carcinoma of the uterine cervix, colorectal carcinoma, esophageal carcinoma, gallbladder carcinoma, non-small cell lung cancer, ovarian carcinoma, and gastric cancer (**Table 2**). 13% (1354/ 10336) of patients harbored PIK3CA mutations in MSK-

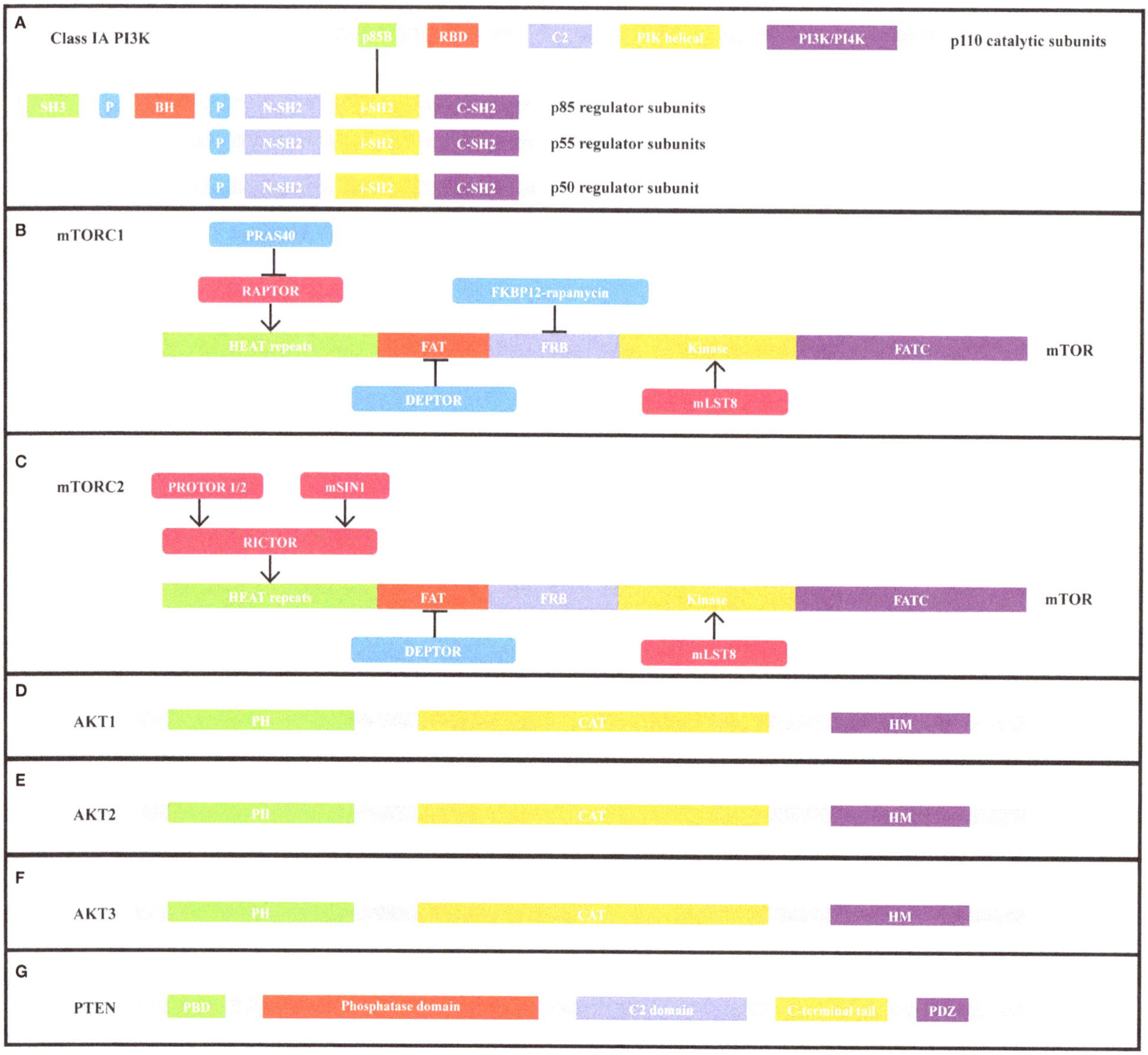

FIGURE 2 | Structure of class IA PI3K, mTORC1, mTORC2, AKT1, AKT2, AKT3, and PTEN from Uniprot.org. **(A)** class IA PI3K consists of catalytic and regulatory subunits. **(B)** mTORC1 subunits and corresponding binding sites on mTOR. **(C)** mTORC2 subunits and corresponding binding sites on mTOR. **(D)** Structure of AKT1. **(E)** Structure of AKT2. **(F)** Structure of AKT3. **(G)** Structure of PTEN. RBD, Ras binding domain; P, proline-rich domain; BH, breakpoint cluster homology domain; C2, membrane-interacting domain; iSH2, inter-SH2 domain; FRB, FKBP12-rapamycin-binding; HEAT, Huntingtin/Elongation factor 3/a subunit of protein phosphatase2A/TOR1; mSIN1, mammalian stress-activated; PH, pleckstrin homology; CAT, catalytic domain; HM, hydrophobic motif.

IMPACT Clinical Sequencing Cohort, while 11% (1143/10194) of patients harbored PIK3CA mutations in China Pan-cancer Cohort (OrigiMed2020) (20, 22). The most common mutations in PIK3CA are in the helix domain (E542/E545) and the kinase domain (H1047) (22–24). PIK3CA mutations are prevalent in breast cancer, with 35.7% (2261/6338) of tumors carrying the mutations, most common in estrogen receptor-positive breast cancer. H1047R (35%), E545K (17%), E542K (11%), N345K (6%), and H1047L (3%) were the five mutations that accounted for 73% of all PIK3CA mutations (25). PIK3CA H1047R and H1047L are hotspot mutations within the PI3K/PI4K kinase domain of the Pik3ca protein. Moreover, the E545K and E542K mutations in the PIK helical domain of the Pik3ca protein are also hotspot mutations. Besides, PIK3CA N345K lies in the Pik3ca protein's C2 PI3K-type domain. H1047R, H1047L, E545K, E542K, and N345K contribute to enhanced Akt and Mek1/2 phosphorylation, cell survival, and transformation (26, 27). PIK3CA amplification is a frequent genetic event in various cancers such as lung squamous cell carcinoma, cervical squamous cell carcinoma, esophageal adenocarcinoma, breast carcinoma, and is usually mutually exclusive with PIK3CA mutations. Increased PIK3CA copy number is strongly

TABLE 2 | Genetic alterations of the PIK3CA, mTOR, PTEN, AKT1, AKT2, and AKT3 genes in human cancers.

PIK3CA **Cancer Type**	**Number of Cases**	**Mutation Frequency**	**Amplification Frequency**
Endometrial Carcinoma	586	44.54%	4.10%
Cervical Squamous Cell Carcinoma	251	22.71%	11.55%
Invasive Breast Carcinoma	1084	30.72%	1.85%
Head and Neck Squamous Cell Carcinoma	523	13.58%	11.85%
Colorectal Adenocarcinoma	594	24.75%	–
Bladder Urothelial Carcinoma	411	20.44%	2.68%
Non-Small Cell Lung Cancer	1053	5.41%	15.95%
Ovarian Epithelial Tumor	584	0.86%	19.35%
Esophagogastric Adenocarcinoma	514	14.20%	5.06%
Diffuse Glioma	513	8.19%	0.78%
Glioblastoma	592	6.25%	2.53%
Melanoma	444	4.73%	0.45%
Prostate Adenocarcinoma	494	2.02%	2.23%
mTOR			
Cancer Type	Number of Cases	Mutation Frequency	Amplification Frequency
Melanoma	444	11.94%	0.90%
Endometrial Carcinoma	586	10.58%	0.85%
Esophagogastric Adenocarcinoma	514	6.42%	1.75%
Colorectal Adenocarcinoma	594	6.73%	–
Renal Clear Cell Carcinoma	511	6.07%	–
Non-Small Cell Lung Cancer	1053	4.18%	0.19%
PTEN			
Cancer Type	Number of Cases	Mutation Frequency	Delation Frequency
Endometrial Carcinoma	586	58.02%	2.56%
Glioblastoma	592	22.13%	8.95%
Prostate Adenocarcinoma	494	2.63%	15.59%
Melanoma	444	9.46%	5.86%
Cervical Squamous Cell Carcinoma	251	7.57%	4.78%
Esophagogastric Adenocarcinoma	514	6.03%	4.28%
Invasive Breast Carcinoma	1084	5.17%	4.98%
Non-Small Cell Lung Cancer	1053	5.60%	4.75%
Sarcoma	255	2.35%	5.88%
Colorectal Adenocarcinoma	594	5.22%	2.36%
Bladder Urothelial Carcinoma	411	3.89%	3.16%
Ovarian Epithelial Tumor	584	1.20%	4.45%
Diffuse Glioma	513	4.68%	0.97%
Hepatocellular Carcinoma	369	1.90%	3.52%
Head and Neck Squamous Cell Carcinoma	523	2.29%	2.87%
AKT1			
Cancer Type	Number of Cases	Mutation Frequency	Amplification Frequency
Endometrial Carcinoma	586	3.24%	1.02%
Ovarian Epithelial Tumor	584	3.94%	0.17%
Invasive Breast Carcinoma	1084	2.49%	1.11%
Melanoma	444	2.70%	–
Cervical Squamous Cell Carcinoma	251	1.59%	1.20%
Non-Small Cell Lung Cancer	1053	0.85%	1.71%
AKT2			
Cancer Type	Number of Cases	Mutation Frequency	Amplification Frequency
Pancreatic Adenocarcinoma	184	0.54%	7.07%
Endometrial Carcinoma	586	3.58%	3.57%
Ovarian Epithelial Tumor	584	0.17%	5.31%
Cervical Squamous Cell Carcinoma	251	1.99%	3.59%
Sarcoma	255	0.39%	3.53%
Non-Small Cell Lung Cancer	1053	1.14%	3.32%
Esophagogastric Adenocarcinoma	514	2.14%	1.17%
Bladder Urothelial Carcinoma	411	0.97%	2.43%
AKT3			
Cancer Type	Number of Cases	Mutation Frequency	Amplification Frequency
Invasive Breast Carcinoma	1084	0.74%	9.78%
Endometrial Carcinoma	586	5.29%	2.73%
Hepatocellular Carcinoma	369	0.27%	5.96%
Melanoma	444	2.48%	2.93%

(Continued)

TABLE 2 | Continued

PIK3CA Cancer Type	Number of Cases	Mutation Frequency	Amplification Frequency
Ovarian Epithelial Tumor	584	5.65%	–
Non-Small Cell Lung Cancer	1053	1.14%	3.51%
Esophagogastric Adenocarcinoma	514	1.75%	1.36%
Pancreatic Adenocarcinoma	184	0.54%	2.17%
Colorectal Adenocarcinoma	594	2.19%	0.51%

The Cancer Genome Atlas (TCGA) PanCancer Atlas Studies included 32 studies selected (10967 samples) (20, 21).

associated with increased PIK3CA expression and PI3K activity in malignancies. In addition, breast cancer patients with high PIK3CA copy numbers have a worse prognosis (22–24, 28).

Genetic Alterations in the mTOR Gene

The mTOR protein, which is encoded by the mTOR gene, belongs to a serine-threonine kinase that controls cell responses to stressors such as growth factors, nutrient deprivation, and DNA damage and regulates tumor growth, survival, and metabolic signaling (**Figures 2B, C**). mTOR activation mutations enhance the kinase activity of mTOR, resulting in the overactivation of downstream pro-proliferative pathways. MTOR mutations are common in malignant tumors, such as endometrial carcinoma, melanoma, esophagogastric adenocarcinoma, colorectal adenocarcinoma, renal cell carcinoma, and bladder cancer (**Table 2**) (29). In MSK-IMPACT Clinical Sequencing Cohort, MTOR is mutated at a rate of 3% (329/10336) in metastatic cancer, which is also observed at the similar rate (2.9%, 292/10194) observed in China Pan-cancer Cohort (OrigiMed2020) (20, 22). Nonsynonymous mTOR mutations are present in 10.4% (N=412) of melanoma patients and are associated with a poor prognosis (30). Besides, 6% of clear-cell renal cell carcinoma patients with mTOR mutation were identified (31). The predicted mutation incidence was 3% (N=8630) for mTOR in head and neck cancer (32). The mTOR missense mutations are found in a wide variety of malignancies, most notably in roughly 7.5% of lung adenocarcinomas, 6% of clear cell renal cell carcinomas, 5% of endometrial carcinomas, and 4% of colorectal carcinomas (33). The most prevalent alterations of MTOR in malignant tumors are E1799K, S2215F, and amplification (29). Mutations in key regions such as HEAT repeat, FAT domain, and kinase domain make the mTOR gene highly tumorigenic. Moreover, mTOR W1456R, M938T, V2284M, T2294I, V2291I, P2273S, G1479N, and E2288K mutants dramatically elevated the activity of protein kinase. Besides, the mTOR/p70S6K pathway was significantly increased in the W1456R, P2273S, and E2288K mutants. In addition, the W1456R, P2273S, and E2288K mutants affected the mTOR/p70S6K and Akt pathways (34).

Genetic Alterations in the AKT Gene

AKT1, AKT2, and AKT3, as members of the AGC kinase family, are serine/threonine protein kinases and downstream effectors of the PI3K signaling pathway (**Figures 2D–F**). Following PI3K activation, cytosolic AKT1 is transported to the membrane where it interacts with PIP3 (PtdIns3,4,5-P3), resulting in AKT1 phosphorylation and activation. AKT1 can stimulate a variety of downstream effectors, including GSK3, FOXO, and mTORC1, all of which are crucial for cell survival, growth, and metabolism. AKT1 can be negatively regulated as a result of PTEN phosphatase activity inhibiting PI3K. Besides, activation of the PI3K pathway or inactivation of PTEN can cause AKT1 activation in cancers. AKT1 activation mutations and AKT1 infrequent amplification enable AKT1 activation independent of phosphoinositide (14, 35, 36). The activating mutations of AKT2 and AKT3 induce disruption of intramolecular pleckstrin homology domain (PH) and kinase domain (KD) interactions, resulting in AKT oncogenic activation (37). AKT1, AKT2, AKT3 aberrations were identified in 1.8% (183/10336), 1.6% (163/10336), and 1.4% (149/10336) of patients in the MSK-IMPACT Clinical Sequencing Cohort, respectively. While AKT1, AKT2, AKT3 aberrations were identified in 1.4% (138/10194), 2% (206/10194), and 1.2% (122/10194) of patients in China Pan-cancer Cohort (OrigiMed2020) (20, 22). AKT1 E17K is a hotspot mutation, the most frequent AKT1 mutation in breast cancer, and a highly recurrent AKT1 mutation in many other cancer types. 6.3% (N=619) of breast cancer patients carry the AKT1 E17K mutation, associated with increased mortality (38). AKT1 E17K mutation boosts the binding of Akt1 to the phosphatidylinositol-3,4,5-trisphosphate (PIP3) ligand, which facilitates Akt transport from the cytoplasm to the cell membrane, and further stimulates Akt phosphorylation on the cell membrane. Activated AKT relocates in the cytoplasm, nucleus, or other intracellular locations phosphorylates a wide variety of substrate proteins and consequently modulates cell activity. Besides, AKT1 E17K mutation accelerates cell migration and resistance to chemotherapeutic treatments in luminal breast cancer cells (39, 40). The oncogene AKT2 is triggered by amplification or overexpression in a variety of malignant tumors, thus facilitating tumor invasion and metastasis (41, 42). More prevalent amplification of the oncogene AKT3 has been detected in many cancers, such as breast carcinoma, endometrial carcinoma, melanoma, ovarian epithelial tumor, cholangiocarcinoma, and non-small cell lung cancer (**Table 2**) (22, 23).

Genetic Alterations in the PTEN Gene

PTEN is a tumor suppressor gene that can negatively regulate the PI3K/AKT/mTOR pathway and is one of the most common mutated genes in cancer (**Figure 2G** and **Table 2**). PTEN functions as a phosphatase on the cell membrane, converting phosphatidylinositol (3–5)-triphosphate (PIP3) to phosphatidylinositol (4, 5)-diphosphate (PIP2). PTEN dysfunction caused by inactivation mutations, homozygous deletions, loss of heterozygosity (LOH), or epigenetic modifications accumulates PIP3 and activates catabolic downstream AKT/mTOR signaling, thereby stimulating cell proliferation and survival. In addition, nuclear PTEN can modulate RAD51 expression, which is tightly associated with homologous recombination (HR) and DNA double-strand breaks (DSBs). Furthermore, PTEN deficiency may also result in increased genomic instability, allowing for the accumulation of deleterious mutations (43). Nedd8 interacts with PTEN at high glucose levels, inducing PTEN neddylation and resulting in nuclear import of PTEN without impairing PTEN stability. Neddylated PTEN mainly aggregates in the nucleus and dephosphorylates the fatty acid synthase (FASN), suppresses FASN ubiquitylation and degradation through TRIM21, and subsequently enhances fatty acid synthesis. Besides, PTEN neddylation was closely associated with tumor development and a worse prognosis in breast cancer (44). Germline PTEN mutations are found in approximately 80% of patients with the cancer predisposition syndrome Cowden, which is associated with a high incidence of breast and thyroid cancer events (45, 46). The PTEN mutation is one of the most prevalent cancer mutations, frequently found in endometrial carcinoma, glioblastoma, and prostate adenocarcinoma. PTEN mutations occurred in 9% (888/10336) of patients in the MSK-IMPACT Clinical Sequencing Cohort, while PTEN was altered in only 5% (534/10194) of patients in China Pan-cancer Cohort (OrigiMed2020) (20, 22). PTEN mutations or deletions are detected in 45% of endometrial cancer and are more frequent in endometrioid endometrial cancer than in other histological subtypes (47). PTEN mutations were found in 29.0% (N=303) of glioblastoma patients, and PTEN deletions were identified in 39.6% (N=260) of glioblastoma cases. 13.5% (N=260) of cases had concomitant PTEN mutation and deletions (48). PTEN mutations and/or deletions are identified in 30% of prostate cancer cases. PTEN silencing lowers H3K27me3 and H3K27Ac enrichment in the Nkx3.1 promoter region and promotes alterations in DNA CpG methylation and transcriptome gene expression, associated with various inflammatory and immunological pathways in the development of prostate cancer (49). PTEN Y240 phosphorylation mediated by FGFR2 prevents cells from DNA damage *via* enabling DNA repair. PTEN Y240 phosphorylation facilitates homologous recombination (HR)-mediated DNA double-strand break (DSB) repair through enhancing RAD51 filament synthesis or stabilization. PTEN Y240 phosphorylation interacts with chromatin and recruits RAD51 to facilitate DNA repair. Inhibiting Y240 phosphorylation can make glioblastoma more sensitive to ionizing radiation (IR), thus extending glioblastoma survival time (50).

THE PI3K/AKT/MTOR PATHWAY AND DIFFERENT CELLULAR PROCESSES IN CANCER

Cell Proliferation

PI3K/Akt/mTOR signaling pathway involved in cell survival, growth, and proliferation is the commonly activated signaling pathway in human cancers. Dysregulated mTOR activation is a frequent observation in cancer and represents a process in cancerogenesis. mTOR interacts with other proteins and is a component of two protein complexes, mTOR complex 1 and mTOR complex 2, that control various cellular activities. Both mTORC1 and mTORC2 contain subunits that mediate different but overlapping activities. mTORC1 is triggered by a variety of nutrients and can be stimulated by PI3K signaling. mTORC1 is an upstream regulator, whereas mTORC2 is a downstream effector of Akt. Akt is an essential substrate of mTORC2, which is often shown to be overactive in malignancies. Akt accumulates signals from the PI3K/mTORC2 and PI3K/PDK1 to enhance cell survival, growth, and proliferation (51). mTORC1 regulates the phosphorylation of downstream translation effectors such as the ribosomal protein S6 kinase B1 (S6K1) and the eukaryotic translation initiation factor 4E (eIF4E)-binding protein 1 (4E-BP1) to control cell growth and proliferation. mTORC2 controls cell survival and proliferation *via* phosphorylating Akt Ser473. Small molecules, such as hormones and growth factors, can activate Akt, mTORC2, and then mTORC1 through an Akt-dependent phosphorylation pathway. Nutrients can activate Akt, mTORC2, and directly stimulate mTORC1 through an Akt-independent phosphorylation pathway. Glycogen synthase kinase-3 beta (GSK3) is a significant Akt substrate, and its deactivation is induced by phosphorylation. GSK3 promotes cell proliferation by modulating the stability and production of proteins involved in the G1/S cell cycle phase transition, such as cyclin D1. FKBP4 enhances cell proliferation in breast cancer by increasing Akt phosphorylation at Ser473 and Thr308 through PI3K/PDK1 and mTORC2 (52). GSK3 collaborates with mTORC1 by increasing p70S6K1 activity by phosphorylating at Ser371 inside the p70S6K1 turn motif, which enhances mTORC1- mediated Thr389 phosphorylation. GSK3 may serve as an inducer of malignant cell growth and survival. Phosphorylation of some GSK3 substrates is critical for cell proliferation or survival and produces a phosphorylated protein recognized by E3 ubiquitin ligase, causing the phosphorylated protein to be degraded by the proteasome. After Rictor is phosphorylated by GSK3 and interacts with FBXW-7, it is degraded through a ubiquitination/proteasome-dependent pathway. When PI3K/Akt signaling inactivates GSK3, Rictor expression, and mTORC2 assembly increase, boosting mTORC2 activity (53). Rictor functions as an upstream kinase for many members of the AGC (cAMP-dependent, cGMP-dependent, and protein kinase C) protein family, such as Akt, SGK, and PKC, and is a critical component of mTORC2. Stimulation of Rictor/mTORC2 affects the structure of actin and enhances cell proliferation by phosphorylating the substrates. When used in conjunction with rapamycin, Rictor down-regulation significantly decreased cell proliferation, increased cell cycle arrest, and induced apoptosis by inhibiting the AktSer473 feedback phosphorylation (54). Activation of the mTORC2 subunit p-AKT (Ser473) and RICTOR stimulate the esophageal squamous cell carcinoma. Inhibiting RICTOR may increase esophageal squamous cell carcinoma cell sensitivity to PP242 (a pan-mTOR inhibitor) as well as RAD001 (a mTORC1 inhibitor) (55).

Autophagy

Autophagy is a critical homeostatic cellular recycling process that degrades damaged or dysfunctional cellular proteins and organelles. As a result of the dysregulation of the PI3K/Akt/

mTOR pathway, autophagy can be triggered in malignancies, allowing them to adapt to low-nutrient environments and proliferate (56). mTOR is a regulator that inhibits autophagy, and anticancer therapies that disrupt the PI3K/Akt/mTOR pathway promote autophagy. mTORC1 inhibits catabolism *via* suppressing autophagy and lysosome formation, which are two processes critical for lysosome-dependent macromolecule degradation. mTORC1 inhibits autophagy and lysosomal degradation *via* phosphorylating ULK1, a critical autophagy modulator, and TFEB, a modulator of lysosomal gene expression. The activity of mTORC1 can be modulated by energy levels, nutrient status, and hypoxic settings *via* the AMPK/TSC pathway, which affects autophagy. The mTORC1 downstream effectors' elongation factor 4E-BP1 and p70S6 kinase control protein synthesis. Stimulated mTORC1 phosphorylates the autophagy protein complex (ULK1/2) to suppress the downstream autophagy cascade. AMPK activated by AMP or LKB1 can promote autophagy by inhibiting the activity of mTORC1 through phosphorylation of TSC1/2. The intracellular flow of essential amino acids may limit autophagy by stimulating mTORC1. Additionally, MEK/ERK signaling promotes starvation-induced autophagy and ROS-dependent ERK activation boosts autophagy and induces cell death (57). PI3KCI stimulates Akt, which can attenuate the inhibitory impact of the TSC1/2 heterodimer on Rheb, thereby activating mTORC1 and inhibiting autophagy. Akt is triggered by mTORC2, which further inhibits autophagy. Moreover, PTEN promotes autophagy by suppressing the production of PIP3, which in turn triggers the PI3K/Akt/mTOR signaling. GTP-Ras suppresses autophagy *via* activating PI3KCI and the RAF/MEK/ERK pathway (58). The cyclin–CDK inhibitor CDKN1B (also known as p27Kip1) enhances starvation-induced autophagy *via* a mTORC1-dependent pathway. A portion of p27Kip1 is transported to lysosomes in amino acid-derived cells, where it cooperates with LAMTOR1, an essential component of the Ragulator complex, to stimulate mTORC1. When p27Kip1 binds to LAMTOR1, regulatory assembly and mTORC1 stimulation are inhibited, thereby facilitating autophagy. In p27 −/− cells, elevated mTORC1 activity contributes to cytoplasmic retention of TFEB, impaired lysosomal function, and decreased autophagy flux, ultimately improving cell survival (59). Gαq, a component of the mTOR/Raptor/p62 complex, regulates autophagy by promoting the assembly of the active mTORC1 complex through PB1-mediated Gαq/p62 interaction in the presence of nutrients (60).

Apoptosis

Apoptosis is a type of programmed cell death that enables the body to clear abnormal or unneeded cells in an orderly manner. Caspases are critical to the apoptotic mechanism as the initiators and executors of apoptosis, which can be activated by the extrinsic death receptor pathway, the intrinsic mitochondrial pathway, and the intrinsic endoplasmic reticulum pathway. The extrinsic death receptor pathway begins with the binding of death ligands (TNF and FasL) to death receptors (TNFR1 and Fas). The binding of the death ligand to the death receptor promotes the formation of the death-inducing signaling complex (DISC), a ligand-receptor-conjugating protein complex that further leads to the assembly and activation of caspase 8. The activated caspase 8 serves as an initiator caspase, which triggers apoptosis by cleaving other downstream caspases. Moreover, internal stimuli such as genetic damage, hypoxia, excessive cytosolic Ca2+ concentrations, and severe oxidative stress may cause elevated mitochondrial permeability and the production of pro-apoptotic substances such as cytochrome-c into the cytoplasm, stimulating the intrinsic mitochondrial pathway. Cytoplasmic release of cytochrome c activates caspase 3 *via* forming an apoptosome complex, composed of cytochrome c, Apaf-1, and caspase 9. The intrinsic mitochondrial pathway is tightly regulated by the Bcl-2 family proteins, mainly composed of pro-apoptotic proteins and anti-apoptotic proteins. Anti-apoptotic proteins such as Bcl-2, Bcl-XL, Bcl-W, BFL-1, and McL-1 regulate apoptosis by inhibiting the release of cytochrome c from mitochondria, while pro-apoptotic proteins such as Bax, Bak, Bad, Bcl-XS, Bid, Bik, Bim, and Hrk enhance the release of cytochrome c from mitochondria. Both extrinsic and intrinsic pathways are closely associated with various signaling proteins, such as NK-kB and p53-MDM2, and converge to caspases. Additionally, the intrinsic endoplasmic reticulum pathway is caspase 12-dependent and mitochondria-independent. Overall, the mechanisms of apoptosis evasion and carcinogenesis are mediated by the imbalance of Bcl-2 family proteins, reduced caspases expression, disrupted death receptor signaling pathway, p53 defects/mutations, and overexpression of inhibitor of apoptosis proteins (IAPs) such as BIRC1 (NAIP), BIRC2 (c-IAP1), BIRC3 (c-IAP2), BIRC4 (XIAP), BIRC5 (Survivin), BIRC6 (Apollon/BRUCE), BIRC7 (Livin/MLIAP) and BIRC8 (ILP2) (61, 62). mTOR inhibitors can rapidly inhibit 4E-BP1 phosphorylation *via* DR5/FADD/Caspase-8 axis and trigger the extrinsic apoptotic pathway in colorectal cancer cells. High dosages of mTOR inhibitors result in a significant reduction of 4E-BP1 phosphorylation and mTOR activity, all of which may be factors in ER stress, C/EBP homologous protein (CHOP), and death receptor 5 (DR5) and consequent cancer cell death. Besides, mTOR inhibitors have a substantial synergistic effect with tumor necrosis factor-related apoptosis-inducing ligand (TRAIL) and chemotherapy in inducing Fas-associated protein with death domain (FADD) and DR5-dependent apoptosis. Generally, mTOR inhibitors may have an anti-tumor effect *via* stimulating the extrinsic apoptotic pathway (63).

Angiogenesis

Angiogenesis is the formation of new blood vessels, enabling oxygen and nutrients to be delivered to the body's tissues. Angiogenesis is critical in the development of cancer, which requires the development of new blood vessels to grow and metastasize. Endogenous angiogenesis regulators mainly include growth factors, cytokines, proteases, protease inhibitors, trace elements, oncogenes, and endogenous modulators. A balance of activators such as vascular endothelial growth factor (VEGF), basic fibroblast growth factor (bFGF), platelet-derived endothelial cell growth factor (PD-ECGF), tumor necrosis factor (TNF)-α, angiogenin, transforming growth factor (TGF)-α, TGF-β, granulocyte colony-stimulating factor (G-

CSF), placental growth factor (PGF), hepatocyte growth factor (HGF), interleukin-8 (IL-8), and epidermal growth factor (EGF) and inhibitors such as angiostatin, interferon, endostatin, platelet factor 4 (PF4), thrombospondin (TSP), and tissue inhibitors of metalloproteinases (TIMPs) regulates angiogenesis (64–66). mTOR, a crucial switch that regulates anabolism and catabolism of endothelial cells, is critical in angiogenesis. Shear stress and coordinated interactions between endothelial growth factors (VEGF, PDGF-B, ANG2, ANG1, bFGF, ephrin-B2, and TGF-beta superfamily), intracellular signaling molecules (NOTCH1 and COUP-TFII), and intercellular connections (VCAM1) contribute to tumor angiogenesis, which may activate the PI3K/Akt/mTOR pathway in cancer cells. Hypoxia stabilizes HIF-1α, which triggers tumor cells to produce more vascular endothelial growth factor (VEGF). Stimulation of the PI3K/AKT pathway in tumor cells may boost the production of VEGF *via* hypoxia-inducible factor 1 (HIF-1) dependent and independent pathways. Besides, the PI3K/AKT pathway also regulates other angiogenic factors such as angiopoietins and nitric oxide. Angiogenic tumor cells release more bFGF and VEGF than non-angiogenic tumor cells. Increased VEGF levels may enhance vascular permeability, resulting in leaky vessels, slow blood flow, and high interstitial pressure. The binding of VEGF to receptors stimulates the PI3K/AKT/mTOR pathway, which is critical for cell migration (67). Suppression of the mTOR pathway prevents VEGF-mediated angiogenesis and cell proliferation by decreasing VEGF production and secretion, and VEGFR2-mediated signaling. Rutacecarpine suppresses angiogenesis *via* targeting VEGFR2 and the Akt/mTOR/p70s6k signaling pathways regulated by VEGFR2 (68). Rapamycin inhibits angiogenesis and lymphangiogenesis in melanoma by inhibiting the expression of VEGF-A/VEGFR-2 and VEGF-C/VEGFR-3 (69). VEGF stimulation increased the expression of Sox7 and Sox17 in angiogenesis through the mTOR pathway. Additionally, Sox7 and Sox17 increased the expression of VEGFR2 in angiogenic vessels (70).

Epithelial-to-Mesenchymal Transition

Epithelial-mesenchymal transition (EMT) refers to the transition of cells from epithelial to mesenchymal phenotypes, which results in functional alterations in cell migration and invasion. EMT is a vital step through which epithelial cells develop mesenchymal, fibroblast-like features characterized by decreased intercellular adhesion and enhanced motility. EMT-like processes play a significant role in tumor growth and malignant transformation, causing cancer cells to become more aggressive and spread (71, 72). During EMT, the expression of epithelial markers (E-cadherin) decreases, and the expression of mesenchymal markers (vimentin and fibronectin) increases. Snail, ZEB, and Twist regulate these markers by blocking the CDH1 gene encoding E-cadherin. Cumulative evidence indicates that the AKT/mTOR pathway is closely associated with the EMT process (73, 74). Phosphorylation and activation of EMT transcription factors are a result of AKT activation. Increased AKT activation causes decreased E-cadherin expression, partly attributable to the Snail accumulation in the nucleus. Besides, AKT may trigger Twist expression, which decreases E-cadherin expression and inhibits cell migration. Activation of NF-kB *via* AKT may cause the accumulation of ZEB-1, which acts as a repressor of E-cadherin expression. Growth factors, specific proteins, and aberrant tumor suppressors may stimulate AKT and regulate EMT transcription factor expression and EMT activation. Cancer cells experience dramatic remodeling of the actin cytoskeleton during the EMT process. mTORC2 modulates the actin cytoskeleton of the cell and EMT *via* regulating the phosphorylation status of Protein Kinase C (PKC) and activating Akt (75). TGF-receptors interact with the regulatory p85 subunit of PI3K, triggering the PI3K/AKT pathway. TGF-β has the potential to cause EMT *via* activating the mTOR pathway (76–79).

Chemoresistance

The druggable metabolic vulnerability is mediated by mTORC1, which inhibits autophagy and enhances resistance to chemotherapy and targeted drugs (80–82). The mTOR pathway regulates FANCD2, which leads to cancer cells' resistance to DNA double-strand breaks (83). The combination of adriamycin/cisplatin and mTOR inhibitor (torisel) blocked 4EBP-1 and p70S6K phosphorylation, elevated γH2AX expression indicative of DNA damage, and induced cell cycle arrest at G2/M and apoptosis, indicating a potential role of mTOR inhibitors in rebuilding chemosensitivity to adriamycin/cisplatin (84). FOXD1-AS1 facilitated the translation of FOXD1 protein *via* the eIF4G-eIF4E-eIF4A translational complex. Moreover, FOXD1-AS1 modulated 4E-BP1 phosphorylation and enhanced eIF4G-eIF4E interaction *via* triggering the PI3K/AKT/mTOR pathway. Overall, FOXD1-AS1 increases FOXD1 translation through PI3K/AKT/mTOR signaling, thereby exacerbating gastric cancer development and resistance to chemotherapy (85). Chemotherapy-resistant epithelial ovarian cancer cells exhibit EMT and increased expression of tumor stem cell markers due to stimulation of the PI3K/Akt/mTOR signaling pathway. In combination with cisplatin, BEZ235, an anti-PI3K/mTOR inhibitor, might be a viable therapeutic approach for epithelial ovarian cancer chemoresistance (86). Aurora-A expression was positively correlated with phosphorylated AKT/4E-BP1 expression in endometrial cancer tissues. Aurora-A triggers the AKT/mTOR pathway in endometrial cancer, which stimulates cell proliferation and causes chemoresistance, suggesting that Aurora-A inhibitor and AKT/mTOR inhibitor in combination with chemotherapy intervention may be a therapeutic strategy for Aurora-A overexpressed endometrial cancer (87).

RECENT ADVANCES IN PI3K/AKT/MTOR INHIBITOR RESEARCH

Because of the significant rise in the number of novel therapeutic drugs that target molecular pathways, targeted therapeutic agents are now more precise than traditional chemotherapy agents. The PI3K/AKT/mTOR pathway is critical for cell growth, proliferation, and survival, and it is one of the most frequently disrupted pathways in malignancies, making it a desirable target for treatment (**Figure 3**). In this review, we reviewed the research progress of PI3K/AKT/mTOR inhibitors and presented the representative PI3K/AKT/mTOR inhibitors in **Table 1**.

PI3K Inhibitors

Phosphatidylinositol 3–kinases (PI3Ks) are a class of lipid kinases that control signaling and intracellular vesicular trafficking *via* phosphorylating intracellular inositol lipids. PI3Ks are classified into three groups based on their structural characteristic and substrate specificity. Class I PI3Ks synthesize 3-phosphoinositide lipids that activate signal transduction pathways directly. Class I PI3Ks are classified into subclasses IA and IB according to their regulatory mechanisms. Class IA PI3Ks are heterodimers with a catalytic subunit of p110 and a regulatory subunit of p85. The class IA catalytic isoforms p110α, p110β, and p110δ are encoded by the PIK3CA, PIK3CB, and PIK3CD genes, respectively. The class IB PI3K are the heterodimers with a catalytic subunit of p110γ and a regulatory subunit of p101 or p87. The class IB isoforms p110γ, p101, or p87 are encoded by the PIK3CG, PIK3R5, and PIK3R6 genes, respectively. The class I PI3Ks are frequently activated in malignant tumors, associated with translation, cell growth, glucose metabolism, cytoskeletal motility, cell survival, transformation. Cellular processes such as growth, cell migration, primary cilium function, glucose metabolism, cell survival, and angiogenesis are modulated by the Class II PI3Ks. The class II catalytic isoforms PI3KC2α, PI3KC2β, and PI3KC2γ are encoded by the PIK3C2A, PIK3C2B, and PIK3C2G genes, respectively. Autophagy, endosomal trafficking, and phagocytosis are dependent on the class III PI3K. The class III PI3Ks are the heterodimers with a catalytic subunit of VPS34 encoded by PIK3C3 and a regulatory and accessory subunit of VPS15 encoded by PIK3R4. Presently, several types of PI3K-specific inhibitors have been developed. PI3K inhibitors are divided into three categories according to their pharmacokinetic characteristics and capacity to interact with ATP-binding clefts: pan-PI3K inhibitors, isoform-selective PI3K inhibitors, and dual PI3K/mTOR inhibitors.

Pan-Class I inhibitors can block catalytic properties of p110 isoforms. The use of pan-PI3K inhibitors was restricted owing to the adverse pharmacological event caused by off-target effects, and on-target consequences of blocking all class I PI3K isoforms, independent of their role in carcinogenesis. PX-866, a derivative

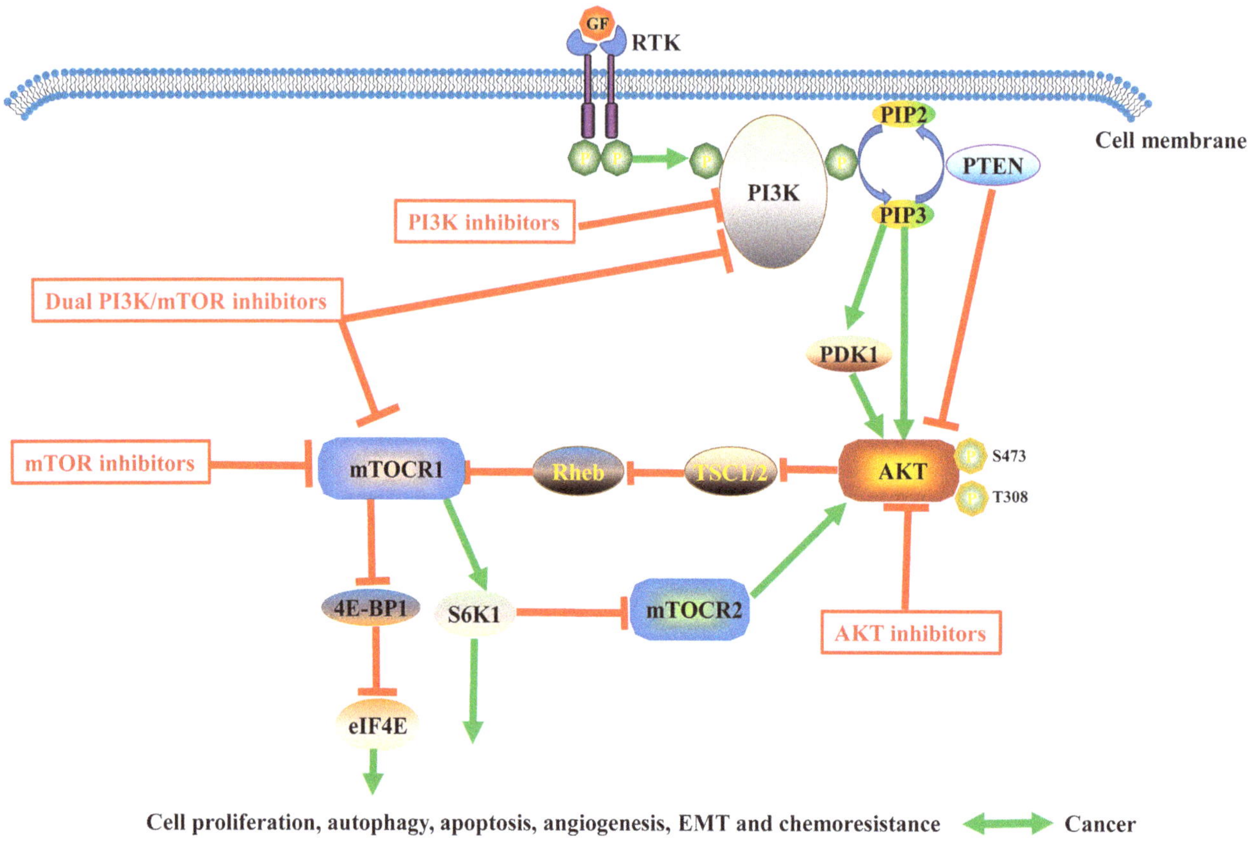

FIGURE 3 | Schematic representation of the PI3K/Akt/mTOR pathway and its related inhibitors in solid tumors. The activation of the PI3K/Akt/mTOR pathway is associated with cell proliferation, autophagy, apoptosis, angiogenesis, EMT, and chemoresistance in solid tumors. GF, growth factor; EMT, epithelial-to-mesenchymal transition; RTK, tyrosine kinase receptor.

of Wortmannin, is a physiologically stable pan-PI3K inhibitor that targets the PI3K pathway and has shown improved antineoplastic activity and favorable pharmacokinetic properties in a variety of tumors (88). In glioblastoma, blockage of the PI3K pathway by PX-866 results in cell growth suppression and reduced stimulation of downstream pathways. PX-866 was generally well tolerated. However, it failed to achieve the efficacy endpoints. 21% of individuals with recurrent glioblastoma had sustained stable disease. However, there are no biomarkers that can distinguish participants (89). Buparlisib (NVP-BKM120) is a pan-PI3K inhibitor targeting all class I PI3K isoforms. Based on the safety profile of buparlisib with fulvestrant in the BELLE-3 trial, further studies on buparlisib with fulvestrant in postmenopausal, hormone-receptor-positive, HER2-negative, advanced breast cancer patients pretreated with endocrine treatment and mTOR inhibitors are not recommended. However, the efficacy of buparlisib with fulvestrant supports the use of PI3K inhibitors combined with endocrine therapy in individuals with PIK3CA mutations, indicating that PIK3CA mutations may be a biomarker of PI3K inhibitor efficacy (90). Buparlisib had limited single-agent efficacy in PI3K-activated recurrent glioblastoma. The lack of efficacy of buparlisib was attributed to inadequate blockage of the PI3K pathway, despite the drug's substantial brain penetration. Further studies on PI3K inhibitors with more pathway blocking are needed (91). In the BERIL-1 study, patients with relapsed or metastatic head and neck squamous cell carcinoma treated with buparlisib in combination with paclitaxel had a median progression-free survival of 1.1 months longer than those treated with placebo plus paclitaxel (4.6 months *vs.* 3.5 months). Although the adverse events were considered manageable, patients treated with buparlisib plus paclitaxel had more grade 3 or 4 adverse events. Buparlisib plus paclitaxel seemed to be an effective second-line therapy for patients with platinum-pretreated recurrent or metastatic head and neck squamous cell carcinoma (92). In 2017, the Food and Drug Administration (FDA) granted approval to copanlisib (a pan-PI3K inhibitor) based on results from the CHRONOS-1 trial for the treatment of adult patients with recurrent follicular lymphoma who have undergone at least two previous systemic therapies (93). In addition to PX-866, buparlisib, and copanlisib, other pan-PI3K inhibitors include CH5132799, pilaralisib, ZSTK474, sonolisib, pictilisib, B591, TG-100-115, and RIDR-PI-103. Further clinical trials are needed to evaluate the efficacy of pan-PI3K inhibitors in solid tumors. The wide activity of pan-PI3K inhibitor may increase the risk of adverse effects and toxicity.

Isoform-selective PI3K inhibitors targeting one of the PI3K isoforms have enhanced, precise targeting and decreased toxicity compared with pan-PI3K inhibitors. Isoform-specific PI3K inhibitors may need appropriate patient identification according to sensitivity and resistance markers. In 2014, Idelalisib (a PI3Kδ inhibitor) is approved by the FDA for the treatment of chronic lymphocytic leukemia, relapsed follicular B-cell non-Hodgkin lymphoma, and relapsed small lymphocytic lymphoma (94). In 2018, the FDA approved duvelisib (an isoform-specific inhibitor targeting PI3Kγ and PI3Kδ) based on results from the DUO and DYNAMO for adult patients with relapsed or refractory chronic lymphocytic leukemia or small lymphocytic lymphoma after more than two previous therapies (95, 96). In 2019, the FDA approved alpelisib (a PI3Kα inhibitor) in combination with fulvestrant for postmenopausal women, and men, with hormone receptor-positive, human epidermal growth factor receptor 2 -negative, PIK3CA-mutated, advanced or metastatic breast cancer based on the results from the SOLAR-1 trial (97). According to the results of the CBYL719X2101 trial, alpelisib exhibited an acceptable safety and promising antitumor activity in patients with PIK3CA-mutant malignancies, indicating that selective PI3K inhibitors in conjunction with additional antineoplastic drugs may be effective for the treatment of PIK3CA-mutant malignancies (98). In 2021, the FDA approved umbralisib (a PI3Kδ/CK1ϵ inhibitor) for the treatment of marginal zone lymphoma and follicular lymphoma based on the results from the UTX-TGR-205 trial (99). In addition to idelalisib (δ), alpelisib (α), duvelisib (δ/γ), and umbralisib (δ), other isoform-selective PI3K inhibitors include serabelisib (a PI3Kα inhibitor), GSK2636771 (a PI3Kβ inhibitor), Zandelisib (a PI3Kδ inhibitor), AMG319 (a PI3Kδ inhibitor), linperlisib (a PI3Kδ inhibitor), parsaclisib (a PI3Kδ inhibitor), leniolisib (a PI3Kδ inhibitor), eganelisib (a PI3Kγ inhibitor), tenalisib (a PI3Kδ/γ inhibitor), taselisib (a PI3Kα/δ/γ inhibitor), AZD8186 (a PI3Kβ/δ inhibitor), and AZD8835 (a PI3Kδ/α inhibitor).

Akt Inhibitors

AKT, an effector of the PI3K/AKT/mTOR pathway to activate tumors, is a promising target. The Akt kinase family comprises the AKT1, AKT2, and AKT3 isoforms. AKT activity is controlled in an Akt-dependent manner *via* phosphorylation and dephosphorylation. Akt inhibitors have been classified into three categories depending on how they impede Akt activity. ATP-competitive inhibitors reduce the phosphorylation of Akt by competing with ATP. Allosteric inhibitors prevent Akt from interacting with its substrate by causing conformational transitions in enzymic structure. Irreversible inhibitors are another less common type of Akt inhibitor. ATP-competitive inhibitors (GSK690693, ipatasertib, uprosertib, and capivasertib) and allosteric inhibitors (MK-2206) have demonstrated the more potent inhibition of Akt in malignant cells. ATP-competitive inhibitors attach to the active conformation of Akt, in which the pleckstrin homology (PH) domain has swung away from the kinase domain and exposed the ATP-binding pocket, thereby blocking the activity of Akt. Allosteric inhibitors can impede the localization of AKT to the plasma membrane and prevent the phosphorylation and activation of AKT.

In the EAY131-Y trial, the objective response rate of single-agent capivasertib (AZD5363) was 28.6% (N=35) in patients with an AKT1 E17K-mutated tumor. One patient with endometrioid endometrial cancer had a complete response and was still on treatment after 35.6 months. Moreover, 46% (N=35) of patients had stable disease, and 6% (N=35) of patients had progressive disease, suggesting that capivasertib shows clinically substantial efficacy in refractory malignant tumors (100). Adding pan-AKT inhibitor capivasertib to docetaxel and prednisolone did not improve a composite progression-free survival in metastatic castration-resistant prostate cancer regardless of whether the PI3K/AKT/PTEN pathway was activated or not in the ProCAID trial (101). After a median follow-up of 4.9 months, median progression-free survival was 10.3 months for patients with metastatic, estrogen-receptor-positive breast cancer treated with capivasertib plus fulvestrant compared with 4.8 months for patients treated with fulvestrant plus placebo in the FAKTION trial (102). The combination of capivasertib and paclitaxel for metastatic triple-negative breast cancer can contribute to significantly prolonged progression-free survival (5.9 months *vs.* 4.2 months) and overall survival (19.1 months *vs.* 12.6 months) compared with paclitaxel plus placebo in the PAKT trial. The results suggested that capivasertib plus paclitaxel has potential as a first-line treatment for metastatic triple-negative breast cancer. In PIK3CA/AKT1/PTEN-altered patients, median progression-free survival with capivasertib plus paclitaxel was 9.3 months while placebo plus paclitaxel was only 3.7 months. Severe adverse events (grade 3-4) were more common in patients treated with capivasertib plus paclitaxel ($P < 0.01$). The most common adverse events with capivasertib plus paclitaxel versus paclitaxel plus placebo were diarrhea (13% *vs.* 1%), infection (4% *vs.* 1%), neutropenia (3% *vs.* 3%), rash (4% *vs.* 0%), and fatigue (4% *vs.* 0%) (103).

Targeting AKT signaling ipatasertib (GDC-0068) exhibited an acceptable safety profile and significant disease control in patients with AKT-activated solid tumors (104). After a median follow-up of 19 months, the inhibition of PI3K/AKT and androgen-receptor dual pathways by ipatasertib (an ATP-competitive AKT inhibitor) plus abiraterone can improve the median radiographical progression-free survival of metastatic prostate cancer patients with PTEN loss compared with placebo plus abiraterone (18·5 months *vs.* 16·5 months) in the IPATential150 trial. 39% (21/546) of patients treated with the placebo plus abiraterone and 70% (386/551) of patients treated with ipatasertib plus abiraterone experienced grade 3 or higher adverse events. Adverse events led to drug discontinuation in 5% (28/546) of patients treated with the placebo plus abiraterone and 21% (116/551) of patients treated with ipatasertib plus abiraterone (105). In the intention-to-treat population, the combination of ipatasertib and paclitaxel for triple-negative breast cancer can result in significantly prolonged median progression-free survival compared with paclitaxel plus placebo (6.2 months *vs.* 4.9 months) in the LOTUS trial. Median progression-free survival in PTEN-low patients with ipatasertib plus paclitaxel was 6.2 months compared to placebo plus paclitaxel in 3.7 months. Serious adverse events occurred in 28% (17/61) of patients in the ipatasertib plus paclitaxel group and 42% (26/62) of patients in the placebo plus paclitaxel group. The ipatasertib plus paclitaxel group was mainly associated with severe adverse reactions related to infections and gastrointestinal effects, while the placebo plus paclitaxel group was mainly associated with severe adverse reactions related to infections (106).

In the I-SPY 2 trial, MK-2206 (an allosteric inhibitor) combined with standard neoadjuvant chemotherapy contributed to higher pathologic complete response rates in human epidermal growth factor receptor 2 (HER2)-positive, hormone receptor (HR)-negative early-stage breast cancer. Substantial skin adverse reactions are observed, but adverse events, such as rash, can be controlled. Although MK-2206 is not currently being explored further in breast cancer, this type of Akt inhibitor is still promising for clinical use (107).

mTOR Inhibitors

The mTOR kinase family mainly consists of three functional components: mTOR1, mTOR2, and mTOR3. mTOR1 and mTOR2 are linked with cancer. mTORC1 serves as a downstream effector for several commonly disrupted oncogenic pathways, including the PI3K/AKT and MAPK pathways, and the mTOR pathway is overactive in various tumor types, making mTOR a target for cancer treatment. mTOR inhibitors are a type of drug that works by selectively inhibiting mTOR activity. Generally, mTOR inhibitors are classified into two categories: rapamycin and its analogs (rapalogs), and ATP-competitive mTOR kinase inhibitors. The former is capable of suppressing mTORC1, and the latter can suppress mTORC1/2.

Rapamycin (Sirolimus), a rapalog, was initially used as an immunosuppressant in patients experiencing organ transplantation and it also has anti-proliferative properties. A phase I/II study of pemetrexed in combination with sirolimus in recurrent, metastatic non-small cell lung cancer revealed synergistic benefits when sirolimus was added to pemetrexed (108). In 2007, temsirolimus (CCI-779) was the first rapalog to be approved by the Food and Drug Administration (FDA) for the treatment of advanced renal cell carcinoma (109). FDA approves everolimus (a rapalog) for treatment of various diseases, such as renal cell carcinoma, progressive neuroendocrine tumors of pancreatic origin (PNET), postmenopausal women with advanced hormone receptor-positive, HER2-negative breast cancer, neuroendocrine tumors (NET) of gastrointestinal (GI) or lung origin, tuberous sclerosis complex (TSC)-associated partial-onset seizures, TSC-associated subependymal giant cell astrocytoma (SEGA) and TSC-associated renal angiomyolipoma. In the MIRACLE study, the progression-free survival of patients with HR-positive, ERBB2-negative premenopausal advanced breast cancer treated with everolimus plus letrozole was substantially longer than that of patients treated with letrozole (19.4 months *vs.* 12.9 months; $P=0.008$), suggesting the effectiveness of everolimus among patients who experienced disease progression and took the same endocrine therapy (110). Compared to fulvestrant plus vistusertib (a dual mTORC1 and mTORC2 inhibitor) or fulvestrant alone, the combination of fulvestrant and everolimus (a mTORC1 inhibitor) resulted in a substantially longer progression-free survival in patients with hormone receptor-positive metastatic breast cancer. Adding vistusertib to fulvestrant failed to show a benefit in the MANTA study (111). In the AcSé-ESMART trial, the CDK4/6 inhibitor ribociclib combined with topotecan and temozolomide (TOTEM) or everolimus was well-tolerated in children with advanced malignancies (112).

The development of resistance to rapamycin analogs seems inevitable due to compensatory activation of the PI3K/Akt pathway. Several drugs have been developed as ATP competitors that block the catalytic activity of mTOR to overcome the ineffectiveness of rapamycin in antitumor therapy. Researchers are now focused on developing mTORC1/2 complex inhibitors such as vistusertib (AZD2014), sapanisertib (TAK-228), AZD8055, and PP242 to overcome this shortcoming of rapamycin analogs (113). 118 postmenopausal women with hormone receptor-positive, human epidermal growth factor receptor 2 negative advanced/metastatic breast cancer participated in a phase IB/II study (NCT02049957) in which the safety, tolerability, and antitumor activity of sapanisertib plus exemestane or fulvestrant were assessed. The combination of sapanisertib with exemestane or fulvestrant has a maximum tolerable dosage of 4 mg once daily. Sapanisertib plus exemestane or fulvestrant showed therapeutic benefit in postmenopausal women with pretreatment everolimus-sensitive or everolimus-resistant breast cancer with clinical benefit rate at 16 weeks (CBR-16) of 45% versus 23% in everolimus-sensitive versus everolimus-resistant subgroups. Molecular analysis revealed a positive correlation between the presence of an AKT1 mutation and improved effectiveness (114). In comparison to the combination of fulvestrant and vistusertib, or to fulvestrant alone, fulvestrant with everolimus showed a substantially longer progression-free survival in patients with hormone receptor-positive metastatic breast cancer. The addition of the dual mTORC1 and mTORC2 inhibitor vistusertib to fulvestrant failed to show any advantage in the MANTA trial (111). Besides, vistusertib was well tolerated in children with advanced malignancies. However, the study arms were discontinued due to the lack of tumor responses and a failure to engage the target (113). Nonetheless, dual mTORC1 and mTORC2 inhibitors targeting the PI3K/AKT/mTOR pathway in the treatment of malignant tumors are still being investigated.

Dual PI3K/mTOR Inhibitors

Dual PI3K/mTOR inhibitors interact with the ATP-binding cleft of both PI3K and mTOR, reducing the kinase activity of both enzymes and impacting pathway activities more effectively than mTOR kinase inhibitors alone. Dual PI3K/mTOR inhibitors have shown some promise in the early-stage trial. Additional research is required to establish whether dual PI3K/mTOR inhibitors are more effective than mTOR inhibitors. Dual PI3K/mTOR inhibitors such as dactolisib (BEZ235), apitolisib (GDC-0980), gedatolisib (PF-05212384), bimiralisib (PQR309), paxalisib (GDC-0084), and voxtalisib (SAR245409, XL765) have shown substantial anticancer efficacy in various tumor xenografts (9, 115–117).

Treatment with dactolisib (BEZ235), when compared to everolimus, has not been shown to improve effectiveness in patients with advanced pancreatic neuroendocrine tumors who have not previously received mTOR inhibitor treatment, and it may have a worse tolerability profile. The limited effectiveness and poor tolerability of dual PI3K/mTOR inhibitors may restrict their potential for clinical applications (118). In a phase Ib trial (NCT01634061), individuals with castration-resistant prostate cancer were administered dactolisib (BEZ235) plus abiraterone acetate. Eighteen individuals (N=25) were randomized to receive dactolisib plus abiraterone acetate at the first dosage level (200 mg bid) in the dactolisib plus abiraterone acetate arm (NCT01634061). Five dose-limiting toxicities were found in nine individuals. Dactolisib plus abiraterone acetate in castration-resistant prostate cancer will not be studied further due to the available pharmacokinetics, safety, and effectiveness evidence (119). A phase Ib dose-escalation trial (NCT01508104) showed that dactolisib with everolimus was neither efficacious nor tolerable enough in patients with advanced malignancies. Systemic exposure to dactolisib increased in a dose-proportional manner, whereas oral bioavailability was poor, perhaps due to gastrointestinal toxicity (120). Additionally, the combination of gedatolisib (dual PI3K/mTOR inhibitor) with carboplatin and paclitaxel was tolerated in patients with advanced solid tumors, and preliminary effectiveness was seen particularly in clear cell ovarian cancer in a phase I dose-escalation trial (121). In a phase II study (MAGGIE), the efficacy of apitolisib (a dual PI3K/mTOR inhibitor) was assessed in patients with advanced endometrial cancer. The anticancer efficacy observed with apitolisib was restricted by its tolerability. A comprehensive molecular profile revealed that 57% (N=46) of patients had at least one PIK3CA, PTEN, or AKT1 mutation. Each of the three individuals who had a confirmed response had at least one PI3K pathway gene mutation, indicating that patients with mutations in the PI3K pathway may have benefited more with apitolisib. The most common grade 3 or higher adverse events were rash (maculopapular, acneiform). Two serious adverse events due to grade 3 rash were associated with MK-2206 (122). In addition, enrichment for PI3K pathway biomarkers may be beneficial for future research of more selective inhibitors in PI3K/mTOR signaling.

CONCLUSION AND PROSPECT

Multiple studies have revealed significant genetic alterations in cancer cases. Due to the heterogeneity and complexity of tumors, the mechanism of carcinogenesis remains undetermined. Targeted treatment is developed as an evolving strategy to improve the survival of cancer patients. The PI3K/AKT/mTOR pathway is the most commonly disrupted in cancer. This hyperactive pathway offers possibilities and opportunities for drug research and discovery. The previous studies have exhibited that significant PI3K/AKT/mTOR axis is significantly altered in cancer and targeting this axis with multiple inhibitors can modulate a variety of cellular processes such as cell proliferation, autophagy, apoptosis, angiogenesis, EMT, and chemoresistance. Pharmaceutical research has contributed to the development of various types of inhibitors that target distinct components of this axis. mTOR inhibitors, PI3K inhibitors, Akt inhibitors, and dual PI3K/mTOR inhibitors have all been studied as monotherapy or in combination with other inhibitors in the treatment and prevention of cancer. Despite substantial advancements, effective management of cancer remains a challenge due to the heterogeneity of cancer and proper patient identification for targeted therapy.

There are still many issues in this review that deserve attention or need to be further explored. For example, most of the data on precision medicine come from developed countries in Europe and the United States, while data from other regions, such as Asia, are relatively rare. Differences in data on precision medicine from different populations need to be explored more widely. Besides, multiple TCGA datasets included more primary tumors, and the genetic profiles of primary tumors may differ from those of advanced or metastatic tumors. Moreover, combination with PARP inhibitors or immune checkpoint inhibitors is a promising direction that needs further exploration. Additionally, multiple combinations of targeted therapy strategies are appropriate only for specific cancer types. For example, dactolisib plus abiraterone acetate (a CYP17 inhibitor) is mainly used to treat castration-resistant prostate cancer. Capivasertib plus fulvestrant (an estrogen receptor antagonist) is primarily used to treat metastatic, estrogen-receptor-positive breast cancer. Furthermore, PI3K/AKT/mTOR inhibitor resistance and its mechanism need to be further elucidated.

Targeted therapy targeting the PI3K/AKT/mTOR pathway may produce a variety of adverse reactions and is prone to progress due to drug resistance. Tumor-specific research should be a severe issue, and appropriate dosing regimens need to be explored to make PI3K/AKT/mTOR inhibitors more tolerable and efficient. Increasing the number of clinical studies is an effective way to tailor treatments for cancer patients. Further research is needed to uncover the resistance mechanisms of PI3K/AKT/mTOR inhibitors, explore how to overcome resistance to PI3K/AKT/mTOR inhibitors, and develop new, more rational therapeutic combinations.

AUTHOR CONTRIBUTIONS

YP, YW, CZ, WM, and CCZ designed the study and supervised. YP, CZ, and YW collected data. YP performed statistical analysis. YP, WM, and YW interpreted data and drafted the manuscript. CCZ contributed to administrative and technical and material support. All authors contributed to the article and approved the submitted version.

REFERENCES

Foster KG, Fingar DC. Mammalian Target of Rapamycin (mTOR): Conducting the Cellular Signaling Symphony. *J Biol Chem* (2010) 285 (19):14071–7. doi: 10.1074/jbc.R109.094003

Kim LC, Cook RS, Chen J. Mtorc1 and Mtorc2 in Cancer and the Tumor Microenvironment. *Oncogene* (2017) 36(16):2191–201. doi: 10.1038/onc.2016.363

Lee BJ, Boyer JA, Burnett GL, Thottumkara AP, Tibrewal N, Wilson SL, et al. Selective Inhibitors of Mtorc1 Activate 4EBP1 and Suppress Tumor Growth. *Nat Chem Biol* (2021) 17(10):1065–74. doi: 10.1038/s41589-021- 00813-7

Luciani A, Stagi M. How Mtorc1 Makes Sense of Nutrients. *Kidney Int* (2021) 99(2):295–8. doi: 10.1016/j.kint.2020.07.052

Wipperman MF, Montrose DC, Gotto AM Jr, Hajjar DP. Mammalian Target of Rapamycin: A Metabolic Rheostat for Regulating Adipose Tissue Function and Cardiovascular Health. *Am J Pathol* (2019) 189(3):492–501. doi: 10.1016/j.ajpath.2018.11.013

Li H, Prever L, Hirsch E, Gulluni F. Targeting PI3K/AKT/mTOR Signaling Pathway in Breast Cancer. *Cancers (Basel)* (2021) 13(14):3517. doi: 10.3390/cancers13143517

Pungsrinont T, Kallenbach J, Baniahmad A. Role of PI3K-AKT-mTOR Pathway as a Pro-Survival Signaling and Resistance-Mediating Mechanism to Therapy of Prostate Cancer. *Int J Mol Sci* (2021) 22(20):11088. doi: 10.3390/ijms222011088

Martorana F, Motta G, Pavone G, Motta L, Stella S, Vitale SR, et al. AKT Inhibitors: New Weapons in the Fight Against Breast Cancer? *Front Pharmacol* (2021) 12:662232. doi: 10.3389/fphar.2021.662232

Vanhaesebroeck B, Perry MWD, Brown JR, Andre F, Okkenhaug K. PI3K Inhibitors are Finally Coming of Age. *Nat Rev Drug Discov* (2021) 20 (10):741–69. doi: 10.1038/s41573-021-00209-1

Hua H, Zhang H, Chen J, Wang J, Liu J, Jiang Y. Targeting Akt in Cancer for Precision Therapy. *J Hematol Oncol* (2021) 14(1):128. doi: 10.1186/s13045- 021-01137-8

Khorasani ABS, Pourbagheri-Sigaroodi A, Pirsalehi A, Safaroghli-Azar A, Zali MR, Bashash D. The PI3K/Akt/mTOR Signaling Pathway in Gastric Cancer; From Oncogenic Variations to the Possibilities for Pharmacologic Interventions. *Eur J Pharmacol* (2021) 898:173983. doi: 10.1016/ j.ejphar.2021.173983

Fusco N, Sajjadi E, Venetis K, Gaudioso G, Lopez G, Corti C, et al. PTEN Alterations and Their Role in Cancer Management: Are We Making Headway on Precision Medicine? *Genes (Basel)* (2020) 11(7):719. doi: 10.3390/genes11070719

Yip HYK, Papa A. Signaling Pathways in Cancer: Therapeutic Targets, Combinatorial Treatments, and New Developments. *Cells* (2021) 10(3):659. doi: 10.3390/cells10030659

Hoxhaj G, Manning BD. The PI3K-AKT Network at the Interface of Oncogenic Signalling and Cancer Metabolism. *Nat Rev Cancer* (2020) 20 (2):74–88. doi: 10.1038/s41568-019-0216-7

Harsha C, Banik K, Ang HL, Girisa S, Vikkurthi R, Parama D, et al. Targeting AKT/mTOR in Oral Cancer: Mechanisms and Advances in Clinical Trials. *Int J Mol Sci* (2020) 21(9):3285. doi: 10.3390/ijms21093285

Duan Y, Haybaeck J, Yang Z. Therapeutic Potential of PI3K/AKT/mTOR Pathway in Gastrointestinal Stromal Tumors: Rationale and Progress. *Cancers (Basel)* (2020) 12(10):2972. doi: 10.3390/cancers12102972

Iksen, Pothongsrisit S, Pongrakhananon V. Targeting the PI3K/AKT/mTOR Signaling Pathway in Lung Cancer: An Update Regarding Potential Drugs and Natural Products. *Molecules* (2021) 26(13):4100. doi: 10.3390/molecules26134100

Zhong L, Li Y, Xiong L, Wang W, Wu M, Yuan T, et al. Small Molecules in Targeted Cancer Therapy: Advances, Challenges, and Future Perspectives. *Signal Transduct Target Ther* (2021) 6(1):201. doi: 10.1038/s41392-021- 00572-w

Bader AG, Kang S, Zhao L, Vogt PK. Oncogenic PI3K Deregulates Transcription and Translation. *Nat Rev Cancer* (2005) 5(12):921–9. doi: 10.1038/nrc1753

Gao J, Aksoy BA, Dogrusoz U, Dresdner G, Gross B, Sumer SO, et al. Integrative Analysis of Complex Cancer Genomics and Clinical Profiles Using the Cbioportal. *Sci Signal* (2013) 6(269):pl1. doi: 10.1126/ scisignal.2004088

Cerami E, Gao J, Dogrusoz U, Gross BE, Sumer SO, Aksoy BA, et al. The Cbio Cancer Genomics Portal: An Open Platform for Exploring Multidimensional Cancer Genomics Data. *Cancer Discov* (2012) 2(5):401– 4. doi: 10.1158/2159-8290.CD-12-0095

Zehir A, Benayed R, Shah RH, Syed A, Middha S, Kim HR, et al. Mutational Landscape of Metastatic Cancer Revealed From Prospective Clinical Sequencing of 10,000 Patients. *Nat Med* (2017) 23(6):703–13. doi: 10.1038/nm.4333

Robinson DR, Wu YM, Lonigro RJ, Vats P, Cobain E, Everett J, et al. Integrative Clinical Genomics of Metastatic Cancer. *Nature* (2017) 548 (7667):297–303. doi: 10.1038/nature23306

Bolton KL, Ptashkin RN, Gao T, Braunstein L, Devlin SM, Kelly D, et al. Cancer Therapy Shapes the Fitness Landscape of Clonal Hematopoiesis. *Nat Genet* (2020) 52(11):1219–26. doi: 10.1038/s41588-020-00710-0

Martinez-Saez O, Chic N, Pascual T, Adamo B, Vidal M, Gonzalez-Farre B, et al. Frequency and Spectrum of PIK3CA Somatic Mutations in Breast Cancer. *Breast Cancer Res* (2020) 22(1):45. doi: 10.1186/s13058-020-01284-9

Dogruluk T, Tsang YH, Espitia M, Chen F, Chen T, Chong Z, et al. Identification of Variant-Specific Functions of PIK3CA by Rapid Phenotyping of Rare Mutations. *Cancer Res* (2015) 75(24):5341–54. doi: 10.1158/0008-5472.CAN-15-1654

Ng PK, Li J, Jeong KJ, Shao S, Chen H, Tsang YH, et al. Systematic Functional Annotation of Somatic Mutations in Cancer. *Cancer Cell* (2018) 33(3):450–62.e10. doi: 10.1016/j.ccell.2018.01.021

Gonzalez-Angulo AM, Chen H, Karuturi MS, Chavez-MacGregor M, Tsavachidis S, Meric-Bernstam F, et al. Frequency of Mesenchymal- Epithelial Transition Factor Gene (MET) and the Catalytic Subunit of Phosphoinositide-3-Kinase

(PIK3CA) Copy Number Elevation and Correlation With Outcome in Patients With Early Stage Breast Cancer. *Cancer* (2013) 119(1):7–15. doi: 10.1002/cncr.27608

Zhang Y, Kwok-Shing Ng P, Kucherlapati M, Chen F, Liu Y, Tsang YH, et al. A Pan-Cancer Proteogenomic Atlas of PI3K/AKT/mTOR Pathway Alterations. *Cancer Cell* (2017) 31(6):820–32.e3. doi: 10.1016/ j.ccell.2017.04.013

Kong Y, Si L, Li Y, Wu X, Xu X, Dai J, et al. Analysis of mTOR Gene Aberrations in Melanoma Patients and Evaluation of Their Sensitivity to PI3K-AKT-mTOR Pathway Inhibitors. *Clin Cancer Res* (2016) 22(4):1018– 27. doi: 10.1158/1078-0432.CCR-15-1110

Brugarolas J. Molecular Genetics of Clear-Cell Renal Cell Carcinoma. *J Clin Oncol* (2014) 32(18):1968–76. doi: 10.1200/JCO.2012.45.2003

Moura AC, Assad DX, Amorim Dos Santos J, Porto de Toledo I, Barra GB, Castilho RM, et al. Worldwide Prevalence of PI3K-AKT-mTOR Pathway Mutations in Head and Neck Cancer: A Systematic Review and Meta- Analysis. *Crit Rev Oncol Hematol* (2021) 160:103284. doi: 10.1016/ j.critrevonc.2021.103284

Kandoth C, McLellan MD, Vandin F, Ye K, Niu B, Lu C, et al. Mutational Landscape and Significance Across 12 Major Cancer Types. *Nature* (2013) 502(7471):333–9. doi: 10.1038/nature12634

Murugan AK, Alzahrani A, Xing M. Mutations in Critical Domains Confer the Human mTOR Gene Strong Tumorigenicity. *J Biol Chem* (2013) 288 (9):6511–21. doi: 10.1074/jbc.M112.399485

Manning BD, Toker A. AKT/PKB Signaling: Navigating the Network. *Cell* (2017) 169(3):381–405. doi: 10.1016/j.cell.2017.04.001

Vivanco I, Sawyers CL. The Phosphatidylinositol 3-Kinase AKT Pathway in Human Cancer. *Nat Rev Cancer* (2002) 2(7):489–501. doi: 10.1038/nrc839

Parikh C, Janakiraman V, Wu WI, Foo CK, Kljavin NM, Chaudhuri S, et al. Disruption of PH-Kinase Domain Interactions Leads to Oncogenic Activation of AKT in Human Cancers. *Proc Natl Acad Sci USA* (2012) 109(47):19368–73. doi: 10.1073/pnas.1204384109

Rudolph M, Anzeneder T, Schulz A, Beckmann G, Byrne AT, Jeffers M, et al. AKT1 (E17K) Mutation Profiling in Breast Cancer: Prevalence, Concurrent Oncogenic Alterations, and Blood-Based Detection. *BMC Cancer* (2016) 16:622. doi: 10.1186/s12885-016-2626-1

Beaver JA, Gustin JP, Yi KH, Rajpurohit A, Thomas M, Gilbert SF, et al. PIK3CA and AKT1 Mutations Have Distinct Effects on Sensitivity to Targeted Pathway Inhibitors in an Isogenic Luminal Breast Cancer Model System. *Clin Cancer Res* (2013) 19(19):5413–22. doi: 10.1158/1078- 0432.CCR-13-0884

Chen Y, Huang L, Dong Y, Tao C, Zhang R, Shao H, et al. Effect of AKT1 (P. E17K) Hotspot Mutation on Malignant Tumorigenesis and Prognosis. *Front Cell Dev Biol* (2020) 8:573599. doi: 10.3389/fcell.2020.573599

Sharma M, Dey CS. Role of Akt Isoforms in Neuronal Insulin Signaling and Resistance. *Cell Mol Life Sci* (2021) 78(23):7873–98. doi: 10.1007/s00018- 021-03993-6

Pereira L, Horta S, Mateus R, Videira MA. Implications of Akt2/Twist Crosstalk on Breast Cancer Metastatic Outcome. *Drug Discov Today* (2015) 20(9):1152–8. doi: 10.1016/j.drudis.2015.06.010

Song MS, Salmena L, Pandolfi PP. The Functions and Regulation of the PTEN Tumour Suppressor. *Nat Rev Mol Cell Biol* (2012) 13(5):283–96. doi: 10.1038/nrm3330

Xie P, Peng Z, Chen Y, Li H, Du M, Tan Y, et al. Neddylation of PTEN Regulates its Nuclear Import and Promotes Tumor Development. *Cell Res* (2021) 31(3):291–311. doi: 10.1038/s41422-020-00443-z

Hollander MC, Blumenthal GM, Dennis PA. PTEN Loss in the Continuum of Common Cancers, Rare Syndromes and Mouse Models. *Nat Rev Cancer* (2011) 11(4):289–301. doi: 10.1038/nrc3037

Moliere S, Mathelin C. The Cowden Syndrome. *N Engl J Med* (2020) 382 (15):e29. doi: 10.1056/NEJMicm1910478

Alexa M, Hasenburg A, Battista MJ. The TCGA Molecular Classification of Endometrial Cancer and Its Possible Impact on Adjuvant Treatment Decisions. *Cancers (Basel)* (2021) 13(6):1478. doi: 10.3390/cancers13061478

Choi SW, Lee Y, Shin K, Koo H, Kim D, Sa JK, et al. Mutation-Specific Non-Canonical Pathway of PTEN as a Distinct Therapeutic Target for Glioblastoma. *Cell Death Dis* (2021) 12(4):374. doi: 10.1038/s41419-021- 03657-0

Wang C, Feng Y, Zhang C, Cheng D, Wu R, Yang Y, et al. PTEN Deletion Drives Aberrations of DNA Methylome and Transcriptome in Different Stages of Prostate Cancer. *FASEB J* (2020) 34(1):1304–18. doi: 10.1096/ fj.201901205RR

Ma J, Benitez JA, Li J, Miki S, Ponte de Albuquerque C, Galatro T, et al. Inhibition of Nuclear PTEN Tyrosine Phosphorylation Enhances Glioma Radiation Sensitivity Through Attenuated DNA Repair. *Cancer Cell* (2019) 35(3):504–18.e7. doi: 10.1016/j.ccell.2019.01.020

Tian T, Li X, Zhang J. mTOR Signaling in Cancer and mTOR Inhibitors in Solid Tumor Targeting Therapy. *Int J Mol Sci* (2019) 20(3):755. doi: 10.3390/ijms20030755

Mange A, Coyaud E, Desmetz C, Laurent E, Beganton B, Coopman P, et al. FKBP4 Connects Mtorc2 and PI3K to Activate the PDK1/Akt-Dependent Cell Proliferation Signaling in Breast Cancer. *Theranostics* (2019) 9 (23):7003–15. doi: 10.7150/thno.35561

Evangelisti C, Chiarini F, Paganelli F, Marmiroli S, Martelli AM. Crosstalks of GSK3 Signaling With the mTOR Network and Effects on Targeted Therapy of Cancer. *Biochim Biophys Acta Mol Cell Res* (2020) 1867 (4):118635. doi: 10.1016/j.bbamcr.2019.118635

Bian YH, Xu J, Zhao WY, Zhang ZZ, Tu L, Cao H, et al. Targeting Mtorc2 Component Rictor Inhibits Cell Proliferation and Promotes Apoptosis in Gastric Cancer. *Am J Transl Res* (2017) 9(9):4317–30.

Lu Z, Shi X, Gong F, Li S, Wang Y, Ren Y, et al. RICTOR/mTORC2 Affects Tumorigenesis and Therapeutic Efficacy of mTOR Inhibitors in Esophageal Squamous Cell Carcinoma. *Acta Pharm Sin B* (2020) 10(6):1004–19. doi: 10.1016/j.apsb.2020.01.010

Yoshida GJ. Therapeutic Strategies of Drug Repositioning Targeting Autophagy to Induce Cancer Cell Death: From Pathophysiology to Treatment. *J Hematol Oncol* (2017) 10(1):67. doi: 10.1186/s13045-017- 0436-9

Al-Bari MAA, Xu P. Molecular Regulation of Autophagy Machinery by mTOR-Dependent and -Independent Pathways. *Ann N Y Acad Sci* (2020) 1467(1):3–20. doi: 10.1111/nyas.14305

Janku F, McConkey DJ, Hong DS, Kurzrock R. Autophagy as a Target for Anticancer Therapy. *Nat Rev Clin Oncol* (2011) 8(9):528–39. doi: 10.1038/ nrclinonc.2011.71

Nowosad A, Jeannot P, Callot C, Creff J, Perchey RT, Joffre C, et al. P27 Controls Ragulator and mTOR Activity in Amino Acid-Deprived Cells to Regulate the Autophagy-Lysosomal Pathway and Coordinate Cell Cycle and Cell Growth. *Nat Cell Biol* (2020) 22(9):1076–90. doi: 10.1038/s41556-020- 0554-4

Cabezudo S, Sanz-Flores M, Caballero A, Tasset I, Rebollo E, Diaz A, et al. Galphaq Activation Modulates Autophagy by Promoting Mtorc1 Signaling. *Nat Commun* (2021) 12(1):4540. doi: 10.1038/s41467-021-24811-4

Wong RS. Apoptosis in Cancer: From Pathogenesis to Treatment. *J Exp Clin Cancer Res* (2011) 30:87. doi: 10.1186/1756-9966-30-87

Carneiro BA, El-Deiry WS. Targeting Apoptosis in Cancer Therapy. *Nat Rev Clin Oncol* (2020) 17(7):395–417. doi: 10.1038/s41571-020-0341-y

He K, Zheng X, Li M, Zhang L, Yu J. mTOR Inhibitors Induce Apoptosis in Colon Cancer Cells *via* CHOP-Dependent DR5 Induction on 4E-BP1 Dephosphorylation. *Oncogene* (2016) 35(2):148–57. doi: 10.1038/ onc.2015.79

Nishida N, Yano H, Nishida T, Kamura T, Kojiro M. Angiogenesis in Cancer. *Vasc Health Risk Manag* (2006) 2(3):213–9. doi: 10.2147/ vhrm.2006.2.3.213

Lugano R, Ramachandran M, Dimberg A. Tumor Angiogenesis: Causes, Consequences, Challenges and Opportunities. *Cell Mol Life Sci* (2020) 77 (9):1745–70. doi: 10.1007/s00018-019-03351-7

Zuazo-Gaztelu I, Casanovas O. Unraveling the Role of Angiogenesis in Cancer Ecosystems. *Front Oncol* (2018) 8:248. doi: 10.3389/fonc.2018.00248

Karar J, Maity A. PI3K/AKT/mTOR Pathway in Angiogenesis. *Front Mol Neurosci* (2011) 4:51. doi: 10.3389/fnmol.2011.00051

Ji L, Wu M, Li Z. Rutacecarpine Inhibits Angiogenesis by Targeting the VEGFR2 and VEGFR2-Mediated Akt/mTOR/p70s6k Signaling Pathway. *Molecules* (2018) 23(8):2047. doi: 10.3390/molecules23082047

Wang M, Xu Y, Wen GZ, Wang Q, Yuan SM. Rapamycin Suppresses Angiogenesis and Lymphangiogenesis in Melanoma by Downregulating VEGF-A/VEGFR-2 and VEGF-C/VEGFR-3 Expression. *Onco Targets Ther* (2019) 12:4643–54. doi: 10.2147/OTT.S205160

Kim K, Kim IK, Yang JM, Lee E, Koh BI, Song S, et al. SoxF Transcription Factors Are Positive Feedback Regulators of VEGF Signaling. *Circ Res* (2016) 119(7):839–52. doi: 10.1161/CIRCRESAHA.116.308483

Roche J. The Epithelial-To-Mesenchymal Transition in Cancer. *Cancers (Basel)* (2018) 10(2):52. doi: 10.3390/cancers10020052

Yang J, Antin P, Berx G, Blanpain C, Brabletz T, Bronner M, et al. Guidelines and Definitions for Research on Epithelial-Mesenchymal Transition. *Nat Rev Mol Cell Biol* (2020) 21(6):341–52. doi: 10.1038/s41580-020-0237-9

Chen HT, Liu H, Mao MJ, Tan Y, Mo XQ, Meng XJ, et al. Crosstalk Between Autophagy and Epithelial-Mesenchymal Transition and its Application in Cancer Therapy. *Mol Cancer* (2019) 18(1):101. doi: 10.1186/s12943-019- 1030-2

Herrerias MM, Budinger GRS. Revisiting mTOR and Epithelial- Mesenchymal Transition. *Am J Respir Cell Mol Biol* (2020) 62(6):669–70. doi: 10.1165/rcmb.2020-0109ED

Annunziata MC, Parisi M, Esposito G, Fabbrocini G, Ammendola R, Cattaneo F. Phosphorylation Sites in Protein Kinases and Phosphatases Regulated by Formyl Peptide Receptor 2 Signaling. *Int J Mol Sci* (2020) 21 (11):3818. doi: 10.3390/ijms21113818

Karimi Roshan M, Soltani A, Soleimani A, Rezaie Kahkhaie K, Afshari AR, Soukhtanloo M. Role of AKT and mTOR Signaling Pathways in the Induction of

Epithelial-Mesenchymal Transition (EMT) Process. *Biochimie* (2019) 165:229–34. doi: 10.1016/j.biochi.2019.08.003

Hao Y, Baker D, Ten Dijke P. TGF-Beta-Mediated Epithelial-Mesenchymal Transition and Cancer Metastasis. *Int J Mol Sci* (2019) 20(11):2767. doi: 10.3390/ijms20112767

Choi D, Kim CL, Kim JE, Mo JS, Jeong HS. Hesperetin Inhibit EMT in TGF-Beta Treated Podocyte by Regulation of mTOR Pathway. *Biochem Biophys Res Commun* (2020) 528(1):154–9. doi: 10.1016/j.bbrc.2020.05.087

Lamouille S, Connolly E, Smyth JW, Akhurst RJ, Derynck R. TGF-Beta- Induced Activation of mTOR Complex 2 Drives Epithelial-Mesenchymal Transition and Cell Invasion. *J Cell Sci* (2012) 125(Pt 5):1259–73. doi: 10.1242/jcs.095299

Gremke N, Polo P, Dort A, Schneikert J, Elmshauser S, Brehm C, et al. mTOR-Mediated Cancer Drug Resistance Suppresses Autophagy and Generates a Druggable Metabolic Vulnerability. *Nat Commun* (2020) 11 (1):4684. doi: 10.1038/s41467-020-18504-7

Murugan AK. mTOR: Role in Cancer, Metastasis and Drug Resistance. *Semin Cancer Biol* (2019) 59:92–111. doi: 10.1016/j.semcancer.2019.07.003

Rascio F, Spadaccino F, Rocchetti MT, Castellano G, Stallone G, Netti GS, et al. The Pathogenic Role of PI3K/AKT Pathway in Cancer Onset and Drug Resistance: An Updated Review. *Cancers (Basel)* (2021) 13(16):3949. doi: 10.3390/cancers13163949

Shen C, Oswald D, Phelps D, Cam H, Pelloski CE, Pang Q, et al. Regulation of FANCD2 by the mTOR Pathway Contributes to the Resistance of Cancer Cells to DNA Double-Strand Breaks. *Cancer Res* (2013) 73(11):3393–401. doi: 10.1158/0008-5472.CAN-12-4282

Gaur S, Chen L, Yang L, Wu X, Un F, Yen Y. Inhibitors of mTOR Overcome Drug Resistance From Topoisomerase II Inhibitors in Solid Tumors. *Cancer Lett* (2011) 311(1):20–8. doi: 10.1016/j.canlet.2011.06.005

Wu Q, Ma J, Wei J, Meng W, Wang Y, Shi M. FOXD1-AS1 Regulates FOXD1 Translation and Promotes Gastric Cancer Progression and Chemoresistance by Activating the PI3K/AKT/mTOR Pathway. *Mol Oncol* (2021) 15(1):299–316. doi: 10.1002/1878-0261.12728

Deng J, Bai X, Feng X, Ni J, Beretov J, Graham P, et al. Inhibition of PI3K/ Akt/ mTOR Signaling Pathway Alleviates Ovarian Cancer Chemoresistance Through Reversing Epithelial-Mesenchymal Transition and Decreasing Cancer Stem Cell Marker Expression. *BMC Cancer* (2019) 19(1):618. doi: 10.1186/s12885-019-5824-9

Wu J, Cheng Z, Xu X, Fu J, Wang K, Liu T, et al. Aurora-A Induces Chemoresistance Through Activation of the AKT/mTOR Pathway in Endometrial Cancer. *Front Oncol* (2019) 9:422. doi: 10.3389/ fonc.2019.00422

Hong DS, Bowles DW, Falchook GS, Messersmith WA, George GC, O'Bryant CL, et al. A Multicenter Phase I Trial of PX-866, an Oral Irreversible Phosphatidylinositol 3-Kinase Inhibitor, in Patients With Advanced Solid Tumors. *Clin Cancer Res* (2012) 18(15):4173–82. doi: 10.1158/1078-0432.CCR-12-0714

Pitz MW, Eisenhauer EA, MacNeil MV, Thiessen B, Easaw JC, Macdonald DR, et al. Phase II Study of PX-866 in Recurrent Glioblastoma. *Neuro Oncol* (2015) 17(9):1270–4. doi: 10.1093/neuonc/nou365

Di Leo A, Johnston S, Lee KS, Ciruelos E, Lonning PE, Janni W, et al. Buparlisib Plus Fulvestrant in Postmenopausal Women With Hormone- Receptor-Positive, HER2-Negative, Advanced Breast Cancer Progressing on or After mTOR Inhibition (BELLE-3): A Randomised, Double-Blind, Placebo-Controlled, Phase 3 Trial. *Lancet Oncol* (2018) 19(1):87–100. doi: 10.1016/S1470-2045(17)30688-5

Wen PY, Touat M, Alexander BM, Mellinghoff IK, Ramkissoon S, McCluskey CS, et al. Buparlisib in Patients With Recurrent Glioblastoma Harboring Phosphatidylinositol 3-Kinase Pathway Activation: An Open- Label, Multicenter, Multi-Arm, Phase II Trial. *J Clin Oncol* (2019) 37 (9):741–50. doi: 10.1200/JCO.18.01207

Soulieres D, Faivre S, Mesia R, Remenar E, Li SH, Karpenko A, et al. Buparlisib and Paclitaxel in Patients With Platinum-Pretreated Recurrent or Metastatic Squamous Cell Carcinoma of the Head and Neck (BERIL-1): A Randomised, Double-Blind, Placebo-Controlled Phase 2 Trial. *Lancet Oncol* (2017) 18(3):323–35. doi: 10.1016/S1470-2045(17)30064-5

Dreyling M, Santoro A, Mollica L, Leppa S, Follows GA, Lenz G, et al. Phosphatidylinositol 3-Kinase Inhibition by Copanlisib in Relapsed or Refractory Indolent Lymphoma. *J Clin Oncol* (2017) 35(35):3898–905. doi: 10.1200/JCO.2017.75.4648

Brown JR, Byrd JC, Coutre SE, Benson DM, Flinn IW, Wagner-Johnston ND, et al. Idelalisib, an Inhibitor of Phosphatidylinositol 3-Kinase P110delta, for Relapsed/ Refractory Chronic Lymphocytic Leukemia. *Blood* (2014) 123 (22):3390–7. doi: 10.1182/blood-2013-11-535047

Flinn IW, Hillmen P, Montillo M, Nagy Z, Illes A, Etienne G, et al. The Phase 3 DUO Trial: Duvelisib vs Ofatumumab in Relapsed and Refractory CLL/ SLL. *Blood* (2018) 132(23):2446–55. doi: 10.1182/blood-2018-05-850461

Flinn IW, Miller CB, Ardeshna KM, Tetreault S, Assouline SE, Mayer J, et al. DYNAMO: A Phase II Study of Duvelisib (IPI-145) in Patients With Refractory Indolent Non-Hodgkin Lymphoma. *J Clin Oncol* (2019) 37 (11):912–22. doi: 10.1200/JCO.18.00915

Andre F, Ciruelos E, Rubovszky G, Campone M, Loibl S, Rugo HS, et al. Alpelisib for PIK3CA-Mutated, Hormone Receptor-Positive Advanced Breast Cancer. *N Engl J Med* (2019) 380(20):1929–40. doi: 10.1056/ NEJMoa1813904

Juric D, Rodon J, Tabernero J, Janku F, Burris HA, Schellens JHM, et al. Phosphatidylinositol 3-Kinase Alpha-Selective Inhibition With Alpelisib (BYL719) in PIK3CA-Altered Solid Tumors: Results From the First-In- Human Study. *J Clin Oncol* (2018) 36(13):1291–9. doi: 10.1200/ JCO.2017.72.7107

Fowler NH, Samaniego F, Jurczak W, Ghosh N, Derenzini E, Reeves JA, et al. Umbralisib, a Dual PI3Kdelta/CK1epsilon Inhibitor in Patients With Relapsed or Refractory Indolent Lymphoma. *J Clin Oncol* (2021) 39 (15):1609–18. doi: 10.1200/JCO.20.03433

Kalinsky K, Hong F, McCourt CK, Sachdev JC, Mitchell EP, Zwiebel JA, et al. Effect of Capivasertib in Patients With an AKT1 E17K-Mutated Tumor: NCI-MATCH Subprotocol EAY131-Y Nonrandomized Trial. *JAMA Oncol* (2021) 7(2):271–8. doi: 10.1001/jamaoncol.2020.6741

Crabb SJ, Griffiths G, Marwood E, Dunkley D, Downs N, Martin K, et al. Pan-AKT Inhibitor Capivasertib With Docetaxel and Prednisolone in Metastatic Castration-Resistant Prostate Cancer: A Randomized, Placebo- Controlled Phase II Trial (ProCAID). *J Clin Oncol* (2021) 39(3):190–201. doi: 10.1200/JCO.20.01576

Jones RH, Casbard A, Carucci M, Cox C, Butler R, Alchami F, et al. Fulvestrant Plus Capivasertib Versus Placebo After Relapse or Progression on an Aromatase Inhibitor in Metastatic, Oestrogen Receptor-Positive Breast Cancer (FAKTION): A Multicentre, Randomised, Controlled, Phase 2 Trial. *Lancet Oncol* (2020) 21(3):345–57. doi: 10.1016/S1470-2045(19)30817-4

Schmid P, Abraham J, Chan S, Wheatley D, Brunt AM, Nemsadze G, et al. Capivasertib Plus Paclitaxel Versus Placebo Plus Paclitaxel As First-Line Therapy for Metastatic Triple-Negative Breast Cancer: The PAKT Trial. *J Clin Oncol* (2020) 38(5):423–33. doi: 10.1200/JCO.19.00368

Saura C, Roda D, Rosello S, Oliveira M, Macarulla T, Perez-Fidalgo JA, et al. A First-In-Human Phase I Study of the ATP-Competitive AKT Inhibitor Ipatasertib Demonstrates Robust and Safe Targeting of AKT in Patients With Solid Tumors. *Cancer Discov* (2017) 7(1):102–13. doi: 10.1158/2159- 8290.CD-16-0512

Sweeney C, Bracarda S, Sternberg CN, Chi KN, Olmos D, Sandhu S, et al. Ipatasertib Plus Abiraterone and Prednisolone in Metastatic Castration- Resistant Prostate Cancer (IPATential150): A Multicentre, Randomised, Double-Blind, Phase 3 Trial. *Lancet* (2021) 398(10295):131–42. doi: 10.1016/S0140-6736(21)00580-8

Kim SB, Dent R, Im SA, Espie M, Blau S, Tan AR, et al. Ipatasertib Plus Paclitaxel Versus Placebo Plus Paclitaxel as First-Line Therapy for Metastatic Triple-Negative Breast Cancer (LOTUS): A Multicentre, Randomised, Double-Blind, Placebo-Controlled, Phase 2 Trial. *Lancet Oncol* (2017) 18 (10):1360–72. doi: 10.1016/S1470-2045(17)30450-3

Chien AJ, Tripathy D, Albain KS, Symmans WF, Rugo HS, Melisko ME, et al. MK-2206 and Standard Neoadjuvant Chemotherapy Improves Response in Patients With Human Epidermal Growth Factor Receptor 2-Positive and/or Hormone Receptor-Negative Breast Cancers in the I-SPY 2 Trial. *J Clin Oncol* (2020) 38(10):1059–69. doi: 10.1200/JCO.19.01027

Komiya T, Memmott RM, Blumenthal GM, Bernstein W, Ballas MS, De Chowdhury R, et al. A Phase I/II Study of Pemetrexed With Sirolimus in Advanced, Previously Treated Non-Small Cell Lung Cancer. *Transl Lung Cancer Res* (2019) 8(3):247–57. doi: 10.21037/tlcr.2019.04.19

Motzer RJ, Hudes GR, Curti BD, McDermott DF, Escudier BJ, Negrier S, et al. Phase I/II Trial of Temsirolimus Combined With Interferon Alfa for Advanced Renal Cell Carcinoma. *J Clin Oncol* (2007) 25(25):3958–64. doi: 10.1200/JCO.2006.10.5916

Fan Y, Sun T, Shao Z, Zhang Q, Ouyang Q, Tong Z, et al. Effectiveness of Adding Everolimus to the First-Line Treatment of Advanced Breast Cancer in Premenopausal Women Who Experienced Disease Progression While Receiving Selective Estrogen Receptor Modulators: A Phase 2 Randomized Clinical Trial. *JAMA Oncol* (2021) 7(10):e213428. doi: 10.1001/ jamaoncol.2021.3428

Schmid P, Zaiss M, Harper-Wynne C, Ferreira M, Dubey S, Chan S, et al. Fulvestrant Plus Vistusertib vs Fulvestrant Plus Everolimus vs Fulvestrant Alone for Women With Hormone Receptor-Positive Metastatic Breast Cancer: The MANTA Phase 2 Randomized Clinical Trial. *JAMA Oncol* (2019) 5(11):1556–64. doi: 10.1001/jamaoncol.2019.2526

Bautista F, Paoletti X, Rubino J, Brard C, Rezai K, Nebchi S, et al. Phase I or II Study of Ribociclib in Combination With Topotecan-Temozolomide or Everolimus in

Children With Advanced Malignancies: Arms A and B of the AcSe-ESMART Trial. *J Clin Oncol* (2021) 39(32):3546–60. doi: 10.1200/ JCO.21.01152

Morscher RJ, Brard C, Berlanga P, Marshall LV, Andre N, Rubino J, et al. First-In-Child Phase I/II Study of the Dual Mtorc1/2 Inhibitor Vistusertib (AZD2014) as Monotherapy and in Combination With Topotecan- Temozolomide in Children With Advanced Malignancies: Arms E and F of the AcSe-ESMART Trial. *Eur J Cancer* (2021) 157:268–77. doi: 10.1016/ j.ejca.2021.08.010

Lim B, Potter DA, Salkeni MA, Silverman P, Haddad TC, Forget F, et al. Sapanisertib Plus Exemestane or Fulvestrant in Women With Hormone Receptor-Positive/ HER2-Negative Advanced or Metastatic Breast Cancer. *Clin Cancer Res* (2021) 27(12):3329–38. doi: 10.1158/1078-0432.CCR-20-4131

Mishra R, Patel H, Alanazi S, Kilroy MK, Garrett JT. PI3K Inhibitors in Cancer: Clinical Implications and Adverse Effects. *Int J Mol Sci* (2021) 22 (7):3464. doi: 10.3390/ijms22073464

Hillmann P, Fabbro D. PI3K/mTOR Pathway Inhibition: Opportunities in Oncology and Rare Genetic Diseases. *Int J Mol Sci* (2019) 20(22):5792. doi: 10.3390/ijms20225792

Yang J, Nie J, Ma X, Wei Y, Peng Y, Wei X. Targeting PI3K in Cancer: Mechanisms and Advances in Clinical Trials. *Mol Cancer* (2019) 18(1):26. doi: 10.1186/ s12943-019-0954-x

Salazar R, Garcia-Carbonero R, Libutti SK, Hendifar AE, Custodio A, Guimbaud R, et al. Phase II Study of BEZ235 Versus Everolimus in Patients With Mammalian Target of Rapamycin Inhibitor-Naive Advanced Pancreatic Neuroendocrine Tumors. *Oncologist* (2018) 23 (7):766–e90. doi: 10.1634/theoncologist.2017-0144

Massard C, Chi KN, Castellano D, de Bono J, Gravis G, Dirix L, et al. Phase Ib Dose-Finding Study of Abiraterone Acetate Plus Buparlisib (BKM120) or Dactolisib (BEZ235) in Patients With Castration-Resistant Prostate Cancer. *Eur J Cancer* (2017) 76:36–44. doi: 10.1016/j.ejca.2017.01.024

Wise-Draper TM, Moorthy G, Salkeni MA, Karim NA, Thomas HE, Mercer CA, et al. A Phase Ib Study of the Dual PI3K/mTOR Inhibitor Dactolisib (BEZ235) Combined With Everolimus in Patients With Advanced Solid Malignancies. *Target Oncol* (2017) 12(3):323–32. doi: 10.1007/s11523-017- 0482-9

Colombo I, Genta S, Martorana F, Guidi M, Frattini M, Samartzis EP, et al. Phase I Dose-Escalation Study of the Dual PI3K-Mtorc1/2 Inhibitor Gedatolisib in Combination With Paclitaxel and Carboplatin in Patients With Advanced Solid Tumors. *Clin Cancer Res* (2021) 27(18):5012–9. doi: 10.1158/1078-0432.CCR-21-1402

Makker V, Recio FO, Ma L, Matulonis UA, Lauchle JO, Parmar H, et al. A Multicenter, Single-Arm, Open-Label, Phase 2 Study of Apitolisib (GDC- 0980) for the Treatment of Recurrent or Persistent Endometrial Carcinoma (MAGGIE Study). *Cancer* (2016) 122(22):3519–28. doi: 10.1002/cncr.30286

14

Role of Small Molecule Targeted Compounds in Cancer: Progress, Opportunities and Challenges

Guoqiang Sun[1†], Dawei Rong[2†], Zhouxiao Li[3†], Guangshun Sun[1], Fan Wu[1], Xiao Li[1], Hongyong Cao[1], Ye Cheng[1*], Weiwei Tang[2*] and Yangbai Sun[4*]*

[1] *Department of General Surgery, Nanjing First Hospital, Nanjing Medical University, Nanjing, China,* [2] *Hepatobiliary/Liver Transplantation Center, The First Affiliated Hospital of Nanjing Medical University, Key Laboratory of Living Donor Transplantation, Chinese Academy of Medical Sciences, Nanjing, China,* [3] *Department of Hand Surgery, Plastic Surgery and Aesthetic Surgery, Ludwig-Maximilians University, Munich, Germany,* [4] *Department of Musculoskeletal Surgery, Fudan University Shanghai Cancer Center, Shanghai, China*

***Correspondence:**
Hongyong Cao
caohongy6167@163.com
Ye Cheng
m18270916389@163.com
Weiwei Tang
1243773473twww@sina.com
Yangbai Sun
drsunyb@fudan.edu.cn

†These authors share first authorship

Research on molecular targeted therapy of tumors is booming, and novel targeted therapy drugs are constantly emerging. Small molecule targeted compounds, novel targeted therapy drugs, can be administered orally as tablets among other methods, and do not draw upon genes, causing no immune response. It is easily structurally modified to make it more applicable to clinical needs, and convenient to promote due to low cost. It refers to a hotspot in the research of tumor molecular targeted therapy. In the present study, we review the current Food and Drug Administration (FDA)-approved use of small molecule targeted compounds in tumors, summarize the clinical drug resistance problems and mechanisms facing the use of small molecule targeted compounds, and predict the future directions of the evolving field.

Keywords: small molecular compounds, carcinoma, drug resistance, target, therapy

INTRODUCTION

The tumor is a neoplastic proliferation of the abnormal cells of the body formed. Usually, it is abnormal tissue mass on parts of the body. It refers to a new organism generated by abnormal proliferation and the differentiating process of body cells based on a range of initiating and promoting elements. If new organisms develop, they continue to proliferate since the restraints are eliminated. Its growth accepts no normal physiological regulation, while damaging normal tissues and organs. From the perspective of the progression of tumor occurrence and development, the difficulties of the tumor treating process are elucidated below. (1) The etiology of primary tumors remains unclear, and tumors are unlikely to be cured completely. (2) Specific to one group of uncontrolled, infinitely proliferating cells, during their proliferation, the structure and function of normal tissues and organs will be destroyed, and the normal physiological function of the body will be affected. For instance, the immune function of most cases subject to malignant tumors will be reduced to various degrees, causing the body's immune system to be unable to initiate the regular immune program for the tumor's inhibiting process. (3) The treating process of the tumor cannot be ended only by the patient's recent recovery after his treating process, since the tumor is significantly prone to relapse and metastasis, and an active treating process is required during its occurrence. On the whole, the treating process of a malignant tumor consists of the surgical treating process, chemotherapeutic process, radiotherapy, immunotherapy, etc.

(Wyld et al., 2015; De Ruysscher et al., 2019; Heinhuis et al., 2019; McLaughlin et al., 2020). The specific treating process plan should be discussed under the diagnosis and treating process mode with the participation of multiple doctors. It should be taken and determined given the nature of the tumor, stage, and the patient's systemic state.

The new drug developing process shifts its focus to identify molecules and target carcinomas. Carcinoma therapeutic process can be targeted primarily by small molecules and antibodies (Diesendruck and Benhar, 2017; Huck et al., 2018). Antibodies usually exhibit high selective properties. Nevertheless, their aims fall generally into the restriction of the cell surface and are unable to exert drug effect in the membrane. In addition, antibodies should be injected intravenously or subcutaneously for their high molecular weight (e.g., molecule weight of antibody PD-1 Pembrolizumab is 146.286 KD, molecule weight of PD-1 inhibitor BMS-1 is 475.58) and influence of gastrointestinal enzymes on protein digestion. As opposed to those mentioned, small molecule targeted compounds have different selective properties and, due to their small sizes (molecule weight <1000), are capable of binding to various intracellular and extracellular aims orally (Moroz et al., 2016; Wu et al., 2016; Roskoski, 2020). Here, we selected 103 anti-cancer small molecule targeted compounds (**Table 1**) from the U.S. Food and Drug Administration (FDA) approved drugs to treat cancer[1]. Many of mentioned approvals have shown advantages compared with the cytotoxic chemotherapeutic process, with fewer side influences from the critical treating process inside a recurrence or metastatic environment. Moreover, there are instances regarding small molecule targeted compounds gaining the approval to treat residual disease or as adjuvant therapeutic processes based on therapeutic intent. This review will review the current FDA-approved use of small molecule targeted compounds in tumors, summarize the clinical drug resistance problems and mechanisms facing the use of molecular inhibitors, and predict the future directions of the evolving field.

CLASSIFICATION OF SMALL MOLECULE TARGETED COMPOUNDS

The principle of small molecule targeted compounds is to target the molecular biology basis of tumorigenesis, usually to regulate the activity of protein targets. Depending on the type of target, small molecule targeted compounds play different roles. At present, the protein targets of small molecule targeted compounds mainly include enzymes, and receptors. Small molecule targeted compounds can be divided into receptor agonists and receptor antagonists while acting on the receptor.

Enzyme Inhibitor

Small molecules that act as inhibiting elements of enzymes reduce their catalytic activity by binding to them. Sunitinib and Sorafenib refer to prototypic instances of small molecule multikinase inhibitors (Ito et al., 2019; Procopio et al., 2019; Verschuur et al., 2019; Zahoor et al., 2019; Mammatas et al., 2020; Ruanglertboon et al., 2020). Consistent with most agents pertaining to the mentioned class, these two drugs suppress PDGFR-α, KIT, VEGFR2, and VEGFR1 in various targets. Sunitinib is a multi-target RTK inhibitor, targeting VEGFR2, and PDGFRβ, which also inhibits c-Kit (Mendel et al., 2003). Sunitinib is approved to treat adults with gastrointestinal stromal tumor, pancreatic neuroendocrine tumor and renal cell carcinoma (RCC). A multinational, randomized, double-blind, placebo-controlled phase 3 trial evaluated the clinical effect of Sunitinib in patients with advanced, well-differentiated pancreatic neuroendocrine tumors. The median progression-free survival (mPFS) was 11.4 months in the Sunitinib group versus 5.5 months in the placebo group. The objective response rate was 9.3% of the Sunitinib group and 0% of the placebo group. Clinical trial results show that Sunitinib improves the mPES and objective remission rate (ORR) of patients with pancreatic neuroendocrine tumors. Clinical trial results show that Sunitinib improves the mPES and ORR of patients with pancreatic neuroendocrine tumors. The adverse reactions caused by Sunitinib in the experiment were diarrhea, nausea, vomiting, weakness, and fatigue (Raymond et al., 2011).

Sorafenib is applied in renal cell cancer, hepatocellular carcinoma and thyroid cancer, based on FDA approval. Sorafenib is a multikinase inhibitor of Raf-1, B-Raf, and VEGFR (Wilhelm et al., 2004). In addition to inhibiting the RAF/MEK/ERK signaling pathway, Sorafenib tosylate significantly inhibits the phosphorylation of eIF4E and down-regulates the level of Mcl-1 in liver cancer (HCC) cells in a MEK/ERK-dependent manner, and induces significant apoptosis (Liu et al., 2006). Due to factors such as hepatitis B virus infection, the incidence of liver cancer remains high in the Asia-Pacific region (Petrick et al., 2016). The application of Sorafenib in liver cancer is prevalent. Therefore, the clinical effect of Sorafenib in patients in the Asia-Pacific region is an important issue. A phase III randomized, double-blind, placebo-controlled trial in patients of the Asia-Pacific region with advanced hepatocellular carcinoma evaluated the efficacy and safety of Sorafenib. A total of 271 patients from China, South Korea, and Taiwan was enrolled in the study. Finally, the median overall survival (MOS) of the sorafenib treatment group was 6.5 months, and that of the placebo group was 4.2 months. The median time to progression was 2.8 months in the Sorafenib group and 1.4 months in the placebo group. The most common grade 3/4 drug-related adverse events were hand-foot skin reactions (10.7%), diarrhea (6.0%), and fatigue (3.4%), and these adverse events rarely lead to discontinuation (Cheng et al., 2009). Dose-restricting toxic influences are consistent in such a drug class and receive the predominant motivation through the VEGFR inhibiting process. One subset of carcinomas is significantly addicted to one oncogene or certain molecular defects capable of exploiting channels selectively (e.g., those impacting DNA repairing or apoptotic process). Selection-related small molecule targeted compounds are capable of effectively antagonizing the expected aim and eliminating the off-aim inhibiting process, probably causing dose decrease or reduction of intolerable side-influences. EGFR inhibitors (e.g., Gefitinib and Erlotinib) received the initial development with no single

[1]https://www.cancer.gov/about-cancer/treatment/drugs

TABLE 1 | The application of small molecule targeted compounds in tumors.

Compound name	Indication of tumor type	Target
Erdafitinib	Urothelial carcinoma	FGFR
Everolimus	Breast cancer, Pancreatic cancer, gastrointestinal cancer, gastrointestinal cancer, and lung cancer, Subependymal giant cell astrocytoma, Renal Cell Cancer	mTOR
Abemaciclib	Breast cancer	CDK4/6
Alpelisib	Breast cancer	PI3Kα
Anastrozole	Breast cancer	Aromatase
Exemestane	Breast cancer	Aromatase
Toremifene	Breast cancer	Estrogen receptor
Fulvestrant	Breast cancer	Estrogen receptor
Letrozole	Breast cancer	Estrogen receptor
Palbociclib	Breast cancer	CDK4/6
Ribociclib	Breast cancer	CDK4/6
Lapatinib ditosylate	Breast cancer	EGFR,ErbB2,ErbB4
Olaparib	Breast cancer, ovarian cancer, Ovarian epithelial, fallopian tube, or primary peritoneal cancer, Pancreatic cancer, Prostate cancer	PARP1/2
Megestrol acetate	Breast cancer, Endometrial cancer	progestogen Receptor, Androgen Receptor
Neratinib maleate	Breast cancer	HER2, EGFR
Tamoxifen citrate	Breast cancer, Ductal carcinoma *in situ*	Estrogen receptor
Talazoparib tosylate	Breast cancer	PARP1
Tucatinib	Breast cancer	HER2, ErbB2
Goserelin acetate	Breast cancer, prostate cancer	LHRH agonist
Topotecan Hydrochloride	Cervical cancer, Ovarian cancer, Ovarian cancer	Topoisomerase I
Irinotecan Hydrochloride	Colorectal cancer, Rectal Cancer	Topoisomerase I
Regorafenib	Colorectal cancer, Gastrointestinal stromal tumor, Hepatocellular carcinoma, Rectal Cancer	Ret, Raf-1,VEGFR2
Ziv-Aflibercept	Colorectal cancer, Rectal Cancer	KIT, PDGFRβ, RAF, RET, VEGFR1/2/3
Lenvatinib mesylate	Endometrial carcinoma, Hepatocellular carcinoma, Renal cell carcinoma, Thyroid cancer	VEGFR1/2/3, c-RET
Avapritinib	Gastrointestinal stromal tumor	PDGFRα, c-Kit
Imatinib mesylate	Acute lymphoblastic leukemia, Chronic eosinophilic leukemia or hypereosinophilic syndrome, Chronic myelogenous leukemia, Dermatofibrosarcoma protuberans, Gastrointestinal stromal tumor, Myelodysplastic/myeloproliferative neoplasms, Systemic mastocytosis	v-Abl,c-Kit, PDGFR
Ripretinib	Gastrointestinal stromal tumor	c-Kit,PDGFRα
Sunitinib malate	Gastrointestinal stromal tumor, Pancreatic cancer, Renal cell carcinoma	VEGFR2, PDGFRβ, c-kit
Axitinib	Renal Cell Cancer	VEGFR1/2/3,PDGFRβ,c-Kit
Tivozanib Hydrochloride	Renal Cell Cancer	VEGFR1/2/3
Sorafenib tosylate	Renal Cell Cancer, Hepatocellular carcinoma, Thyroid cancer	Raf-1, VEGFR2, B-Raf
Pazopanib Hydrochloride	Renal Cell Cancer	VEGFR1/2/3
Temsirolimus	Renal Cell Cancer	mTOR
Dasatinib	Acute Lymphoblastic Leukemia (ALL), Chronic myelogenous leukemia (CML)	Abl, Src, c-Kit
Ponatinib Hydrochloride	Acute lymphoblastic leukemia, Chronic myelogenous leukemia (CML)	Abl,PDGFRα,VEGFR2,FGFR1, Src
Enasidenib mesylate	Acute myeloid leukemia (AML)	IDH2
Gilteritinib fumarate	Acute myeloid leukemia (AML)	FLT3/AXL
Glasdegib maleate	Acute myeloid leukemia	Smoothened (Smo)
Ivosidenib	Acute myeloid leukemia (AML)	IDH1
Midostaurin	Acute myeloid leukemia (AML), mast cell leukemia	PKCα/β/γ, Syk, Flk-1
Mitoxantrone Hydrochloride	Acute non-lymphocytic leukemia, Acute non-lymphocytic leukemia, Prostate cancer	Topoisomerase II, PKC

(Continued)

TABLE 1 | Continued

Compound name	Indication of tumor type	Target
Venetoclax	Acute myeloid leukemia, Chronic lymphocytic leukemia (CLL) or small lymphocytic lymphoma (SLL)	Bcl-2
Acalabrutinib	Chronic lymphocytic leukemia or small lymphocytic lymphoma, Mantle cell lymphoma	BTK
Duvelisib	Chronic lymphocytic leukemia or small lymphocytic lymphoma, Follicular lymphoma	PI3K δ/γ
Ibrutinib	Chronic lymphocytic leukemia and small lymphocytic lymphoma, Mantle cell lymphoma, Mantle cell lymphoma, Waldenström macroglobulinemia	BTK, Bmx, CSK, FGR, BRK
Idelalisib	Chronic lymphocytic leukemia (CLL), Non-Hodgkin lymphoma (NHL), Follicular B-cell non-Hodgkin lymphoma, Small lymphocytic lymphoma	p110δ
Bosutinib	Chronic myelogenous leukemia (CML)	Src/Abl
Nilotinib	Chronic myelogenous leukemia (CML)	BCR-ABL
Cabozantinib-S-Malate	Hepatocellular carcinoma, Medullary thyroid cancer, Renal cell carcinoma	VEGFR2, c-Met, c-RET, c-Kit
Pemigatinib	Cholangiocarcinoma	FGFR
Afatinib dimaleate	Non-small cell lung cancer (NSCLC)	EGFR, HER2
Alectinib	Non-small cell lung cancer	ALK
Brigatinib	Non-small cell lung cancer	ALK,IGF-1R,FLT3,FLT3, EGFR
Capmatinib Hydrochloride	Non-small cell lung cancer	c-Met
Ceritinib	Non-small cell lung cancer	ALK
Crizotinib	Anaplastic large cell lymphoma, Non-small cell lung cancer	ROS1, c-Met, ALK
Dabrafenib mesylate	Anaplastic thyroid cancer, Melanoma, Non-small cell lung cancer	B-Raf
Dacomitinib	Non-small cell lung cancer	EGFR, ErbB2, ErbB4
Entrectinib	Non-small cell lung cancer, Solid tumors	TrkA/B/C,ROS1, ALK
Erlotinib Hydrochloride	Non-small cell lung cancer, Pancreatic cancer	EGFR
Pralsetinib	Medullary thyroid cancer, Non-small cell lung cancer, Thyroid cancer	RET
Gefitinib	Non-small cell lung cancer	EGFR
Lorlatinib	Non-small cell lung cancer	ALK, ROS1
Trametinib dimethyl sulfoxide	Anaplastic thyroid cancer, Melanoma, Non-small cell lung cancer	MEK
Osimertinib mesylate	Non-small cell lung cancer	EGFR
Selpercatinib	Medullary thyroid cancer, Non-small cell lung cancer, Thyroid cancer	c-RET
Tepotinib Hydrochloride	Non-small cell lung cancer	c-Met
Binimetinib	Melanoma	MEK
Encorafenib	Colorectal cancer, Melanoma	RAF
Vemurafenib	Melanoma	B-Raf^{V600E}
Plerixafor	Multiple myeloma, Non-Hodgkin lymphoma (NHL)	CXCR4, CXCL12
Panobinostat lactate	Multiple myeloma	HDAC
Selinexor	Diffuse large B-cell lymphoma, Multiple myeloma	CRM1
Fedratinib Hydrochloride	Myelofibrosis	JAK2
Ruxolitinib phosphate	Myelofibrosis, Polycythemia vera	JAK1/2
Copanlisib Hydrochloride)	Follicular lymphoma	PI3K$\alpha/\beta/\gamma/\delta$
Belinostat	Peripheral T-cell lymphoma	HDAC
Zanubrutinib	Mantle cell lymphoma	BTK
Romidepsin	Cutaneous T-cell lymphoma, Peripheral T-cell lymphoma	HDAC1, HDAC2
Tazemetostat Hydrobromide	Epithelioid sarcoma, Follicular lymphoma	EZH2
Umbralisib tosylate	Marginal zone lymphoma, Follicular lymphoma	PI3Kδ
Vorinostat	Cutaneous T-cell lymphoma	HDAC
Rucaparib camsylate	Ovarian epithelial, fallopian tube, or primary peritoneal cancer, Prostate cancer	PARP1

(Continued)

TABLE 1 | Continued

Compound name	Indication of tumor type	Target
Niraparib tosylate monohydrate	Ovarian epithelial, fallopian tube, or primary peritoneal cancer	PARP1/PARP2
Propranolol hydrochloride	Infantile hemangioma	β-Adrenoceptor
Apalutamide	Prostate cancer	androgen receptor
Bicalutamide	Prostate cancer	Androgen Receptor
Darolutamide	Prostate cancer	androgen receptor
Degarelix	Prostate cancer	GnRH receptor
Leuprolide acetate	Prostate cancer	GnRHR agonist
Enzalutamide	Prostate cancer	androgen-receptor
Flutamide	Prostate cancer	androgen-receptor
Nilutamide	Prostate cancer	androgen-receptor
Relugolix	Prostate cancer	GnRHR
Vismodegib	Basal cell carcinoma	Hedgehog
Sonidegib	Basal cell carcinoma	Smo
Cobimetinib	Melanoma	MEK
Larotrectinib sulfate	Solid tumors	TRK
Imiquimod	Basal cell carcinoma	TLR7
Vandetanib	Medullary thyroid cancer	VEGFR2
Abiraterone acetate	Prostate cancer	CYP17
Tretinoin	Acute promyelocytic leukemia	Retinoic acid receptor, Retinoid X receptor
Sotorasib	Non-small cell lung cancer	K-Ras (G12C)

case selecting method and exhibited appropriate efficacy in cases subjected to non-small-cell lung carcinoma undergoing the pretreating process using the normal cytotoxic chemotherapeutic process (Shepherd et al., 2005; Kim et al., 2008).

Receptor Antagonist

In normal scenarios, the receptor is activated after binding to its ligand (signal), and the signal is transmitted down, producing certain biological phenomena. Some compounds can bind to the receptor, act in the identical role as the ligand and activate the receptor. Such compounds are receptor agonists. In the presence of an agonist, an antagonist antagonizes the agonistic effect of the agonist on the receptor, and the antagonist alone exerts no effect on the receptor (Pease, 2017; Arena et al., 2018). Prostate carcinoma is the most common carcinoma among aged males in western countries and more aggressive and lethal castration-resistant prostate carcinoma (CRPC) often occurs after the androgen deprivation therapeutic process (ADT). The high expression of androgens and androgen receptors (AR) is closely related to prostate carcinoma. Efficient AR antagonists, such as Enzalutamide and ARN-509, could be employed as potent anti-prostate carcinoma agents (Ge et al., 2018). Selinexor, combined with Dexamethasone, has gained approval for patients with Penta-refractory multiple myeloma (MM) by FDA. As we all know, transcription takes place in the nucleus, separated from the translation of cytoplasm. Nuclear pore complex (NPC) assures adequate cell function of transmission of genetic information, acting as a connection bridge. Large molecule (40 kDa) cargo requires a specific transport receptor protein to pass through NPC, such as chromosome region maintenance-1 (CRM-1) which is the target site to selinexor. Selinexor is a slow reversible, oral and selective Inhibitor of Nuclear Export compound, binding covalently to cysteine 528 in the cargo-binding nuclear export slot of CRM-1 and forcing the nuclear to retain and activate tsp, GR and IkBa; as well as a nuclear-cytoplasmic export limitation and mRNA translation of eIF4E-bound oncoprotein (Sun et al., 2013; Neggers et al., 2015). Consequently, Selinexor triggers cell cycle arrest and apoptosis in the solid and hematologic tumor cells. The part II of phase 2b Selinexor Treatment of Refractory Myeloma (STORM) trial (NCT02336815, part II) enrolled 122 heavily pretreated patients with TCR/Penta- exposed MM. ORR was observed in 26.2% of patients; ORR was observed in 25.3% of the five refractory patients. The clinical benefit rate (CBR) was 39%, the median remission period was 4.4 months, and the most prolonged remission periods exceeded 18 months. mPFS was 3.7 months for all patients, and 2.1 months for non-responders. MOS was 8.6 months for all patients, and 1.9 months for non-responders (Chari et al., 2019; Podar et al., 2020). Lenvatinib inhibits vascular endothelial growth factor receptor 1–3, fibroblast growth factor receptor 1–4, platelet-derived growth factor receptorα, and KIT, approved for Endometrial carcinoma, hepatocellular carcinoma, RCC, thyroid cancer (Matsui et al., 2008). In hepatocellular carcinoma, it is used as a first-line treatment for patients whose disease cannot be removed by surgery. Kudo et al. (2018) concluded that the overall survival rate of Lenvatinib is not inferior to Sorafenib in untreated advanced hepatocellular carcinoma through an open, phase 3, multi-center, non-inferior quality trial. In the study, 954 qualified patients were randomly assigned to Lenvatinib group (n = 478) or sorafenib group (n = 476). The median survival time of Lenvatinib is 13.6 months and not less than the median survival time of Sorafenib 12.3 months, which meets the criteria of non-inferiority. The most common adverse events of any grade in the Lenvatinib group were hypertension [201 cases (42%)], diarrhea [184 cases (39%)], loss of appetite [162 cases (34%)], weight loss [147 cases (31%)]. Palmar and plantar red sensory disturbances [249 cases (52%)], diarrhea [220 cases (46%)], hypertension [144 cases (30%)], and decreased appetite [127 cases (27%)] in the Sorafenib group. These results show that Lenvatinib has a better clinical benefit than Sorafenib (Al-Salama et al., 2019).

Receptor Agonist

Although enzyme inhibitors and receptor antagonists show superior clinical efficacy of various cancers in small molecule targeted compounds, receptor agonists exert a specific effect in cancer endocrine therapy. Androgen deprivation therapy is an essential treatment of advanced and metastatic prostate cancer, including surgical castration and medical castration (Singer et al., 2008) [e.g., Bicalutamide and Nilutamide, Ketoconazole, or Corticosteroids (Teo et al., 2019)], and its purpose is to remove the role of nutrition androgen for prostate cancer. Luteinizing hormone-releasing hormone (LHRH) agonists are a type of androgen deprivation therapy. Goserelin acetate and Leuprolide acetate are LHRH agonists, continuous application can down-regulate the LHRH receptor and cause desensitization of the gonadotropin cell receptor after a short period of high stimulation, resulting in the obstruction of the secretion of testosterone in the testicular stromal cells (Stojilkovic et al., 1994; Shim et al., 2019). Compared with LHRH agonists, anti-androgen drugs show poor survival results, so LHRH agonists have a more comprehensive range of applications in the treatment of prostate cancer (Seidenfeld et al., 2000). A retrospective study showed that, unlike single antiandrogen therapy, LHRH agonist monotherapy provides long-term and durable control of localized prostate cancer. For those anti-androgen monotherapy ineffective patients, LHRH agonist is also an effective treatment option (Raina et al., 2007). In addition to prostate cancer, LHRH agonist Goserelin Acetate is also approved by FDA for the treatment of breast cancer.

THE APPLICATION OF SMALL MOLECULE TARGETED COMPOUNDS IN CANCERS

In this review, we classify the existing small molecule targeted compounds for the carcinoma therapeutic process into the following four categories according to the different channels targeted. We have screened out 103 small molecule targeted compounds for cancer treatment from the drugs approved by the FDA. Specific targets and detailed information are shown in **Table 1**.

Targeting DNA Damage/Repair Channel

DNA undergoes continuous exposure to various damages of endogenous and exogenous elements. Their repairing process is critical to maintain genomic integrity for a long, safe life. An incomplete or unsuccessful DNA repairing process causes genomic instability and cellular transforming process. The DNA damage response (DDR) is a complex cellular network activated by DNA damage with the final aim to repair the DNA damage and restore genomic integrity, through the involvement of many intracellular channels (Ciccia and Elledge, 2010; O'Connor, 2015). DDR is vital for maintaining genomic integrity, as suggested by the fact that germline mutations in DDR genes are associated with an increased risk of tumors (Klinakis et al., 2020). Given its effect on DDR and DNA repairing, DNA-dependent protein kinase (DNA-PK) inhibitors are expedited to be developed. According to **Figure 1**, several potential modes of small molecular parts pertaining to DNA helicases are presented. Olaparib refers to one potent poly adenosine diphosphate ribose polymerase (PARP) inhibitor, inducing synthetic lethality in BRCA1/2-lacking tumor cells. In December 2014, Olaparib gained approval from the European Medicines Agency for its application in the therapeutic maintenance process of cases under the effect of BRCA1/2-mutated ovarian carcinomas (OC) in respondence to platinum-related chemotherapeutic process. Moreover, in the US, Olaparib gained expedited approval from the US FDA as a monotherapy agent for cases subjected to deleterious or suspected deleterious germline BRCA-mutated advanced OC and those administrated using three or more prior lines of chemotherapeutic process (Musella et al., 2015). Moore et al. (2018) have completed a phase III trial that was random and, double-blind to assess the Olaparib efficacy in patients of newly diagnosed advanced ovarian cancer primary peritoneal cancer, or fallopian tube cancer (or a combination thereof) with a mutation in BRCA1, BRCA2, or both (BRCA1/2). Of the 391 randomized patients, 260 were assigned to receive Olaparib treatment and 131 accepted placebo treatment. A total of 388 patients have concentratedly confirmed germline BRCA1/2 mutations, and two patients have concentratedly confirmed systemic BRCA1/2 mutations. After a median follow-up of 41 months, disease progression or death risk Olaparib lower than placebo 70% (Kaplan Meier estimated 3-year probability of freedom from disease progression and death was 60% vs. 27%). Specific to phase II clinical trials, covering cases subjected to advanced CRPC, Olaparib seems to be efficacious and well-tolerated (De Felice et al., 2017). And de Bono et al. (2020) finished a randomized, open-label, phase III trial, evaluating Olaparib in metastatic CRPC patients who had disease progression after receiving a novel hormonal drug. In cohort A of at least one alteration in BRCA1, BRCA2, or ATM, the imaging-based progression-free survival of the Olaparib group was significantly longer than that of the control group (median, 7.4 vs. 3.6 months), objective response rate and the time to pain progression were confirmed to obtained a significant benefit. In cohort A, the MOS of the Olaparib group and the control group were 18.5 and 15.1 months, respectively, and 81% of progressing patients switched to Olaparib treatment. The overall population of cohort A and cohort B acquired an apparent benefit of Olaparib for imaging-based progression-free survival.

Inhibitors of topoisomerase I (Top1) that result in stalled Top1 cleavage complexes (Top1cc) are commonly employed against carcinoma. Combination chemotherapeutic process with DNA repair inhibitors can potentially improve response to

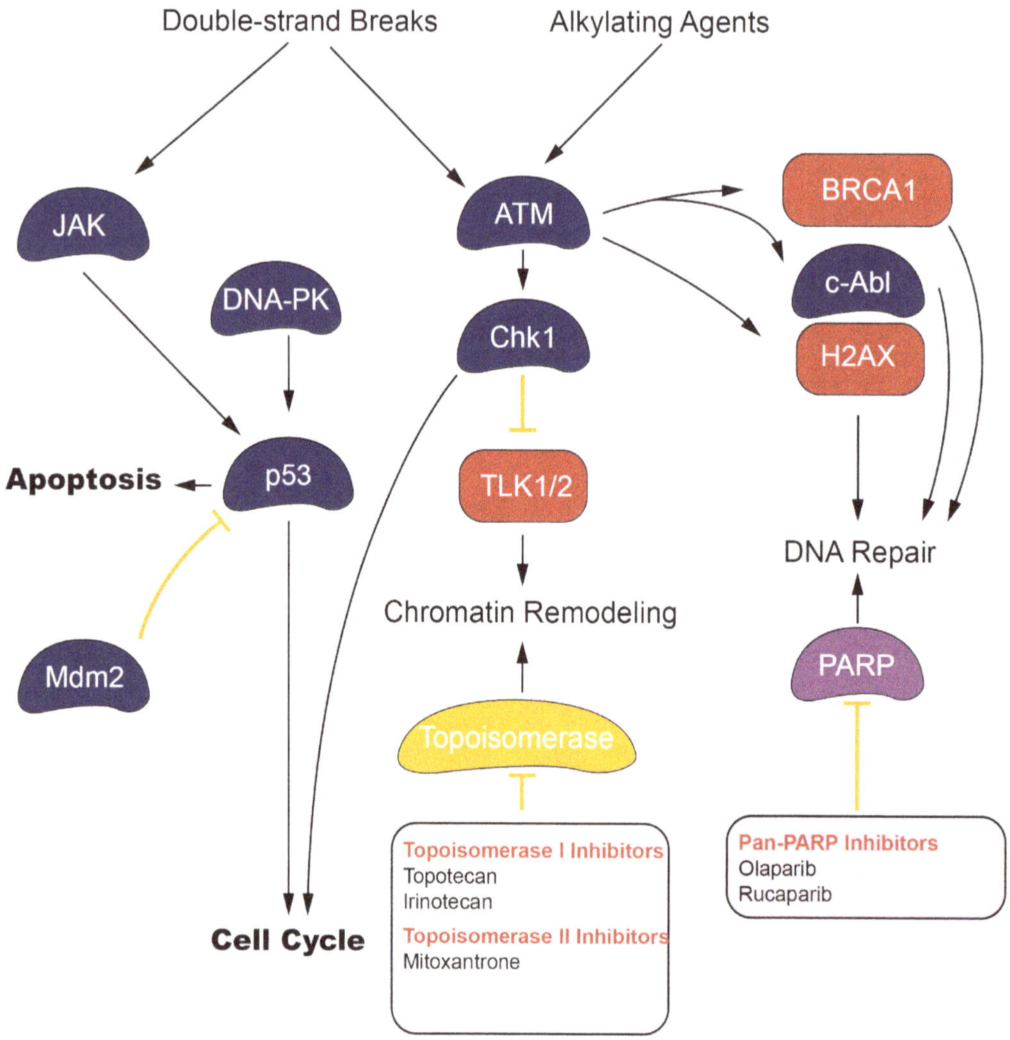

FIGURE 1 | Small molecule targeted compounds targeting DNA damage/repair channel in cancers.

the mentioned widely used chemotherapeutics. One line of inquiry focuses on inhibitors of tyrosyl-DNA phosphodiesterase 1 (Tdp1), a repair enzyme for Top1cc. Tdp1 catalyzes the hydrolysis of DNA adducts covalently linked to the 3'-phosphate of DNA, including Top1-derived peptides and 3'-phosphoglycolates. Tdp1 inhibitors (Topotecan Hydrochloride Irinotecan Hydrochloride) should synergize not only with Top1-targeting drugs (Camptothecins, Indenoisoquinolines), but also with bleomycin, topoisomerase II (Top2) inhibitors (Etoposide, Doxorubicin) and DNA alkylating agents (Huang et al., 2011).

Targeting Endocrinology and Hormones Channel

Inhibitors targeting estrogen and AR are of great significance for the treating process of endocrine tumors (**Figure 2**). Fulvestrant, a selective estrogen receptor down-regulator (SERD), which blocks the proliferation of breast carcinoma cells (Wakeling et al., 1991), is an effective endocrine treating process for women with hormone-sensitive advanced breast carcinoma. Fulvestrant is approved as a first-line treating process for metastatic breast carcinoma. Still, its use in this setting may be limited to situations where the combination with CDK4/6 inhibitors is not available. Response to Fulvestrant was particularly durable in cases subjected to bone-only metastatic disease (Soleja et al., 2019). The combination of Fulvestrant with CDK4/6 inhibitors has shown superior efficacy compared to the monotherapy process in cases subjected to metastatic hormone receptor-positive breast carcinoma who have progressed or relapsed on prior Tamoxifen or Aromatase inhibitor therapeutic process (Sledge et al., 2017). On the whole, resistance to hormonal therapy displays an association with PIK3CA and ESR1 mutations. Alternative hormone resistance channels may be mediated by upregulation of PI3K/AKT, HER2, FGFR, and IGF channels (Beeram et al., 2007; Zhang et al., 2011). Fulvestrant regimens in combination with emerging targeted agents are being developed to overcome endocrine-resistant breast carcinoma. Most recently, Fulvestrant with Alpelisib, an α-selective PI3K inhibitor, has been recently approved for cases who have progressed on an endocrine therapeutic process with PIK3CA mutated breast carcinoma (Soleja et al., 2019). The FDA approval is based on a randomized, double-blind, placebo-controlled SOLAR-1 study of Alpelisib plus Fulvestrant and placebo plus Fulvestrant. The median PFS of the Alperizil combined with Fulvestrant group was 11.0 months, while the median PFS of the placebo plus Fulvestrant group was 5.7 months. The MOS of the Alpelisib plus Fulvestrant group has not been reached, while the MOS of the Fulvestrant control group is 26.9 months. The most common adverse reactions are increased blood sugar, increased creatinine, decreased lymphocyte count, increased gamma-glutamyl transferase and other laboratory abnormalities (Narayan et al., 2021).

Androgen receptor signaling refers to one critical channel in prostate carcinoma, and cases receive the initial administration with ADT. Cases that stopped responding to ADT process were recognized as having CRPC, which is still dependent on AR signaling. Enzalutamide, an orally available AR inhibitor, was initially approved by the US FDA for the treating process of cases subjected to metastatic CRPC that have previously received docetaxel. The indication was subsequently extended to include all cases subjected to metastatic CRPC, and most recently to include cases subjected to non-metastatic CRPC (Sternberg, 2019).

Targeting Metabolism Channel

Inhibiting the process of metabolic channels also brings a new dawn to the carcinoma treating process (**Figure 3**). Cytochrome CYP450 cyclooxygenase catalyzes the epoxidation of polyunsaturated fatty acids, including arachidonic acid, eicosapentaenoic acid, and docosahexaenoic acid. The product of arachidonic acid refers to one feasible lipid facilitating angiogenesis and facilitates tumors developing and growing processes. Besides, derivatives of eicosapentaenoic acid and docosahexaenoic acid limit angiogenesis and have protecting effects under certain pathological conditions covering carcinoma (Sausville et al., 2019; Guengerich, 2020). Inhibitors against the CYP450 family came into being. Since androgen signaling critically impacts the proliferating and metastatic processes of prostate carcinoma, ADT or castration therapeutic process is recognized as the backbone of the treatment process for newly diagnosed metastatic prostate carcinoma. Nevertheless, all men experience disease progression on ADT to a state known as metastatic castration-resistant prostate carcinoma (mCRPC), as driven by AR signaling or intratumoral androgen synthesis continuously. For this reason, the extragonadal ablation of androgen synthesis from pregnane precursors holds much promise. One inhibitor of cytochrome P450 17α-hydroxy/17,20-lyase (CYP17) enzymes, Abiraterone Acetate, has already been approved for men with mCRPC. Newer CYP17 inhibitors continue to be developed, which are either more selective or have concomitant inhibiting actions on AR signaling. The mentioned include VT-464, Orteronel, and Galeterone (Alex et al., 2016).

Retinoids and their naturally metabolized and synthetic products [All-trans retinoic acid (ATRA), 13-cis retinoic acid and Bexarotene] induce differentiating processes in various cell types. Retinoids exert their actions primarily through binding to the nuclear retinoic acid receptors (α, β, γ), which are transcriptional and homeostatic regulators with functions that are often compromised early in the neoplastic transforming process (Alvarez et al., 2007).

All-trans retinoic acid combined with chemotherapy is the standard treatment for acute promyelocytic leukemia (APL), with a cure rate of more than 80% (Lo-Coco et al., 2013). Tretinoin is approved by FDA to be used with arsenic trioxide to treat APL in patients whose cancer has a certain type of chromosome mutation that affects the PML gene and RARA gene.

Besides, the retinoids have been investigated broadly for carcinoma prevention and treatment, primarily attributed to their capacity for inducing cellular differentiating process and arrest proliferating process. RA-regulated tumor suppressor genes, when expressed, can inhibit tumor growth (Houle et al., 1993). Among the three RARs, RARβ has been well known for its tumor suppressive effects in epithelial cells (Tang and Gudas, 2011). It is also becoming increasingly clear that RARβ expression is lost early in carcinogenesis or is epigenetically silenced in many solid tumors (Sirchia et al., 2000), providing an opportunity for emerging treating strategic processes to be investigated with the use of retinoids as well as epigenetically-related modifying elements promoting silenced genes to be re-expressed.

As revealed from Ai et al. (2018) the proliferating and migrating processes were inhibited and the apoptosis of Non-small cell lung cancer (NSCLC) cells was accelerated by Bexarotene (Retinoic acid). Moreover, overexpressed slc10a2 in NSCLC cells can more significantly limit the proliferating and migrating processes, and promote apoptosis under the treating process of bexarotene. As opposed to those mentioned, the opposite results were obtained after the slc10a2 gene was silenced in NSCLC cells administrated with Bexarotene. Furthermore, TSC2, LKB1, P53, P21, PTEN, caspase 7, caspase 3 expressing states were increased and the expression of Bcl-2, cyclin D1, c-FLIP were declined in NSCLC cells and slc10a2 overexpressed NSCLC cells with the treating process of Bexarotene. The opposite situations were seen after the slc10a2 gene was silenced in NSCLC cells. Further studies revealed the increased expression of slc10a2 activated the expression of peroxisome. The mentioned results suggest that Bexarotene inhibits the viability of lung carcinoma cells via slc10a2/PPARγ/PTEN/mTOR signaling channel (Sirchia et al., 2000).

Targeted Angiogenesis Channel

Angiogenesis is considered the forming process of novel blood vessels from vessels that exist in advance. It refers to one complicated multiple-step process, showing tight regulation under a delicate balance between inducers and inhibitors that act together to maintain physiological homeostasis (Hanahan and Folkman, 1996). Nevertheless, tumor under proliferation will activate angiogenesis through the shift of the balance of

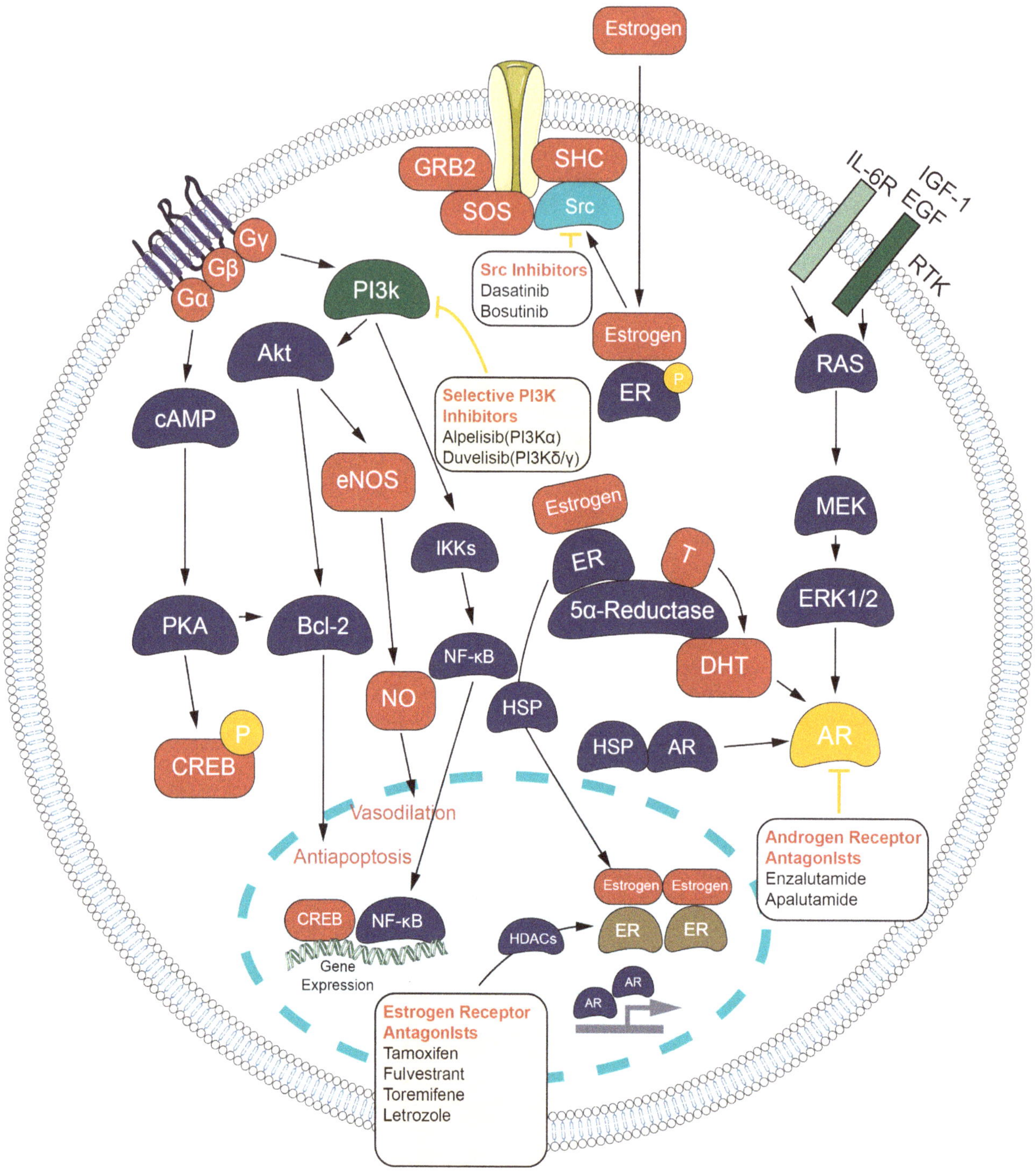

FIGURE 2 | Small molecule targeted compounds targeting endocrinology and hormones channel in cancers.

inducers and inhibitors to one pro-angiogenic result, to fulfill its increased demand of oxygen and nutrients (Carmeliet, 2005). Environmental hypoxia in tumors appears as one primary element that turns on an 'angiogenic switch' by enhancing expression and activation of transcription element hypoxia-inducible-element-1 (HIF-1) channel or HIF-1-independent channels, and it induces the expression of multiple genes contributing to the angiogenic process (Pugh and Ratcliffe, 2003). In Folkman (1972) proposed anti-angiogenesis as a new anticarcinomaous strategy initially. Seventeen years later, vascular endothelial growth element A's (VEGFA) isolation and cloning became one landmark to clarify angiogenic mechanism (Keck et al., 1989), and underpinned the emerging field of research into anti-angiogenic treating processes for

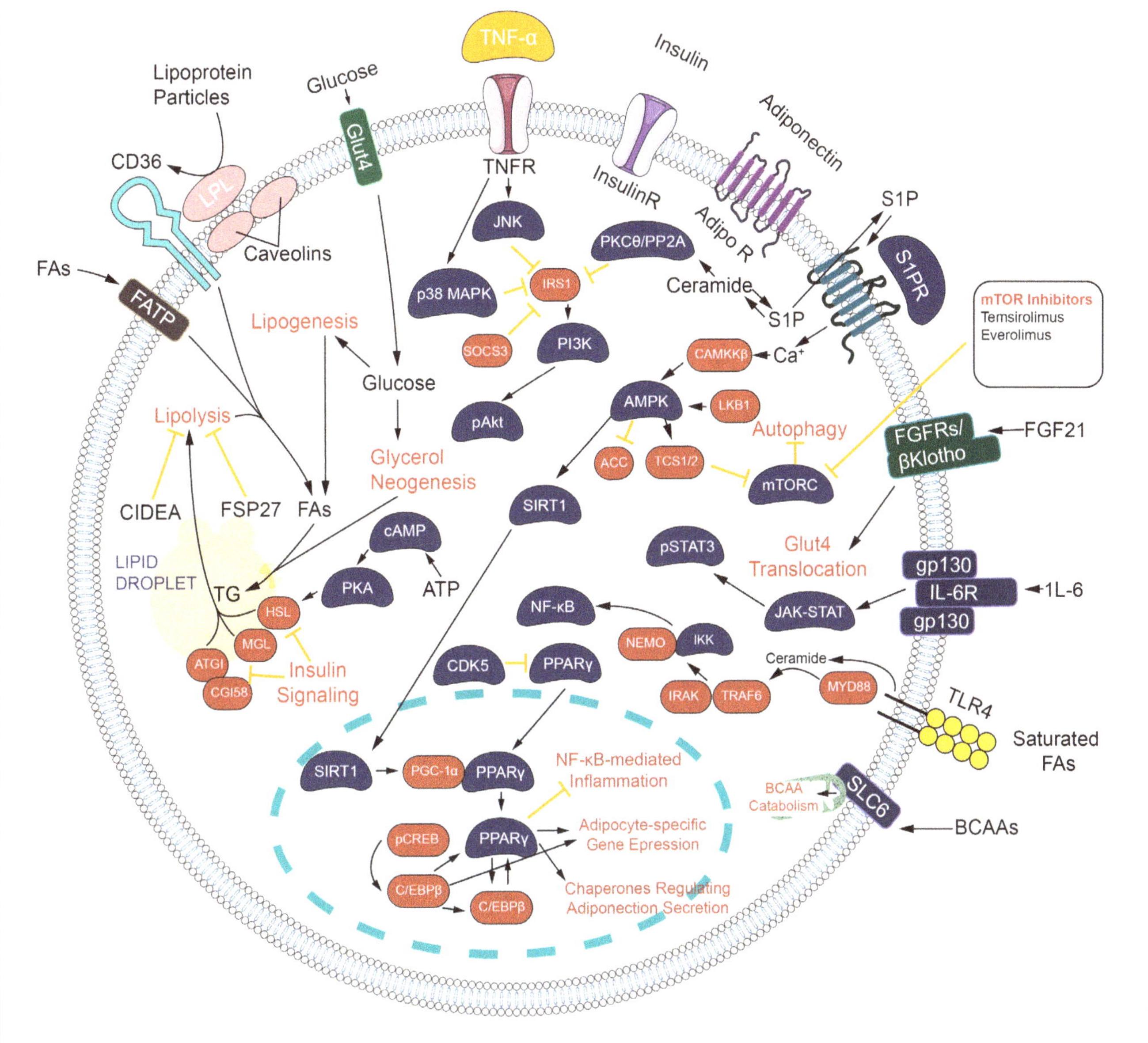

FIGURE 3 | Small molecule targeted compounds targeting metabolism channel in cancers.

carcinoma. The active relevant studies resulted in FDA approval of Bevacizumab (a monoclonal antibody for VEGFA) as the initial anti-angiogenic drug for colorectal carcinoma in 2004 (Hurwitz et al., 2004). Over the last decade, numerous potential anti-angiogenic targets have been identified in sequence, covering cell adhesion molecule, tumor-associated stromal cell, matrix metalloproteinase, and fibroblast growth element. To be specific, VEGFs and their receptors (VEGF receptor-1, VEGF receptor-2, and VEGF receptor-3), exhibiting tyrosine kinase activity, play critical roles in angiogenesis (Ferrara et al., 2003). Therefore, most of the angiogenesis inhibitors are developed targeting VEGFs or their receptors. To date, a large number of angiogenesis inhibitors have been discovered and developed, ranging from monoclonal antibodies, endogenous angiogenesis peptide inhibitors, to small molecule drugs (**Figure 4**). In the past few years, many emerging small molecule inhibitors have been synthesized, covering phosphatidylinositol 3-kinase, benzoxazines targeting receptor tyrosine kinase, 6-(pyrimidine-r-acyloxy)-naphthalene-1-carboxamides, and indoline-2-one group and noreremophilane-based inhibitors, respectively (Al-Rawi et al., 2015; Muthukumarasamy et al., 2016). The mentioned emerging series of compounds showed potential for treating solid tumors in pre-clinical experiments. Furthermore, natural products from marine, bacteria, or herb received the development and demonstration of anti-angiogenic properties (Wang and Miao, 2013; Ehlers et al., 2016). Advanced RCC is usually treated with targeted drugs that block blood vessels. Sorafenib and Axitinib are two commonly used drugs. The mechanism of action of Sorafenib has been described above. Axitinib is an inhibitor of VEGFR-1,

VEGFR-2, VEGFR-3, PDGFR-β, and c-KIT. Axitinib can block the autophosphorylation of VEGFR, endothelial cell viability regulated by VEGF, microtubule formation, and downstream signals (Rössler et al., 2011). There are related studies on the comparison of the effects and safety of these two drugs. Brian I Rini et al. (2011) conducted a randomized phase 3 study to compare the clinical efficacy and safety of Axitinib and Sorafenib as a second-line treatment for patients with metastatic RCC. Among the 723 patients enrolled, they were randomly divided into the Axitinib group (361 cases) and the Sorafenib group (362 cases). The result was that the mPES with Axitinib was 6.7 months, and the mPES with Sorafenib was 4.7 months. In terms of safety, 14 of 359 patients (4%) who received Axitinib and 29 (8%) of 355 patients who received Sorafenib stopped treatment due to side effects. The most common adverse events were diarrhea, hypertension, and fatigue of Axitinib group, and diarrhoea, palmar-plantar erythrodysesthesia, and alopecia of sorafenib group. Therefore, Axinitinib shows better clinical benefit in the treatment of advanced renal cancer compared with Sorafenib.

Targeted Immune Checkpoint Blockers

Since the FDA approved Ipilimumab which is a human CTLA-4 blocking antibody and alters the adaptive immune system (Carreau and Pavlick, 2019) for the treatment of melanoma in 2011, cancer immunotherapy has become an epoch-making achievement and has achieved some exciting clinical applications. Tumor evolution is to avoid immune attack. The tumor microenvironment is immunosuppressive and can be suppressed by immune checkpoints (Baumeister et al., 2016; Hoos, 2016). Immunotherapy aims at reactivating repressive immune cells of cancer patients and acquires exciting results, especially for immune checkpoint blockers of immune monoclonal antibodies, such as PD-1 antibody, PD-L1 antibody, as well as CTLA-4 antibody (Carbone et al., 2017). The most significant benefit of immune checkpoint inhibitor therapy is to restore the function of the immune system, use immune function to clear the specificity of the tumor, and form a lasting memory similar to the antigen. In addition to mentioned agents, molecule inhibitors of immunity are gradually becoming the focus of immunotherapy due to the advantages that they can be absorbed orally, have a small molecular weight and can penetrate cell membranes to act in cells. PD-1, PD-L1, and CTLA-4 are the three most popular immune targets. PD-1 is a member of the CD28 family and is an inhibitory receptor expressed on activated T cells, B cells, macrophages, regulatory T cells (Tregs) and natural killer (NK) cells. It has two binding ligands PD-L1 and PD-L2 (B7 family) expressed on normal cells. The combination of PD-1 with either ligand can inhibit T cell activity, induce T cell tolerance, and inhibit Proliferate, reduce the immune response of T cells and induce cell death, thereby preventing immune cell activation and killing normal cells, and inhibiting the proliferation, differentiation and secretion of antibodies of B cells. CTLA-4 has the same ligand as CD28, but CTLA-4 transmits inhibitory signals. The affinity of CTLA-4 to the ligand is significantly higher than CD28 (Greaves and Gribben, 2013; Kuzume et al., 2020). Some tumor cells will use this mechanism to secrete a large amount of PD-L1/L2 to reduce T cell activation and antigen-specific T cell response, result in evading immune surveillance (Zou et al., 2016). Although no related small molecule targeted compounds have been approved for marketing, some drugs have shown certain therapeutic prospects. In 2016, CA170 was the first to obtain a new drug research application for small molecule immune checkpoint inhibitors. CA-170 is the only small molecule modulator that can be taken orally for PD-L1 and VISTA proteins in clinical trials, and is an essential immune activation negative checkpoint modulator. According to reports, the treatment results are similar to FDA-approved monoclonal antibodies to a specific extent, and overcome the latter's high production cost and side effects (Musielak et al., 2019). In 2016, CA-170 became the first small molecule immunotherapy to enter the Phase I clinical trial of advanced solid tumors and lymphomas (Shaabani et al., 2018). Stimulator of interferon genes (STING) is an immunostimulatory small molecule target, mainly distributed in immune-related tissue cells, such as thymus, spleen, and peripheral blood leukocytes. STING activation leads to nuclear translocation of transcription factors, induces the expression of interferon (INF) and cytokines, promotes the aggregation and activation of T cells, and then kills tumor cells. Zaidi et al. (2021) evaluated ADU-S100 anticarcinoma effect on esophageal adenocarcinoma, which is a STING agonist. The tumor volume in the ADU-S100 and ADU-S100 plus irradiation groups decreased by 30.1 and 50.8%, respectively, and the tumor volume in the placebo group and placebo plus irradiation group increased by 76.7 and 152.4%, respectively. INFβ tumor necrosis factor-α IL-6 and CCL-2 were significantly upregulated in the treatment group compared with placebo. Currently, ADU-S100 is being evaluated in clinical trials (NCT03172936) (Zaidi et al., 2021).

Others

In recent years, small molecule targeted compounds have targeted drug-resistant mutation sites to solve the drug-resistant problem of targeted drugs. NSCLC is the focus of targeted therapy with small molecule inhibitors, but the problem of drug resistance is a complex problem to solve. KRAS p.G12C mutation occurs in 13% of NSCLC and 1 to 3% colorectal cancer and other cancers. Sotorasib is a selective and irreversible KRASG12C targeted small molecule, and has exciting effects. Hong et al. (2020) conducted a phase 1 trial of Sotorasib in patients of advanced solid tumors with KRAS p.G12C mutations. In the subgroup of patients with NSCLC, 32.2% (19 patients) had a clear objective response (complete or partial response), and 88.1% (52 patients) had disease control (objective response or stable disease); The mPES time was 6.3 months. In the colorectal cancer subgroup, 7.1% (3 patients) received a confirmed response, 73.8% (31 patients) received disease control, and the mPES was 4.0 months. Reactions have also been observed in patients with pancreatic cancer, endometrial cancer, appendix cancer, and melanoma. And in the CodeBreak 100 phase II trial, Sotorasib elicited a response in more than one-third of patients and resulted in a mPES of nearly 7 months. Amgen has submitted an application for approval of the drug to the FDA and the European Medicines Agency (No author list, 2021). On May 29, 2021, the FDA announced the accelerated

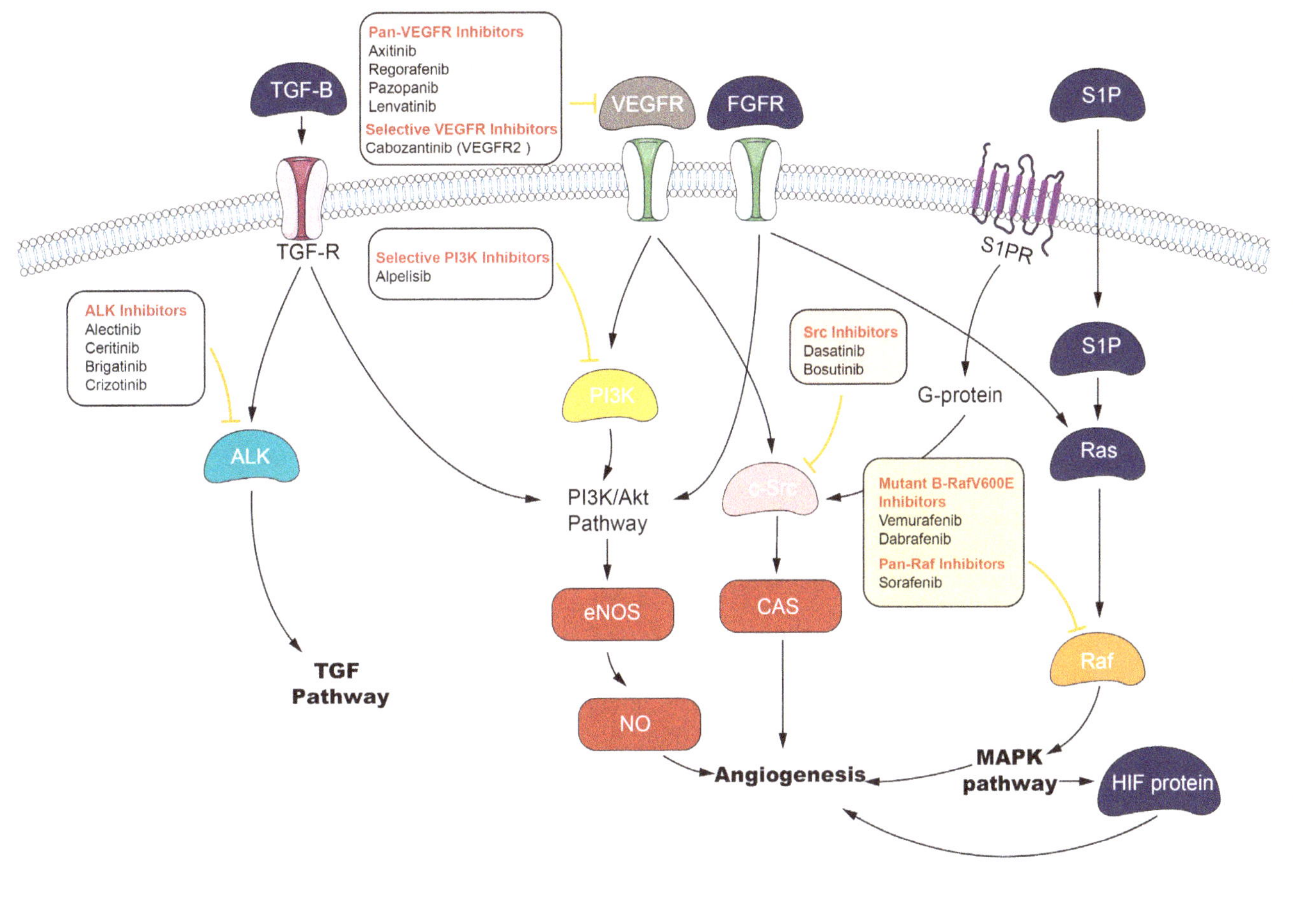

FIGURE 4 | Small molecule targeted compounds targeting angiogenesis channel in cancers.

approval of Sotorasib (Lumakras) for the treatment of NSCLC patients with KRAS G12C mutations. These patients receive at least one pre-systemic treatment. Sotorasib is the world's first anti-tumor drug targeting mutant KRAS protein. T790M mutation and MET mutation are the secondary drug resistance mutations of EGFR in lung cancer patients after receiving EGFR inhibitor treatment (Suda et al., 2017). Small molecule targeting compounds that target T790M, such as Osimertinib, have been approved for marketing and have achieved better efficacy than chemotherapeutic drugs (Mok et al., 2017). Until the revolutionary anti-cancer drug Tepotinib was approved for the market, the gap that there was no small molecule drug for MET mutations was broken. In an open-label phase 2 study, Tepotinib was used in advanced NSCLC patients with skipping mutations in exon 14 of MET, and about half of the patients had an objective response. Peripheral edema was the main toxic reaction of grade 3 and above (Paik et al., 2020). The FDA has approved Tivozanib of VEGFR inhibitor for the treatment of adult patients with relapsed or refractory advanced RCC who have received two or more systemic therapies. Tivozanib has become the first therapy approved for this indication. ATP-binding cassette (ABC) transporter can mediate multidrug resistance of tumor cells. Yang et al. (2014) reported that Tivozanib had the activity of reversing multidrug resistance mediated by ABCB1 and ABCG2 transporters. Therefore, Tivozanib has revolutionized the treatment of kidney cancer. A phase 3, multicenter, randomized, controlled, open-label study compared Tivozanib and Sorafenib in the treatment of advanced renal cell carcinoma (TiVo-3). The results of the study show that Tivozanib as a third-line or fourth-line treatment can improve the progression-free survival rate of patients with metastatic kidney cancer, and it is better tolerated than Sorafenib (Rini et al., 2020).

MECHANISM OF RESISTANCE OF SMALL MOLECULE INHIBITORS

Drug resistance is a common phenomenon in the treatment of cancer, which is divided into acquired resistance and natural resistance. In cancer chemotherapy, many cancer patients begin to be sensitive to chemotherapeutic drugs. As the treatment progresses, cancer cells will develop resistance through some mechanisms, leading to treatment failure, and the same phenomenon will occur with small molecule inhibitors. Drug resistance includes drug inactivation, drug target alteration, drug efflux, DNA damage repair and epithelial-mesenchymal transition (EMT). The development of drug resistance in the treatment of acute myeloid leukemia with cytarabine is an example of drug inactivation. Cytarabine is activated by multiple phosphorylation, mutation or down-regulation of the phosphorylation pathway will inactivate cytarabine and cause drug resistance (Sampath et al., 2006). Small molecule inhibitors for the treatment of signal kinases will cause changes in drug targets, for example, certain lung cancer patients with EGFR mutations developed resistance to EGFR inhibitors within one year, and EGFR-T790M gatekeeper mutation was reported in half of the cases (Bell et al., 2005). Drug efflux is a most interesting mechanism for researchers to study, involving the enhanced efflux to reduce drug content. ABC transporter is not only a normal physiological phenomenon, but also a mechanism of cancer cell resistance. Multidrug resistance protein 1 (MDRl) is a transporter with extensive substrate specificity and the ability to excrete many exogenous substances from the cell, including Vinblastine, podophyllotoxin, Anthracycline, Taxanes, and kinase inhibitors (Gottesman et al., 2002; Szakács et al., 2004). Hence, MDRl protects cancer cells from drugs.

DNA damage response plays a vital role in resisting drugs that induce DNA damage to kill cancer cells. Though PARP inhibitors target DDR to prevent DNA repair and display a predominant effect with chemotherapy, other DDR mechanisms can be adjusted up to compensate for dysfunctional pathways (Housman et al., 2014). In addition to EMT being an essential mechanism of solid tumor metastasis, EMT is also the cause of drug resistance. It is reported that in head and neck squamous cell carcinoma (HNSCC) cells, the NGF/TrkA axis confers resistance to the EGFR inhibitor Erlotinib through the EMT process. *In vitro* and *in vivo* models, blocking TrkA signaling significantly reverses EMT and makes HNSCC cells sensitive to Erlotinib (Lin et al., 2020). There are still many questions about the drug resistance mechanism of inhibitors, which urgently need to be studied and elucidated, so that the clinical application of the drug can be better.

THE COMBINED THERAPY OF SMALL MOLECULE TARGETED COMPOUNDS

The purpose of combination therapy is to overcome and reverse the drug resistance of inhibitors, reduce side effects and achieve better therapeutic results through the combination of multiple pathway inhibitors. Single-use of small molecule inhibitors to treat cancer often has mutation sites that affect drug treatment. Although few inhibitor combinations are approved by FDA, the combination of inhibitors can solve this problem. MEK inhibitor AZD6244 inhibits the activation of ERK of colon cancer cells, while AZD6244 promotes JAK2-STAT3 signaling activation which induces colon cancer cell resistance to inhibitor. Jin et al. (2019) have shown that the combined effect of MEK inhibitor AZD6244 and JAK2-STA T3 inhibitor AG490 can significantly inhibit cell viability, induce cell apoptosis, and ultimately inhibit the activation of ERK and JAK2-STAT3 signals. The combination of AZD6244 and AG490 has shown better effects than single drugs *in vivo* and *in vitro*. Bruton's tyrosine kinase (BTK) inhibitor Ibrutinib and Acalabrutinib appear to be highly effective. However, BTK inhibition enhances the reliance of mitochondria on BCL-2 without significantly changing the overall activation of mitochondria. The selective BCL-2 inhibitor Venotclax treatment improves the overall mitochondrial activation without increasing dependence on BCL-2. Therefore, BCL-2 inhibitor and BTK inhibitor have synergistic and complementary therapeutic effects (Deng et al., 2017). Toxicity and side effects, including fatigue, skin, mucous membrane, and gastrointestinal adverse reactions, limit the use of different drug dosages and treatment schedules. In some combinations of inhibitors, the combination group shows lower side effects and better therapeutic effects than the single-use group. The phase III clinical trial of patients with metastatic melanoma with BRAF V600E or V600K mutations completed by Robert et al. (2015) confirmed that the combination of the BRAF inhibitor Dabrafenib/Vemurafenib and the MEK inhibitor Trametinib has a better therapeutic effect and Unelevated overall toxicity. The 12-month overall survival rate in the combined treatment group was 72%, and the overall survival rate in the Vemurafenib group was 65%. The mPES was 11.4 months in the combined treatment group, and 7.3 months in the Vemurafenib group. The objective effective rate was 64% in the combined group and 51% in the Vemurafenib group. The rates of serious adverse events and drug discontinuation were similar in the two groups. Cutaneous squamous cell carcinoma and keratoacanthomas were 1% and 18% in the combination treatment group and Vemurafenib group, respectively.

CONCLUSION AND PERSPECTIVES

Small molecule targeted compounds have been developed in clinical medicine for decades, prolonging the survival time of cases subjected to advanced or refractory tumors. However, there are still insufficient approved drugs for practical use for several reasons. Even if a variety of enzymes are identified, inhibitors only target specific kinase targets for EGFRs, FGFRs, VEGFRs, JAK, PI3K, and CDK and other new drugs, resulting in most of the drugs studied having similar structures and mechanisms compared with the inhibitors used. Our detailed use of new gene-editing techniques to construct more comprehensive and effective protein kinase gene knockout libraries and to screen new key kinase targets involved in tumor development could provide new strategies for the developmental process pertaining to small targeted molecule inhibitors. While scientists are working on the next generation of drugs to overcome resistance, they cannot declare their frustration with targeted drugs. As opposed to those mentioned, resistance will promote better inhibitor synthesis. Desirable properties for further development of next-generation compounds include better safety indicators, improved pharmacologic indicators, access to brain metastases or other shelters, and reversal of primary tumors. We expect small molecule targeted compounds to bring good news to cases subjected to advanced carcinoma and open a bright way to solve carcinoma.

AUTHOR CONTRIBUTIONS

All authors listed have made a substantial, direct and intellectual contribution to the work, and approved it for publication.

ACKNOWLEDGMENTS

We sincerely thank Selleck for providing a lot of information for this review.

REFERENCES

Ai, X., Mao, F., Shen, S., Shentu, Y., Wang, J., and Lu, S. (2018). Bexarotene inhibits the viability of non-small cell lung cancer cells via slc10a2/PPARγ/PTEN/mTOR signaling pathway. *BMC Cancer* 18:407. doi: 10.1186/s12885-018-4224-x

Alex, A. B., Pal, S. K., and Agarwal, N. (2016). CYP17 inhibitors in prostate cancer: latest evidence and clinical potential. *Ther. Adv. Med. Oncol.* 8, 267–275. doi: 10.1177/1758834016642370

Al-Rawi, S., Meehan-Andrews, T., Bradley, C., and Al-Rawi, J. (2015). Novel benzoxazines as inhibitors of angiogenesis. *Invest. New Drugs* 33, 45–52. doi: 10.1007/s10637-014-0172-8

Al-Salama, Z. T., Syed, Y. Y., and Scott, L. J. (2019). Lenvatinib: a review in hepatocellular carcinoma. *Drugs* 79, 665–674. doi: 10.1007/s40265-019-01116-x

Alvarez, S., Germain, P., Alvarez, R., Rodríguez-Barrios, F., Gronemeyer, H., and de Lera, A. R. (2007). Structure, function and modulation of retinoic acid receptor beta, a tumor suppressor. *Int. J. Biochem. Cell Biol.* 39, 1406–1415. doi: 10.1016/j.biocel.2007.02.010

Arena, E., Dichiara, M., Floresta, G., Parenti, C., Marrazzo, A., Pittalà, V., et al. (2018). Novel Sigma-1 receptor antagonists: from opioids to small molecules: what is new? *Fut. Med. Chem.* 10, 231–256. doi: 10.4155/fmc-2017-0164

Baumeister, S. H., Freeman, G. J., Dranoff, G., and Sharpe, A. H. (2016). Coinhibitory pathways in immunotherapy for cancer. *Annu. Rev. Immunol.* 34, 539–573. doi: 10.1146/annurev-immunol-032414-112049

Beeram, M., Tan, Q. T., Tekmal, R. R., Russell, D., Middleton, A., and DeGraffenried, L. A. (2007). Akt-induced endocrine therapy resistance is reversed by inhibition of mTOR signaling. *Ann. Oncol.* 18, 1323–1328. doi: 10.1093/annonc/mdm170

Bell, D. W., Gore, I., Okimoto, R. A., Godin-Heymann, N., Sordella, R., Mulloy, R., et al. (2005). Inherited susceptibility to lung cancer may be associated with the T790M drug resistance mutation in EGFR. *Nat. Genet.* 37, 1315–1316. doi: 10.1038/ng1671

Carbone, D. P., Reck, M., Paz-Ares, L., Creelan, B., Horn, L., Steins, M., et al. (2017). First-line nivolumab in stage IV or recurrent non-small-cell lung cancer. *N. Engl. J. Med.* 376, 2415–2426.

Carmeliet, P. (2005). Angiogenesis in life, disease and medicine. *Nature* 438, 932–936. doi: 10.1038/nature04478

Carreau, N. A., and Pavlick, A. C. (2019). Nivolumab and ipilimumab: immunotherapy for treatment of malignant melanoma. *Fut. Oncol.* 15, 349–358.

Chari, A., Vogl, D. T., Gavriatopoulou, M., Nooka, A. K., Yee, A. J., Huff, C. A., et al. (2019). Oral selinexor-dexamethasone for triple-class refractory multiple myeloma. *N. Engl. J. Med.* 381, 727–738.

Cheng, A.-L., Kang, Y.-K., Chen, Z., Tsao, C.-J., Qin, S., Kim, J. S., et al. (2009). Efficacy and safety of sorafenib in patients in the Asia-Pacific region with advanced hepatocellular carcinoma: a phase III randomised, double-blind, placebo-controlled trial. *Lancet Oncol.* 10, 25–34.

Ciccia, A., and Elledge, S. J. (2010). The DNA damage response: making it safe to play with knives. *Mol. Cell* 40, 179–204. doi: 10.1016/j.molcel.2010.09.019

de Bono, J., Mateo, J., Fizazi, K., Saad, F., Shore, N., Sandhu, S., et al. (2020). Olaparib for metastatic castration-resistant prostate cancer. *N. Engl. J. Med.* 382, 2091–2102.

De Felice, F., Tombolini, V., Marampon, F., Musella, A., and Marchetti, C. (2017). Defective DNA repair mechanisms in prostate cancer: impact of olaparib. *Drug Des. Dev. Ther.* 11, 547–552. doi: 10.2147/dddt.s110264

De Ruysscher, D., Niedermann, G., Burnet, N. G., Siva, S., Lee, A. W. M., and Hegi-Johnson, F. (2019). Radiotherapy toxicity. *Nat. Rev. Dis. Primers* 5:13.

Deng, J., Isik, E., Fernandes, S. M., Brown, J. R., Letai, A., and Davids, M. S. (2017). Bruton's tyrosine kinase inhibition increases BCL-2 dependence and enhances sensitivity to venetoclax in chronic lymphocytic leukemia. *Leukemia* 31, 2075–2084.

Diesendruck, Y., and Benhar, I. (2017). Novel immune check point inhibiting antibodies in cancer therapy-Opportunities and challenges. *Drug Resist. Update* 30, 39–47. doi: 10.1016/j.drup.2017.02.001

Ehlers, T., Furness, S., Robinson, T. P., Zhong, H. A., Goldsmith, D., Aribser, J., et al. (2016). Methionine aminopeptidase type-2 inhibitors targeting angiogenesis. *Curr. Top. Med. Chem.* 16, 1478–1488. doi: 10.2174/1568026615666150915121204

Ferrara, N., Gerber, H. P., and LeCouter, J. (2003). The biology of VEGF and its receptors. *Nat. Med.* 9, 669–676. doi: 10.1038/nm0603-669

Folkman, J. (1972). Anti-angiogenesis: new concept for therapy of solid tumors. *Ann. Surg.* 175, 409–416. doi: 10.1097/00000658-197203000-00014

Ge, R., Xu, X., Xu, P., Li, L., Li, Z., and Bian, J. (2018). Degradation of androgen receptor through small molecules for prostate cancer. *Curr. Cancer Drug Targets* 18, 652–667. doi: 10.2174/1568009617666171107103936

Gottesman, M. M., Fojo, T., and Bates, S. E. (2002). Multidrug resistance in cancer: role of ATP-dependent transporters. *Nat. Rev. Cancer* 2, 48–58. doi: 10.1038/nrc706

Greaves, P., and Gribben, J. G. (2013). The role of B7 family molecules in hematologic malignancy. *Blood* 121, 734–744. doi: 10.1182/blood-2012-10-385591

Guengerich, F. P. (2020). Cytochrome P450 2E1 and its roles in disease. *Chem. Biol. Interact.* 322:109056. doi: 10.1016/j.cbi.2020.109056

Hanahan, D., and Folkman, J. (1996). Patterns and emerging mechanisms of the angiogenic switch during tumorigenesis. *Cell* 86, 353–364. doi: 10.1016/s0092-8674(00)80108-7

Heinhuis, K. M., Ros, W., Kok, M., Steeghs, N., Beijnen, J. H., and Schellens, J. H. M. (2019). Enhancing antitumor response by combining immune checkpoint inhibitors with chemotherapy in solid tumors. *Ann. Oncol.* 30, 219–235. doi: 10.1093/annonc/mdy551

Hong, D. S., Fakih, M. G., Strickler, J. H., Desai, J., Durm, G. A., Shapiro, G. I., et al. (2020). KRAS(G12C) inhibition with sotorasib in advanced solid tumors. *N. Engl. J. Med.* 383, 1207–1217.

Hoos, A. (2016). Development of immuno-oncology drugs - from CTLA4 to PD1 to the next generations. *Nat. Rev. Drug Discov.* 15, 235–247. doi: 10.1038/nrd.2015.35

Houle, B., Rochette-Egly, C., and Bradley, W. E. (1993). Tumor-suppressive effect of the retinoic acid receptor beta in human epidermoid lung cancer cells. *Proc. Natl. Acad. Sci. U.S.A.* 90, 985–989. doi: 10.1073/pnas.90.3.985

Housman, G., Byler, S., Heerboth, S., Lapinska, K., Longacre, M., Snyder, N., et al. (2014). Drug resistance in cancer: an overview. *Cancers* 6, 1769–1792.

Huang, S. N., Pommier, Y., and Marchand, C. (2011). Tyrosyl-DNA Phosphodiesterase 1 (Tdp1) inhibitors. *Expert Opin. Ther. Pattern* 21, 1285–1292.

Huck, B. R., Kötzner, L., and Urbahns, K. (2018). Small molecules drive big improvements in immuno-oncology therapies. *Angew. Chem. Int. Ed. Engl.* 57, 4412–4428. doi: 10.1002/anie.201707816

Hurwitz, H., Fehrenbacher, L., Novotny, W., Cartwright, T., Hainsworth, J., Heim, W., et al. (2004). Bevacizumab plus irinotecan, fluorouracil, and leucovorin for metastatic colorectal cancer. *N. Engl. J. Med.* 350, 2335–2342.

Ito, T., Tori, M., Hashigaki, S., Kimura, N., Sato, K., Ohki, E., et al. (2019). Efficacy and safety of sunitinib in Japanese patients with progressive, advanced/metastatic, well-differentiated, unresectable pancreatic neuroendocrine tumors: final analyses from a Phase II study. *Jpn J. Clin. Oncol.* 49, 354–360. doi: 10.1093/jjco/hyz009

Jin, J., Guo, Q., Xie, J., Jin, D., and Zhu, Y. (2019). Combination of MEK inhibitor and the JAK2-STAT3 pathway inhibition for the therapy of colon cancer. *Pathol. Oncol. Res.* 25, 769–775. doi: 10.1007/s12253-019-00592-6

Keck, P. J., Hauser, S. D., Krivi, G., Sanzo, K., Warren, T., Feder, J., et al. (1989). Vascular permeability factor, an endothelial cell mitogen related to PDGF. *Science* 246, 1309–1312. doi: 10.1126/science.2479987

Kim, E. S., Hirsh, V., Mok, T., Socinski, M. A., Gervais, R., Wu, Y. L., et al. (2008). Gefitinib versus docetaxel in previously treated non-small-cell lung cancer (INTEREST): a randomised phase III trial. *Lancet* 372, 1809–1818. doi: 10.1016/s0140-6736(08)61758-4

Klinakis, A., Karagiannis, D., and Rampias, T. (2020). Targeting DNA repair in cancer: current state and novel approaches. *Cell. Mol. Life Sci.* 77, 677–703. doi: 10.1007/s00018-019-03299-8

Kudo, M., Finn, R. S., Qin, S., Han, K. H., Ikeda, K., Piscaglia, F., et al. (2018). Lenvatinib versus sorafenib in first-line treatment of patients with unresectable hepatocellular carcinoma: a randomised phase 3 non-inferiority trial. *Lancet* 391, 1163–1173. doi: 10.1016/s0140-6736(18)30207-1

Kuzume, A., Chi, S., Yamauchi, N., and Minami, Y. (2020). Immune-checkpoint blockade therapy in lymphoma. *Int. J. Mol. Sci.* 21:5456. doi: 10.3390/ijms21155456

Lin, C., Ren, Z., Yang, X., Yang, R., Chen, Y., Liu, Z., et al. (2020). Nerve growth factor (NGF)-TrkA axis in head and neck squamous cell carcinoma triggers EMT and confers resistance to the EGFR inhibitor erlotinib. *Cancer Lett.* 472, 81–96. doi: 10.1016/j.canlet.2019.12.015

Liu, L., Cao, Y., Chen, C., Zhang, X., McNabola, A., Wilkie, D., et al. (2006). Sorafenib blocks the RAF/MEK/ERK pathway, inhibits tumor angiogenesis, and induces tumor cell apoptosis in hepatocellular carcinoma model PLC/PRF/5. *Cancer Res.* 66, 11851–11858. doi: 10.1158/0008-5472.can-06-1377

Lo-Coco, F., Avvisati, G., Vignetti, M., Thiede, C., Orlando, S. M., Iacobelli, S., et al. (2013). Retinoic acid and arsenic trioxide for acute promyelocytic leukemia. *N. Engl. J. Med.* 369, 111–121.

Mammatas, L. H., Zandvliet, A. S., Rovithi, M., Honeywell, R. J., Swart, E. L., Peters, G. J., et al. (2020). Sorafenib administered using a high-dose, pulsatile regimen in patients with advanced solid malignancies: a phase I exposure escalation study. *Cancer Chemother. Pharmacol.* 85, 931–940. doi: 10.1007/s00280-020-04065-5

Matsui, J., Yamamoto, Y., Funahashi, Y., Tsuruoka, A., Watanabe, T., Wakabayashi, T., et al. (2008). E7080, a novel inhibitor that targets multiple kinases, has potent antitumor activities against stem cell factor producing human small cell lung cancer H146, based on angiogenesis inhibition. *Int. J. Cancer* 122, 664–671. doi: 10.1002/ijc.23131

McLaughlin, M., Patin, E. C., Pedersen, M., Wilkins, A., Dillon, M. T., Melcher, A. A., et al. (2020). Inflammatory microenvironment remodelling by tumour cells after radiotherapy. *Nat. Rev. Cancer* 20, 203–217. doi: 10.1038/s41568-020-0246-1

Mendel, D. B., Laird, A. D., Xin, X., Louie, S. G., Christensen, J. G., Li, G., et al. (2003). In vivo antitumor activity of SU11248, a novel tyrosine kinase inhibitor targeting vascular endothelial growth factor and platelet-derived growth factor receptors: determination of a pharmacokinetic/pharmacodynamic relationship. *Clin. Cancer Res.* 9, 327–337.

Mok, T. S., Wu, Y. L., Ahn, M. J., Garassino, M. C., Kim, H. R., Ramalingam, S. S., et al. (2017). Osimertinib or platinum-pemetrexed in EGFR T790M-positive lung cancer. *N. Engl. J. Med.* 376, 629–640.

Moore, K., Colombo, N., Scambia, G., Kim, B. G., Oaknin, A., Friedlander, M., et al. (2018). Maintenance olaparib in patients with newly diagnosed advanced ovarian cancer. *N. Engl. J. Med.* 379, 2495–2505.

Moroz, E., Matoori, S., and Leroux, J. C. (2016). Oral delivery of macromolecular drugs: where we are after almost 100years of attempts. *Adv. Drug Deliv. Rev.* 101, 108–121. doi: 10.1016/j.addr.2016.01.010

Musella, A., Marchetti, C., Gasparri, M. L., Salerno, L., Casorelli, A., Domenici, L., et al. (2015). PARP inhibition: a promising therapeutic target in ovarian cancer. *Cell. Mol. Biol.* 61, 44–61.

Musielak, B., Kocik, J., Skalniak, L., Magiera-Mularz, K., Sala, D., Czub, M., et al. (2019). CA-170 - a potent small-molecule PD-L1 inhibitor or not? *Molecules* 24:2804. doi: 10.3390/molecules24152804

Muthukumarasamy, K. M., Handore, K. L., Kakade, D. N., Shinde, M. V., Ranjan, S., Kumar, N., et al. (2016). Identification of noreremophilane-based inhibitors of angiogenesis using zebrafish assays. *Org. Biomol. Chem.* 14, 1569–1578. doi: 10.1039/c5ob01594d

Narayan, P., Prowell, T. M., Gao, J. J., Fernandes, L. L., Li, E., Jiang, X., et al. (2021). FDA approval summary: alpelisib plus fulvestrant for patients with HR-positive, HER2-negative, PIK3CA-mutated, advanced or metastatic breast cancer. *Clin. Cancer Res.* 27, 1842–1849.

Neggers, J. E., Vercruysse, T., Jacquemyn, M., Vanstreels, E., Baloglu, E., Shacham, S., et al. (2015). Identifying drug-target selectivity of small-molecule CRM1/XPO1 inhibitors by CRISPR/Cas9 genome editing. *Chem. Biol.* 22, 107–116. doi: 10.1016/j.chembiol.2014.11.015

O'Connor, M. J. (2015). Targeting the DNA damage response in cancer. *Mol. Cell* 60, 547–560.

Paik, P. K., Felip, E., Veillon, R., Sakai, H., Cortot, A. B., Garassino, M. C., et al. (2020). Tepotinib in non-small-cell lung cancer with MET Exon 14 skipping mutations. *N. Engl. J. Med.* 383, 931–943.

Pease, J. E. (2017). Designing small molecule CXCR3 antagonists. *Expert Opin. Drug Discov.* 12, 159–168. doi: 10.1080/17460441.2017.1268597

Petrick, J. L., Braunlin, M., Laversanne, M., Valery, P. C., Bray, F., and McGlynn, K. A. (2016). International trends in liver cancer incidence, overall and by histologic subtype, 1978-2007. *Int. J. Cancer* 139, 1534–1545. doi: 10.1002/ijc.30211

Podar, K., Shah, J., Chari, A., Richardson, P. G., and Jagannath, S. (2020). Selinexor for the treatment of multiple myeloma. *Expert Opin. Pharmacother.* 21, 399–408. doi: 10.1080/14656566.2019.1707184

Procopio, G., Apollonio, G., Cognetti, F., Miceli, R., Milella, M., Mosca, A., et al. (2019). Sorafenib versus observation following radical metastasectomy for clear-cell renal cell carcinoma: results from the phase 2 randomized open-label RESORT study. *Eur. Urol. Oncol.* 2, 699–707. doi: 10.1016/j.euo.2019.08.011

Pugh, C. W., and Ratcliffe, P. J. (2003). Regulation of angiogenesis by hypoxia: role of the HIF system. *Nat. Med.* 9, 677–684. doi: 10.1038/nm0603-677

Raina, R., Pahalajani, G., Agarwal, A., and Zippe, C. (2007). Long-term effectiveness of luteinizing hormone-releasing hormone agonist or antiandrogen monotherapy in elderly men with localized prostate cancer (T1-2): a retrospective study. *Asian J. Androl.* 9, 253–258. doi: 10.1111/j.1745-7262.2007.00074.x

Raymond, E., Dahan, L., Raoul, J. L., Bang, Y. J., Borbath, I., Lombard-Bohas, C., et al. (2011). Sunitinib malate for the treatment of pancreatic neuroendocrine tumors. *N. Engl. J. Med.* 364, 501–513.

Rini, B. I., Escudier, B., Tomczak, P., Kaprin, A., Szczylik, C., Hutson, T. E., et al. (2011). Comparative effectiveness of axitinib versus sorafenib in advanced renal cell carcinoma (AXIS): a randomised phase 3 trial. *Lancet* 378, 1931–1939. doi: 10.1016/s0140-6736(11)61613-9

Rini, B. I., Pal, S. K., Escudier, B. J., Atkins, M. B., Hutson, T. E., Porta, C., et al. (2020). Tivozanib versus sorafenib in patients with advanced renal cell carcinoma (TIVO-3): a phase 3, multicentre, randomised, controlled, open-label study. *Lancet Oncol.* 21, 95–104. doi: 10.1016/s1470-2045(19)30735-1

Robert, C., Karaszewska, B., Schachter, J., Rutkowski, P., Mackiewicz, A., Stroiakovski, D., et al. (2015). Improved overall survival in melanoma with combined dabrafenib and trametinib. *N. Engl. J. Med.* 372, 30–39.

Roskoski, R. Jr. (2020). Properties of FDA-approved small molecule protein kinase inhibitors: a 2020 update. *Pharmacol. Res.* 152:104609. doi: 10.1016/j.phrs.2019.104609

Rössler, J., Monnet, Y., Farace, F., Opolon, P., Daudigeos-Dubus, E., Bourredjem, A., et al. (2011). The selective VEGFR1-3 inhibitor axitinib (AG-013736) shows antitumor activity in human neuroblastoma xenografts. *Int. J. Cancer* 128, 2748–2758. doi: 10.1002/ijc.25611

Ruanglertboon, W., Sorich, M. J., Rowland, A., and Hopkins, A. M. (2020). Effect of early adverse events resulting in sorafenib dose adjustments on survival outcomes of advanced hepatocellular carcinoma patients. *Int. J. Clin. Oncol.* 25, 1672–1677. doi: 10.1007/s10147-020-01698-7

Sampath, D., Cortes, J., Estrov, Z., Du, M., Shi, Z., Andreeff, M., et al. (2006). Pharmacodynamics of cytarabine alone and in combination with 7-hydroxystaurosporine (UCN-01) in AML blasts in vitro and during a clinical trial. *Blood* 107, 2517–2524. doi: 10.1182/blood-2005-08-3351

Sausville, L. N., Williams, S. M., and Pozzi, A. (2019). Cytochrome P450 epoxygenases and cancer: a genetic and a molecular perspective. *Pharmacol. Ther.* 196, 183–194. doi: 10.1016/j.pharmthera.2018.11.009

Seidenfeld, J., Samson, D. J., Hasselblad, V., Aronson, N., Albertsen, P. C., Bennett, C. L., et al. (2000). Single-therapy androgen suppression in men with advanced prostate cancer: a systematic review and meta-analysis. *Ann. Intern. Med.* 132, 566–577. doi: 10.7326/0003-4819-132-7-200004040-00009

Shaabani, S., Huizinga, H. P. S., Butera, R., Kouchi, A., Guzik, K., Magiera-Mularz, K., et al. (2018). A patent review on PD-1/PD-L1 antagonists: small molecules, peptides, and macrocycles (2015-2018). *Expert Opin. Ther. Pattern* 28, 665–678. doi: 10.1080/13543776.2018.1512706

Shepherd, F. A., Rodrigues Pereira, J., Ciuleanu, T., Tan, E. H., Hirsh, V., Thongprasert, S., et al. (2005). Erlotinib in previously treated non-small-cell lung cancer. *N. Engl. J. Med.* 353, 123–132.

Shim, M., Bang, W. J., Oh, C. Y., Lee, Y. S., and Cho, J. S. (2019). Effectiveness of three different luteinizing hormone-releasing hormone agonists in the chemical castration of patients with prostate cancer: Goserelin versus triptorelin versus leuprolide. *Invest. Clin. Urol.* 60, 244–250. doi: 10.4111/icu.2019.60.4.244

Singer, E. A., Golijanin, D. J., Miyamoto, H., and Messing, E. M. (2008). Androgen deprivation therapy for prostate cancer. *Expert Opin. Pharmacother.* 9, 211–228.

Sirchia, S. M., Ferguson, A. T., Sironi, E., Subramanyan, S., Orlandi, R., Sukumar, S., et al. (2000). Evidence of epigenetic changes affecting the chromatin state of the retinoic acid receptor beta2 promoter in breast cancer cells. *Oncogene* 19, 1556–1563. doi: 10.1038/sj.onc.1203456

Sledge, G. W. Jr., Toi, M., Neven, P., Sohn, J., Inoue, K., Pivot, X., et al. (2017). MONARCH 2: abemaciclib in combination with fulvestrant in women with HR+/HER2- advanced breast cancer who had progressed while receiving endocrine therapy. *J. Clin. Oncol.* 35, 2875–2884. doi: 10.1200/jco.2017.73.7585

Soleja, M., Raj, G. V., and Unni, N. (2019). An evaluation of fulvestrant for the treatment of metastatic breast cancer. *Expert Opin. Pharmacother.* 20, 1819–1829. doi: 10.1080/14656566.2019.1651293

No author list (2021). Sotorasib closer to approval. *Cancer Discov.* 11:Of2. doi: 10.1158/2159-8290.cd-nb2021-0309

Sternberg, C. N. (2019). Enzalutamide, an oral androgen receptor inhibitor for treatment of castration-resistant prostate cancer. *Fut. Oncol.* 15, 1437–1457. doi: 10.2217/fon-2018-0940

Stojilkovic, S. S., Reinhart, J., and Catt, K. J. (1994). Gonadotropin-releasing hormone receptors: structure and signal transduction pathways. *Endocr. Rev.* 15, 462–499. doi: 10.1210/edrv-15-4-462

Suda, K., Bunn, P. A. Jr., Rivard, C. J., Mitsudomi, T., and Hirsch, F. R. (2017). Primary double-strike therapy for cancers to overcome EGFR kinase inhibitor resistance: proposal from the bench. *J. Thorac. Oncol.* 12, 27–35. doi: 10.1016/j.jtho.2016.09.003

Sun, Q., Carrasco, Y. P., Hu, Y., Guo, X., Mirzaei, H., Macmillan, J., et al. (2013). Nuclear export inhibition through covalent conjugation and hydrolysis of Leptomycin B by CRM1. *Proc. Natl. Acad. Sci. U.S.A.* 110, 1303–1308. doi: 10.1073/pnas.1217203110

Szakács, G., Annereau, J. P., Lababidi, S., Shankavaram, U., Arciello, A., Bussey, K. J., et al. (2004). Predicting drug sensitivity and resistance: profiling ABC transporter genes in cancer cells. *Cancer Cell* 6, 129–137. doi: 10.1007/978-1-59259-745-1_9

Tang, X. H., and Gudas, L. J. (2011). Retinoids, retinoic acid receptors, and cancer. *Annu. Rev. Pathol.* 6, 345–364. doi: 10.1146/annurev-pathol-011110-130303

Teo, M. Y., Rathkopf, D. E., and Kantoff, P. (2019). Treatment of advanced prostate cancer. *Annu. Rev. Med.* 70, 479–499.

Verschuur, A. C., Bajèiová, V., Mascarenhas, L., Khosravan, R., Lin, X., Ingrosso, A., et al. (2019). Sunitinib in pediatric patients with advanced gastrointestinal stromal tumor: results from a phase I/II trial. *Cancer Chemother. Pharmacol.* 84, 41–50. doi: 10.1007/s00280-019-03814-5

Wakeling, A. E., Dukes, M., and Bowler, J. A. (1991). potent specific pure antiestrogen with clinical potential. *Cancer Res.* 51, 3867–3873.

Wang, Y. Q., and Miao, Z. H. (2013). Marine-derived angiogenesis inhibitors for cancer therapy. *Mar. Drugs* 11, 903–933. doi: 10.3390/md11030903

Wilhelm, S. M., Carter, C., Tang, L., Wilkie, D., McNabola, A., Rong, H., et al. (2004). BAY 43-9006 exhibits broad spectrum oral antitumor activity and targets the RAF/MEK/ERK pathway and receptor tyrosine kinases involved in tumor progression and angiogenesis. *Cancer Res.* 64, 7099–7109. doi: 10.1158/0008-5472.can-04-1443

Wu, P., Nielsen, T. E., and Clausen, M. H. (2016). Small-molecule kinase inhibitors: an analysis of FDA-approved drugs. *Drug Discov. Today* 21, 5–10. doi: 10.1016/j.drudis.2015.07.008

Wyld, L., Audisio, R. A., and Poston, G. J. (2015). The evolution of cancer surgery and future perspectives. *Nat. Rev. Clin. Oncol.* 12, 115–124. doi: 10.1038/nrclinonc.2014.191

Yang, D., Kathawala, R. J., Chufan, E. E., Patel, A., Ambudkar, S. V., Chen, Z. S., et al. (2014). Tivozanib reverses multidrug resistance mediated by ABCB1 (P-glycoprotein) and ABCG2 (BCRP). *Fut. Oncol.* 10, 1827–1841. doi: 10.2217/fon.13.253

Zahoor, H., Mir, M. C., Barata, P. C., Stephenson, A. J., Campbell, S. C., Fergany, A., et al. (2019). Phase II trial of continuous treatment with sunitinib in patients with high-risk (BCG-refractory) non-muscle invasive bladder cancer. *Invest. New Drugs* 37, 1231–1238. doi: 10.1007/s10637-018-00716-w

Zaidi, A. H., Kelly, R. J., Gorbunova, A., Omstead, A. N., Salvitti, M. S., Zheng, P., et al. (2021). Intratumoral immunotherapy with STING agonist, ADU-S100, induces CD8+ T-cell mediated anti-tumor immunity in an esophageal adenocarcinoma model. *Oncotarget* 12, 292–303. doi: 10.18632/oncotarget.27886

Zhang, Y., Moerkens, M., Ramaiahgari, S., de Bont, H., Price, L., Meerman, J., et al. (2011). Elevated insulin-like growth factor 1 receptor signaling induces antiestrogen resistance through the MAPK/ERK and PI3K/Akt signaling routes. *Breast Cancer Res.* 13:R52.

Zou, W., Wolchok, J. D., and Chen, L. (2016). PD-L1 (B7-H1) and PD-1 pathway blockade for cancer therapy: mechanisms, response biomarkers, and combinations. *Sci. Transl. Med.* 8:328rv4. doi: 10.1126/scitranslmed.aad7118

15

PNA-Modified Liposomes Improve the Delivery Efficacy of CAPIRI for the Synergistic Treatment of Colorectal Cancer

Wenbin Diao [1,2], Ben Yang [1,2], Sipeng Sun [1,2], Anping Wang [1,2], Rongguan Kou [1], Qianyun Ge [1,2], Mengqi Shi [1,2], Bo Lian [1,2], Tongyi Sun [1,2], Jingliang Wu [1,2], Jingkun Bai [1,2], Meihua Qu [3], Yubing Wang [1,2], Wenjing Yu [1,2]* and Zhiqin Gao [1,2]**

[1]School of Life Science and Technology, Weifang Medical University, Weifang, China, [2]Shandong Universities Key Laboratory of Biopharmaceuticals, Weifang, China, [3]Translational Medical Center, Second People's Hospital of Weifang, Weifang, China

***Correspondence:**
Yubing Wang
ybwang@wfmc.edu.cn
Wenjing Yu
yuwjwf@163.com
Zhiqin Gao
zhiqingao2013@163.com

Tumor-associated antigen mucin 1 (MUC1) is highly expressed in colorectal cancer and is positively correlated with advanced stage at diagnosis and poor patient outcomes. The combination of irinotecan and capecitabine is standard chemotherapy for metastatic colorectal cancer and is known as XELIRI or CAPIRI, which significantly prolongs the progression-free survival and overall survival of colorectal cancer patients compared to a single drug alone. We previously reported that peanut agglutinin (PNA)-conjugated liposomes showed enhanced drug delivery efficiency to MUC1-positive liver cancer cells. In this study, we prepared irinotecan hydrochloride (IRI) and capecitabine (CAP)-coloaded liposomes modified by peanut agglutinin (IRI/CAP-PNA-Lips) to target MUC1-positive colorectal cancer. The results showed that IRI/CAP-PNA-Lips showed an enhanced ability to target MUC1-positive colorectal cancer cells compared to unmodified liposomes. Treatment with IRI/CAP-PNA-Lips also increased the proportion of apoptotic cells and inhibited the proliferation of colorectal cancer cells. The targeting specificity for tumor cells and the antitumor effects of PNA-modified liposomes were significantly increased in tumor-bearing mice with no severe cytotoxicity to normal tissues. These results suggest that PNA-modified liposomes could provide a new delivery strategy for the synergistic treatment of colorectal cancer with clinical chemotherapeutic agents.

Keywords: colorectal cancer, liposomes, peanut agglutinin, combination therapy, irinotecan, capecitabine

INTRODUCTION

The 2020 Global Cancer Report showed that the incidence of colorectal cancer ranks third among all cancers (Engstrand et al., 2018; Xu, Fan, et al., 2019; Sung et al., 2021). The main treatment for colorectal cancer is surgical resection combined with chemotherapy (Chau and Cunningham, 2002). The topoisomerase I inhibitor irinotecan (IRI) mainly relies on its active metabolite SN-38 to exert tumor-suppressive effects and is widely used in the treatment of colorectal and pancreatic cancers but with toxic effects of neutrophil reduction and diarrhea (de Man et al., 2018). IRI is often used in combination with 5-FU and its derivatives in the clinical treatment of cancer (Paulík et al., 2020). Studies have shown that capecitabine (CAP) is a precursor of 5-FU, and its combination with irinotecan (XELIRI or CAPIRI) is as effective as other synergistic treatments in colorectal cancer patients. The therapy is well tolerated with fewer toxic side effects and a higher safety profile at the same level of efficacy (Goldberg, 2005; Walko and Lindley, 2005; Lam et al., 2016). Due to the limitations of conventional chemotherapeutic drugs, such as poor targeting, short drug clearance half-life, low bioavailability, and poor solubility, there is much room to improve the efficacy of chemotherapy. Liposomes are ideal carriers to encapsulate chemotherapy drugs, not only to reduce drug toxicity and improve drug stability but also to enhance antitumor efficacy through surface modifications for active targeting and precise drug delivery (Harashima et al., 1999; Barenholz, 2012; Mitragotri et al., 2015).

Mucin 1 (MUC1) is a type of tumor-associated carbon antigen (TACA), which is a highly glycosylated mucin, and studies have shown that it is an important biomarker in colorectal cancer (Nabavinia et al., 2017; Gao et al., 2020). Altered expression of MUC1 glycosyltransferase results in a Thomsen–Friedenreich (TF) structure, which reduces the adhesion between tumor cells. Studies have shown that high expression of MUC1 promotes tumor cell proliferation and metastasis, and its expression is proportional to tumor malignancy and is associated with poor prognosis in patients (Li et al., 2019). Thus, using MUC1-specific ligands to modify liposomes could enable targeted delivery of drugs to MUC1-positive colorectal cancer tissue. Peanut agglutinin (PNA) is a homotetrameric plant agglutinin extracted from peanuts that can bind to a variety of disaccharides containing β-D-galactosyl-(1–3)-N-acetyl-D-galactosamine [Gal-β(1–3)GalNAc]. Studies have found that the core component of the TF structure is Gal-β(1–3)GalNAc, which is the core structure of MUC1 (Beack et al., 2017; Kumagai et al., 2019). Therefore, PNA-modified liposomes can actively target MUC1-positive colorectal cancers to deliver drugs centrally. Previously, we reported that PNA-modified liposomes showed enhanced drug delivery efficiency toward MUC1-positive liver cancer cells, which suggested the feasibility of using PNA-modified liposomes targeting MUC1 as a means to enhance its antitumor effects (Li, Diao, et al., 2020).

In this study, we prepared PNA-modified liposomes coloaded with IRICAP (IRI/CAP-PNA-Lips), achieved targeted codelivery of drugs, and improved the effectiveness of the anti-colorectal cancer effect. PNA-modified liposomes coloaded with drugs are important as a novel drug delivery strategy to enhance the efficacy of the clinical synergistic treatment of colorectal cancer.

MATERIALS AND METHODS

Synthesis and Identification of DSPE-PEG2K-PNA

Ten milligrams of peanut agglutinin (PNA, Medicago, Uppsala, Sweden) was weighed and dissolved in 2 ml of pH 7.4 PBS, and 0.2 ml (5.0 eq.) of DSPE-PEG2K-NHS (Xi'an Rui Xi Biotechnology Corporation, Xi'an, China) was added to DMSO solution. The reaction solution was transferred to a dialysis bag (cutoff molecular weight 8,000–14,000 Da) after 4 h of reaction at room temperature and then dialyzed with pure water for 12 h. The dialysate was collected and freeze-dried to obtain DSPE-PEG2K-PNA.

SDS–polyacrylamide gel electrophoresis (SDS–PAGE) was used for the analysis of PNA and DSPE-PEG2K-PNA. The gel was stained with 0.25% Coomassie Brilliant Blue solution for 3 h and then decolorized with the decolorizing solution until the bands were clear. The successful linkage of PNA and DSPE-PEG2K was determined using infrared spectroscopy analysis.

Analysis of the Optimal Synergistic Ratio of Irinotecan Hydrochloride (IRI) and Capecitabine (CAP) Using the Combination Index Method

The CI method was used to analyze the optimal synergistic ratio of irinotecan hydrochloride (IRI, Yuanye Biotechnology Corporation, Shanghai, China) and capecitabine (CAP, Ark Pharm, Chicago, United States) (Meng et al., 2015). Four colorectal cancer cell lines, Caco-2, HCT116, HT29, and SW620 (Cell Resource Center, Institute of Basic Medical Sciences, Chinese Academy of Medical Sciences, Beijing, China), were treated with different concentrations of IRI or CAP alone for 72 h to obtain the half-maximal inhibitory concentration (IC50) of IRI and CAP, respectively. The concentrations of the main drug, IRI, were determined as 1 μg/ml, 3 μg/ml, 9 μg/ml, 27 μg/ml, and 81 μg/ml, and the amounts of CAP were added at ratios of IRI:CAP equal to 8:1, 4:1, 3:1, 2:1, 1:1, 1:2, 1:3, 1:4, and 1:8 to obtain forty-five different concentrations and ratios of IRI and CAP mixture. Concentrations of IRI equal to 1 μg/ml, 3 μg/ml, 9 μg/ml, 27 μg/ml, and 81 μg/ml, and equivalent concentrations of CAP alone were used as controls. The four cell lines were treated with forty-five different concentration conditions for 72 h, and the IC50 values were calculated for the combination of the two drugs at different ratios. Six replicate wells were used in each group.

Based on the IC50 values, CI at different IRI/CAP ratios was calculated using the following equation:

$$CI = IC_1/IC_{m1} + IC_2/IC_{m2}.$$

IC_1 and IC_2 represent the IC50 values of IRI and CAP when the two drugs are combined to treat cells. IC_{m1} and IC_{m2} represent the IC50 values of IRI and CAP when they are treated alone (Guo et al., 2020). If the CI is greater than 1, it means that the two drugs have an antagonistic effect, less than 1 means that the two drugs have a synergistic effect, and equal to 1 means that the two drugs have an additive effect.

Preparation of PNA-Modified Liposomes Coloaded With IRICAP

Blank liposomes (Lips) were prepared by a thin-film dispersion method (Gao et al., 2021). Lecithin and cholesterol (Avet Pharmaceutical Corporation, Shanghai, China) were dissolved in 4 ml of chloroform at a mass ratio of 4:1, and the organic solvent was removed by heating and evaporating in a rotary evaporator (Yarmato Technology & Trading Corporation, Shanghai, China) to form lipid films. Then, 70 mg/ml ammonium sulfate was hydrated and homogenized for particle size using an ultrasonic cell crusher (Sonics & Materials,

United States). The liposome extruders were passed over 0.2 and 0.1 μm filter membranes, repeatedly extruded 10 times, and dialyzed with ddH_2O for 6 h to obtain unmodified blank liposomes.

Liposomes coloaded with IRICAP (IRI/CAP-Lips) and PNA-modified liposomes coloaded with IRICAP (IRI/CAP-PNA-Lips) were prepared by thin-film dispersion combined with the ammonium sulfate gradient method (Abraham et al., 2005; Zhang and Yao, 2012). Capecitabine was dissolved in chloroform according to the mass ratio (phospholipid:CAP = 1.3:1) to obtain loaded capecitabine liposomes (CAP-Lips). Then, CAP-Lips were mixed with IRI according to the mass ratio (phospholipid:IRI = 10:1), and IRI/CAP-Lips were obtained after hydration and dialysis. DSPE-PEG2K-PNA was used according to the mass ratio (phospholipid:PNA = 10:1) in chloroform, and IRI/CAP-PNA-Lips were obtained based on the IRI/CAP-Lip preparation procedure.

Characterization of PNA-Modified Liposomes Coloaded With IRICAP

The liposomes of each type were ultrasonically crushed for 10 min and then passed through 0.2 and 0.1 μm membrane filters ten times, diluted 10-fold with ddH_2O, and prepared for use. The morphological observation was performed using transmission electron microscopy (HITACHI High-Tech Corporation, Japan) after phosphotungstic acid staining (Feng et al., 2019). Particle size and potential were determined using a Malvern particle size meter (Malvern Panalytical Corporation, UK) (Sarisozen et al., 2012).

The encapsulation efficiency (EE) and drug loading (DL) of the coloaded liposomes were measured by using high-performance liquid chromatography (HPLC, Thermo Fisher Scientific, Massachusetts, United States) (Wang et al., 2019). After 6.8 g of potassium dihydrogen phosphate was dissolved in 800 ml of water, 10 ml of triethylamine was added, and the pH was adjusted to 4.0 with phosphoric acid. Water was then added to 1,000 ml to configure the phosphate buffer with a mobile phase ratio of methanol:acetonitrile:phosphate buffer equal to 55:5:45. After diluting the liposomes 10-fold, 0.2% Triton X-100 was added to permeabilize the membrane for 15 min, and the absorption peaks of IRI and CAP were detected at 254 and 307 nm, respectively. The EE and DL of liposomes were calculated using the following equations:

Encapsulation efficiency (EE) % = Mass of the drug loaded/ Total mass of the drug used × 100%

Drug loading (DL) % = Mass of the drug loaded/Total mass of liposomes × 100%

Stability and Drug Release Analysis of PNA-Modified Liposomes Coloaded With IRICAP

Each type of liposome was stored in saline and 3% BSA at 4°C for 16 days. The changes in particle size and potential over 16 days were measured using a Malvern particle size meter.

The *in vitro* dialysis method was used for the drug release analysis of liposomes (Liu et al., 2017; Li, Hou, et al., 2020). For this, 2 ml of each type of liposome was placed in a dialysis bag (with molecular weight cutoff at 8,000–14,000 Da), placed in a conical flask containing 100 ml of phosphate-buffered saline (PBS), and incubated at 37°C on a shaker at 100 rpm. At each time point (15 min, 30 min, 1, 8, 12, and 24 h), samples (2 ml) were taken from the PBS and immediately replenished with an equal volume of fresh PBS. The levels of IRI and CAP in the samples and the cumulative drug release were analyzed by HPLC.

Identification of MUC1-Positive Colorectal Cancer Cell Lines

Caco-2, HCT116, HT29, and SW620 cells were cultured overnight in 6-well plates (3×10^5 cells/well). Total RNA that had been extracted by the TRIzol method was used as the template to produce cDNA by using an RT-PCR kit (Toyobo Life Science, Shanghai, China). Furthermore, the cDNA was used as a template for real-time quantitative PCR, using a program that was set to 95°C, 30 s→95°C, 5 s; 60°C, 10 s; and 72°C, 15 s (40 cycles). The Ct values of each group were recorded, and the relative expression of each group was calculated by the 2^(-Delta Delta C(T)) method.

The four cell lines were cultured overnight in 6-well plates (3×10^5 cells/well), and RIPA lysis was performed to extract cellular protein. Western blot analysis identified MUC1 expression in the four cell lines.

Furthermore, all four cell lines were inoculated into cell crawls (5×10^4 cells/well) for 24 h, fixed in 4% tissue cell fixative for 10 min, permeabilized with 0.1% Triton X-100 for 10 min, blocked with 3% BSA for 2 h, incubated overnight at 4°C with MUC1-specific antibody (Cell Signaling Technology, Danvers, Massachusetts, United States), and further incubated with fluorescent secondary antibody for 1 h. DAPI was used to stain the nuclei. The four cell lines were then visualized with a confocal laser scanning microscope (CLSM, Leica Microscope Imaging System, Germany) to observe MUC1 expression. After each step of the aforementioned treatment, the cells were rinsed with PBS three times.

Targeting Property Analysis of PNA-Modified Liposomes *In Vitro*

To study the cellular uptake of liposomes by cells *in vitro*, FITC and rhodamine (Rhb) were used to replace the CAP and IRI to prepare liposomes coloaded with FITCRhb (FITC/Rhb-Lips) and PNA-modified liposomes coloaded with FITCRhb (FITC/Rhb-PNA-Lips). Caco-2, HCT116, HT29, and SW620 cells were inoculated into cell crawls (5×10^4 cells/well) overnight. The cells were incubated for 4 h with the addition of complete medium containing equal concentrations of FITC/Rhb, FITC/Rhb-Lips, and FITC/Rhb-PNA-Lips (Khan et al., 2020). We used 0.1% Triton X-100 to permeabilize the cell membrane and nuclear membrane. DAPI was utilized to stain the nucleus and an anti-fluorescence quencher as a sealant. Images were taken to observe the fluorescence distribution and intensity of different cells with CLSM. Each of the aforementioned steps was performed in the dark, and the cells were rinsed with PBS three times after the treatment (Xu et al., 2019).

Cytotoxicity Analysis of PNA-Modified Liposomes Coloaded With IRICAP *In Vitro*

Caco-2, HCT116, HT29, and SW620 cells were inoculated into 96-well plates (1×10^4 cells/well) overnight. The old medium was discarded, and Lips, IRI/CAP, IRI/CAP-Lips, and IRI/CAP-PNA-Lips were added to a 1.5-fold concentration gradient of IRI for 72 h. The old medium was replaced with a medium containing MTS and incubated for 15 min at 37°C. Enzyme-linked immunoassay (BIO-RAD, Hercules, California, United States) was used to detect optical density (OD) values. Inhibition of cell viability and IC50 values were calculated after 72 h of treatment with PNA-modified liposomes.

The four cell lines were treated with complete medium containing Lips, IRI/CAP, IRI/CAP-Lips, and IRI/CAP-PNA-Lips (C_{IRI} = 25 μg/ml, 50 μg/ml, 100 μg/ml) for 24 h. The MTS assay was used to analyze the inhibition of cell viability (Wang et al., 2015; Thapa et al., 2017).

$$\text{Cell Viability}(\%) = OD_{sample} - OD_{blank}/OD_{control} - OD_{blank} \times 100\%$$

Analysis of the Targeting Property of PNA-Modified Liposomes Coloaded With IRICAP *In Vivo*

To study the targeting property of liposomes *in vivo*, fluorescent-labeled liposomes were prepared by using Cy7 (Meilun Biotechnology Corporation, Dalian, China) at a mass ratio of phospholipid:Cy7 of 50:1 instead of the drugs encapsulated into the hydrophilic phase of liposomes.

BALB/C-nu mice (male, 4–5 weeks old, 14 ± 2 g, Viton River Laboratory Animal Technology Corporation, Beijing, China) were selected. All experiments met the institution's animal care standards and were approved by the Ethical Review Committee of Weifang Medical College. SW620 cells in the logarithmic growth phase were resuspended to 5×10^7cells/mL with saline and subcutaneously injected with 0.2 ml of cell suspension to construct a subcutaneous tumor-bearing nude mouse model.

When the mean tumor volume reached 100 mm^3, tumor-bearing nude mice were divided equally into three groups ($n = 6$) for targeted property analysis *in vivo* (Jiang et al., 2016). The distribution of fluorescence signals was observed at 1, 2, 4, 8, 12, 24, and 48 h after tail vein injection of Cy7, Cy7-Lips, and Cy7-PNA-Lips (2.5 mg/kg) by using a small animal imaging system *in vivo* (PerkinElmer Inc., United States) (Song et al., 2014; Xiong et al., 2017). Nude mice were euthanized 48 h after injection, and the heart, liver, spleen, lung, and kidney tumors were photographed to analyze the distribution of fluorescence in vital organs and tumor tissues.

Analysis of the Antitumor Ability of PNA-Modified Liposomes Coloaded With IRICAP *In Vivo*

Tumor-bearing nude mice were separated equally into 4 groups ($n = 6$) for antitumor experiments *in vivo*. Normal saline, IRI/CAP, IRI/CAP-Lips, and IRI/CAP-PNA-Lips (C_{IRI} = 20 mg/kg) were injected intraperitoneally every 4 days starting from the first day of grouping, and the body weight and tumor volume of nude mice were measured every other day (Guichard et al., 2001). After 20 days of treatment, tumor-bearing nude mice were euthanized; vital organs and tumor tissues were taken, photographed, and weighed; and the tumor inhibition rate (TIR) was calculated for each treatment group. The tumor tissues were fixed, embedded, and sectioned, and Ki-67 staining was performed to analyze the inhibitory ability of different treatments on the proliferation of tumor cells.

$$\text{Tumor volume}(mm^3) = \text{length} \times \text{width}^2 \times 0.5$$

$$\text{Tumor inhibition rate}(TIR) = 1 - V_{\text{treatment group}}/V_{\text{control group}} \times 100\%$$

Systemic Toxicity Assessment of PNA-Modified Liposomes Coloaded With IRICAP

Heart, liver, spleen, lung, and kidney tumors from the euthanized tumor-bearing nude mice were fixed, paraffin-embedded, and sectioned. H&E staining was performed on the tissue sections, and the sections were observed under a 20× microscope to determine whether obvious organic lesions appeared in each vital organ.

Heart blood was drawn from the SW620 tumor-bearing nude mouse model after 20 days of treatment, and the plasma was centrifuged for serum biochemical parameter analysis (Yu et al., 2019).

RESULTS

Synthesis and Characterization of DSPE-PEG2K-PNA

DSPE-PEG2K was bonded to peanut agglutinin (PNA) through an amide bond (-CO-NH-). The presence of the characteristic peaks of both DSPE-PEG2K and PNA in the infrared spectroscopy (IR) spectrum of DSPE-PEG2K-PNA (**Figure 1B**) indicated that DSPE-PEG2K-PNA was successfully synthesized. The SDS–PAGE results also indicated that PNA was ligated to DSPE-PEG2K. PNA is a homotetramer with a molecular weight of approximately 120 kDa and a monomeric molecular weight of approximately 32 kDa, which was consistent with the band on the SDS–PAGE gel. The band of DSPE-PEG2K-PNA showed that the molecular weight was heavier than the molecular weight of PNA. In addition, PEG-specific staining clearly marked the DSPE-PEG2K-PNA band in yellow, while the PNA band had no color. These results suggest that we successfully synthesized DSPE-PEG2K-PNA (**Figure 1C**; **Supplementary Figure S1D**).

The Optimal Synergistic Ratio of Irinotecan Hydrochloride and Capecitabine Is 3:1

The ratio of irinotecan hydrochloride (IRI) and capecitabine (CAP) in clinical synergistic treatment is approximately 1:8 (Kerr, 2002). To evaluate the optimal synergistic ratio of IRI

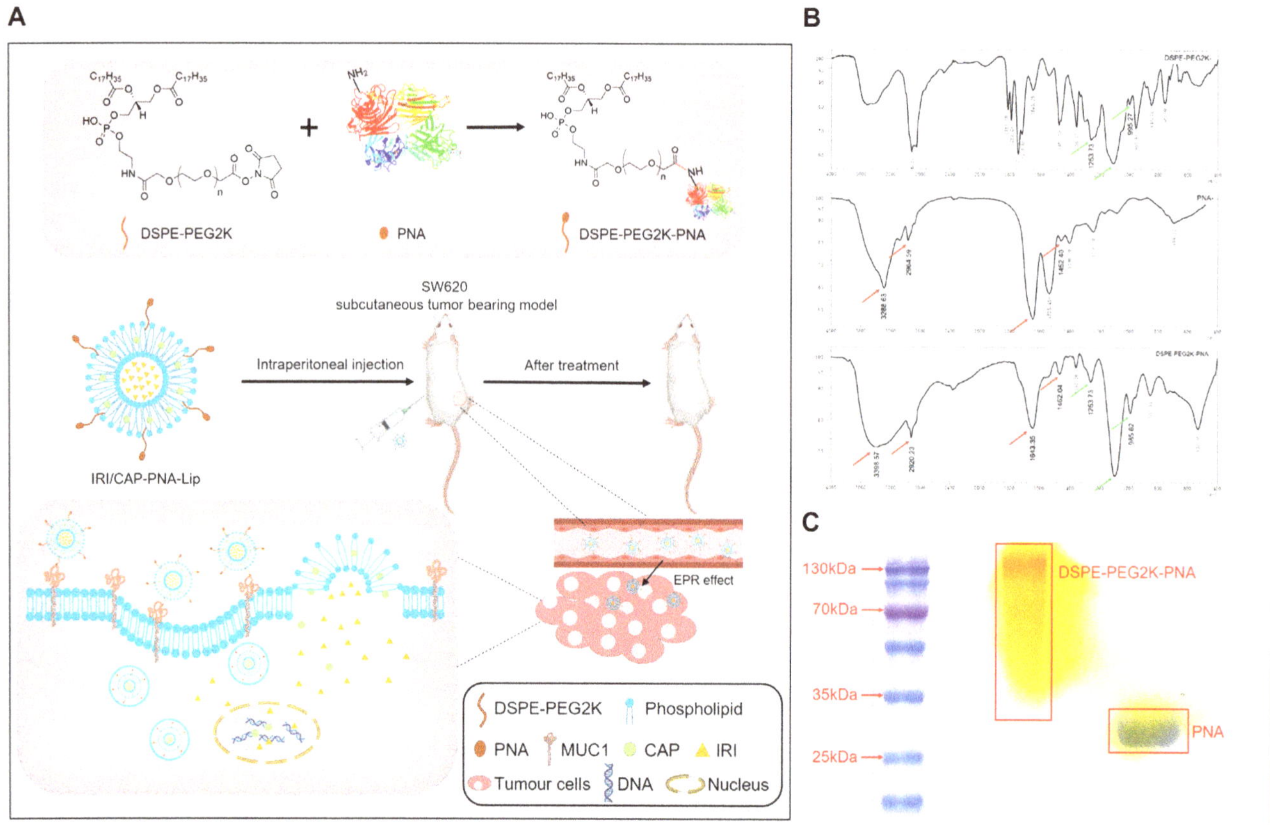

FIGURE 1 | (A) Schematic diagram of the preparation of PNA-modified liposomes and ligand–receptor-mediated targeting mechanisms for tumor tissue recognition. Liposomes loaded with IRICAP were modified with PNA as the ligand. PNA specifically interacts with MUC1, which is highly expressed in colorectal cancer cells. IRI and CAP are released into cells and bind to DNA to inhibit nucleic acid synthesis, thus enhancing the efficacy of anti-colorectal cancer. **(B)** Infrared spectroscopy identified the successful synthesis of DSPE-PEG2K-PNA. **(C)** SDS–PAGE to identify PNA was ligated to DSPE-PEG2K.

and CAP in the four colorectal cancer cell lines *in vitro*, the cell viability assay was performed by the MTS assay, and the combination index (CI) was compared (**Figure 2**). The CI of the four cell lines at different ratios was less than 1, suggesting that the combination of IRI and CAP exerted a synergistic effect. Caco-2, HT29, and SW620 had the lowest CI values when IRI: CAP was 3:1. The low CI values of HCT116 were 0.52 and 0.58 at IRI:CAP of 1:8 and 3:1, respectively (**Table 1**). The lowest CI values for Caco-2, HT29, and SW620 cells were observed at IRI: CAP of 3:1, and the lowest CI values were observed in HCT116 cells. We determined this ratio as the optimal synergistic ratio of the two drugs.

Characterization of PNA-Modified Liposomes Coloaded With CAPIRI

The particle size of PNA-modified liposomes coloaded with IRICAP (IRI/CAP-PNA-Lips) was 122.6 ± 0.58 nm. The polymer dispersity index (PDI) of coloaded PNA-modified liposomes was less than 0.2, which indicated that the particle size was dispersed equally (**Figures 3A,B**). For IRI/CAP-PNA-Lips, the encapsulation efficiency (EE) of IRI and CAP was 89.45 ± 0.015% and 7.56 ± 0.014%, respectively. The drug load (DL) of IRI and CAP was 17.98 ± 0.003% and 6.18 ± 0.013%, respectively (**Table 2**; **Supplementary Figures S1A–C**). The DL ratio of IRI and CAP in the coloaded PNA-modified liposomes was 3:1, which was consistent with the optimal synergistic ratio.

A drug release assay was performed *in vitro* to evaluate the sustained release effect and maximum cumulative release of coloaded liposomes. The maximum cumulative release of free drugs was achieved at 8 h, with over 80% of IRI and 60% of CAP. The cumulative release curves of IRI and CAP in coloaded liposomes can be divided into two phases: initial rapid release and sustained release. IRI in IRI/CAP-PNA-Lips and IRI/CAP-Lips had a rapid release in the first 8 h, and the rapid release phase of CAP in IRI/CAP-PNA-Lips and IRI/CAP-Lip was reached in the first hour. After that, the curve gradually changed to a sustained release phase. Finally, the maximum cumulative release of IRI was reached at 24 h in IRI/CAP-PNA-Lips and IRI/CAP-Lips, with maximum release rates of 72.9 ± 5.3% and 64.6 ± 2.9%, respectively. The maximum cumulative release of CAP in IRI/CAP-PNA-Lips and IRI/CAP-Lips had maximum release rates of 50.7 ± 3.2% and 53.6 ± 5.5%, respectively (**Figures 3C,D**). The particle size and potential of each type of liposome were stable, and no significant changes were observed after

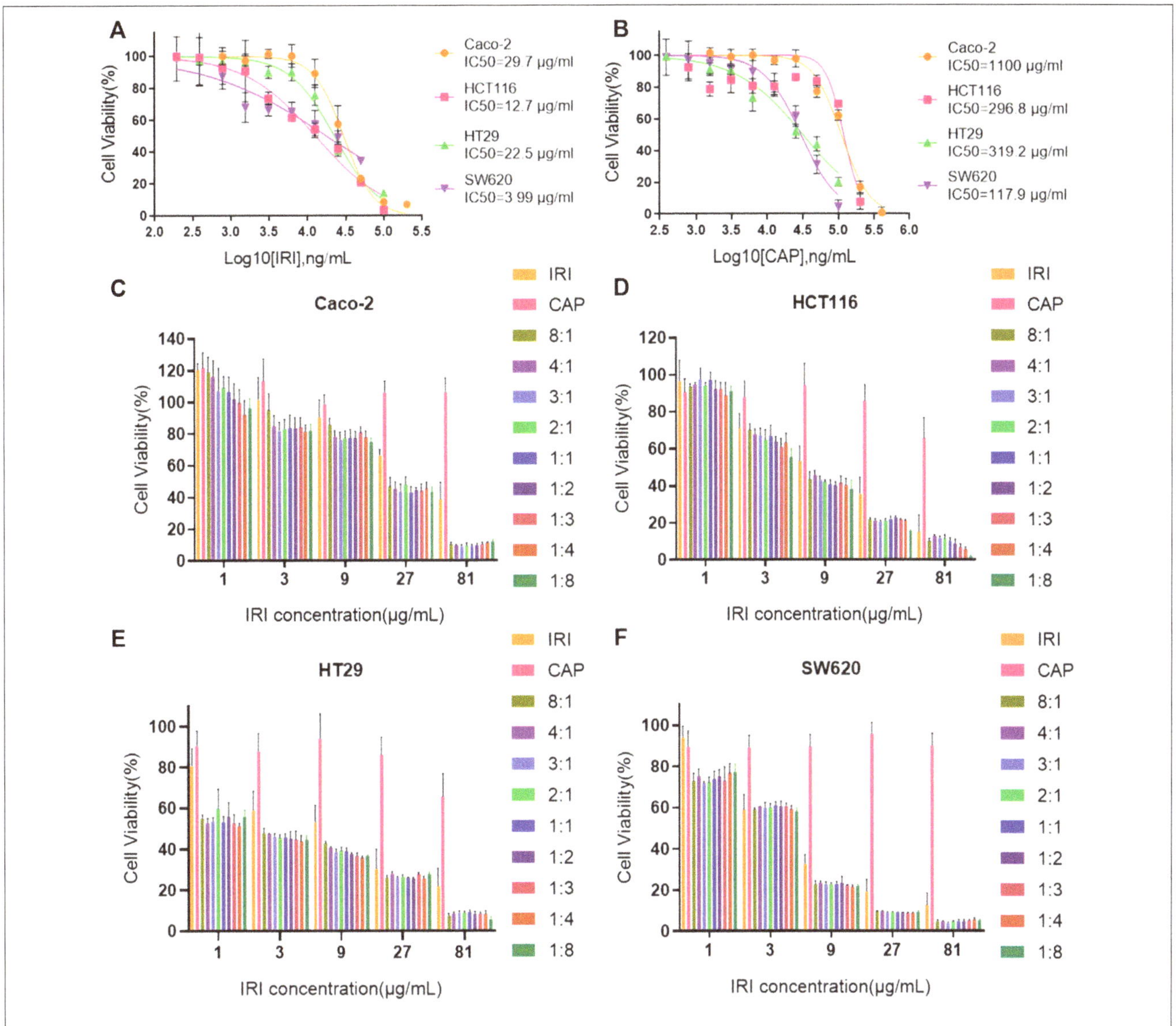

FIGURE 2 | The optimal synergistic ratio of irinotecan hydrochloride and capecitabine was 3:1. **(A,B)** IC50 value analysis of CAP and IRI alone in Caco-2, HCT116, HT29, and SW620 cell lines. **(C–F)** Effect of IRI and CAP on the viability of Caco-2, HCT116, HT29, and SW620 cells at different ratios.

TABLE 1 | CI values for four colorectal cancer cell lines at different combination ratios of IRI/CAP.

	Caco-2			HCT116			HT29			SW620		
	IC50 (IRI)	IC50 (CAP)	CI	IC50 (IRI)	IC50 (CAP)	CI	IC50 (IRI)	IC50 (CAP)	CI	IC50 (IRI)	IC50 (CAP)	CI
IRI	29.69	–	–	12.6	–	–	22.5	–	–	9.35	–	–
CAP	–	1100	–	–	296.8	–	–	319.2	–	–	117.9	–
8:01	26.3	3.29	0.89	7.44	0.93	0.59	5.01	0.63	0.22	3.2	0.4	0.35
4:01	22.1	5.53	0.75	7.57	1.9	0.61	5.11	1.28	0.23	2.9	0.725	0.32
3:01	20.1	6.7	0.68	7.22	2.41	0.58	4.89	1.63	0.22	2.7	0.9	0.29
2:01	22.2	11.1	0.76	6.78	3.39	0.55	4.98	2.49	0.22	3.1	1.55	0.34
1:01	20.4	20.4	0.71	6.94	6.94	0.57	5.08	5.08	0.24	2.7	2.7	0.31
1:02	20.6	41.2	0.73	6.44	12.88	0.55	5.12	10.24	0.26	2.7	5.4	0.33
1:03	21.4	64.2	0.78	6.17	18.51	0.55	4.96	14.88	0.26	2.5	7.5	0.33
1:04	20.6	82.4	0.77	6.03	24.12	0.56	4.89	19.56	0.27	2.3	9.2	0.32
1:08	19.5	156	0.8	4.9	39.2	0.52	4.86	38.88	0.33	2.6	20.8	0.45

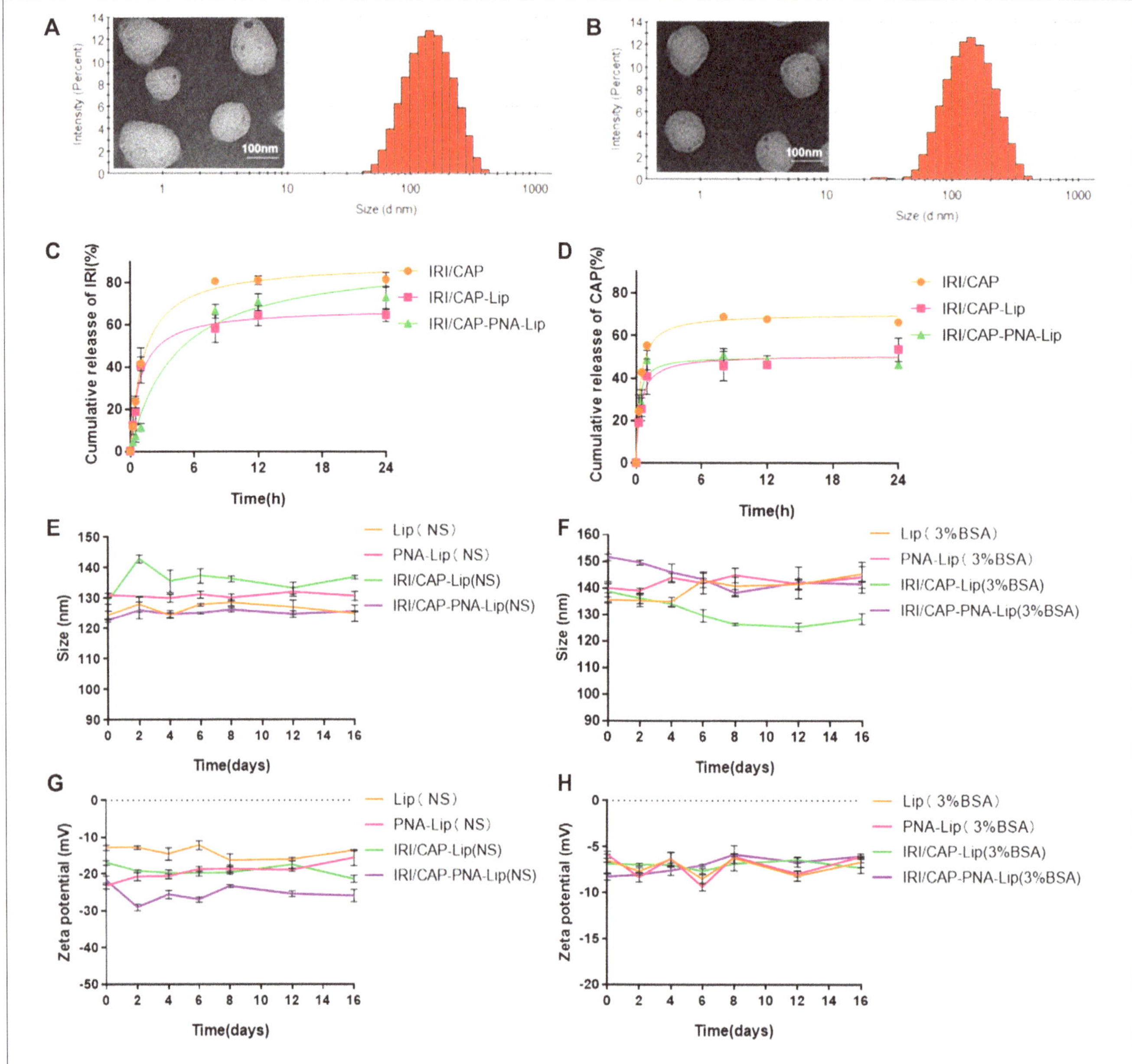

FIGURE 3 | Analysis of the drug release capacity and stability of different types of drug-loaded liposomes. **(A,B)** Particle size histograms and transmission electron microscopy (TEMik) images of IRI/CAP-Lips and IRI/CAP-PNA-Lips. **(C)** Cumulative drug release profiles of IRI-loaded liposomes in PBS at 37°C. **(D)** Cumulative release curves of CAP-loaded liposomes in PBS at 37°C. **(E,F)** Folding graphs of particle size changes of different types of liposomes stored in saline or 3% BSA at 4°C for 16 days. **(G,H)** Folding graphs of potential changes of different types of liposomes stored in saline or 3% BSA at 4°C for 16 days. The data are presented as the mean ± SD (n = 3).

TABLE 2 | Characteristics of different types of liposomes (mean ± SD, n = 3).

	Size (nm)	PDI	Zeta (mV)	EE IRI (%)	EE CAP (%)	DL IRI (%)	DL CAP (%)
Lips	126.6 ± 1.58	0.16 ± 0.04	−12.9 ± 0.70	–	–	–	–
PNA-Lips	130.9 ± 0.80	0.12 ± 0.02	−23.3 ± 0.81	–	–	–	–
IRI/CAP-Lips	126.7 ± 2.51	0.18 ± 0.05	−15.5 ± 0.56	57.67 ± 0.090	4.63 ± 0.020	11.53 ± 0.020	3.79 ± 0.010
IRI/CAP-PNA-Lips	122.6 ± 0.58	0.17 ± 0.03	−21.3 ± 0.49	89.45 ± 0.015	7.56 ± 0.014	17.98 ± 0.003	6.18 ± 0.013

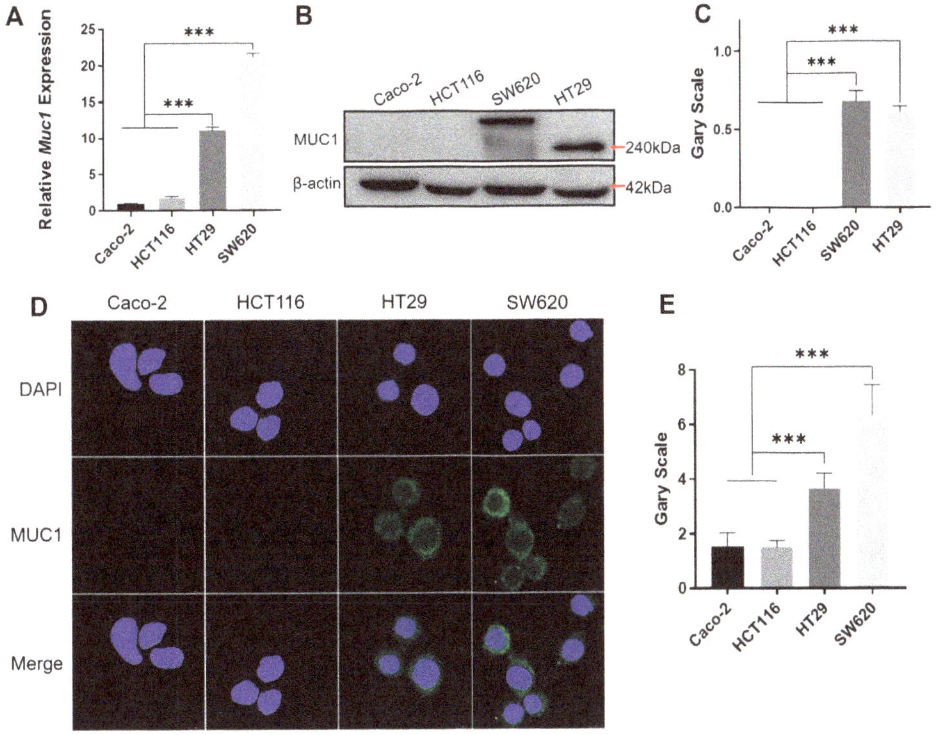

FIGURE 4 | Identification of MUC1 expression in colorectal cancer cells. **(A)** Real-time quantitative PCR analysis of MUC1 expression at the mRNA level in Caco-2, HCT116, HT29, and SW620 cell lines. **(B)** Western blot analysis of MUC1 expression in four cell lines. **(C)** Quantitative histogram of Western blot results. **(D)** Cellular immunofluorescence assay for the identification of MUC1 expression in four cell lines. **(E)** Quantitative histogram of cellular immunofluorescence results. ***$p < 0.001$.

storage in physiological saline or 3% BSA for half a month at 4°C (**Figures 3E–H**).

MUC1 Was Highly Expressed in the Colorectal Cancer Cell Lines HT29 and SW620

The results of real-time quantitative PCR and Western blotting showed that MUC1 was highly expressed in HT29 and SW620 cells (**Figures 4A–C**). Furthermore, immunofluorescence using a MUC1-specific antibody showed that the green fluorescence intensity was significantly higher in HT29 and SW620 cells than in Caco-2 and HCT116 cells (**Figures 4D,E**). The experiments showed that MUC1 was not expressed in the colorectal cancer cell lines Caco-2 and HCT116, while it was highly expressed in the colorectal cancer cell lines HT29 and SW620.

Enhanced Cellular Uptake of PNA-Modified Liposomes by MUC1-Positive Colorectal Cancer Cell Lines

To explore the targeting efficiency of PNA-modified liposomes to MUC1-positive cells, PNA-modified liposomes loaded with FITC and rhodamine (Rhb) were prepared. The cellular uptake of FITC and Rhb in the four cell lines showed distinct results. Two MUC1-negative cell lines, Caco-2 and HCT116, showed no significant difference in the cellular uptake of FITC and Rhb in the FITC/Rhb-PNA-Lip groups compared to the FITC/Rhb-Lip groups. The fluorescence signals of the FITC/Rhb-PNA-Lip groups were significantly enhanced in HT29 and SW620 cells, which are MUC1-positive cell lines (**Figure 5**; **Supplementary Figures S2A–D**). The aforementioned results suggest that PNA-modified liposomes exhibit effective MUC1-targeting properties in colorectal cancer cells and could work as efficient drug delivery carriers to MUC1-positive colorectal cancer.

PNA-Modified Liposomes Coloaded With IRICAP Significantly Inhibited the Viability of MUC1-Positive Colorectal Cancer Cell Lines *In Vitro*

Based on the effectiveness of cellular uptake, the MTS assay was used to further evaluate the inhibitory effect of PNA-modified liposomes coloaded with IRICAP on the viability of colorectal cancer cell lines. The results showed that in the MUC1-positive colorectal cancer cell line HT29, the IC50 values for the IRI/CAP-Lip and IRI/CAP-PNA-Lip groups were 5.8 μg/ml and 5.1 μg/ml, respectively. Another MUC1-positive colorectal cancer cell line, SW620, had IC50 values for the IRI/CAP-Lip and IRI/CAP-PNA-Lip groups of 5.4 μg/ml and 4.7 μg/ml, respectively. There was no significant difference in the cytotoxicity of the IRI/CAP-Lip and IRI/CAP-PNA-Lip treatment groups (**Figures 6A–D**).

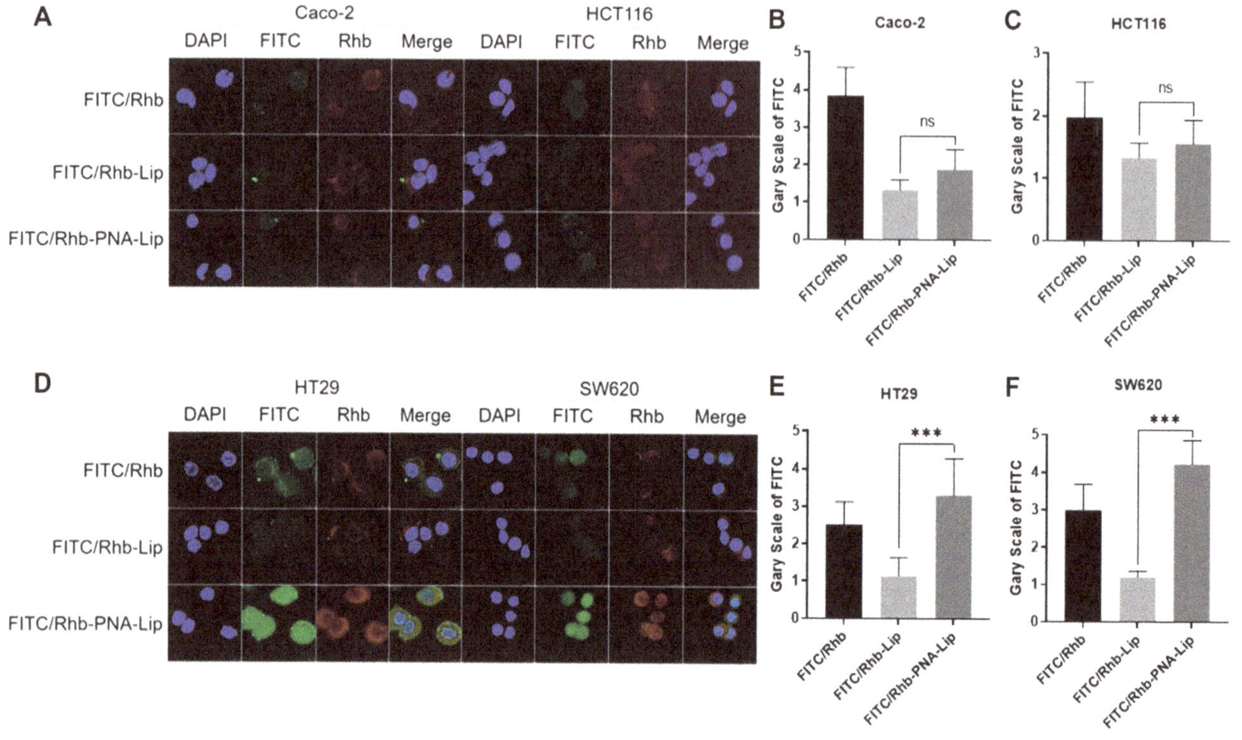

FIGURE 5 | CLSM analysis showed that PNA-modified liposomes enhance the cellular uptake of drugs by MUC1-positive cells. **(A)** CLSM observation of the distribution of fluorescence signals in Caco-2 and HCT116 cells. **(B,C)** Quantitative histograms of FITC fluorescence signals in Caco-2 and HCT116 cells. **(D)** CLSM observation of the distribution of fluorescence signals in HT29 and SW620 cells. **(E,F)** Quantitative histograms of FITC fluorescence signals in HT29 and SW620 cells. The data are presented as the mean ± SD (n = 3). $^{***}p < 0.001$.

This result may be due to the complete cellular uptake of the liposomes coloaded with CAPIRI by all cells after 72 h. Therefore, HT29 and SW620 cells were treated individually for 24 h, and we discovered that IRI/CAP-PNA-Lips had a stronger inhibitory effect at IRI concentrations up to 50 μg/ml (**Supplementary Figures S3A,B**).

When a single concentration of coloaded liposomes (C_{IRI} = 50 μg/ml) was used to treat cells for 24 h, the viability of HT29 and SW620 cells was significantly inhibited by PNA-modified liposomes coloaded with IRICAP compared to unmodified liposomes, which was consistent with the result of 100 μg/ml IRI in coloaded liposomes (**Figures 6E–H**; **Supplementary Figures S3C–J**).

PNA-Modified Liposomes Coloaded With IRICAP Promote Apoptosis in MUC1-Positive Colorectal Cancer Cells *In Vitro*

Based on the results of the MTS assays, we treated Caco-2, HCT116, HT29, and SW620 cells with coloaded liposomes at an IRI concentration of 50 μg/ml for 24 h. The effect of coloaded liposomes on the apoptosis of cells was evaluated using the Annexin V/PI double-staining method. The effects of IRI/CAP-Lips and IRI/CAP-PNA-Lips on the apoptosis of MUC1-negative Caco-2 and HCT116 cells were not significant. For MUC1-positive HT29 and SW620 cells, the apoptosis rate in the IRI/CAP-PNA-Lip group was 1.3-fold and 1.9-fold higher than that in the IRI/CAP-Lip group, respectively. The results suggested that PNA-modified liposomes coloaded with IRICAP significantly upregulated the apoptosis in MUC1-positive colorectal cancer cell lines (**Figure 7**).

PNA-Modified Liposomes Significantly Increase MUC1-Targeting Properties in Colorectal Cancer Tumors *In Vivo*

Small animal live-imaging techniques were used to observe the distribution of Cy7 in tumor uptake to assess the targeting ability of PNA-modified liposomes *in vivo*. Fluorescence signals could be observed in the whole body 1 h after tail vein injection of Cy7, which barely disappeared after 12 h in the tumor tissue. For the Cy7-Lip and Cy7-PNA-Lip groups, fluorescence signals were observed in the whole body between 1 and 2 h after injection. However, there was slower decay of fluorescence signals in the tumor tissue, which was different from the free drug conditions. After 2 h, the fluorescence signals of the Cy7-Lip and Cy7-PNA-Lip groups were consistently stronger than those of the Cy7 group, and the fluorescence signal of the Cy7-PNA-Lip group was consistently stronger than that of the Cy7-Lip group.

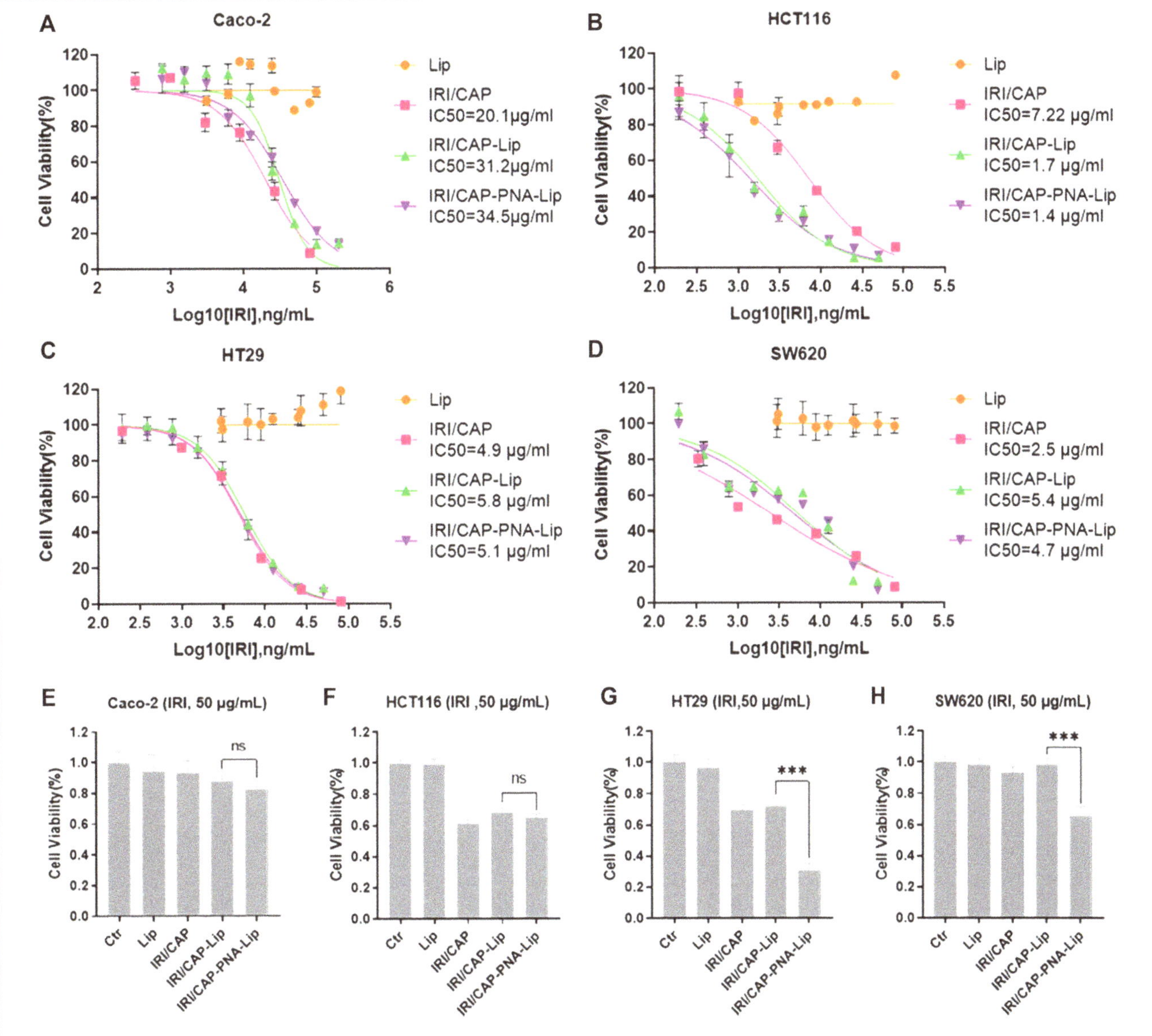

FIGURE 6 | IRI/CAP-PNA-Lips significantly inhibited the viability of MUC1-positive colorectal cancer cell lines *in vitro*. **(A–D)** Cytotoxicity analysis of coloaded liposomes in Caco-2, HCT116, HT29, and SW620 cell lines. **(E–H)** Effect of an IRI concentration of 50 μg/ml on cell viability after treatment of Caco-2, HCT116, HT29, and SW620 cell lines for 24 h. The data are presented as the mean ± SD (n = 3). ***p < 0.001.

The Cy7-PNA-Lip group showed the strongest fluorescence signals in the tumor tissue at 4 h after injection, which persisted in the tumor tissues up to 48 h after injection (**Figure 8B**). To verify that Cy7-PNA-Lips could improve the accumulation of drugs in tumor tissues and the targeted delivery efficiency, tumor-bearing nude mice were euthanized 48 h after injection (**Figure 8C**; **Supplementary Figure S2E**). Fluorescence accumulation was observed in the primary organs and tumor tissues. The Cy7-PNA-Lip group showed the strongest signals (**Figure 8D**). The results were consistent with the trend observed with cellular uptake, which suggested that PNA-modified liposomes could deliver targets and improve cellular uptake to improve drug accumulation in tumor tissues.

PNA-Modified Liposomes Coloaded With IRICAP Have Shown Improved Antitumor Ability *In Vivo*

Four groups of tumor-bearing nude mice were treated with physiological saline, IRI/CAP, IRI/CAP-Lips, or IRI/CAP-PNA-Lips to evaluate the antitumor ability of PNA-modified liposomes coloaded with IRICAP *in vivo*. There was no significant variation in the bodyweight of mice in the four groups after treatment (**Figure 9C**). All three dosing groups exhibited antitumor properties, but the tumor volume and weight of the IRI/CAP-PNA-Lip group were the lowest and were even lower than those of the IRI/CAP-Lip group (**Figures 9B,D**). The results showed that the IRI/CAP-PNA-

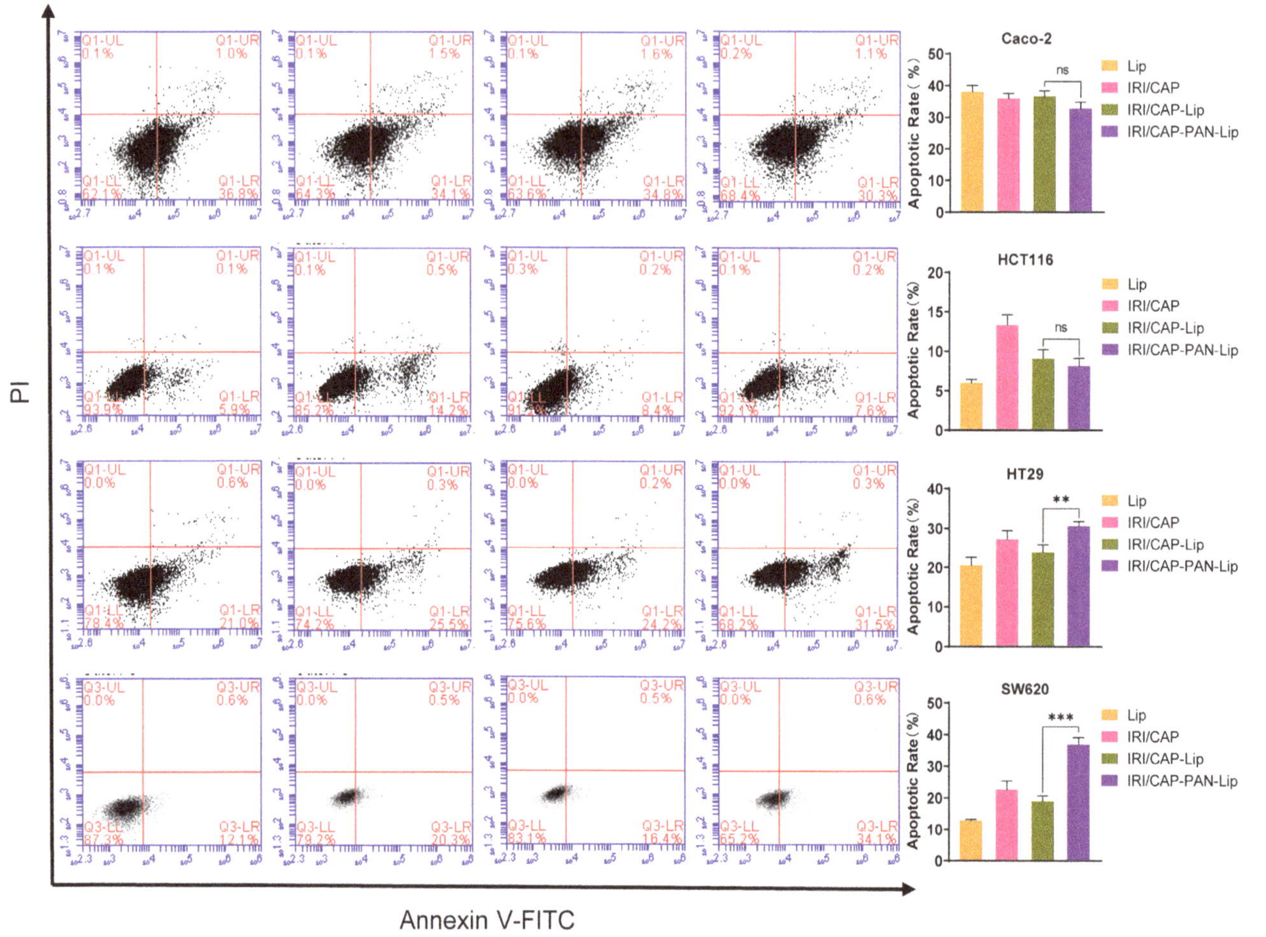

FIGURE 7 | IRI/CAP-PNA-Lips significantly induced apoptosis compared to IRI/CAP-Lips in HT29 and SW620 cell lines. The effects of Lips, IRI/CAP, IRI/CAP-Lips, and IRI/CAP-PNA-Lips on the apoptosis of colorectal cancer cell lines and their quantitative histograms. The data are presented as the mean ± SD ($n = 3$). **$p < 0.01$. ***$p < 0.001$.

Lip group had the strongest antitumor effect, with the tumor inhibition rate (TIR) reaching 12.69%, which was 9.6-fold better than that of the free drug group (**Figures 9E,F**).

Systemic Toxicity of PNA-Modified Liposomes Coloaded With IRICAP *In Vivo*

To evaluate the systemic toxicity of IRI/CAP-PNA-Lips *in vivo*, H&E staining was performed on the heart, liver, spleen, lung, and kidney. No histopathological abnormalities were observed in the four groups (**Figure 10A**). The tumor tissues of the saline group were closely arranged with large nuclei, while the tumor tissues of the IRI/CAP-PNA-Lip group presented the highest degree of apoptosis and necrosis, reduced cytokinesis, agglutination of chromatin in the nuclei, and a large number of vacuoles. Immunohistochemistry results showed that Ki-67 expression was decreased in the tumor tissues of the IRI/CAP-PNA-Lip group compared to the IRI/CAP-Lip group, which suggested that PNA-modified liposomes coloaded with IRICAP had a stronger antitumor cell proliferative effect (**Figure 10B**).

Plasma biochemical analyses were used to assess the effects of PNA-modified liposomes coloaded with IRICAP on the major metabolic organs of tumor-bearing mice. The results showed that except for the creatinine (Cr) value in the free drug group, which was slightly higher than that in the saline group ($p < 0.01$), the biochemical indices of urea, alanine aminotransferase (ALT), alkaline phosphatase (ALP), and aspartate aminotransferase (AST) showed no significant variation. The aforementioned results suggest that PNA-modified liposomes coloaded with IRICAP do not produce any systemic toxicity in the experimental mice (**Figures 10C–G**).

DISCUSSION

The desired synergistic effect relies on well-controlled drug dose matching and duration of effect. Peng et al. (2021) used liposomes to codeliver adriamycin and sorafenib, and the results showed that liposomes could achieve codelivery of the drugs and effectively improve the synergistic effect of the drugs.

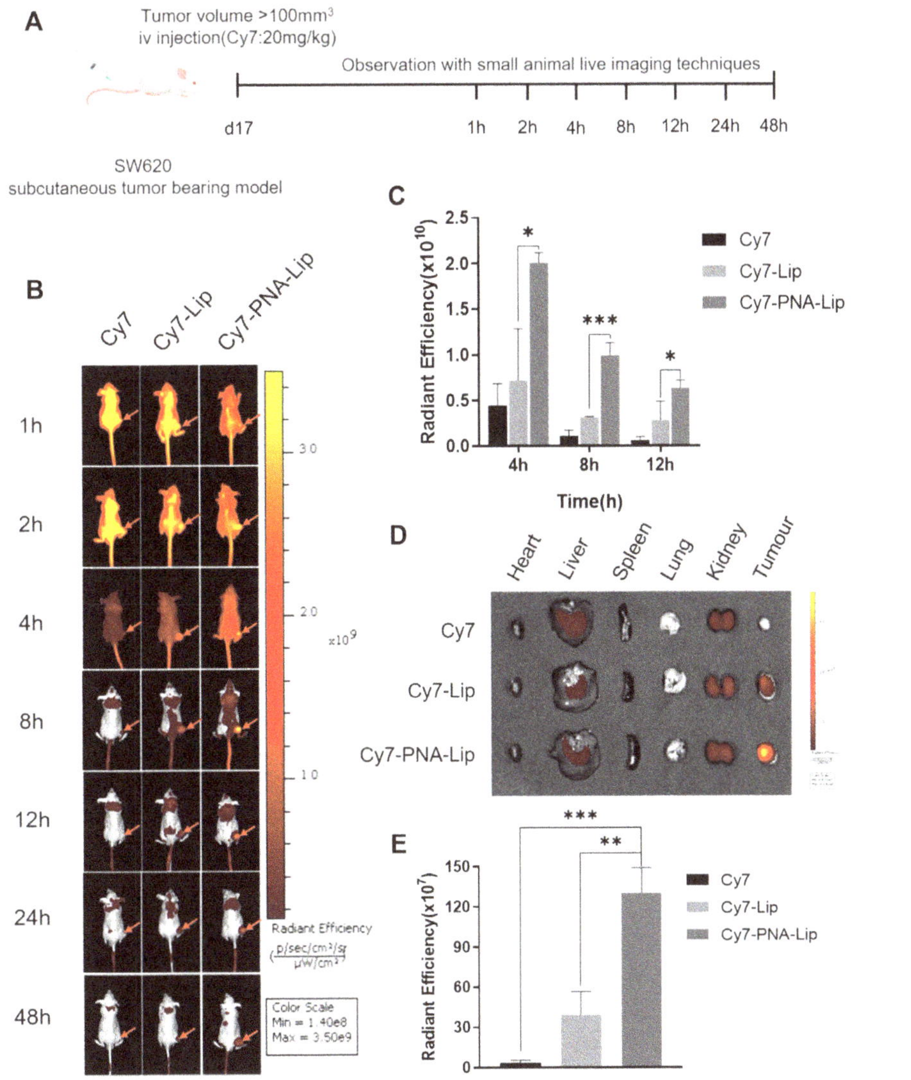

FIGURE 8 | PNA-modified liposomes exhibited effective MUC1-targeting properties in colorectal cancer tumors. **(A)** Design principles for the analysis of the targeting ability of PNA-modified liposomes *in vivo*. **(B)** Distribution of Cy7 in tumor-bearing nude mice after tail vein injection. **(C)** Quantitative histogram of fluorescence signals at tumor sites at different points in time. **(D)** Distribution of Cy7 in vital organs and tumor tissues after 48 h. **(E)** Quantitative histograms of fluorescence signals in tumors. The data are presented as the mean ± SD (n = 3). $^{*}p < 0.05$. $^{**}p < 0.01$. $^{***}p < 0.001$.

Although coloaded liposomes could improve drug efficacy, they are not specific for tumor tissue. Therefore, ligand-modified liposomes for active targeted drug delivery to enhance antitumor ability can be synthesized. IRI and CAP are synergistic chemotherapies approved by the FDA for treating colorectal cancer, but ligand-modified liposomes coloaded with IRICAP have not been reported (Chiorean et al., 2020). In this study, PNA-modified liposomes coloaded with IRICAP were prepared to specifically and actively target MUC1-positive colorectal cancer tumor tissue to further improve the synergistic efficacy. This drug delivery system can improve drug efficacy and reduce drug dosage while reducing drug concentrations in normal tissues and toxic side effects (Caliskan et al., 2019).

Taking into account the different water solubilities of CAP and IRI, they were encapsulated in hydrophobic or hydrophilic phases. This construction contributed to protecting the chemical stability of the two drugs during preparation, preservation, and blood transport while facilitating the stability of coloaded liposomes (Huang et al., 2019). Nanomedicines with particle size less than 200 nm can accumulate in tumor tissues through the enhanced permeability and retention effect (EPR). In this study, the particle size of each type of liposome fluctuated within approximately 120–130 nm, which is also close to the range reported in other studies (Kalyane et al., 2019; Park et al., 2019; Tan et al., 2019). The PDI of drug-loaded liposomes was between 0.1 and 0.3 in most studies, and the PDI of the liposomes in this study ranged between 0.12 and 0.18 (<0.2), indicating a

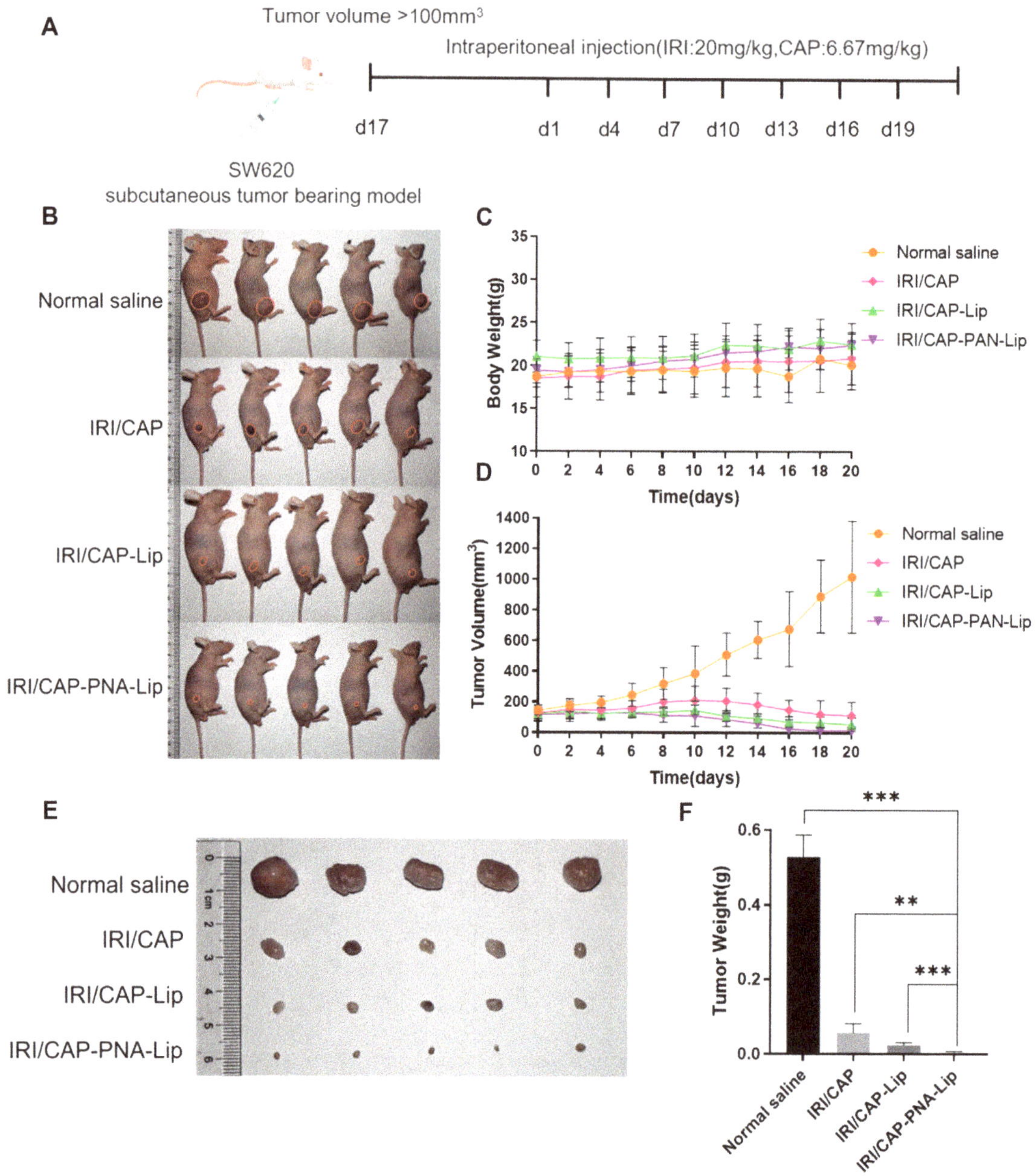

FIGURE 9 | PNA-modified liposomes significantly enhance the antitumor efficacy of the drug. **(A)** Design principles for the analysis of the antitumor abilities of PNA-modified liposomes *in vivo*. **(B)** Photos of tumor-bearing nude mice in each group after 20 days of treatment. **(C)** Changes in the bodyweight of the tumor-bearing nude mice. **(D)** Folding line graph of the change in tumor volume. **(E)** Photographs of tumors. **(F)** Histograms of tumor weights. The data are presented as the mean ± SD (n = 5). $^{**}p < 0.01$. $^{***}p < 0.001$.

good dispersion of the liposomes (Yang et al., 2015; Li et al., 2017). To enhance the efficacy of coloaded liposomes, we prepared negative potential liposomes that can protect liposomes from the reticuloendothelial system (RES) and effectively improve the circulation time in the blood (Ghosh et al., 2021). In addition, we hoped that the coloaded liposomes will accumulate and release as much of the drug as possible in the tumor tissue during circulation in blood. The 24-h maximum cumulative drug release of IRI and CAP in IRI/CAP-PNA-Lips was less than 60%, and sustained drug release was successfully achieved compared to the free drug *in vitro*, which reduced unnecessary drug release during circulation in blood (Allen and Cullis, 2013; Yalcin et al., 2018).

By Western blotting, we found that the molecular weight of MUC1 in HT29 and SW620 cells was not consistent, which was consistent with other studies showing that the different degrees of extracellular glycosylation of MUC1 cause the molecular weight to range from 240 to 500 kDa (Nath and Mukherjee, 2014; Apostolopoulos et al., 2015). Subsequently, cellular uptake experiments showed that the coloaded liposomes achieved

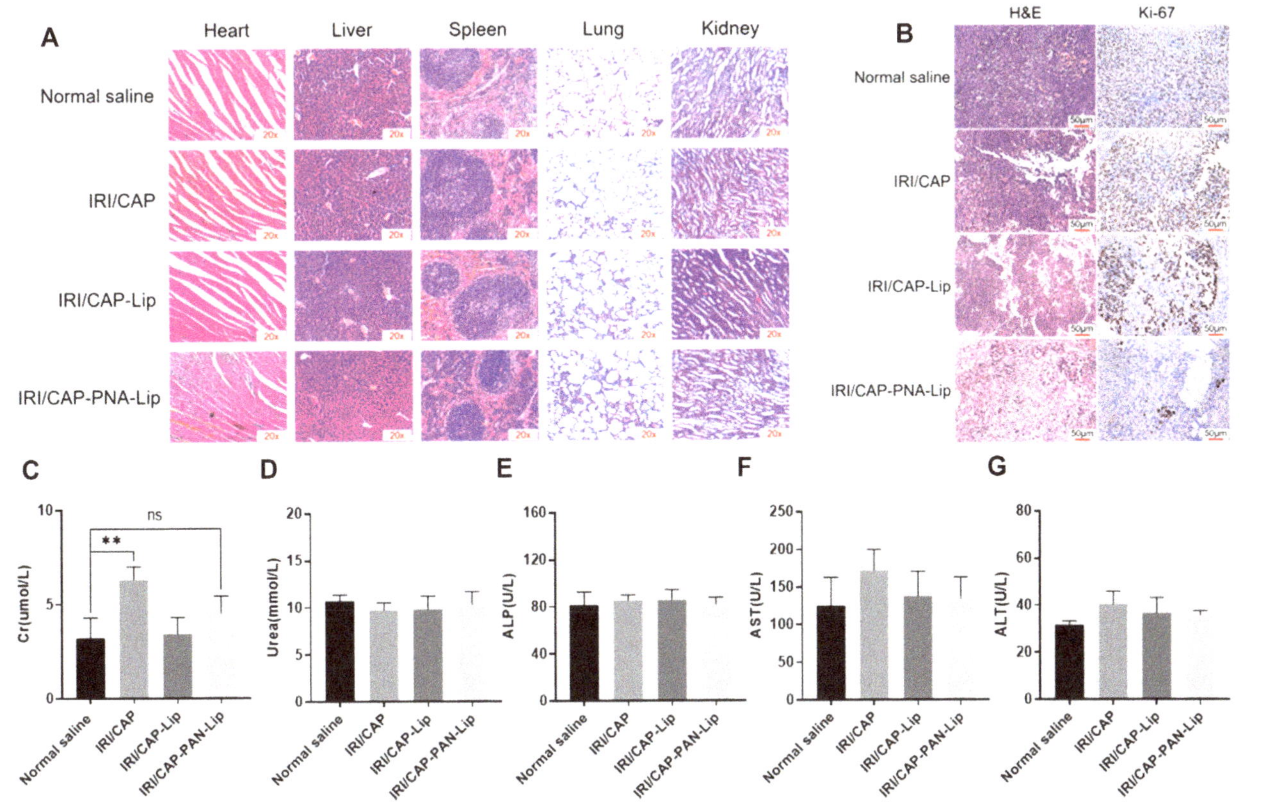

FIGURE 10 | PNA-modified liposomes had no systemic toxicity and enhanced the antiproliferative ability of drugs on MUC1-positive tumors. **(A)** H&E staining of vital organs. No significant pathological changes were observed in any group except for the tumor tissue. 20x **(B)** Ki-67 staining of tumors in different treatment groups. The plasma biochemical analysis of the tumor-bearing nude mice showed no significant difference compared with the saline group except for Cr. **(C)** Creatinine, Cr. **(D)** Urea. **(E)** Alkaline phosphatase, ALP. **(F)** Aspartate aminotransferase, AST. **(G)** Alanine aminotransferase, ALT. $^{**}p < 0.01$.

same-time and same-place drug delivery, which was beneficial in improving the synergistic drug efficacy (Zhang et al., 2017; Du et al., 2020). Meanwhile, the fluorescence signals of FITC/Rhb-PNA-Lips were significantly higher than those of the FITC/Rhb-Lip group due to the specific binding of PNA-modified liposomes to MUC1, which enhanced the cellular uptake of liposomes, and the *in vivo* targeting analyses were consistent with the results *in vitro* (Tang et al., 2020). When we further analyzed the ability of PNA-modified liposomes coloaded with IRICAP to inhibit cell viability *in vitro*, interestingly there was no significant difference in MUC1-positive cells in the IRI/CAP-PNA-Lip group compared to the IRI/CAP-Lip group, which has also been reported in other studies (Zhang et al., 2018). Based on the analysis of the cellular uptake results, we reduced the drug treatment time to 24 h after each group, and IRI/CAP-PNA-Lips showed significant cell viability inhibition compared to the control group. The IRI/CAP-PNA-Lip group showed excellent results in the antitumor assay *in vivo*, with a continuous decrease in tumor volume with a tendency to completely disappear. As a result, we had to euthanize the nude mice no longer than 20 days after treatment. Combined with our previous studies, we suggest that the potential antitumor mechanism of IRI/CAP-PNA-Lips is that colorectal cancer cells improve their uptake of liposomes through receptor-mediated endocytosis, promoting drug entry into the nucleus and inhibiting DNA replication and synthesis, which specifically blocks the S phase of the cell cycle, thereby inhibiting the proliferation of colorectal cancer cells (Li et al., 2020).

There are some limitations of IRI/CAP-PNA-Lips in this study. CAP can be classified as both a water-soluble and a fat-soluble drug, which leads to a lower encapsulation rate in the hydrophobic phase compared to other studies. In this study, we were unable to fully mimic the dose and dosing cycle of IRI in combination with CAP as in clinical treatment. The administration was through intraperitoneal injection for the *in vivo* experiments, and although other studies have shown that small molecules with particle size less than 300 nm can be absorbed through the intestine and IRI/CAP-PNA-Lips exert excellent antitumor effects, there is still a gap in comparison with the effectiveness of clinical intravenous drug administration (Eloy et al., 2016; Kopeckova et al., 2019).

In summary, well-characterized PNA-modified liposomes loaded with IRICAP (IRI/CAP-PNA-Lips) were successfully prepared to achieve synergistic drug delivery and enhanced the synergistic treatment effect in this study. The local drug concentrations and retention times in tumor tissues are increased through targeting ability that further enhances the antitumor effect of the drugs. Both *in vitro* and *in vivo* experiments are suggestive of the excellent antitumor effect of IRI/CAP-PNA-Lips. Therefore, this study is important for optimizing clinical combination treatment protocols, improving the antitumor effect of drugs, and reducing the drug delivery concentration required to achieve beneficial tumor treatment effects. PNA-modified liposomes could be a potential strategy for the treatment of colorectal cancer.

AUTHOR CONTRIBUTIONS

WD designed the research and participated in the experimental performance, data analysis, and drafting of the manuscript. BY participated in the experimental performance of HPLC. SS and AW participated in the assessment of cellular uptake and data analysis. RK, QG, and MS participated in the construction of the tumor-bearing nude mouse model. BL, TS, JW, and JB provided guidance on experimental techniques. MQ, YW, and WJ participated in the research design and revised the manuscript. ZG provided technical support and all of the reagents and chemicals. All authors have read and approved the final manuscript.

REFERENCES

Abraham, S. A., Waterhouse, D. N., Mayer, L. D., Cullis, P. R., Madden, T. D., and Bally, M. B. (2005). The Liposomal Formulation of Doxorubicin. *Methods Enzymol.* 391, 71–97. doi:10.1016/S0076-6879(05)91004-5

Allen, T. M., and Cullis, P. R. (2013). Liposomal Drug Delivery Systems: from Concept to Clinical Applications. *Adv. Drug Deliv. Rev.* 65 (1), 36–48. doi:10.1016/j.addr.2012.09.037

Apostolopoulos, V., Stojanovska, L., Gargosky, S. E., Muc, Á., and Muc, Á. (2015). MUC1 (CD227): a Multi-Tasked Molecule, *Cell. Mol. Life Sci.* 72, 4475, 4500. doi:10.1007/s00018-015-2014-z

Barenholz, Y. (2012). Doxil®--the First FDA-Approved Nano-Drug: Lessons Learned. *J. Control Release* 160 (2), 117–134. doi:10.1016/j.jconrel.2012.03.020

Beack, S., Cho, M., Kim, Y. E., Ahn, G. O., and Hahn, S. K. (2017). Hyaluronate-Peanut Agglutinin Conjugates for Target-specific Bioimaging of Colon Cancer. *Bioconjug Chem.* 28 (5), 1434–1442. doi:10.1021/acs.bioconjchem.7b00126

Caliskan, Y., Dalgic, A. D., Gerekci, S., Gulec, E. A., Tezcaner, A., Ozen, C., et al. (2019). A New Therapeutic Combination for Osteosarcoma: Gemcitabine and Clofazimine Co-loaded Liposomal Formulation. *Int. J. Pharm.* 557, 97–104. doi:10.1016/j.ijpharm.2018.12.041

Chau, I., and Cunningham, D. (2002). Chemotherapy in Colorectal Cancer: New Options and New Challenges. *Br. Med. Bull.* 64, 159–180. doi:10.1093/bmb/64.1.159

Chiorean, E. G., Nandakumar, G., Fadelu, T., Temin, S., Alarcon-Rozas, A. E., Bejarano, S., et al. (2020). Treatment of Patients with Late-Stage Colorectal Cancer: ASCO Resource-Stratified Guideline. *JCO Glob. Oncol.* 6, 414–438. doi:10.1200/JGO.19.00367

de Man, F. M., Goey, A. K. L., van Schaik, R. H. N., Mathijssen, R. H. J., and Bins, S. (2018). Individualization of Irinotecan Treatment: A Review of Pharmacokinetics, Pharmacodynamics, and Pharmacogenetics. *Clin. Pharmacokinet.* 57 (10), 1229–1254. doi:10.1007/s40262-018-0644-7

Du, C., Li, S., Li, Y., Galons, H., Guo, N., Teng, Y., et al. (2020). F7 and Topotecan Co-loaded Thermosensitive Liposome as a Nano-Drug Delivery System for Tumor Hyperthermia. *Drug Deliv.* 27 (1), 836–847. doi:10.1080/10717544.2020.1772409

Eloy, J. O., Petrilli, R., Topan, J. F., Antonio, H. M. R., Barcellos, J. P. A., Chesca, D. L., et al. (2016). Co-loaded Paclitaxel/rapamycin Liposomes: Development, Characterization and *In Vitro* and *In Vivo* Evaluation for Breast Cancer Therapy. *Colloids Surf. B Biointerfaces* 141, 74–82. doi:10.1016/j.colsurfb.2016.01.032

Engstrand, J., Nilsson, H., Strömberg, C., Jonas, E., and Freedman, J. (2018). Colorectal Cancer Liver Metastases - a Population-Based Study on Incidence, Management and Survival. *BMC Cancer* 18 (1), 78–11. doi:10.1186/s12885-017-3925-x

Feng, C., Zhang, H., Chen, J., Wang, S., Xin, Y., Qu, Y., et al. (2019). Ratiometric Co-encapsulation and Co-delivery of Doxorubicin and Paclitaxel by Tumor-Targeted Lipodisks for Combination Therapy of Breast Cancer. *Int. J. Pharm.* 560, 191–204. doi:10.1016/j.ijpharm.2019.02.009

Gao, B., Luo, J., Liu, Y., Su, S., Fu, S., Yang, X., et al. (2021). Intratumoral Administration of Thermosensitive Hydrogel Co-loaded with Norcantharidin Nanoparticles and Doxorubicin for the Treatment of Hepatocellular Carcinoma. *Int. J. Nanomedicine* 16, 4073–4085. doi:10.2147/IJN.S308057

Gao, T., Cen, Q., and Lei, H. (2020). A Review on Development of MUC1-Based Cancer Vaccine. *Biomed. Pharmacother.* 132, 110888. doi:10.1016/j.biopha.2020.110888

Ghosh, S., Lalani, R., Maiti, K., Banerjee, S., Bhatt, H., Bobde, Y. S., et al. (2021). Synergistic Co-loading of Vincristine Improved Chemotherapeutic Potential of Pegylated Liposomal Doxorubicin against Triple Negative Breast Cancer and Non-small Cell Lung Cancer. *Nanomedicine* 31, 102320. doi:10.1016/j.nano.2020.102320

Goldberg, R. M. (2005). Advances in the Treatment of Metastatic Colorectal Cancer. *Oncologist* 10 (S3), 40–48. doi:10.1634/theoncologist.10-90003-40

Guichard, S., Arnould, S., Hennebelle, I., Bugat, R., and Canal, P. (2001). Combination of Oxaliplatin and Irinotecan on Human Colon Cancer Cell Lines: Activity *In Vitro* and *In Vivo*. *Anticancer Drugs* 12 (9), 741–751. doi:10.1097/00001813-200110000-00006

Guo, W., Song, Y., Song, W., Liu, Y., Liu, Z., Zhang, D., et al. (2020). Co-delivery of Doxorubicin and Curcumin with Polypeptide Nanocarrier for Synergistic Lymphoma Therapy. *Sci. Rep.* 10 (1), 7832–7848. doi:10.1038/s41598-020-64828-1

Harashima, H., Tsuchihashi, M., Iida, S., Doi, H., and Kiwada, H. (1999). Pharmacokinetic/pharmacodynamic Modeling of Antitumor Agents Encapsulated into Liposomes. *Adv. Drug Deliv. Rev.* 40 (1–2), 39–61. doi:10.1016/s0169-409x(99)00039-3

Huang, M., Liang, C., Tan, C., Huang, S., Ying, R., Wang, Y., et al. (2019). Liposome Co-encapsulation as a Strategy for the Delivery of Curcumin and Resveratrol. *Food Funct.* 10 (10), 6447–6458. doi:10.1039/c9fo01338e

Jiang, H., Geng, D., Liu, H., Li, Z., and Cao, J. (2016). Co-delivery of Etoposide and Curcumin by Lipid Nanoparticulate Drug Delivery System for the Treatment of Gastric Tumors. *Drug Deliv.* 23 (9), 3665–3673. doi:10.1080/10717544.2016.1217954

Kalyane, D., Raval, N., Maheshwari, R., Tambe, V., Kalia, K., and Tekade, R. K. (20192018). Employment of Enhanced Permeability and Retention Effect (EPR): Nanoparticle-Based Precision Tools for Targeting of Therapeutic and Diagnostic Agent in Cancer. *Mater Sci. Eng. C Mater Biol. Appl.* 98, 1252–1276. doi:10.1016/j.msec.2019.01.066

Kerr, D. J. (2002). Capecitabine/irinotecan Combination Regimens in Colorectal Cancer. *Oncol. Willist. Park)* 16 (4), 27–29.

Khan, M. M., Madni, A., Tahir, N., Parveen, F., Khan, S., Jan, N., et al. (2020). Co-delivery of Curcumin and Cisplatin to Enhance Cytotoxicity of Cisplatin Using Lipid-Chitosan Hybrid Nanoparticles. *Int. J. Nanomedicine* 15, 2207–2217. doi:10.2147/IJN.S247893

Kopeckova, K., Eckschlager, T., Sirc, J., Hobzova, R., Plch, J., Hrabeta, J., et al. (2019). Nanodrugs Used in Cancer Therapy. *Biomed. Pap. Med. Fac. Univ. Palacky. Olomouc Czech Repub.* 163 (2), 122–131. doi:10.5507/bp.2019.010

Kumagai, H., Yamada, K., Nakai, K., Kitamura, T., Mohri, K., Ukawa, M., et al. (2019). Tumor Recognition of Peanut Agglutinin-Immobilized Fluorescent Nanospheres in Biopsied Human Tissues. *Eur. J. Pharm. Biopharm.* 136, 29–37. doi:10.1016/j.ejpb.2019.01.007

Lam, S. W., Guchelaar, H. J., and Boven, E. (2016). The Role of Pharmacogenetics in Capecitabine Efficacy and Toxicity. *Cancer Treat. Rev.* 50, 9–22. doi:10.1016/j.ctrv.2016.08.001

Li, C., Zuo, D., Liu, T., Yin, L., Li, C., and Wang, L. (2019). Prognostic and Clinicopathological Significance of MUC Family Members in Colorectal Cancer: A Systematic Review and Meta-Analysis. *Gastroenterology Res. Pract.* 2019, 1–16. doi:10.1155/2019/2391670

Li, R., Deng, L., Cai, Z., Zhang, S., Wang, K., Li, L., et al. (2017). Liposomes Coated with Thiolated Chitosan as Drug Carriers of Curcumin. *Mater Sci. Eng. C Mater Biol. Appl.* 80, 156–164. doi:10.1016/j.msec.2017.05.136

Li, X., Diao, W., Xue, H., Wu, F., Wang, W., Jiang, B., et al. (2020). Improved Efficacy of Doxorubicin Delivery by a Novel Dual-Ligand-Modified Liposome in Hepatocellular Carcinoma. *Cancer Lett.* 489, 163–173. doi:10.1016/j.canlet.2020.06.017

Li, Y., Hou, H., Zhang, P., and Zhang, Z. (2020). Co-delivery of Doxorubicin and Paclitaxel by reduction/pH Dual Responsive Nanocarriers for Osteosarcoma Therapy. *Drug Deliv.* 27 (1), 1044–1053. doi:10.1080/10717544.2020.1785049

Liu, K., Chen, W., Yang, T., Wen, B., Ding, D., Keidar, M., et al. (2017). Paclitaxel and Quercetin Nanoparticles Co-loaded in Microspheres to Prolong Retention Time for Pulmonary Drug Delivery. *Int. J. Nanomedicine* 12, 8239–8255. doi:10.2147/IJN.S147028

Meng, H., Wang, M., Liu, H., Liu, X., Situ, A., Wu, B., et al. (2015). Use of a Lipid-Coated Mesoporous Silica Nanoparticle Platform for Synergistic Gemcitabine and Paclitaxel Delivery to Human Pancreatic Cancer in Mice. *ACS Nano* 9 (4), 3540–3557. doi:10.1021/acsnano.5b00510

Mitragotri, S., Anderson, D. G., Chen, X., Chow, E. K., Ho, D., Kabanov, A. V., et al. (2015). Accelerating the Translation of Nanomaterials in Biomedicine. *ACS Nano* 9 (7), 6644–6654. doi:10.1021/acsnano.5b03569

Nabavinia, M. S., Gholoobi, A., Charbgoo, F., Nabavinia, M., Ramezani, M., and Abnous, K. (2017). Anti-MUC1 Aptamer: A Potential Opportunity for Cancer Treatment. *Med. Res. Rev.* 37 (6), 1518–1539. doi:10.1002/med.21462

Nath, S., and Mukherjee, P. (2014). MUC1: A Multifaceted Oncoprotein with a Key Role in Cancer Progression. *Trends Mol. Med.* 20 (6), 332–342. doi:10.1016/j.molmed.2014.02.007

Park, J., Choi, Y., Chang, H., Um, W., Ryu, J. H., and Kwon, I. C. (2019). Alliance with EPR Effect: Combined Strategies to Improve the EPR Effect in the Tumor Microenvironment. *Theranostics* 9 (26), 8073–8090. doi:10.7150/thno.37198

Paulík, A., Nekvindová, J., and Filip, S. (2020). Irinotecan Toxicity during Treatment of Metastatic Colorectal Cancer: Focus on Pharmacogenomics and Personalized Medicine. *Tumori* 106 (2), 87–94.

Peng, Y., Su, Z., Wang, X., Wu, T., Xiao, H., Shuai, X., et al. (2021). Near-Infrared Light Laser-Triggered Release of Doxorubicin and Sorafenib from TemperatureSensitive Liposomes for Synergistic Therapy of Hepatocellular Carcinoma. *J. Biomed. Nanotechnol.* 16 (9), 1381–1393.

Sarisozen, C., Vural, I., Levchenko, T., Hincal, A. A., and Torchilin, V. P. (2012). Long-circulating PEG-PE Micelles Co-loaded with Paclitaxel and Elacridar (GG918) Overcome Multidrug Resistance. *Drug Deliv.* 19 (8), 363–370. doi:10.3109/10717544.2012.724473

Song, W., Tang, Z., Zhang, D., Zhang, Y., Yu, H., Li, M., et al. (2014). Anti-tumor Efficacy of c(RGDfK)-Decorated Polypeptide-Based Micelles Co-loaded with Docetaxel and Cisplatin. *Biomaterials* 35 (9), 3005–3014. doi:10.1016/j.biomaterials.2013.12.018

Sung, H., Ferlay, J., Siegel, R. L., Laversanne, M., Soerjomataram, I., Jemal, A., et al. (2021). Global Cancer Statistics 2020: GLOBOCAN Estimates of Incidence and Mortality Worldwide for 36 Cancers in 185 Countries. *CA A Cancer J. Clin.* 71 (3), 209–249. doi:10.3322/caac.21660

Tan, X., Fang, Y., Ren, Y., Li, Y., Wu, P., Yang, X., et al. (2019). D-α-tocopherol Polyethylene Glycol 1000 Succinate-Modified Liposomes with an siRNA Corona Confer Enhanced Cellular Uptake and Targeted Delivery of Doxorubicin via Tumor Priming. *Int. J. Nanomedicine* 14, 1255–1268. doi:10.2147/IJN.S191858

Tang, H., Chen, J., Wang, L., Li, Q., Yang, Y., Lv, Z., et al. (2020). Co-delivery of Epirubicin and Paclitaxel Using an Estrone-Targeted PEGylated Liposomal Nanoparticle for Breast Cancer. *Int. J. Pharm.* 573, 118806. doi:10.1016/j.ijpharm.2019.118806

Thapa, R. K., Byeon, J. H., Choi, H. G., Yong, C. S., and Kim, J. O. (2017). PEGylated Lipid Bilayer-Wrapped Nano-Graphene Oxides for Synergistic Co-delivery of Doxorubicin and Rapamycin to Prevent Drug Resistance in Cancers. *Nanotechnology* 28 (29), 295101. doi:10.1088/1361-6528/aa7997

Walko, C. M., and Lindley, C. (2005). Capecitabine: A Review. *Clin. Ther.* 27 (1), 23–44. doi:10.1016/j.clinthera.2005.01.005

Wang, B., Yu, X. C., Xu, S. F., and Xu, M. (2015). Paclitaxel and Etoposide Co-loaded Polymeric Nanoparticles for the Effective Combination Therapy against Human Osteosarcoma. *J. Nanobiotechnology* 13 (1), 22–11. doi:10.1186/s12951-015-0086-4

Wang, Y., Qian, J., Yang, M., Xu, W., Wang, J., Hou, G., et al. (2019). Doxorubicin/cisplatin Co-loaded Hyaluronic Acid/chitosan-Based Nanoparticles for *In Vitro* Synergistic Combination Chemotherapy of Breast Cancer. *Carbohydr. Polym.* 225, 115206. doi:10.1016/j.carbpol.2019.115206

Xiong, Q., Cui, M., Bai, Y., Liu, Y., Liu, D., and Song, T. (2017). A Supramolecular Nanoparticle System Based on β-cyclodextrin-conjugated Poly-L-Lysine and Hyaluronic Acid for Co-delivery of Gene and Chemotherapy Agent Targeting Hepatocellular Carcinoma. *Colloids Surf. B Biointerfaces* 155, 93–103. doi:10.1016/j.colsurfb.2017.04.008

Xu, C., Wang, Y., Guo, Z., Chen, J., Lin, L., Wu, J., et al. (2019). Pulmonary Delivery by Exploiting Doxorubicin and Cisplatin Co-loaded Nanoparticles for Metastatic Lung Cancer Therapy. *J. Control Release* 295, 153–163. doi:10.1016/j.jconrel.2018.12.013

Xu, J., Fan, J., Qin, X., Cai, J., Gu, J., Wang, S., et al. (2019). Chinese Guidelines for the Diagnosis and Comprehensive Treatment of Colorectal Liver Metastases (Version 2018). *J. Cancer Res. Clin. Oncol.* 145 (3), 725–736. doi:10.1007/s00432-018-2795-1

Yalcin, T. E., Ilbasmis-Tamer, S., Ibisoglu, B., Özdemir, A., Ark, M., and Takka, S. (2018). Gemcitabine Hydrochloride-Loaded Liposomes and Nanoparticles: Comparison of Encapsulation Efficiency, Drug Release, Particle Size, and Cytotoxicity. *Pharm. Dev. Technol.* 23 (1), 76–86. doi:10.1080/10837450.2017.1357733

Yang, Z., Liu, J., Gao, J., Chen, S., and Huang, G. (2015). Chitosan Coated Vancomycin Hydrochloride Liposomes: Characterizations and Evaluation. *Int. J. Pharm.* 495 (1), 508–515. doi:10.1016/j.ijpharm.2015.08.085

Yu, T., Huang, X., Liu, J., Fu, Q., Wang, B., and Qian, Z. (2019). Polymeric Nanoparticles Encapsulating α-mangostin Inhibit the Growth and Metastasis in Colorectal Cancer. *Appl. Mater. Today* 16, 351–366. doi:10.1016/j.apmt.2019.06.014

Zhang, B., Song, Y., Wang, T., Yang, S., Zhang, J., Liu, Y., et al. (2017). Efficient Co-delivery of Immiscible Hydrophilic/hydrophobic Chemotherapeutics by Lipid Emulsions for Improved Treatment of Cancer. *Int. J. Nanomedicine* 12, 2871–2886. doi:10.2147/IJN.S129091

Zhang, Z., Qian, H., Huang, J., Sha, H., Zhang, H., Yu, L., et al. (2018). Anti-EGFR-iRGD Recombinant Protein Modified Biomimetic Nanoparticles Loaded with Gambogic Acid to Enhance Targeting and Antitumor Ability in Colorectal Cancer Treatment. *Int. J. Nanomedicine* 13, 4961–4975. doi:10.2147/IJN.S170148

Zhang, Z., and Yao, J. (2012). Preparation of Irinotecan-Loaded Folate-Targeted Liposome for Tumor Targeting Delivery and its Antitumor Activity. *AAPS PharmSciTech* 13 (3), 802–810. doi:10.1208/s12249-012-9776-5

16

Targeting TMEM88 as an Attractive Therapeutic Strategy in Malignant Tumors

Ming Cai[1,2†], Wei-Jian Ni[3,4†], Ying-Hong Wang[5], Jing-Ji Wang[2] and Hong Zhou[5*]*

[1] Department of Pharmacy, The Second Affiliated Hospital of Anhui University of Chinese Medicine, Hefei, China, [2] Anhui Acupuncture and Moxibustion Clinical Medicine Research Center, The Second Affiliated Hospital of Anhui University of Chinese Medicine, Hefei, China, [3] Inflammation and Immune Mediated Diseases Laboratory of Anhui Province, The Key Laboratory of Anti-inflammatory of Immune Medicines, Ministry of Education, Anhui Institute of Innovative Drugs, School of Pharmacy, Anhui Medical University, Hefei, China, [4] Anhui Provincial Hospital, The First Affiliated Hospital of USTC, Division of Life Sciences and Medicine, University of Science and Technology of China, Hefei, China, [5] Department of Pharmacy, Anhui Provincial Cancer Hospital, The First Affiliated Hospital of USTC, Division of Life Sciences and Medicine, University of Science and Technology of China, Hefei, China

***Correspondence:**
Wei-Jian Ni
niweijian@ustc.edu.cn
Hong Zhou
zhouhong@ahmu.edu.cn

†These authors have contributed equally to this work and share first authorship

According to authoritative surveys, the overall morbidity and mortality of malignant tumors show an upward trend, and it is predicted that this trend will not be well contained in the upcoming new period. Since the influencing factors, pathogenesis, and progression characteristics of malignant tumors have not been fully elucidated, the existing treatment strategies, mainly including surgical resection, ablation therapy and chemotherapy, cannot achieve satisfactory results. Therefore, exploring potential therapeutic targets and clarifying their functions and mechanisms in continuous research and practice will provide new ideas and possibilities for the treatment of malignant tumors. Recently, a double-transmembrane protein named transmembrane protein 88 (TMEM88) was reported to regulate changes in downstream effectors by mediating different signaling pathways and was confirmed to be widely involved in cell proliferation, differentiation, apoptosis and tumor progression. At present, abnormal changes in TMEM88 have been found in breast cancer, ovarian cancer, lung cancer, thyroid cancer and other malignant tumors, which has also attracted the attention of tumor research and attempted to clarify its function and mechanism. However, due to the lack of systematic generalization, comprehensive and detailed research results have not been comprehensively summarized. In view of this, this article will describe in detail the changes in TMEM88 in the occurrence and development of malignant tumors, comprehensively summarize the corresponding molecular mechanisms, and explore the potential of targeting TMEM88 in the treatment of malignant tumors to provide valuable candidate targets and promising intervention strategies for the diagnosis and cure of malignant tumors.

Keywords: malignant tumor, transmembrane protein 88 (Tmem88), Wnt/β-catenin, target, therapeutic strategy

INTRODUCTION

In recent years, membrane proteins have been studied and have become a research hotspot because they are widely distributed in tissues and play important and complex roles in various physiological processes and multiple diseases. Authoritative studies have shown that membrane proteins are distributed in the membranes of various cells and organelles, accounting for approximately 25% of the human proteome (1, 2), and exert undeniable effects on signal transduction in the cell-external environment and cell-cell interactions (3). Several studies have pointed out that membrane proteins can be classified into peripheral membrane proteins, lipid-anchored membrane proteins and integral membrane proteins according to their own structure and how they bind to biological membranes. The integral membrane protein contains at least one transmembrane fragment, which is also a transmembrane protein. These transmembrane proteins are not only involved in the body's metabolism and functional regulation (4–7) but also perform considerable regulatory roles in the tumorigenesis and progression of several tumors (8–11). For example, ATG9A, the only transmembrane protein currently in the core machinery of autophagy, can affect pathophysiological events such as cell growth, proliferation, stress and injury by regulating autophagy (12). In addition, endoplasmic reticulum-associated transmembrane protein 166 (TMEM166) was found not only in a variety of normal tissues and organs but also involved in multiple pathological processes, including cancer, infection, neurodegeneration, autoimmune disease, and sexually transmitted diseases, by regulating programmed cell death (13). Moreover, a transmembrane protein called the tyrosine kinase receptor may be abnormally activated to affect tumor cell growth, metastasis, invasion and malignant transformation by regulating multiple subprotein families and downstream signaling pathways (14). The aforementioned findings have made the transmembrane protein family a research focus that has received extensive attention. As an indispensable transmembrane protein family member, transmembrane protein 88 (TMEM88) has also been found to affect the growth and development of the body in normally expressed tissues, such as the development of cardiomyocytes and the activation of hematopoietic stem cells, while abnormal expression can affect the progression of various diseases, such as the inflammatory response, extracellular matrix secretion and drug resistance (15–21) (**Figure 1**). As an important tumor suppressor gene, TMEM88 benefits from the regulation of the Wnt signaling pathway and its downstream target genes and is widely involved in various biological events of malignant tumor cells, which has potential research value (22, 23). However, the current research on TMEM88 is still in its infancy, and there is no complete summary to help researchers fully understand the important role of TMEM88 in tumor research and prevention. In these circumstances, exploring TMEM88 as a new biomarker for tumor diagnosis and confirming that TMEM88 has become a promising target will be the research and prevention of tumors. In view of this, this review comprehensively describes the structure and function of TMEM88 and discusses its progress in the study of malignant tumors to provide important references and directions for subsequent research.

GENERAL STRUCTURE AND BIOLOGICAL FUNCTION OF TMEM88

The TMEM88 gene is a plus strand gene consisting of 1214 bases located at the p13.1 position on chromosome 17, and the corresponding TMEM88 protein is a 159 amino acid residue with a molecular weight of 17251 Da. An initial study found that the TMEM88 molecule is expressed on the Xenopus embryonic cell membrane (24). Meanwhile, the study also found that when the expression of TMEM88 was significantly upregulated in human embryonic kidney cells, the downstream Wnt/β-catenin signal transduction process was inhibited, while silencing TMEM88 could activate the Wnt/β-catenin signal transduction process. Another study found that TMEM88 can inhibit Wnt/β-catenin signal activation in human embryonic stem cells to a certain extent, thereby regulating the differentiation and development of embryonic stem cells into cardiomyocytes (21). With the progress of research, it was found that the TMEM88 protein is widely present in a variety of tumors, but its functions are different due to the different tissue and subcellular locations (**Table 1**). One study found that cytoplasmic localization of TMEM88 was positively correlated with TNM stage and lymph node metastasis in triple-negative breast cancer, whereas nuclear localization was negatively correlated with lymph node metastasis in nontriple-negative breast cancer (30); in ovarian cancer, TMEM88 was found to downregulate the levels of c-Myc and Cyclin D1, thereby inhibiting the proliferation of ovarian cancer cells (19). In non-small-cell lung cancer (NSCLC), the high expression of TMEM88 is positively correlated with a better prognosis of patients, but the detailed mechanism needs to be further clarified (28).

ROLE AND MECHANISM OF TMEM88 IN MALIGNANT TUMORS

In recent years, an increasing number of research results have shown that abnormal expression of TMEM88 exists in several malignant tumors (ovarian cancer, breast cancer, lung cancer, etc.) and has actively participated in the abnormality of tumor cell proliferation, invasion, metastasis and apoptosis. Meanwhile, with the development of structural biology, biochemistry and other disciplines, breakthroughs and progress have been made in the isolation and characterization of transmembrane proteins, which indicates that it may become a promising molecular marker and valuable intervention target for tumor diagnosis, therapy and prognosis (**Figure 2**).

TMEM88 in Ovarian Cancer

Ovarian cancer has become a malignant tumor in the female germline that seriously threatens women's health, with its third incidence rate (after cervical cancer and endometrial cancer) and

TABLE 1 | The landscape of the roles of TMEM88 in various human tissues.

Tissue localization	Disease types	Associated tissues or cells	Alterations	Target	Function	References
Human embryo	cell development	Human embryonic stem cells	Upregulation	DVL	Regulate cardiomyocyte specification	Lee, Heejin et al. (22) Lee, Ho-Jin et al. (24) Palpant, Nathan J et al. (21)
Ovarian	ovarian cancer	CP70 and PEO4 A2780 and PEO1	Upregulation Downregulation	JUN, PTIX2, β-catenin, c-Myc and cyclin-D1	Regulate platinum resistance	de Leon, Maria et al. (19)
Thyroid	thyroid cancer	BCPAP, TPC1, K1 and NPA87	Downregulation	TCF/LEF, c-Myc and cyclin D1	Suppress tumor process	Geng, Qianqian et al. (25)
Lung	Lung cancer	A549, H1299, H460, H292, SPC-A-1 and LTEP-A-2	Downregulation	DVL, FZD and ROR1	Suppress tumor process	Zhang, Xiupeng et al. (26) Stewart, David J. (27) Ma, Rongna etal. (28)
Skin	keloids	Keloid fibroblasts	Downregulation	β-catenin, c-Myc and cyclin D1	Inhibit extracellular matrix expression	Zhao, Huafei et al. (16)
Bladder	bladder cancer	5637, UM-UC-3, T24 and SW780	Downregulation	GSK-3β, β-catenin and TCF/LEF	Suppress tumor process	Zhao, Xu et al. (29)
Breast	triple-negative breast cancer	MCF-7, HER18, MDA-MB-231 and MDA-MB-468	Upregulation	DVL, Snail, Occludin and Zo-1	Promote tumor process	Yu, Xinmiao et al. (30)
Liver	liver fibrosis	LX-2 and human liver fibrotic tissues	Downregulation	β-catenin, Wnt3a, Wnt2b, Wnt10b, p-JNK and p-P38	Regulate proinflammatory cytokine secretion and inhibit HSC excitation	Xu, Tao et al. (17) Xu, Tao et al. (31)

c-Myc, c-Myc proto-oncogene; DVL, PDZ domain of Dishevelled-1; FZD, Wnt receptor Frizzled; GSK-3β, glycogen synthase kinase-3β; HSC, hepatic stellate cell; JNK, c-Jun N-terminal kinase; JUN, jun proto-oncogene; >PITX2, paired-like homeodomain 2; ROR1, receptor tyrosine kinase-like orphan receptor 1; TCF/LEF, T-cell factor/lymphoid enhancer-binding factor; TMEM88, transmembrane protein 88.

the highest mortality rate. On the one hand, due to the lack of typical clinical manifestations in the early stage, a large proportion of patients are already in the middle and late stages when they are diagnosed, and even the tumor cells have metastasized far away. On the other hand, platinum-based chemotherapy is the main means to maintain the survival of such patients, but many patients suffer from drug resistance, tumor recurrence and metastasis after chemotherapy (32). Based on this, exploring the pathogenesis and drug resistance mechanism of ovarian cancer and finding effective targets are of great significance for improving treatment and improving the 5-year survival rate of ovarian cancer patients. Maria de Leon et al. used an Illumina 450k DNA methylation array to detect methylated genes and levels in ovarian cancer xenografts and found that compared with platinum-sensitive transplanted tumors, the promoter region of the TMEM88 gene in platinum-resistant transplanted tumors in nude mice was significantly hypomethylated, while TMEM88 mRNA showed a substantial increase (19). Meanwhile, the application of the DNA methyltransferase inhibitor SGI-110 can significantly increase the TMEM88 mRNA level and corresponding protein expression in platinum-sensitive ovarian cancer cells. Both *in vitro, in vivo* and clinical studies have shown that the level of TMEM88 is significantly increased in platinum-resistant ovarian cancer xenograft nude mice, platinum-resistant ovarian cancer cells and recurrent ovarian cancer tissue, while knockdown or decrease the expression of TMEM88 can resensitize tumor cells to platinum drugs. Mechanistic studies found that silencing TMEM88 alleviated the inhibition of canonical Wnt/β-catenin signaling by reducing the interaction of the C-terminal VWV (Val-Trp-Val) sequence with the PDZ domain of Dishevelled-1 (Dvl-1) (19, 23). The activation of Wnt/β-catenin signaling increased the expression of the downstream target genes c-Myc and β-catenin to increase ovarian cancer cell proliferation and the proportion of S-phase cells throughout the cell cycle and reincreased platinum sensitivity. Meanwhile, the aforementioned studies also found that TMEM88 overexpression induced cell dormancy to help it evade the lethal effects of chemotherapy and trigger recurrent tumors. These studies suggest that TMEM88 may have an important regulatory role in the process of ovarian cancer resistance and may also be used to identify epigenetic modifiers associated with platinum resistance, which may provide new clues and insights for predicting ovarian cancer recurrence and overall cancer patient survival.

TMEM88 in Breast Cancer

Authoritative research estimates that breast cancer has become the most prevalent cancer type among female cancer patients in the United States, and death also ranks second among female cancer-related death types, with a true proportion of 15% in 2022

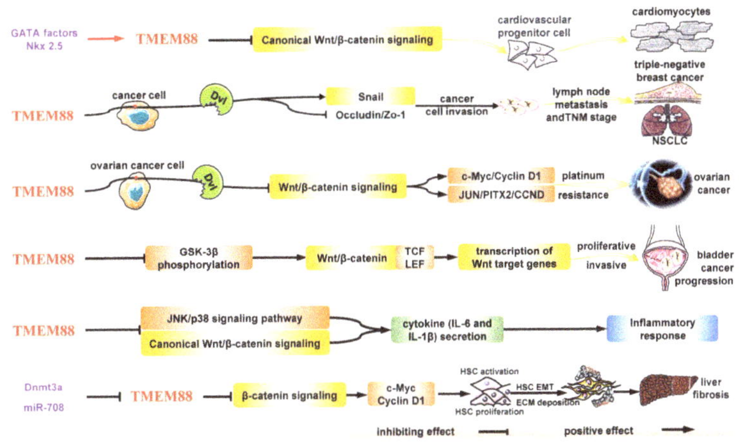

FIGURE 1 | The structure and general biological functions of TMEM88 in humans. As a secondary transmembrane protein, TMEM88 is widely distributed in many types of cells and tissues and plays an important regulatory role in various diseases and pathological processes, such as cancers, fibrosis, and inflammatory responses. Under stimulation, including DNA methylation, noncoding RNA and the inflammatory environment, the mRNA and protein levels of TMEM88 changed significantly. Subsequently, the significantly changed TMEM88 regulates the classical and noncanonical Wnt/β-catenin signaling pathways through different mechanisms in the cytoplasm and nucleus, such as the interaction with DVL proteins, thereby affecting the transcription and expression of downstream target genes. Ultimately, these effector target molecules affect the growth and development of tissues and organs and the progression of diseases, such as tumors by regulating various cellular life activities, such as cell proliferation, migration, invasion, and drug resistance. CCND, Cyclin D1; c-Myc, c-Myc proto-oncogene; Dnmt3a, DNA (cytosine-5)-methyltransferase 3a; DVL, PDZ domain of Dishevelled-1; ECM, extracellular matrix; EMT, epithelial-mesenchymal transition; GATA, GATA transcription factor; GSK-3β, glycogen synthase kinase-3β; HSC, hepatic stellate cell; JNK, c-Jun N-terminal kinase; JUN, jun proto-oncogene; NSCLC, non-small-cell lung cancer; PITX2, paired-like homeodomain 2; TCF/LEF, T-cell factor/lymphoid enhancer-binding factor; TMEM88, transmembrane protein 88; TNM, tumor node metastasis.

(33). According to the latest data released by the National Cancer Center, the incidence of breast cancer in China is 7.11%, and the mortality rate is 2.81%, ranking fifth and seventh, respectively (34). Based on the above statistical results, breast cancer is a serious public health issue in current society and needs to be given great attention. Although great progress has been made in clinical treatment strategies, including surgery, chemotherapy, radiotherapy and hormone therapy, the long-term clinical

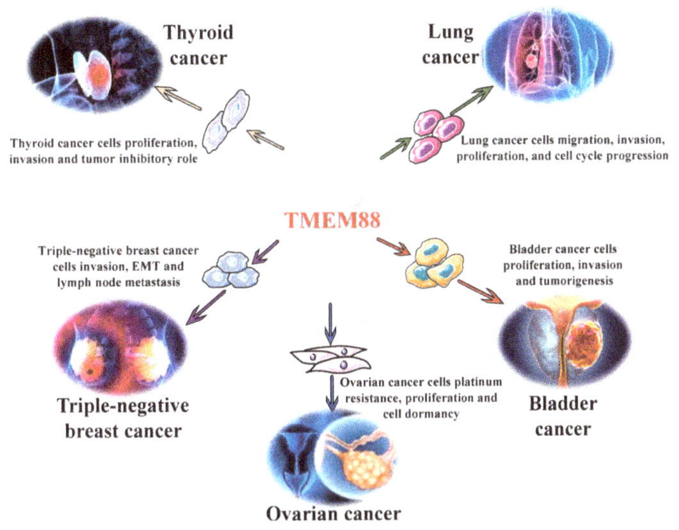

FIGURE 2 | Regulatory effects of TMEM88 in malignant tumors. Different tumor microenvironments, such as inflammation and oxidative stress, can cause significant changes in the levels of TMEM88 in tissues and cells, which will affect tumor cell properties, including abnormal cell proliferation, invasion, migration, and epithelial-mesenchymal transition (EMT), through canonical and noncanonical Wnt/β-catenin signaling and other signal transduction pathways. These tumor cell properties lead to the occurrence, growth, invasion, and metastasis of various tumors, including ovarian cancer, thyroid cancer, triple-negative breast cancer, bladder cancer, and lung cancer, and ultimately affect tumor progression and poor prognosis.

prognosis and the survival rate of patients are still not satisfactory (35, 36). Therefore, it has become an urgent problem to be solved in breast cancer research to explore new therapeutic targets and develop effective intervention strategies. During the process of exploring new targets for breast cancer, Yu et al. conducted a study that first performed a correlation analysis between 139 breast cancer tissues and normal breast tissues. The results showed that the overall expression level of TMEM88 in breast cancer tissues (71.22%, 99/139) was significantly higher than that in normal tissue (11.4%, 4/35; $P < 0.001$), and the specific expression differences were not the same. Specifically, expression and localization analysis revealed that TMEM88 was moderately elevated in breast cancer *in situ* and highly elevated in invasive breast ductal carcinoma compared with negative or low expression in normal breast tissue, which suggests that the expression of TMEM88 has potential as a marker for breast cancer classification. In addition, the study also found that the cytoplasmic localization of TMEM88 was positively correlated with advanced TNM stage ($P = 0.038$) and lymph node metastasis ($P = 0.01$), while nuclear localization was inversely related to lymph node metastasis ($P = 0.046$). These results indicate that TMEM88 plays different functions depending on different subcellular localizations in the development of breast cancer (cytoplasmic TMEM88 promotes tumors, while nuclear TMEM88 suppresses tumors), suggesting that TMEM88 has important research value and needs to be considered (30). When using breast cancer cells (MDA-MB-231 and MCF-7) as the object to explore the mechanism, Yu et al. also found that TMEM88 and Dvl colocalized in the cytoplasm and TMEM88 can interact with Dvl to promote the expression of Snail protein and inhibit the expression of Zo-1 and Occludin, thereby reducing the invasion and metastasis of breast cancer cells. The above results show that the expression level of TMEM88 has certain differences in different types of breast cancer, and the cytoplasmic level and nuclear expression of TMEM88 have obvious tissue distribution specificity, which may facilitate TMEM88 becoming a promising therapeutic target for the treatment of breast cancer; however, the specific mechanism and intervention potential need further research to clarify.

TMEM88 in Lung Cancer

Lung cancer has become the malignant tumor with the greatest threat to human health and life worldwide due to its higher incidence and mortality than other malignant tumors, accounting for 11.6% of cancer patients and 18.4% of total cancer deaths (37, 38). Among all lung cancer patients, NSCLC accounts for approximately 80%-85% of the total population. Although surgical resection is an effective treatment for early-stage lung cancer, the 5-year survival rate is still unsatisfactory (approximately 30-60%) (39, 40). What is even more regrettable is that most patients are already in the middle stage when they are diagnosed, most are even in the advanced stage, and they have lost the opportunity for surgical treatment, which accounts for one of the main reasons for the poor prognosis and high mortality of lung cancer patients (41). Therefore, exploring new targets and researching new treatment methods are urgently needed and will also provide a large number of theoretical and research foundations for the development of clinical treatments for lung cancer. In a study of 214 cases of NSCLC, Zhang et al. found that the expression of TMEM88 in the adjacent tissue was negative or weakly positive compared with the tissue of NSCLC patients by immunohistochemical analysis. The correlation analysis results of clinicopathological characteristics showed that high expression of TMEM88 in the cytoplasm was directly correlated with the tissue differentiation, lymph node metastasis and tumor stage of NSCLC patients ($P < 0.001$, $P = 0.032$ and $P = 0.012$), but there was no obvious correlation with sex, age, or histological type ($P = 1$, $P = 0.884$ and $P = 1$). Kaplan-Meier survival analysis showed that the overall survival of lung cancer patients (38.8 ± 4.83 months) with high TMEM88 expression was significantly lower than that of patients (58.64 ± 4.24 months) with low TMEM88 expression (26). This study preliminarily demonstrated the potential role and promising research value of TMEM88 in the development and exploration of NSCLC, but the specific pathogenesis needs to be further clarified. Subsequently, Zhang et al. used Western blotting to analyze the changes in TMEM88 in 40 fresh NSCLC specimens and found that TMEM88 expression was higher than that in normal lung tissue, which is also consistent with previous findings. Immunofluorescence staining of 7 types of lung cancer cells (A549, LTE, SPC, H292, H1299, BE1 and LH7 cells) found that the content of TMEM88 was significantly higher than that in human bronchial epithelial cells (HBE), while TMEM88 was found in the other two lung cancer cell types (LK2 and H460 cells) and was interestingly lower than that in HBE cells, and TMEM88 was predominantly located on the cell membrane in all types of lung cancer cells studied. Taking LK2 cells as the research object to study the effect of TMEM88, it was found that overexpression of TMEM88 can inhibit the excessive proliferation, invasion and migration of LK2 cells, thus preventing the growth of transplanted tumors in nude mice (26). Another study analyzed the NSCLC tissues and adjacent normal tissues of 12 patients and found that the degree of TMEM88 methylation in NSCLC tissues (82.2% ± 10.3%) was higher than that in normal tissues (65.9% ± 7.2%, $P < 0.01$), which was negatively correlated with overall survival ($P = 0.021$) (28). Subsequently, researchers used 5-aza-2'-deoxycytidine (DAC) to treat A549 and H1299 cells to further evaluate the functional alterations of TMEM88 methylation in lung cancer. The experimental results show that the degree of methylation of TMEM88 decreases while the expression level of TMEM88 increases after treatment with DAC. Scratch experiments, migration experiments and cell cycle experiments have found that TMEM88 can potently inhibit abnormal lung cancer cell proliferation, invasion and migration (26, 28), indicating that TMEM88 can exert a tumor suppressor effect and can be considered a candidate therapeutic target for the prognosis and cure of lung cancer, opening up a new avenue for the prevention of lung cancer.

TMEM88 in Thyroid Cancer

Thyroid cancer (TC) has become one of the most common malignancies of the endocrine system over the past few decades, with a steady increase in global morbidity and mortality and a strong female predominance, which is well validated by the finding that the incidence in women in most populations is approximately three times that in men (42). Since 2003, the incidence of thyroid cancer in China has suddenly started to rise rapidly and has maintained an annual percentage change of approximately 14.51 from 2003 to 2007, while urban women have witnessed a faster rate of change, and by 2012, thyroid cancer had become one of the ten most common cancers (43–45). Meanwhile, one study also predicts that thyroid cancer may become the fourth most common malignant tumor in the world by 2030 (46). From a pathological point of view, thyroid cancer is mainly divided into papillary carcinoma, follicular carcinoma, anaplastic carcinoma and medullary carcinoma, among which papillary carcinoma is the most common (47). Most papillary thyroid carcinomas have a good prognosis, but local recurrence or distant metastasis after treatment is also common, and some patients die due to disease progression. Many studies have shown that various factors, such as radiation exposure, environmental and industrial pollution, and family inheritance, may promote the occurrence and development of thyroid cancer, but its pathogenesis is still unclear (43, 48). Therefore, exploring the pathogenesis of thyroid cancer and finding potential targets will provide an important basis for the preclinical study and clinical treatment of thyroid cancer. In one study, the researchers found that TMEM88 was significantly reduced in thyroid cancer by analyzing the gene expression profile interactive analysis database (25). In addition, Geng et al. also showed that the expression levels of TMEM88 were significantly decreased in 8 thyroid cancer patient specimens as well as in 4 thyroid cancer cell lines, BCPAP, TPC1, K1 and NPA87. Various experimental methods, such as Western blotting, qRT-PCR, cell counting kit-8 assay and colony formation experiments, found that restoration of TMEM88 by vector transfection can markedly suppress the proliferation, colony formation and invasion ability of thyroid cancer cells. In contrast, depletion of TMEM88 can accelerate the proliferation and invasion ability of thyroid cancer cells. The results of tumor formation experiments in nude mice also suggested that TMEM88 overexpression can significantly inhibit the growth of thyroid cancer, which is associated with the downregulation of active β-catenin expression. The above results show that TMEM88 exerts a nonnegligible role in the occurrence and development of thyroid cancer, and in-depth research on the mechanism of TMEM88 will offer new targets and ideas for the research and prevention of thyroid cancer.

TMEM88 in Bladder Cancer

An authoritative analysis found that bladder cancer, the fifth most common cancer in Western countries, has an increasing incidence with age and is found in the highest proportion in individuals over the age of 65 (49). In China, the incidence of bladder cancer ranks second among male genitourinary malignancies and 7th among all malignant tumors (50). Clinical studies have shown that bladder cancer is a highly malignant tumor that is prone to recurrence and progresses rapidly, especially muscle-invasive BC (MIBC), which often recurs after the first resection and has a poor prognosis (51, 52). Therefore, it is particularly urgent to explore the possible pathogenesis and potential therapeutic targets of bladder cancer. In one study, research found that TMEM88 is closely relevant to the pathogenesis and development of bladder cancer, and inhibition of the TMEM88/Wnt axis can significantly affect abnormal bladder cancer cell proliferation and the regulation of the cell cycle (29), which suggests that targeting TMEM88 for bladder cancer research will be a new strategy and direction. Moreover, the study conducted bioinformatic analysis of the GEPIA2 and ENCORI databases and found that the expression of TMEM88 in bladder cancer tissues was significantly reduced compared to that in normal tissues. In the detection of 6 bladder cancer patient tissues, it was found that the expression of TMEM88 in patient tissues indeed showed a downward trend compared with adjacent normal tissues. *In vitro*, depletion of TMEM88 in bladder cancer cells, such as UM-UC-3 and T24 cells, can enhance their invasive and proliferative capacity, while restoring TMEM88 levels can reverse these effects. In *in vivo* experiments in nude mice, overexpression of TMEM88 exhibited a certain inhibitory action on bladder cancer cell growth and tumor formation (53). The above results show that TMEM88 is most likely to become the specific target and that targeting TMEM88 may effectively treat bladder cancer.

Possible Mechanism of TMEM88 in Malignant Tumors

The relatively conserved Wnt signaling pathway is one of the major factors regulating development across the animal kingdom and is a key driver of stem cells in most types of tissues (54, 55). While regulating embryonic development and maintaining tissue homeostasis, it mediates downstream signals to participate in various biological/pathological processes and the genesis and development of cancer (53, 56, 57). During the research process of TMEM88, studies have pointed out that the C-terminal tripeptide Val-Trp-Val sequence of a subtype of TMEM88 CRA-a can bind to the PDZ domain of the scrambled protein and prohibit the Wnt/β-catenin signaling pathway, which exerts a nonnegligible effect in regulating tumor cell proliferation, metastasis and host antitumor immunity (22, 27, 58). For example, it can be coexpressed in the cytoplasm with scattered proteins in NSCLC and breast cancer to elevate the levels of Snail and thereby promote tumor progression. Analysis of the transcriptome information of ovarian cancer patients in the TCGA database shows that TMEM88 is closely correlated with the mRNA expression levels of c-Myc and β-catenin mRNA (P = 0.01252 and 0.0128) (19). In addition, Geng et al. found that the overexpression of TMEM88 significantly reduced the transcriptional activity of TCF/LEF and inhibited the expression of the downstream target genes c-Myc and cyclin D1 of the Wnt/β-catenin signaling pathway (25). Furthermore, reactivation of Wnt/β-catenin signaling by transfection of the pENTRN90-β-catenin vector partially reversed the inhibitory effect of TMEM88 on the proliferation and invasion of thyroid cancer cells, indicating that TMEM88 exerts an anti-thyroid cancer effect in the presence of Wnt/β-catenin protein signaling. A study in bladder cancer found that overexpression of TMEM88 also inhibited the activation of the Wnt/β-catenin signaling pathway by reducing the phosphorylation level of GSK-3β (Ser9 site) (29). However, in a study of triple-negative breast cancer, transfection of MCF-7 and MDA-MB-231 cells to overexpress or silence TMEM88 did not affect the activity of the canonical Wnt signaling pathway or the expression of corresponding target genes such as MMP-7, c-Myc and cyclin D1 (30). Taken together, the above studies suggest that TMEM88, as an important linker in the genesis and development of various cancer diseases, can function by regulating different downstream oncogenic signals and effector molecules. It transmits upstream signals and regulates downstream signal transduction, such as Wnt signaling pathways, to interfere with the occurrence and progression of tumors and then has an anticancer effect. Based on this, TMEM88 should be considered a novel and important research target in cancer research, which needs to be deeply explored for its potential.

TARGETING TMEM88 POTENTIAL FOR TREATING MALIGNANT TUMORS

With the deepening of people's understanding of tumor research and clinical, molecular targeted therapy has also received increasing attention and aroused the interest of researchers. At present, the most common molecular targeted therapeutic drugs mainly include small molecular epidermal kinase inhibitors, such as gefitinib (AstraZeneca, UK) (59); anti-EGFR monoclonal antibodies, such as cetuximab (Merck & Leone Pharmaceutical Co, Germany) (60); anti-HER-2 monoclonal antibodies, such as trastuzumab (Roche Group, Switzerland) (61); Bcr-Abl tyrosine kinase inhibitors, such as imatinib (Novartis, Switzerland) (62); anti-CD20 monoclonal antibodies, such as rituximab (Roche Group, Switzerland) (63); and vascular endothelial growth factor receptor inhibitors, such as bevacizumab (Roche Group, Switzerland) (64). When the above drugs exert antitumor effects, they can significantly reduce the toxicity to normal cells, which provides a new direction for molecular targeted therapy of tumors. However, due to the heterogeneity of cancers, the current targeted therapeutic drugs benefit only a portion of cancer patients, which forces us to explore a broader spectrum of malignant tumor therapeutic targets and develop promising therapeutic drugs to address the urgent issue in tumor research and current clinical practice.

To date, a variety of transmembrane proteins have become powerful targets for drug development and have even entered clinical trials and clinical applications. As a representative, the G protein coupled receptor (GPCR) family is the largest transmembrane protein family in humans and is also an important target of many drugs (65). Currently, 475 drugs targeting GPCR have been approved by the FDA, accounting for 34% of all FDA approved drugs. Meanwhile, 321 drugs targeting GPCRs are in clinical studies (66, 67). The above drugs are mainly distributed in small molecule drugs, polypeptide drugs, monoclonal antibodies, and recombinant proteins. Four-transmembrane proteins, CD20 and Claudin 18.2, are important targets for disease treatment and drug development. CD20 is a transmembrane phosphorin located on the surface of B lymphocytes, mainly in the preceding B-cell to mature B-cell stage (68). Currently, the antitumor drug antibody and inflammatory immune regulatory antibody drugs that target CD20 have entered the fast lane developed by the product (69). Claudin18.2 is the most important member of the Claudin transmembrane protein family. In the normal physiological state, Claudin18.2 protein is only expressed on the surface of human gastric epithelial shorthearter cells. However, in the pathological state, Claudin18.2 protein is highly expressed in gastric cancer, esophageal cancer, pancreatic cancer, and other solid tissues (15, 70–72). The significant differences and high tissue specificity make Claudin 18.2 an ideal target for solid tumor immunotherapy(2016). Currently, it has been close to 20 drugs targeting Claudin18.2 in the clinical phase, such as zolbetuximab (Phase III: NCT03653507, Astellas Pharma Inc., Japan), TST001 (Phase I: NCT04495296, MabSpace Biosciences, China) and AMG910 (Phase I: NCT04260191, Amgen Inc., USA), and these drugs are primarily concentrated on monoclonal antibody and bispecific antibody, antibody-drug conjugate (ADC), and chimeric antigen receptor T-cell immunotherapy (CAR-T) (72–75). The abovementioned drug development of transmembrane proteins has laid a solid foundation for the research and exploration of targeted TMEM88 to treat malignant tumors. Meanwhile, we should be more aware of the current gaps in the development of drugs targeting TMEM88 for the treatment of tumors: 1. Insufficient analysis of the three-dimensional and crystal structure of the TMEM88 protein makes the structural information of the protein lacking. 2. Research on the full length of the TMEM88 protein polypeptide and the recognition epitope is insufficient, and information on the active site and affinity is lacking. We believe that the resolution of these problems will greatly promote the development of drugs targeting TMEM88.

However, due to the surface area of the transmembrane protein structure, its expression level is difficult to meet the requirements. Furthermore, it is difficult for us to achieve high-purity multitransmembrane proteins with natural conformations and activity. These difficulties make targeted TMEM88 antitumor drug development difficult. Based on this, various strategies can be considered to increase the development of antitumor drugs targeting TMEM88: 1. Novel protein purification, isolation and characterization systems and techniques need to be applied; 2. Artificial intelligence and computer simulation need to be more invested; 3. Drug diversity needs to be constantly tried, such as antibody drugs, nanodrugs, small-molecule drugs, traditional Chinese medicines and proteolysis targeting-chimeras (PROTAC). In any case, as a two-transmembrane protein, TMEM88 has significant differences and specificities between multiple malignant tumor and adjacent tissues and tumor and normal cells, which makes TMEM88 a potential therapeutic target through different strategies during tumor treatment.

PROSPECTIVE AND CONCLUSIONS

In recent years, tumors have been the main cause of human death, and the occurrence and development of many kinds of tumors are closely related to the imbalance of signal transduction in the body (76). Therefore, it is extremely important to clarify the signal transduction mechanism and find potential new tumor therapeutic targets. In the current literature, TMEM88 is considered to play an important role in the development of breast cancer, lung cancer, thyroid cancer and other tumors by inhibiting Wnt signal transduction and participates in the occurrence and development of tumors, but it needs to be pointed out that TMEM88 research is not deep enough, and many issues remain to be studied. Specifically, TMEM88 has different expression levels in different tumors and has tissue specificity, but what are the specific characteristics; when there are multiple influencing factors, will the role of TMEM88 in malignant tumors be different? TMEM88 methylation affects tumor biology However, what is the specific mechanism? In the process of cancer development, TMEM88 not only regulates the Wnt/β-catenin signaling pathway and participates in it but also affects other signal transduction processes. Therefore, more basic research needs to be carried out to further confirm the specific role of TMEM88 in tumor development, improve its credibility as a potential therapeutic target, and prove its potential to transform from basic research to clinical application in tumor treatment. In any case, the results of multiple studies have shown that TMEM88 may be a tumor diagnosis and prognostic indicator, which will provide new clues and directions for the diagnosis and treatment of clinical malignant tumors. We look forward to using advanced technologies for in-depth research, such as microarray analysis, tissue sample sequencing, high-throughput DNA methylation analysis and other new technologies, revealing the function of TMEM88 regulation in more malignant tumors and elucidating the pathogenesis of TMEM88 in tumors. This will further promote the progress of the diagnosis and treatment of malignant tumors.

AUTHOR CONTRIBUTIONS

HZ, W-JN, and MC designed the “idea”; MC and W-JN wrote the manuscript; Y-HW and J-JW collected the information; W-JN and HZ revised the manuscript. All authors read and approved the final manuscript.

ACKNOWLEDGMENTS

We thank American Journal Experts (AJE) for their guidance on the grammar and language of this article.

REFERENCES

Li C, Ou R, Chen Y, Gu X, Wei Q, Cao B, et al. Mutation Analysis of TMEM Family Members for Early-Onset Parkinson's Disease in Chinese Population. *Neurobiol Aging* (2021) 101:299.e1-6. doi: 10.1016/j.neurobiolaging.2020.11.005

Marx S, Dal Maso T, Chen JW, Bury M, Wouters J, Michiels C, et al. Transmembrane (TMEM) Protein Family Members: Poorly Characterized Even If Essential for the Metastatic Process. *Semin Cancer Biol* (2020) 60:96- 106. doi: 10.1016/j.semcancer.2019.08.018

Liu Y, Zheng Q, He G, Zhang M, Yan X, Yang Z, et al. Transmembrane Protein 215 Promotes Angiogenesis by Maintaining Endothelial Cell Survival. *J Cell Physiol* (2019) 234(6):9525-34. doi: 10.1002/jcp.27641

Zhang Z, Luo S, Barbosa GO, Bai M, Kornberg TB, Ma DK. The Conserved Transmembrane Protein TMEM-39 Coordinates With COPII to Promote Collagen Secretion and Regulate ER Stress Response. *PloS Genet* (2021) 17(2): e1009317. doi: 10.1371/journal.pgen.1009317

Fuhrmann DC, Wittig I, Brune B. TMEM126B Deficiency Reduces Mitochondrial SDH Oxidation by LPS, Attenuating HIF-1alpha Stabilization and IL-1beta Expression. *Redox Biol* (2019) 20:204-16. doi: 10.1016/j.redox.2018.10.007

Beasley HK, Rodman TA, Collins GV, Hinton AJ, Exil V. TMEM135 Is a Novel Regulator of Mitochondrial Dynamics and Physiology With Implications for Human Health Conditions. *Cells* (2021) 10(7):1750-66. doi: 10.3390/cells10071750

Picotto G, Morse LR, Nguyen N, Saltzman J, Battaglino R. TMEM176A and TMEM176B Are Candidate Regulators of Inhibition of Dendritic Cell Maturation and Function After Chronic Spinal Cord Injury. *J Neurotrauma* (2020) 37(3):528-33. doi: 10.1089/neu.2019.6498

Xu J, Su Z, Ding Q, Shen L, Nie X, Pan X, et al. Inhibition of Proliferation by Knockdown of Transmembrane (TMEM) 168 in Glioblastoma Cells *via* Suppression of Wnt/beta-Catenin Pathway. *Oncol Res* (2019) 27(7):819-26. doi: 10.3727/096504018X15478559215014

Shen K, Yu W, Yu Y, Liu X, Cui X. Knockdown of TMEM45B Inhibits Cell Proliferation and Invasion in Gastric Cancer. *Biomed Pharmacother* (2018) 104:576-81. doi: 10.1016/j.biopha.2018.05.016

Li Y, Guo W, Liu S, Zhang B, Yu BB, Yang B, et al. Silencing Transmembrane Protein 45b (TNEM45B) Inhibits Proliferation, Invasion, and Tumorigenesis in Osteosarcoma Cells. *Oncol Res* (2017) 25(6):1021-6. doi: 10.3727/096504016X14821477992177

Zhang X, Wan JX, Ke ZP, Wang F, Chai HX, Liu JQ. TMEM88, CCL14 and CLEC3B as Prognostic Biomarkers for Prognosis and Palindromia of Human Hepatocellular Carcinoma. *Tumour Biol* (2017) 39(7):1010428317708900. doi: 10.1177/1010428317708900

Guardia CM, Tan XF, Lian T, Rana MS, Zhou W, Christenson ET, et al. Structure of Human ATG9A, the Only Transmembrane Protein of the Core Autophagy Machinery. *Cell Rep* (2020) 31(13):107837. doi: 10.1016/ j.celrep.2020.107837

Yang Y, Zhou L, Xue F, An L, Jin M, Li L. Transmembrane Protein 166 and Its Significance. *Protein Pept Lett* (2021) 28(4):382-7. doi: 10.2174/0929866527666201002150316

Du Z, Lovly CM. Mechanisms of Receptor Tyrosine Kinase Activation in Cancer. *Mol Cancer* (2018) 17(1):58. doi: 10.1186/s12943-018-0782-4

Xu B, Liu F, Liu Q, Shi T, Wang Z, Wu N, et al. Highly Expressed Claudin18.2 as a Potential Therapeutic Target in Advanced Gastric Signet-Ring Cell Carcinoma (SRCC). *J Gastrointest Oncol* (2020) 11(6):1431-9. doi: 10.21037/jgo-20-344

Zhao H, Lu F, Cui S, Zhang X, Wang W, Si E, et al. TMEM88 Inhibits Extracellular Matrix Expression in Keloid Fibroblasts. *Biomed Pharmacother* (2017) 95:1436-40. doi: 10.1016/j.biopha.2017.09.047

Xu T, Pan LX, Ge YX, Li P, Meng XM, Huang C, et al. TMEM88 Mediates Inflammatory Cytokines Secretion by Regulating JNK/P38 and Canonical Wnt/beta-Catenin Signaling Pathway in LX-2 Cells. *Inflammopharmacology* (2018) 26(5):1339-48. doi: 10.1007/s10787-017-0419-z

Li LY, Yang CC, Li SW, Liu YM, Li HD, Hu S, et al. TMEM88 Modulates the Secretion of Inflammatory Factors by Regulating YAP Signaling Pathway in Alcoholic Liver Disease. *Inflamm Res* (2020) 69(8):789-800. doi: 10.1007/s00011-020-01360-y

de Leon M, Cardenas H, Vieth E, Emerson R, Segar M, Liu Y, et al.). Transmembrane Protein 88 (TMEM88) Promoter Hypomethylation Is Associated With Platinum Resistance in Ovarian Cancer. *Gynecol Oncol* (2016) 142(3):539-47. doi: 10.1016/j.ygyno.2016.06.017

Cai SP, Cheng XY, Chen PJ, Pan XY, Xu T, Huang C, et al. Transmembrane Protein 88 Attenuates Liver Fibrosis by Promoting Apoptosis and Reversion of Activated Hepatic Stellate Cells. *Mol Immunol* (2016) 80:58-67. doi: 10.1016/j.molimm.2016.11.002

Palpant NJ, Pabon L, Rabinowitz JS, Hadland BK, Stoick-Cooper CL, Paige SL, et al. Transmembrane Protein 88: A Wnt Regulatory Protein That Specifies

Cardiomyocyte Development. *Development* (2013) 140(18):3799–808. doi: 10.1242/dev.094789

Lee H, Evans T.). TMEM88 Inhibits Wnt Signaling by Promoting Wnt Signalosome Localization to Multivesicular Bodies. *iScience* (2019) 19:267–80. doi: 10.1016/j.isci.2019.07.039

Ge YX, Wang CH, Hu FY, Pan LX, Min J, Niu KY, et al. New Advances of TMEM88 in Cancer Initiation and Progression, With Special Emphasis on Wnt Signaling Pathway. *J Cell Physiol* (2018) 233(1):79–87. doi: 10.1002/ jcp.25853

Lee HJ, Finkelstein D, Li X, Wu D, Shi DL, Zheng JJ. Identification of Transmembrane Protein 88 (TMEM88) as a Dishevelled-Binding Protein. *J Biol Chem* (2010) 285(53):41549–56. doi: 10.1074/jbc.M110.193383

Geng Q, Chen X, Chen N. Transmembrane Protein 88 Exerts Tumorinhibitory Role Thyroid Cancer Through Restriction Wnt/beta- Catenin Signaling *Exp Cell Res* (2020) 395(2):112193. doi: 10.1016/ j.yexcr.2020.112193

Zhang X, Yu X, Jiang G, Miao Y, Wang L, Zhang Y, et al. Cytosolic TMEM88 Promotes Invasion and Metastasis in Lung Cancer Cells by Binding DVLS. *Cancer Res* (2015) 75(21):4527–37. doi: 10.1158/0008-5472.CAN-14-3828

Stewart DJ. Wnt Signaling Pathway in Non-Small Cell Lung Cancer. *J Natl Cancer Inst* (2014) 106(1):djt356. doi: 10.1093/jnci/djt356

Rongna M, Nannan F, Xiao Y, Hongyan L, Xiaohong Z, Oumin S, et al. Promoter Methylation of Wnt/**b**-Catenin Signal Inhibitor TMEM88 Is Associated With Unfavorable Prognosis of Non-Small Cell Lung Cancer. *Cancer Biol Med* (2017) 14(4):377–86. doi: 10.20892/j.issn.2095-3941.2017.0061

Zhao X, Li G, Chong T, Xue L, Luo Q, Tang X, et al. TMEM88 Exhibits an Antiproliferative and Anti-Invasive Effect in Bladder Cancer by Downregulating Wnt/beta-Catenin Signaling. *J Biochem Mol Toxicol* (2021) 35(8):e22835. doi: 10.1002/jbt.22835

Yu X, Zhang X, Zhang Y, Jiang G, Mao X, Jin F. Cytosolic TMEM88 Promotes Triple-Negative Breast Cancer by Interacting With Dvl. *Oncotarget* (2015) 6 (28):25034–45. doi: 10.18632/oncotarget.4379

Xu T, Pan L, Li L, Hu S, Zhou H, Yang C, et al. MicroRNA-708 Modulates Hepatic Stellate Cells Activation and Enhances Extracellular Matrix Accumulation *via* Direct Targeting TMEM88. *J Cell Mol Med* (2020) 24 (13):7127–40. doi: 10.1111/jcmm.15119

Zhou F, Yang X, Zhao H, Liu Y, Feng Y, An R, et al. Down-Regulation of OGT Promotes Cisplatin Resistance by Inducing Autophagy in Ovarian Cancer. *Theranostics* (2018) 8(19):5200–12. doi: 10.7150/thno.27806

Siegel RL, Miller KD, Fuchs HE, Jemal A. Cancer Statistic. *CA Cancer J Clin* (2022) 72(1):7–33. doi: 10.3322/caac.21708

Zhang SZ, Zhang L, Xie L. Cancer Burden in China During 1990-2019: Analysis of the Global Burden of Disease. *BioMed Res Int* (2022) 2022:3918045. doi: 10.1155/2022/3918045

Liang Y, Zhang H, Song X, Yang Q. Metastatic Heterogeneity of Breast Cancer: Molecular Mechanism and Potential Therapeutic Targets. Semin. *Cancer Biol* (2020) 60:14–27. doi: 10.1016/j.semcancer.2019.08.012

Tray N, Taff J, Adams S. Therapeutic Landscape of Metaplastic Breast Cancer. *Cancer Treat Rev* (2019) 79:101888. doi: 10.1016/j.ctrv.2019.08.004

Bray F, Ferlay J, Soerjomataram I, Siegel RL, Torre LA, Jemal A. Global Cancer Statistics 2018: GLOBOCAN Estimates of Incidence and Mortality Worldwide for 36 Cancers in 185 Countries. *CA Cancer J Clin* (2018) 68(6):394–424. doi: 10.3322/caac.21492

Kibudde S, Kirenga BJ, Nabwana M, Okuku F, Walusansa V, Orem J. Clinical Profile and Initial Treatment of Non-Small Cell Lung Cancer: A Retrospective Cohort Study at the Uganda Cancer Institute. *Afr Health Sci* (2021) 21 (4):1739–45. doi: 10.4314/ahs.v21i4.30

Hirsch FR, Scagliotti GV, Mulshine JL, Kwon R, Curran WJ, Wu YL, et al. Lung Cancer: Current Therapies and New Targeted Treatments. *Lancet* (2017) 389(10066):299–311. doi: 10.1016/S0140-6736(16)30958-8

Blandin KS, Crosbie PA, Balata H, Chudziak J, Hussell T, Dive C. Progress and Prospects of Early Detection in Lung Cancer. *Open Biol* (2017) 7(9):170070. doi: 10.1098/rsob.170070

Duma N, Santana-Davila R, Molina JR. Non-Small Cell Lung Cancer: Epidemiology, Screening, Diagnosis, and Treatment. *Mayo Clin Proc* (2019) 94(8):1623–40. doi: 10.1016/j.mayocp.2019.01.013

Pizzato M, Li M, Vignat J, Laversanne M, Singh D, La Vecchia C, et al. The Epidemiological Landscape of Thyroid Cancer Worldwide: GLOBOCAN Estimates for Incidence and Mortality Rates in 2020. *Lancet Diabetes Endocrinol* (2022) 10(4):264–72. doi: 10.1016/S2213-8587(22)00035-3

Fei X, Chen W, Zhang S, Liu Q, Zhang Z, Pei Q. The Spatio-Temporal Distribution and Risk Factors of Thyroid Cancer During Rapid Urbanization- A Case Study in China. *Sci Total Environ* (2018) 630:1436–45. doi: 10.1016/ j.scitotenv.2018.02.339

Liu Y, Lai F, Long J, Peng S, Wang H, Zhou Q, et al. Screening and the Epidemic of Thyroid Cancer in China: An Analysis of National Representative Inpatient and Commercial Insurance Databases. *Int J Cancer* (2021) 148 (5):1106–14. doi: 10.1002/ijc.33298

Mammen J, Cappola AR. Autoimmune Thyroid Disease in Women. *JAMA* (2021) 325(23):2392–3. doi: 10.1001/jama.2020.22196

Rahib L, Smith BD, Aizenberg R, Rosenzweig AB, Fleshman JM, Matrisian LM. Projecting Cancer Incidence and Deaths to 2030: The Unexpected Burden of Thyroid, Liver, and Pancreas Cancers in the United States. *Cancer Res* (2014) 74(11):2913–21. doi: 10.1158/0008-5472.CAN-14-0155

Dabravolski SA, Nikiforov NG, Zhuravlev AD, Orekhov NA, Mikhaleva LM, Orekhov AN. The Role of Altered Mitochondrial Metabolism in Thyroid Cancer Development and Mitochondria-Targeted Thyroid Cancer Treatment. *Int J Mol Sci* (2021) 23(1):460–75. doi: 10.3390/ijms23010460

Sandler JE, Huang H, Zhao N, Wu W, Liu F, Ma S, et al. Germline Variants in DNA Repair Genes, Diagnostic Radiation, and Risk of Thyroid Cancer. *Cancer Epidemiol Biomarkers Prev* (2018) 27(3):285–94. doi: 10.1158/1055- 9965.EPI-17-0319

Adeyelu TT, Moya-Garcia AA, Orengo C. Exploiting Protein Family and Protein Network Data to Identify Novel Drug Targets for Bladder Cancer. *Oncotarget* (2022) 13:105–17. doi: 10.18632/oncotarget.28175

Li HZ, Zheng RS, Du LB, Zhang SW, Zhu C, Wei WW, et al. Bladder Cancer Incidence, Mortality and Temporal Trends in China. *Zhonghua Zhong Liu Za Zhi* (2021) 43(3):293–8. doi: 10.3760/cma.j.cn112152- 20200421-00362

Wang Q, Zhang T, Wu J, Wen J, Tao D, Wan T, et al. Prognosis and Risk Factors of Patients With Upper Urinary Tract Urothelial Carcinoma and Postoperative Recurrence of Bladder Cancer in Central China. *BMC Urol* (2019) 19(1):24. doi: 10.1186/s12894-019-0457-5

Ghandour R, Singla N, Lotan Y. Treatment Options and Outcomes in Nonmetastatic Muscle Invasive Bladder Cancer. *Trends Cancer* (2019) 5 (7):426–39. doi: 10.1016/j.trecan.2019.05.011

Nusse R, Clevers H. Wnt/beta-Catenin Signaling, Disease, and Emerging Therapeutic Modalities. *Cell* (2017) 169(6):985–99. doi: 10.1016/ j.cell.2017.05.016

Qu Y, Olsen JR, Yuan X, Cheng PF, Levesque MP, Brokstad KA, et al. Small Molecule Promotes Beta-Catenin Citrullination and Inhibits Wnt Signaling in Cancer. *Nat Chem Biol* (2018) 14(1):94–101. doi: 10.1038/nchembio.2510

Russell JO, Monga SP. Wnt/beta-Catenin Signaling in Liver Development, Homeostasis, and Pathobiology. *Annu Rev Pathol* (2018) 13:351–78. doi: 10.1146/annurev-pathol-020117-044010

Eubelen M, Bostaille N, Cabochette P, Gauquier A, Tebabi P, Dumitru AC, et al. A Molecular Mechanism for Wnt Ligand-Specific Signaling. *Science* (2018) 361(6403):eaat1178. doi: 10.1126/science.aat1178

Galluzzi L, Spranger S, Fuchs E, Lopez-Soto A. WNT Signaling in Cancer Immunosurveillance. *Trends Cell Biol* (2019) 29(1):44–65. doi: 10.1016/ j.tcb.2018.08.005

Sun Z, Ning Q, Li H, Hu T, Tang L, Wen Q, et al. Transmembrane Protein 88 Inhibits Transforming Growth Factor-Beta1-Induced-Extracellular Matrix Accumulation and Epithelial-Mesenchymal Transition Program in Human Pleural Mesothelial Cells Through Modulating TGF-Beta1/Smad Pathway. *J Recept Signal Transd Res* (2022) 42(1):60–6. doi: 10.1080/10799893. 2020.1843493

Noronha V, Patil VM, Joshi A, Menon N, Chougule A, Mahajan A, et al. Gefitinib Versus Gefitinib Plus Pemetrexed and Carboplatin Chemotherapy in EGFR-Mutated Lung Cancer. *J Clin Oncol* (2020) 38(2):124–36. doi: 10.1200/ JCO.19.01154

Pietrantonio F. Encorafenib, Binimetinib, and Cetuximab in BRAF V600E-Mutated Colorectal Cancer. *N Engl J Med* (2020) 382(9):876–7. doi: 10.1056/ NEJMc1915676

Altundag K. Association Between HER2 Status in Residual Disease and Sensitivity to Trastuzumab Emtansine. *Ann Oncol* (2021) 32(9):1191. doi: 10.1016/j. annonc.2021.05.794

Cohen P, Cross D, Janne PA. Kinase Drug Discovery 20 Years After Imatinib: Progress and Future Directions. *Nat Rev Drug Discov* (2021) 20(7):551–69. doi: 10.1038/s41573-021-00195-4

Nair R, Radhakrishnan VS, Mallath MK. Rituximab Biosimilars for B-Cell Lymphomas: A Decade of Real-World Experience From India. *Lancet Haematol* (2021) 8(8):e548–9. doi: 10.1016/S2352-3026(21)00212-X

Garcia-Romero N, Palacin-Aliana I, Madurga R, Carrion-Navarro J, Esteban-Rubio S, Jimenez B, et al. Bevacizumab Dose Adjustment to Improve Clinical Outcomes of Glioblastoma. *BMC Med* (2020) 18(1):142. doi: 10.1186/s12916-020-01610-0

Shimada I, Ueda T, Kofuku Y, Eddy MT, Wuthrich K. GPCR Drug Discovery:

Integrating Solution NMR Data With Crystal and Cryo-EM Structures. *Nat Rev Drug Discov* (2019) 18(1):59–82. doi: 10.1038/nrd.2018.180

Insel PA, Sriram K, Gorr MW, Wiley SZ, Michkov A, Salmeron C, et al. GPCRomics: An Approach to Discover GPCR Drug Targets. *Trends Pharmacol Sci* (2019) 40(6):378–87. doi: 10.1016/j.tips.2019.04.001

Hauser AS, Attwood MM, Rask-Andersen M, Schioth HB, Gloriam DE. Trends in GPCR Drug Discovery: New Agents, Targets and Indications. *Nat Rev Drug Discov* (2017) 16(12):829–42. doi: 10.1038/nrd.2017.178

Kumar A, Planchais C, Fronzes R, Mouquet H, Reyes N. Binding Mechanisms of Therapeutic Antibodies to Human CD20. *Science* (2020) 369(6505):793–9. doi: 10.1126/science.abb8008

Pavlasova G, Mraz M. The Regulation and Function of CD20: An "Enigma" of B-Cell Biology and Targeted Therapy. *Haematologica* (2020) 105(6):1494– 506. doi: 10.3324/haematol.2019.243543

Arnold A, Daum S, von Winterfeld M, Berg E, Hummel M, Rau B, et al. Prognostic Impact of Claudin 18.2 in Gastric and Esophageal Adenocarcinomas. *Clin Transl Oncol* (2020) 22(12):2357–63. doi: 10.1007/ s12094-020-02380-0

Türeci, Mitnacht-Kraus R, Woll S, Yamada T, Sahin U. Characterization of Zolbetuximab in Pancreatic Cancer Models. *Oncoimmunology* (2019) 8(1): e1523096. doi: 10.1080/2162402X.2018.1523096

Katoh M, Katoh M. Precision Medicine for Human Cancers With Notch Signaling Dysregulation (Review). *Int J Mol Med* (2020) 45(2):279–97. doi: 10.3892/ ijmm.2019.4418

Kyuno D, Takasawa A, Takasawa K, Ono Y, Aoyama T, Magara K, et al. Claudin-18.2 as a Therapeutic Target in Cancers: Cumulative Findings From Basic Research and Clinical Trials. *Tissue Barriers* (2022) 10(1):1967080. doi: 10.1080/21688370.2021.1967080

Jiang H, Shi Z, Wang P, Wang C, Yang L, Du G, et al. Claudin18.2- Specific Chimeric Antigen Receptor Engineered T Cells for the Treatment of Gastric Cancer. *J Natl Cancer Inst* (2019) 111(4):409–18. doi: 10.1093/jnci/ djy134

Zhang J, Dong R, Shen L. Evaluation and Reflection on Claudin 18.2 Targeting Therapy in Advanced Gastric Cancer. *Chin J Cancer Res* (2020) 32(2):263–70. doi: 10.21147/j.issn.1000-9604.2020.02.13

Feng RM, Zong YN, Cao SM, Xu RH. Current Cancer Situation in China: Good or Bad News From the 2018 Global Cancer Statistics? *Cancer Commun (Lond)* (2019) 39(1):22. doi: 10.1186/s40880-019-0368-6

Permissions

All chapters in this book were first published by Frontiers; hereby published with permission under the Creative Commons Attribution License or equivalent. Every chapter published in this book has been scrutinized by our experts. Their significance has been extensively debated. The topics covered herein carry significant findings which will fuel the growth of the discipline. They may even be implemented as practical applications or may be referred to as a beginning point for another development.

The contributors of this book come from diverse backgrounds, making this book a truly international effort. This book will bring forth new frontiers with its revolutionizing research information and detailed analysis of the nascent developments around the world.

We would like to thank all the contributing authors for lending their expertise to make the book truly unique. They have played a crucial role in the development of this book. Without their invaluable contributions this book wouldn't have been possible. They have made vital efforts to compile up to date information on the varied aspects of this subject to make this book a valuable addition to the collection of many professionals and students.

This book was conceptualized with the vision of imparting up-to-date information and advanced data in this field. To ensure the same, a matchless editorial board was set up. Every individual on the board went through rigorous rounds of assessment to prove their worth. After which they invested a large part of their time researching and compiling the most relevant data for our readers.

The editorial board has been involved in producing this book since its inception. They have spent rigorous hours researching and exploring the diverse topics which have resulted in the successful publishing of this book. They have passed on their knowledge of decades through this book. To expedite this challenging task, the publisher supported the team at every step. A small team of assistant editors was also appointed to further simplify the editing procedure and attain best results for the readers.

Apart from the editorial board, the designing team has also invested a significant amount of their time in understanding the subject and creating the most relevant covers. They scrutinized every image to scout for the most suitable representation of the subject and create an appropriate cover for the book.

The publishing team has been an ardent support to the editorial, designing and production team. Their endless efforts to recruit the best for this project, has resulted in the accomplishment of this book. They are a veteran in the field of academics and their pool of knowledge is as vast as their experience in printing. Their expertise and guidance has proved useful at every step. Their uncompromising quality standards have made this book an exceptional effort. Their encouragement from time to time has been an inspiration for everyone.

The publisher and the editorial board hope that this book will prove to be a valuable piece of knowledge for researchers, students, practitioners and scholars across the globe.

List of Contributors

Mingming Zhang, Huize Liang and Huaping Jia
Strategic Support Force Characteristic Medical Center of Chinese People's Liberation Army, Beijing, China

Jianqin Liang
The 8th Medical Center, General Hospital of the Chinese People's Liberation Army, Beijing, China

Yanyu Yang
College of Materials Science and Engineering, Zhengzhou University, Zhengzhou, China

Dawei Li
The 4th Medical Center, General Hospital of the Chinese People's Liberation Army, Beijing, China

Tao Wang, Peng Zhang, Chengguo Li, Weizhen Liu, Qian Shen, Lei Yang, Gengchen Xie, Jie Bai, Ruidong Li, Kaixiong Tao and Yuping Yin
Department of Gastrointestinal Surgery, Union Hospital, Tongji Medical College, Huazhong University of Science and Technology, Wuhan, China

Timur Fetisov, Elena Antoshina, Lubov Trukhanova, Tatiana Gor'kova, Olga Vlasova, Irina Khitrovo, Nataliya Kulbachevskaya, Gennady Belitsky and Marianna Yakubovskaya
Blokhin Cancer Research Center, Moscow, Russia

Kirill Kirsanov
Blokhin Cancer Research Center, Moscow, Russia
Peoples' Friendship University of Russia, Moscow, Russia

Ekaterina Lesovaya
Blokhin Cancer Research Center, Moscow, Russia
Pavlov Ryazan State Medical University, Ryazan, Russia

Tatiana Shcherbakova and Dmitry Nilov
Belozersky Institute of Physicochemical Biology, Lomonosov Moscow State University, Moscow, Russia

Vytas Švedas
Belozersky Institute of Physicochemical Biology, Lomonosov Moscow State University, Moscow, Russia
Faculty of Bioengineering and Bioinformatics, Lomonosov Moscow State University, Moscow, Russia

Wei Wang, Yue Sun, Xiaobo Liu and Yun Dai
Laboratory of Cancer Precision Medicine, The First Hospital of Jilin University, Changchun, China

Shaji K. Kumar
Division of Hematology, Mayo Clinic College of Medicine, Rochester, MN, United States

Fengyan Jin
Department of Hematology, The First Hospital of Jilin University, Changchun, China

Hui Zhang
Tianjin Cancer Institute, Key Laboratory of Cancer Prevention and Therapy, National Clinical Research Center for Cancer, Tianjin Medical University Cancer Institute and Hospital, Tianjin's Clinical Research Center for Cancer, Tianjin Medical University, Tianjin, China
Department of Medical Oncology, Shandong Cancer Hospital and Institute, Shandong First Medical University and Shandong Academy of Medical Science, Jinan, China

Rongjie Tao
Department of Medical Oncology, Shandong Cancer Hospital and Institute, Shandong First Medical University and Shandong Academy of Medical Science, Jinan, China

Yong Wang, Shizhen Zhou and Xiangji Meng
Department of Neurosurgery, Shandong Cancer Hospital and Institute, Shandong First Medical University and Shandong Academy of Medical Science, Jinan, China

Huaguo Wu
Department of Head and Neck Surgery, Shandong Cancer Hospital and Institute, Shandong First Medical University and Shandong Academy of Medical Science, Jinan, China

Shuo Li
School of Medicine and Life Science, University of Jinan-Shandong Academy of Medical Science, Jinan, China

Jinming Yu
Tianjin Cancer Institute, Key Laboratory of Cancer Prevention and Therapy, National Clinical Research Center for Cancer, Tianjin Medical University Cancer Institute and Hospital, Tianjin's Clinical Research Center for Cancer, Tianjin Medical University, Tianjin, China
Department of Radiation Oncology, Shandong Cancer Hospital and Institute, Shandong First Medical University and Shandong Academy of Medical Science, Jinan, China

Ying Xia
Center for Clinical Laboratories, The Affiliated Hospital of Guizhou Medical University, Guiyang, China
Department of Pathophysiology, School of Basic Medical Science, Guizhou Medical University, Guiyang, China
Department of Clinical Laboratory, The First Affiliated Hospital of Guizhou University of Traditional Chinese Medicine, Guiyang, China
School of Clinical Laboratory Science, Guizhou Medical University, Guiyang, China

Yong Jin and Hai Huang
Center for Clinical Laboratories, The Affiliated Hospital of Guizhou Medical University, Guiyang, China
School of Clinical Laboratory Science, Guizhou Medical University, Guiyang, China

Daxiang Cui and Cunfeng Song
Shanghai Engineering Research Center for Intelligent Diagnosis and Treatment Instrument, Department of Instrument Science and Engineering, School of Electronic Information and Electrical Engineering, Institute of Nano Biomedicine and Engineering, Shanghai Jiao Tong University, Shanghai, China

Xia Wu
Guizhou Provincial People's Hospital, Guiyang, China

Weilin Jin
Shanghai Engineering Research Center for Intelligent Diagnosis and Treatment Instrument, Department of Instrument Science and Engineering, School of Electronic Information and Electrical Engineering, Institute of Nano Biomedicine and Engineering, Shanghai Jiao Tong University, Shanghai, China
Institute of Cancer Neuroscience, Medical Frontier Innovation Research Center, The First Hospital of Lanzhou University, The First Clinical Medical College of Lanzhou University, Lanzhou, China

Bingjie Fu, Xiaojing Dou, Miao Zou, Hao Lu, Kaixuan Wang, Qingxia Liu, Meihua Jin and Dexin Kong
Tianjin Key Laboratory of Technologies Enabling Development of Clinical Therapeutics and Diagnostics, School of Pharmacy, Key Laboratory of Immune Microenvironment and Diseases (Ministry of Education), Tianjin Medical University, Tianjin, China

Yao Liu and Wei Wang
Department of Otorhinolaryngology Head and Neck Surgery, Key Laboratory of Auditory Speech and Balance Medicine, Institute of Otolaryngology of Tianjin, Tianjin First Central Hospital, Tianjin, China

Jida Guo, Shengqiang Zhang, Jun Wang, Pengfei Zhang, Tong Lu and Linyou Zhang
Department of Thoracic Surgery, The Second Affiliated Hospital of Harbin Medical University, Harbin Medical University, Harbin, China

Jiacheng Wu and Hao Ji
Department of Urology, The Affiliated Tumor Hospital of Nantong University, Nantong, China

Tao Li
Department of Medical Oncology, The Affiliated Tumor Hospital of Nantong University, Nantong, China

Zhi Chen
Department of Pathology, The First People's Hospital of Longquanyi District, Chengdu, China

Baoqian Zhai
Department of Oncology Radiotherapy, Yancheng No. 1 People's Hospital, Yancheng, China

Bingteng Xie and Aiqin Luo
School of Life Science, Beijing Institute of Technology, Beijing, China
Key Laboratory of Molecular Medicine and Biological Diagnosis and Treatment, Beijing Institute of Technology, Ministry of Industry and Information Technology, Beijing, China

Haiping Jiang, Junyi Ye, Lixiang Wang, Xiaofeng Chen, Ming Gao, Xinzhuang Wang, Tao Yan, He Yang, Enzhou Lu, Wenwu Liu, Zhixing Zheng and Xin Chen
Department of Neurosurgery, The First Affiliated Hospital of Harbin Medical University, Harbin, China
Department of Neurosurgery, Key Colleges and Universities Laboratory of Neurosurgery in Heilongjiang Province, Harbin, China
Institute of Neuroscience, Sino-Russian Medical Research Center, Harbin Medical University, Harbin, China

Dongzhi Zhang
Department of Neurosurgery, The First Affiliated Hospital of Harbin Medical University, Harbin, China
Department of Neurosurgery, Key Colleges and Universities Laboratory of Neurosurgery in Heilongjiang Province, Harbin, China
Institute of Neuroscience, Sino-Russian Medical Research Center, Harbin Medical University, Harbin, China
Department of Neurosurgery, The Affiliated Cancer Hospital of Harbin Medical University, Harbin, China

Karpov Denis Aleksandrovich and Sokhatskii Andrei Timofeevich
Department of Neurosurgery, The First Affiliated Hospital of Harbin Medical University, Harbin, China
Department of Neurosurgery, Key Colleges and Universities Laboratory of Neurosurgery in Heilongjiang Province, Harbin, China
Institute of Neuroscience, Sino-Russian Medical Research Center, Harbin Medical University, Harbin, China
Department of Neurosurgery and Medical Rehabilitation, Bashkir State Medical University, Ufa, Russia

Safin Shamil Mahmutovich
Department of Neurosurgery and Medical Rehabilitation, Bashkir State Medical University, Ufa, Russia

Cheng Zhang
Department of Undergraduate, Suffolk University, Boston, MA, United States

Jianing Wu, Penglei Yao, Zhenying Sun and Xuan Rong
Department of Neurosurgery, Shenzhen University General Hospital, Shenzhen, China

Shiguang Zhao
Department of Neurosurgery, The First Affiliated Hospital of Harbin Medical University, Harbin, China
Department of Neurosurgery, Key Colleges and Universities Laboratory of Neurosurgery in Heilongjiang Province, Harbin, China
Institute of Neuroscience, Sino-Russian Medical Research Center, Harbin Medical University, Harbin, China
Department of Neurosurgery, Shenzhen University General Hospital, Shenzhen, China

Prashant Kesharwani, Rahul Chadar and Afsana Sheikh
Department of Pharmaceutics, School of Pharmaceutical Education and Research, Jamia Hamdard, New Delhi, India

Waleed Y. Rizg
Department of Pharmaceutics, Faculty of Pharmacy, King Abdulaziz University, Jeddah, Saudi Arabia

Awaji Y Safhi
Department of Pharmaceutics, Faculty of Pharmacy, Jazan University, Jazan, Saudi Arabia

Yan Peng
Department of Obstetrics, Longhua District Central Hospital, Shenzhen, China

Yuanyuan Wang and Wuxuan Mei
Xianning Medical College, Hubei University of Science and Technology, Xianning, China

Cheng Zhou and Changchun Zeng
Department of Medical Laboratory, Shenzhen Longhua District Central Hospital, Guangdong Medical University, Shenzhen, China

Guoqiang Sun, Guangshun Sun, Fan Wu, Xiao Li, Hongyong Cao and Ye Cheng
Department of General Surgery, Nanjing First Hospital, Nanjing Medical University, Nanjing, China

Dawei Rong and Weiwei Tang
Hepatobiliary/Liver Transplantation Center, The First Affiliated Hospital of Nanjing Medical University, Key Laboratory of Living Donor Transplantation, Chinese Academy of Medical Sciences, Nanjing, China

Zhouxiao Li
Department of Hand Surgery, Plastic Surgery and Aesthetic Surgery, Ludwig-Maximilians University, Munich, Germany

Yangbai Sun
Department of Musculoskeletal Surgery, Fudan University Shanghai Cancer Center, Shanghai, China

Wenbin Diao, Ben Yang, Sipeng Sun, Anping Wang, Qianyun Ge, Mengqi Shi, Bo Lian, Tongyi Sun, Jingliang Wu, Jingkun Bai, Yubing Wang, Wenjing Yu and Zhiqin Gao
School of Life Science and Technology, Weifang Medical University, Weifang, China
Shandong Universities Key Laboratory of Biopharmaceuticals, Weifang, China

Rongguan Kou
School of Life Science and Technology, Weifang Medical University, Weifang, China

Meihua Qu
Translational Medical Center, Second People's Hospital of Weifang, Weifang, China

Ming Cai
Department of Pharmacy, The Second Affiliated Hospital of Anhui University of Chinese Medicine, Hefei, China
Anhui Acupuncture and Moxibustion Clinical Medicine Research Center, The Second Affiliated Hospital of Anhui University of Chinese Medicine, Hefei, China

Jing-Ji Wang
Anhui Acupuncture and Moxibustion Clinical Medicine Research Center, The Second Affiliated Hospital of Anhui University of Chinese Medicine, Hefei, China

Wei-Jian Ni
Inflammation and Immune Mediated Diseases Laboratory of Anhui Province, The Key Laboratory of Anti-inflammatory of Immune Medicines, Ministry of Education, Anhui Institute of Innovative Drugs, School of Pharmacy, Anhui Medical University, Hefei, China
Anhui Provincial Hospital, The First Affiliated Hospital of USTC, Division of Life Sciences and Medicine, University of Science and Technology of China, Hefei, China

Ying-Hong Wang and Hong Zhou
Department of Pharmacy, Anhui Provincial Cancer Hospital, The First Affiliated Hospital of USTC, Division of Life Sciences and Medicine, University of Science and Technology of China, Hefei, China

Index

O

P

R

S

T

U

V

X

www.ingramcontent.com/pod-product-compliance
Lightning Source LLC
LaVergne TN
LVHW082158200926
848484LV00008B/2184